Managing Epilepsy and Co-Existing Disorders

Managing Epilepsy and Co-Existing Disorders

Edited by

Alan B. Ettinger, M.D.

Associate Professor of Clinical Neurology, Albert Einstein College of Medicine of Yeshiva University, Bronx, New York; Chief, EEG Division, and Director, Comprehensive Epilepsy Center, Department of Neurology, Long Island Jewish Medical Center, New Hyde Park, New York; Director, Huntington Hospital Epilepsy Program, Huntington, New York

Orrin Devinsky, M.D.

Professor of Neurology, Neurosurgery, and Psychiatry, New York University School of Medicine, New York; Director, New York University–Mount Sinai Comprehensive Epilepsy Center, New York; Director, Saint Barnabas Institute of Neurology, Livingston, New Jersey

With Forewords by

Frederick Andermann, M.D.

Professor of Neurology and Pediatrics, McGill University Faculty of Medicine, Montreal, Quebec; Director of Epilepsy Service, Montreal Neurological Hospital and Institute

Steven C. Schachter, M.D.

Associate Professor of Neurology, Harvard Medical School, Boston; Medical Director, Office of Clinical Trials and Research, Beth Israel Deaconess Medical Center, Boston

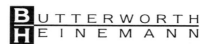

BUTTERWORTH HEINEMANN

Boston   Oxford   Auckland   Johannesburg   Melbourne   New Delhi

BS

Library of Congress Cataloging-in-Publication Data
Managing epilepsy and co-existing disorders / edited by Alan B. Ettinger, Orrin Devinsky ; with forewords by Frederick Andermann and Steven C. Schachter.
    p. ; cm.
  Includes bibliographical references and index.
  ISBN 0-7506-7241-2 (alk. paper)
    1. Epilepsy—Complications. I. Ettinger, Alan B. II. Devinsky, Orrin.
    [DNLM: 1. Epilepsy—complications. 2. Epilepsy—therapy. WL 385 M2665 2002]
  RC372 .M2625 2001
  616.8'53—dc21

                                                                2001037919

British Library Cataloguing-in-Publication Data
A catalogue record for this book is available from the British Library.

The publisher offers special discounts on bulk orders of this book.
For information, please contact:
Manager of Special Sales
Butterworth–Heinemann
225 Wildwood Avenue
Woburn, MA 01801-2041
Tel: 781-904-2500
Fax: 781-904-2620

For information on all Butterworth–Heinemann publications available,
contact our World Wide Web home page at: http://www.bh.com

10 9 8 7 6 5 4 3 2 1

Printed in the United States of America

10/29/03

I dedicate this book to my wife, Deborah, a devoted physician who taught me to look beyond surveys and statistics to truly understand the challenges faced by my patients. I also dedicate this book to my children, Joshua and Jonathan, who didn't mind that they had the only father on the soccer field sidelines with his head immersed in manuscripts.

—A.B.E.

For Deborah, Janna, and Julie

—O.D.

Contents

Contributing Authors

Jane Boggs, M.D.
Associate Professor of Neurology, University of South Alabama College of Medicine, Mobile

Edward B. Bromfield, M.D.
Assistant Professor of Neurology, Harvard Medical School, Boston; Chief, Division of Epilepsy and EEG, Brigham and Women's Hospital, Boston

Thomas R. Browne, M.D.
Professor of Neurology, Boston University School of Medicine; Neurologist, Boston Medical Center

Deborah T. Combs Cantrell, M.D.
Co-Director, North Texas Epilepsy Center, North Texas Neuroscience Center, Irving; Director, Epilepsy Monitoring Unit, Baylor Hospital, Irving

E. Cruz-Martinez, M.D.
University of Miami School of Medicine and Jackson Memorial Medical Center, Florida

Orrin Devinsky, M.D.
Professor of Neurology, Neurosurgery, and Psychiatry, New York University School of Medicine, New York; Director, New York University–Mount Sinai Comprehensive Epilepsy Center, New York; Director, Saint Barnabas Institute of Neurology, Livingston, New Jersey

Susan Duncan, M.R.C.P.I., M.D.
Consultant Neurologist, Hope Hospital, Greater Manchester, United Kingdom

Alan B. Ettinger, M.D.
Associate Professor of Clinical Neurology, Albert Einstein College of Medicine of Yeshiva University, Bronx, New York; Chief, EEG Division, and Director, Comprehensive Epilepsy Center, Department of Neurology, Long Island Jewish Medical Center, New Hyde Park, New York; Director, Huntington Hospital Epilepsy Program, Huntington, New York

Edward Faught, M.D.
Professor and Vice Chairman of Neurology, University of Alabama School of Medicine, Birmingham

Ross B. FineSmith, M.D.
Clinical Instructor of Neurology, New York University Medical School, New York

Mark N. Friedman, D.O.
Harvard Neuroendocrine Unit, Beth Israel Deaconess Medical Center, Boston; Staff Neurologist and Neuroendocrinologist, The NEW Center, Orlando Regional Medical Center, Florida

William R. Garnett, Pharm.D.
Professor of Pharmacy and Neurology, Virginia Commonwealth University School of Medicine and Medical College of Virginia, Richmond

Robin L. Gilmore, M.D.
Professor of Neurology, Pediatrics, and Neuroscience, Evelyn F. and William L. McKnight Brain Institute of the University of Florida, Gainesville; Director of Epilepsy Monitoring Program and Attending Physician, Department of Neurology, Shands Hospital of the University of Florida, Gainesville

Martin Adam Goldstein, M.D.
Department of Neurology and Neuroscience, New York Hospital–Cornell Medical Center, New York

Adarsh K. Gupta, M.D.
Attending Psychiatrist (Neuropsychiatrist), Department of Consultation Liaison Psychiatry, Long Island Jewish Medical Center, New Hyde Park, New York

Cynthia L. Harden, M.D.
Associate Professor of Neurology and Neuroscience, Weill Medical College of Cornell University, New York; Department of Neurology, New York Presbyterian Hospital, New York

Galen V. Henderson, M.D.
Instructor in Neurology, Harvard Medical School, Boston; Director, Neuroscience Intensive Care Unit and Stroke Service, Department of Neurology, Brigham and Women's Hospital, Boston

Andrew G. Herzog, M.D., M.Sc.
Associate Professor of Neurology, Harvard Medical School, Boston; Director, Harvard Neuroendocrine Unit, Beth Israel Deaconess Medical Center, Boston

Andres M. Kanner, M.D.
Associate Professor of Neurological Sciences and Psychiatry, Rush Medical College of Rush University, Chicago; Director, Laboratories of Electroencephalography and Video-EEG Telemetry, Rush–Presbyterian–St. Luke's Medical Center, Chicago

Peter W. Kaplan, M.B.B.S., F.R.C.P.
Associate Professor of Neurology, The Johns Hopkins University School of Medicine and Johns Hopkins Hospital, Baltimore; Chairman of Neurology, Johns Hopkins Bayview Medical Center, Baltimore

Stephen J. Kolb, M.D., Ph.D.
Neurology Resident, University of Pennsylvania Medical Center, Philadelphia; Resident, Department of Neurology, Hospital of the University of Pennsylvania, Philadelphia

Barbara S. Koppel, M.D.
Professor of Clinical Neurology, New York Medical College, Valhalla, New York; Attending Neurologist, Westchester Medical Center, Valhalla; Metropolitan Hospital Center, New York

Allan Krumholz, M.D.
Professor of Neurology, University of Maryland School of Medicine, Baltimore; Director, Maryland Epilepsy Center, University of Maryland Medical Center, Baltimore

Nita A. Limdi, Pharm.D.
Clinical Pharmacist of Neurosciences, University of Alabama at Birmingham Hospital

Richard B. Lipton, M.D.
Professor of Neurology, Epidemiology, and Social Medicine, Albert Einstein College of Medicine of Yeshiva University, New York; Attending Physician, Department of Neurology, Montefiore Medical Center, Bronx, New York

Brian Litt, M.D.
Assistant Professor of Neurology and Bioengineering, University of Pennsylvania School of Medicine, Philadelphia; Director, EEG Laboratory, Department of Neurology, Hospital of the University of Pennsylvania, Philadelphia

María Raquel Lopez, M.D.
Clinical Epilepsy Fellow, Department of Neurology, Beth Israel Deaconess Medical Center and Harvard Medical School, Boston

Daniel J. Luciano, M.D.
Assistant Professor of Clinical Neurology, New York University School of Medicine and Mount Sinai School of Medicine of the City University of New York, New York; Co-Director New York University–Mount Sinai Comprehensive Epilepsy Center, New York; Attending Physician, New York University School of Medicine and Mount Sinai School of Medicine of the City University of New York, New York

Beth A. Malow, M.D., M.S.
Assistant Professor of Neurology, University of Michigan Medical School, Ann Arbor, Michigan

Francesco T. Mangano, M.D.
Resident, Department of Surgery, Division of Neurological Surgery, Long Island
Jewish Medical Center and New York College of Osteopathic Medicine, New Hyde
Park, New York

Alexandra E. McBride, M.D.
Attending Neurologist, Long Island Jewish Medical Center, New Hyde Park,
New York

Daniel K. Miles, M.D.
Assistant Professor of Neurology, New York University School of Medicine, New
York; Director, Pediatric Epilepsy Program, New York University Medical Center,
New York

Souhel Najjar, M.D.
Assistant Professor of Neurology, New York University School of Medicine, New
York; Director, EEG Laboratory, New York University–Mount Sinai Epilepsy Cen-
ter, New York

Douglas R. Nordli, Jr., M.D.
Associate Professor of Pediatrics and Neurology, Northwestern University Medical
School, Chicago; Lorna S. and James P. Langdon Chair of Pediatric Epilepsy,
Department of Neurology and Children's Memorial Epilepsy Center, Children's
Memorial Hospital, Chicago

Gerald Novak, M.D.
Clinical Associate Professor of Neurology and Pediatrics, Albert Einstein College of
Medicine of Yeshiva University, Bronx, New York; Attending Physician, Pediatrics,
Schneider Children's Hospital, New Hyde Park, New York

Susan M. Palac, M.D.
Assistant Professor and Attending Epileptologist, Department of Neurological Sciences, Section of Epilepsy, Rush–Presbyterian–St. Luke's Medical Center, Chicago

Andrew D. Rosenberg, M.D.
Associate Professor of Clinical Anesthesiology, New York University School of
Medicine, New York; Chairman, Department of Anesthesiology, Hospital for Joint
Diseases, New York

A. James Rowan, M.D.
Professor of Neurology, Mount Sinai School of Medicine of the City University of
New York; Chief of Neurology Service, Bronx Veterans Affairs Medical Center,
Bronx, New York

Steven C. Schachter, M.D.
Associate Professor of Neurology, Harvard Medical School, Boston; Medical Direc-
tor, Office of Clinical Trials and Research, Beth Israel Deaconess Medical Center,
Boston

Steven J. Schneider, M.D., F.A.C.S.
Clinical Assistant Professor of Neurosurgery, Albert Einstein College of Medicine of Yeshiva University, Bronx, New York, and New York University Medical Center, New York; Head of Pediatric Neurosurgery Section, North Shore University Hospital, Manhasset, New York; Associate Attending, Division of Neurosurgery, Long Island Jewish Medical Center, New Hyde Park, New York

Lawrence Seiden, M.D.
Assistant Professor of Neurology, University of Maryland School of Medicine, Baltimore

Jehuda P. Sepkuty, M.D.
Assistant Professor of Neurology, The Johns Hopkins University School of Medicine, Baltimore; Neurophysiology and Epileptologist, John Hopkins Hospital, Baltimore

Stephen D. Silberstein, M.D.
Professor of Neurology, Jefferson Medical College of Thomas Jefferson University, Philadelphia; Director, Jefferson Headache Center, Thomas Jefferson University Hospital, Philadelphia

Candace Smith, Pharm.D.
Associate Clinical Professor, Department of Clinical Pharmacy, St. John's University, Jamaica, New York; Director, Pharmacokinetics, Long Island Jewish Medical Center, New Hyde Park, New York

Bradley V. Vaughn, M.D.
Associate Professor of Neurology, University of North Carolina at Chapel Hill School of Medicine

Deborah M. Weisbrot, M.D.
Assistant Professor of Psychiatry, Division of Child and Adolescent Psychiatry, and Director, Child Psychiatry Outpatient Clinic, State University of New York Health Sciences Center at Stony Brook School of Medicine

L. James Willmore, M.D.
Associate Dean and Professor of Neurology, Saint Louis University School of Medicine, St. Louis, Missouri

Foreword

In recent years, we have witnessed a veritable explosion of books on epilepsy, most of them describing general aspects of the topic with varying degrees of detail. Yet, when faced with specific problems related to the association of seizures with other disorders, the information is often fragmentary and hard to access. In clinical practice, only a fraction of seizures occur in otherwise healthy individuals and, even then, specific problems related to their age and gender are present. Providing state-of-the-art information about co-existence of seizures with systemic disorder is thus of great importance. This volume is a valuable source of clarification, especially on the interrelationship between the disorders, factors triggering seizures, and, above all, on the necessity for modifying treatment. Focusing on these associations becomes an important component of the standard of care.

Dr. Ettinger, with his particular interest in emotional and psychiatric aspects of epilepsy, and Dr. Devinsky, with his wide range of experience, are ideally suited to consider these issues. They have brought together appropriate and timely reviews that are highly informative and will no doubt lead to improved care and treatment of people with seizures. Thus, this book has far greater than average usefulness both for the clinician and the investigator. It provides a background and a baseline that hopefully will lead to further study of the numerous issues raised by the co-existence of epilepsy and other disorders.

Frederick Andermann

Foreword

The concept of the mind-body connection is widely accepted in popular culture. Yet among physicians—particularly neurologists—the brain is viewed as walled off from the rest of the body by the blood-brain barrier, as if housed in a sanctuary.

This model of anatomic, physiologic, and pathologic compartmentalization requires revision. An expanding body of evidence suggests that epilepsy is a multi-system, mutually interactive syndrome involving central nervous system structures besides the cortex, as well as non–central nervous system structures. This book comprehensively describes these interactions, revealing an intimate physiologic connection between brain and body.

The contributors show that seizures and seizurelike behaviors in patients with or without epilepsy result from—and, in turn, influence—an extraordinary diversity of systemic perturbations. They detail the frequency, presentation, evaluation, differential diagnosis, treatment, and prognosis of numerous systemic disorders that cause seizures by a pathologic response to illness culminating in tissue or vascular damage and dysfunction in the brain, or as an indirect consequence of end-organ dysfunction and resulting metabolic disruption or cerebral hypoxemia. Other chapters discuss toxins present in the circulation; deficiencies of essential nutrients; and pathologies restricted to the brain, but not necessarily to the cerebral cortex, that may be associated with seizures. Additional sections stress that seizures may impact the heart as well as reproductive endocrine function and suggest that patients may also be predisposed to infection, migraine headaches, and psychiatric conditions by seizures.

As illustrated throughout, these interactions vary as a function of age, gender, genetic susceptibility, and the presence of developmental disabilities, and are further complicated by treatment with antiepileptic drugs, because pharmacokinetics and pharmacodynamics may be altered in the setting of systemic illness and brain dysfunction.

The editors are to be congratulated for creating a single volume that encompasses information that ordinarily must be pieced together from a variety of sources. This book will help neurologists work more productively with their medical colleagues, thereby enabling patients to lead a lifestyle free from the medical and psychosocial complications of seizures.

Steven C. Schachter

Preface

What are the optimal antiepileptic drugs (AEDs) for use in epilepsy patients with hepatic failure? How does one alter AED dosage in patients receiving dialysis? Should prophylactic AEDs be prescribed after moderate head trauma? How does one distinguish seizures from migraines, transient ischemic attacks, movement disorders, or other paroxysmal symptoms?

These are the questions confronting clinicians every day in their evaluation and management of patients with seizures and related disorders. Although many texts review epilepsy, most focus on the epileptic condition itself and devote little attention to the commonly encountered problem of diagnosing and treating seizures in the context of another medical condition. This book addresses the compelling need for a consolidated and comprehensive reference on this subject. With contributions from nationally renowned epilepsy specialists, we have aimed to create a reference source for neurologists and other clinicians that emphasizes practical clinical information not easily accessible elsewhere.

In Chapter 1, Luciano focuses on the clinical features that distinguish epileptic from nonepileptic paroxysmal symptoms.

The next section (Chapters 2–15) covers the evaluation and management of epilepsy in relation to comorbid medical conditions. Each chapter emphasizes causes and risk factors for seizures; medical complications of epilepsy and its treatments; and information on a detailed history, physical examination, and laboratory testing, including neuroimaging, differential diagnosis, treatment, and prognosis.

In Chapter 2, Boggs highlights the emerging field of neurocardiology and demonstrates how seizures influence cardiac function, how cardiac symptoms mimic seizures, how cardiovascular disease precipitates seizures, and how AEDs interact with anticoagulant/antiplatelet therapies. Clinical pearls for distinguishing seizures from convulsive syncope are discussed, and the clinician is advised to watch for hemodynamic instability with parenteral AED administration.

In Chapter 3, Browne reveals strategies for treating epilepsy in the face of renal disease. This chapter helps the clinician select the optimal AED for seizure patients with renal failure on or off dialysis and illustrates how to modify dosing to accommodate renal insufficiency.

With a similar approach, Garnett (Chapter 4) addresses the therapeutic issues specific to epilepsy patients with gastrointestinal or hepatic disease. This topic is of crucial importance because most AEDs have some degree of liver metabolism, protein binding may be altered in hepatic disorders, and gastrointestinal conditions can reduce AED absorption.

In our modern age of renal, hepatic, lung, cardiac, bone marrow, and even pancreatic transplantation procedures, clinicians should be prepared to manage epilepsy in this ever-expanding patient population. Cruz-Martinez and Gilmore (Chapter 5) provide the clinician with advice for managing epilepsy in transplant patients.

In Chapter 6, Goldstein and Harden describe the complex but frequently encountered relationships between infectious diseases and seizures. Although infections may provoke acute or chronic seizures, seizures may also predispose the patient to infection. This chapter also describes the evaluation and treatment of many infectious conditions.

Seiden and Krumholz (Chapter 7) contribute a comprehensive chapter on noninfectious inflammatory disorders. They elaborate on the clinical features of specific potentially epileptogenic conditions such as systemic lupus erythematosus, Sjögren's syndrome, and central nervous system vasculitis.

Chapter 8 by Koppel deals with the relationship between drugs (prescribed, over the counter, and illicit) and seizures. Concerns about prescribing agents with the potential to lower the seizure threshold are clarified for many commonly used drugs. Epilepsy resulting from substance use is also described in detail.

In Chapter 9, Mangano, McBride, and Schneider characterize the relationship between brain tumors and epilepsy. They emphasize the importance of excluding neoplasms in the differential diagnosis of seizures, advanced neuroimaging techniques for enhanced brain tumor detection, treatment issues (e.g., heightened risks of AED-induced allergic reactions), and controversies surrounding electrocorticography in guiding surgical resections. Specific neoplasms are described.

Clinicians commonly encounter diverse metabolic aberrations, including alterations in sodium, glucose, calcium, and magnesium levels. These, together with metabolic enzyme deficiencies and endocrinopathies (e.g., thyroid or parathyroid disease), represent the spectrum of metabolic disorders that may cause seizures, and are the subject of Chapter 10 by Schachter and Lopez.

Sepkuty and Kaplan (Chapter 11) discuss two different medical topics: hematologic and pulmonary disorders. They review important clinical considerations, such as AED effects on folate and associated red blood cell morphology, AED effects on platelet function, and hematologic diseases associated with seizures. Among pulmonary disorders, respiratory dysfunction and its treatments can lower seizure thresholds, whereas seizures and their therapies may be associated with significant respiratory compromise.

Head trauma induces a series of pathophysiologic changes that may result in acute or chronic seizures. Willmore (Chapter 12) reviews the established risk factors for post-traumatic epilepsy, controversies surrounding AED prophylaxis in head trauma patients, and speculated mechanisms for the development of seizures. This chapter culminates in a specific list of recommendations for prophylactic AED therapy after head injury.

Epidemiologic studies demonstrate high rates of headache comorbidity with epilepsy. Migraine may trigger seizures, whereas seizures may initiate headaches. Headaches and seizures may also be independently elicited by underlying central nervous system abnormalities. These complex interrelationships are clarified by Silberstein and Lipton in Chapter 13. Differential diagnosis between headaches and seizures is also discussed, and suggestions for treating combined syndromes are offered.

Malow and Vaughn (Chapter 14) identify sleep disorders as conditions that commonly co-exist with epilepsy. Recognition and treatment of a sleep disorder can improve seizure control and daytime alertness. Alternatively, seizures and AED therapy can adversely affect normal sleep and result in reduced daytime alertness. Diverse types of sleep disorders such as rapid eye movement behavior disorder and somnambulism should be considered in the differential diagnosis of paroxysmal events, as explained in this chapter.

Relationships between cerebrovascular disease and seizures are extensively discussed by Bromfield and Henderson in Chapter 15. Although transient paroxysmal neurologic events raise the differential diagnosis of transient ischemic attack versus seizure, ischemic and hemorrhagic cerebrovascular events are an important cause of seizures, especially in the elderly. This chapter highlights the importance of a detailed history and the strategic use of ancillary testing modalities, including selective neuroimaging and video-electroencephalogram, in patient assessments. Pragmatic recommendations are made regarding treatment of seizures in this setting.

The next section (Chapters 16–18) deals with sexuality and pregnancy in epilepsy. Duncan (Chapter 16) and Friedman and Herzog (Chapter 17) convey opposing viewpoints on whether epilepsy patients are at increased risk for sexual dysfunction. Duncan argues that few adequate studies have been performed in non-institutionalized settings, and that this commonly assumed relationship remains unproven. Friedman and Herzog cite evidence of an adverse impact of the epileptic condition and antiepileptic therapies on reproductive hormone secretion.

According to Cantrell (Chapter 18), managing epilepsy during pregnancy is fraught with many challenges due to seizures, increased maternal complications, and increased risk of adverse outcomes in the newborn. Nevertheless, 90% of women with epilepsy have uncomplicated pregnancies and give birth to healthy children. Following the recommendations outlined in this chapter, such as avoiding polytherapy and prescribing folic acid, will help the clinician optimize management of the pregnant epilepsy patient.

The next section (Chapters 19–21) deals with the interface of epilepsy with psychiatric and behavioral issues. Palac and Kanner (Chapter 19) discuss psychogenically induced nonepileptic seizures (pseudoseizures) and bring the reader up to date on techniques of assessment and management. These authors point out that although many advances have been made in diagnosing pseudoseizures, the most effective treatments have not yet been determined.

Chapter 20 by Gupta, Ettinger, and Weisbrot takes the reader through a whirlwind tour of the complex literature of psychiatric issues in adults with epilepsy. This chapter clarifies numerous biologic, medication-related, and psychosocial etiologies for psychiatric disturbance in epilepsy, and summarizes current knowledge of mood disorders, psychosis, and personality aberrations in epilepsy. It also reviews the role psychotropic properties play in the selection of an AED. A discussion about risks of lowering seizure threshold with the use of psychotropic agents complements the discussion by Koppel in Chapter 8. A brief summary of AED–psychotropic agent interactions included here is elaborated on by Smith in Chapter 26.

Novak (Chapter 21) provides a similar discussion of psychiatric disorders in pediatric epilepsy patients. He addresses key questions asked by physicians caring for these patients, including

What is the prevalence of psychiatric disorders in children with epilepsy?
What is the best way to screen for them?
What kinds of behavioral problems predominate?
What factors are associated with increased risk?
What is the long-term outcome?
What measures should be taken to treat these problems?

The fifth section (Chapters 22–24) focuses on the unique diagnostic and treatment issues of special populations. Miles (Chapter 22) describes a diverse assortment of medical conditions associated with seizures that are unique to pediatric age groups. He covers a wide spectrum of conditions, including nutritional, cardiac, metabolic, infectious, and rheumatologic disorders.

Chapter 23 by FineSmith is devoted to developmental disabilities and epilepsy. Clinical challenges include distinguishing paroxysmal behavioral changes from seizure activity and accomplishing crucial neuroimaging or electroencephalogram studies in poorly cooperative patients. Epileptic issues specific to individual disorders, such as neurofibromatosis or Sturge-Weber, are also reviewed.

Rowan (Chapter 24) contends that epilepsy is a major health problem in another special population, namely, the elderly. With an incidence of epilepsy increasing dramatically after age 60 years, clinicians should be prepared to deal with the unique considerations of epilepsy diagnosis and management in this population. Therefore, Chapter 24 is especially invaluable in its discussion of such topics as seizure etiologies, treating epilepsy in view of altered pharmacodynamic and pharmacokinetic properties in the elderly, and unique comorbid conditions.

The next section of the text is a general reference on AEDs. Chapter 25 by Faught and Limdi examines general categories of AED side effects, which clinicians can use as a quick reference when prescribing individual agents. Although detailed surveys of idiosyncratic and dose-related adverse effects are described, the authors remind us that "The best instrument for detecting drug side effects is the ear. Neither the neurologic examination nor any battery of laboratory tests is as sensitive as a good interview with patient and family."

Chapter 26 by Smith comprehensively reviews AED-related drug interactions. When combining any drug with an AED, the clinician can use this chapter to make dosing adjustments when indicated to accommodate anticipated drug interactions.

The final section (Chapters 27 and 28) is entitled Procedures and Emergency Situations in Epilepsy. Chapter 27 offers suggestions for ensuring safety for epilepsy patients undergoing medical and dental procedures. This chapter is an excellent guide on the risks of lowering seizure thresholds among various anesthetic agents. Furthermore, this chapter advises clinicians on how to provide neurologic clearance for epilepsy patients scheduled for surgery.

Chapter 28 by Kolb and Litt completes the text with a discussion of practical approaches for the management of epilepsy patients in the emergency department and intensive care unit settings. Status epilepticus is discussed, and this chapter also reviews more commonly encountered clinical situations, including managing new-onset seizures or recurrent self-limited seizures in patients presenting to the emergency department and managing other comorbid conditions in patients who also have epilepsy. In the intensive care unit, abundant comorbid medical disorders make the treatment of seizures particularly difficult, and this chapter is therefore an invaluable reference for addressing assessment and treatment in this setting.

We hope that this overview of diagnosis and treatment of epilepsy and its coexisting disorders provides the clinician with a comprehensive but practical guide for daily management. We also hope that this book inspires further research into the interface between seizures and comorbid medical conditions.

Alan B. Ettinger
Orrin Devinsky

Section A

Disorders That Mimic Epilepsy

Chapter 1

Nonepileptic Paroxysmal Disorders

Daniel J. Luciano

There are a number of paroxysmal medical, neurologic, and psychiatric disorders that may be mistaken for epilepsy. Correct diagnosis of such episodes is crucial in providing appropriate treatment and rests initially on an accurate clinical history, particularly because physicians rarely witness the actual event. In rare instances, treatment of these disorders may precipitate a seizure, possibly clouding the diagnostic picture. Similarly, although less commonly, the treatment of seizures may cause the appearance or exacerbation of these other disorders. Many of the nonepileptic disorders mentioned in this chapter are dealt with more extensively in other chapters. This chapter concentrates on phenomenology and the clinical differentiation of seizures from these other paroxysmal disorders. Table 1-1, which is provided for rapid reference, categorizes seizure types and the nonepileptic paroxysmal disorders with which they may be confused.

Overview

The spectrum of ictal semiology is broad, and nonepileptic episodes may be confused with virtually any seizure type. Paroxysmal events that may be mistaken for seizures are termed *nonepileptic seizures* (NESs). NESs may be physiologic or psychological. Examples of physiologic NESs include syncope, migraine, sleep disorders, movement disorders, endocrine or toxic-metabolic disturbances, and cerebrovascular events, such as transient ischemic attacks (TIAs). Of emergency room patients with seizurelike symptoms, the most common diagnoses are syncope, cardiac disturbances, drug use, and metabolic disturbances.[1] Psychological NESs include entities such as panic, dissociation, intermittent explosive disorder, psychosis, conversion disorder ("pseudoseizures"), and malingering. The last two entities differ from other NESs in their intention, conscious or unconscious, to present the appearance of an epileptic seizure. This point is discussed further in the section on psychiatric disorders.

When approaching the differential diagnosis of paroxysmal symptoms, one's greatest tool is a thorough familiarity with epileptic ictal semiology, as well as the clinical characteristics of nonepileptic disorders that can imitate epilepsy. In arriving at the correct diagnosis, there are several historic features that may be helpful.

Ascertaining the nature of any provoking circumstances for an episode may be helpful in differential diagnosis. Although some seizures may be precipitated by certain circumstances (e.g., photosensitive epilepsy triggered by flashing lights), such a causal relationship is more commonly seen with nonepileptic episodes. For example, although patients with epilepsy may report that emotional stress triggers seizures, such stress may be more likely to cause neurocardiogenic (vasovagal) syncope, panic attacks, or hyperventilation. Coughing may trigger tussive syncope, whereas standing precipitates orthostatic syncope. Sudden movement precipitates attacks of paroxysmal kinesigenic

Table 1-1. Nonepileptic Disorders Confused with Various Seizure Types

Seizure Type	Nonepileptic Disorder	Seizure Type	Nonepileptic Disorder	Seizure Type	Nonepileptic Disorder
Simple partial sensory	**Elementary visual hallucinations:**	Simple partial motor (continued)	Nonepileptic myoclonus	Simple partial autonomic (continued)	Panic attacks
	Ocular disorders		Hemiballismus		Nocturnal anxiety attacks
	Disorders of optic pathway		Tic disorders		Post-traumatic stress disorder
	Occipital lobe lesions		Blepharospasm		Hypoglycemia
	Classic migraine		Hemifacial spasm		Pheochromocytoma
	Drug use		Palatal myoclonus		Carcinoid syndrome
	Hypnagogic/hypnopompic hallucinations		Periodic limb movements in sleep		Mastocytosis
	Transient ischemic attacks (TIAs)		Limb-shaking carotid TIA	Simple partial psychic	**Depersonalization/derealization:**
	Elementary auditory hallucinations:		Unilateral asterixis		Dissociative disorder
	Otic disorders		Hyperglycemia		Hyperventilation/panic disorder
	Cranial bruits		**Tonic/dystonic:**		Drug use
	Palatal myoclonus		Paroxysmal choreoathetosis		**Forced thinking:**
	Drug use		Torticollis		Obsessive-compulsive disorder
	Alcoholic hallucinosis		Hypnogenic paroxysmal dystonia		Psychotic disorders
	Brain stem auditory hallucinosis		Hemifacial spasm		**Affective:**
	Vertigo:		Meige's syndrome		Anxiety/panic disorder
	Benign paroxysmal vertigo (children)		Alternating hemiplegia		Depressive disorders
	Vestibular disorders (e.g., Ménière's)		Spasmus nutans	Complex partial	**Amnesia:**
	Brain stem disorders		**Paralysis:**		Transient global amnesia
	Vertebrobasilar insufficiency		TIAs		Dissociative amnesia
	Basilar artery migraine		Hemiplegic migraine		Dissociative fugue
	Camphor poisoning		Alternating hemiplegia		Daydreaming
	Somatic sensations:		Moyamoya hemiplegia		Sleep attack (narcolepsy)
	TIAs		Sleep paralysis		Alcoholic blackout
	Multiple sclerosis		Hypoglycemia		Drug intoxication
	Peripheral neuropathy		**Speech arrest:**		Automatic behavior (sleep disorders)
	Restless legs syndrome		TIAs		**Confusion:**
	Hyperventilation/panic disorder	Simple partial autonomic	**Abdominal sensations:**		Confusional migraine
	Amyloid angiopathy		Migraine		Basilar artery migraine
Simple partial motor	**Focal clonic:**		Gastroesophageal reflux		Confusional arousal
	Tremor		Drug side effects		Parasomnias
	Paroxysmal choreoathetosis		Panic attacks		Drugs/alcohol
	Paroxysmal torticollis (children)		Acute intermittent porphyria		Toxic/metabolic encephalopathy
			Camphor poisoning		Wernicke's encephalopathy
			Sympathetic outflow:		Hypo- or hyperglycemia
			Presyncope		Porphyria

Seizure type	Disorders
Complex partial (continued)	Flumazenil-responsive stupor Camphor poisoning Rabies **Complex hallucinations:** Drugs Alcoholic hallucinosis Delirium tremens Peduncular hallucinosis Sensory deficits Hypnagogic hallucinations Psychosis Camphor poisoning Rabies **Fear and aggression:** Temper tantrums Panic attacks Intermittent explosive disorder Pathologic intoxication Rapid eye movement (REM) behavior disorder Night terrors (pavor nocturnus) Camphor poisoning Rabies **Complex motor activity:** Night terrors (pavor nocturnus) Sleep walking (somnambulism) REM behavior disorder Paroxysmal nocturnal dystonia Automatic behavior (sleep disorders) Stereotypies
Absence	Daydreaming Attention deficit disorder
Myoclonic	Jitteriness of the newborn Benign neonatal myoclonus Benign myoclonus of infancy Shuddering attacks Paroxysmal ataxia
Myoclonic (continued)	Hypnic jerks Tic disorders Periodic limb movements in sleep Hyperexplexia
Tonic	Paroxysmal torticollis Sandifer's syndrome Spasmus nutans Alternating hemiplegia Breath-holding spells Hyperexplexia Infantile masturbation Syncope Pontine hemorrhage Paroxysmal dystonia or chore-oathetosis Hyperventilation syndrome Hypocalcemia Multiple sclerosis Decerebrate/decorticate rigidity Tetanus Strychnine poisoning Breath-holding spells Spasmus nutans
Atonic	Benign paroxysmal vertigo Alternating hemiplegia Syncope Basilar migraine Cataplexy Drop attacks of the elderly Vertebrobasilar TIA Carotid TIA with transient paraparesis Anterior–spinal artery TIA Periodic paralysis Hyperexplexia
Tonic-clonic	Jitteriness of the newborn Jactatio capitis nocturna
Tonic-clonic (continued)	Breath-holding spells Infantile masturbation Syncope Pseudoseizure* Decerebrate/decorticate rigidity Tetanus Strychnine poisoning Camphor poisoning Enuresis Bruxism **Motor:** Palatal myoclonus Hemifacial spasm Tetanus **Non-convulsive:** Akinetic mutism Catatonia Toxic/metabolic encephalopathy Drug intoxication Wernicke's encephalopathy Porphyria Flumazenil-responsive stupor
Status epilepticus	

*Pseudoseizures may appear similar to virtually any seizure type.

choreoathetosis and may also precipitate positional vertigo.

The duration, nature, and ability to modify prodromal symptoms are also important factors in differential diagnosis. In general, epileptic auras tend to be brief, lasting only seconds, whereas the prodrome of many nonepileptic episodes is more protracted. In addition, various episodes have fairly characteristic prodromes. For example, syncope is often preceded by light-headed dizziness, clamminess, nausea, graying of vision, "seeing stars," and distancing of sounds. Migraines are preceded by scintillating scotomata and visual obscuration that typically last much longer than epileptic auras. Prodromes of NESs are also more likely to be modifiable than ictal prodromes, for example, by sitting down, slowing respiration, or consuming glucose.

A crucial general guiding principle in differentiating seizures from other types of events is the stereotypical nature of seizures. Seizures are usually of similar duration, and the same phenomena occur in the same order from event to event in the same patient. In addition, seizures are generally brief, lasting 1–2 minutes on average, whereas nonepileptic episodes often persist longer and may also have a greater temporal variability.

The standard tool of seizure diagnosis has always been the electroencephalogram (EEG), but there is at times an over-reliance on EEG findings. It is important to realize that a given routine EEG will be normal in 50% of patients with definite epilepsy.[2] In addition, even ictal EEGs are normal during the majority of simple partial seizures and 25% of complex partial seizures of frontal origin.[3] Diagnostic confusion can further derive from the fact that up to 10% of normal patients have epileptiform abnormalities in their EEGs.[4] There are also benign EEG variants with epileptiform characteristics that may fool clinicians who are unfamiliar with these patterns. Thus, in differentiating epilepsy from its imitators, the clinical history and a sound knowledge of the characteristics of various paroxysmal disorders are of paramount importance.

See Table 1-1, which lists the nonepileptic disorders that may be confused with various seizure types. For a more detailed discussion of these disorders, please refer to the appropriate portions of the text in this chapter, as well as other pertinent chapters within this text.

Syncope

Syncope is a common problem with an incidence of approximately 3%.[5] Of all paroxysmal physiologic NESs, syncope is the entity most commonly confused with seizures, particularly given the presence of antecedent symptoms suggesting an aura and associated motor activity. Syncope may be mistaken for atonic, tonic, or tonic-clonic events. Most bouts of syncope are benign, isolated, and neurocardiogenic (vasovagal) in nature. However, when cardiac in etiology, this disorder can be potentially life threatening. In some instances, syncope can result in seizures, although seizures may at times resemble syncope or may result in cardiac arrhythmias that may lead to syncope. When patients happen to have both disorders, management can be difficult, as there may be uncertainty as to the nature of a particular episode. In evaluating such patients, the history is of prime importance in arriving at an accurate diagnosis.

In this section, an emphasis is placed on clinical phenomenology and the differentiation of syncope from seizures. Please refer to Chapter 2 for a broader discussion of this topic.

Syncope is a loss of consciousness and postural tone due to cerebral hypoperfusion. Table 1-2 describes historical and clinical features that are helpful in differentiating syncope from seizures. Syncope generally has a slower onset than seizures and a more prolonged prodrome and often occurs when standing. However, Stokes-Adams attacks, representing transient heart block, may occur with no warning. At the beginning of a bout of syncope, patients often feel light-headed and weak and experience pallor, sweating, sensations of heat or cold, and blurry vision. Alterations in perception may occur, such as graying of vision and distancing or echoing of sounds. Such phenomena may at times be mistaken for partial seizures. Nausea is common before or after syncope and should not be confused with the "rising epigastric sensation" that is a very common symptom during the aura of temporal lobe seizures. As opposed to simple nausea, the epileptic aura is a sensation of the stomach rising, as is experienced when an elevator moves downward rapidly. Loss of consciousness then occurs, usually associated with a loss of postural tone and pallor. On the basis of ischemia and release of subcortical cen-

Table 1-2. Differentiation of Syncope and Seizures

Syncope	Seizure
On standing, cough, micturition, blood drawing	Any circumstances
Often, antecedent dizziness, visual obscuration	Various auras that are brief (secs)
Usually 10–15 secs	Usually 1–2 mins
Usually limp, may have tonic or myoclonic activity briefly	Staring or rigidity with clonic activity
Incontinence rare but can occur	Incontinence common
Tongue biting rare	Tongue biting common
Injury rare	Injury common
Pallor	Cyanosis
Postictal state absent	Postictal confusion and lethargy

ters, motor phenomena, such as tonic posturing or myoclonic jerks, may occur during syncope, resulting in the impression of a tonic-clonic seizure.[6] This is known as *convulsive syncope* due to its similarity to a seizure. Such convulsive activity may be seen in as many as 40% of patients with syncope.[6] Rarely, a true epileptic seizure may be precipitated if hypoperfusion persists, such as might occur with a sustained arrhythmia.

Although generally associated with seizures, urinary incontinence may occur during syncope if the bladder is full. Tongue biting is more characteristic of seizures but may occur during syncope if the patient falls and hits his or her chin. However, this tends to occur on the anterior tongue, as opposed to the posterolateral aspect, which is typically bitten during seizures. Patients typically recover rapidly from syncope once reperfusion is established, usually once the patient is supine and there is little in the way of a postictal state. However, in the elderly there may be transient postictal confusion. After a seizure, heart rate and blood pressure are usually increased, whereas they are often lower after a bout of syncope.

The primary causes of syncope include decreased cardiac output (e.g., arrhythmias), decreased blood volume, decreased total peripheral resistance, or a combination of these factors. These states may be reached via various pathophysiologic mechanisms, and there are thus several types of syncope: reflex, respiratory, cardiac, vascular, and areflexic or paralytic.[6] The nature of the precipitating factors for a patient's event and a detailed description of the event itself may suggest the occurrence of syncope and also help to classify the episode among these subtypes. In 50% of cases, no etiology is identified, but in the

remainder, the main cause is cardiovascular or neurocardiogenic.[7]

Reflex and neurocardiogenic (vasovagal) syncope results from a loss of vasomotor tone with pooling of blood in muscles and a paradoxical increase in vagal tone with decreased heart rate, leading to hypotension. Neurocardiogenic syncope is the most common cause of syncope, accounting for 44% of all episodes with an identified etiology.[8] It tends to be familial, recurrent, and frequently precipitated by stress, fear, fatigue, or pain. Blood drawing is a common precipitant. Psychiatric disorders, such as generalized anxiety and panic, may be associated. Postmicturition syncope occurs in elderly men during or shortly after urination and may represent a variant of neurocardiogenic syncope with diminished intravesicular pressure leading to vasodilatation and vagally mediated bradycardia. Carotid sinus hypersensitivity syndrome is another type of reflex syncope that should be suspected when syncope occurs after head turning or wearing of a tight collar.

Respiratory syncope occurs as a result of acutely increased intrathoracic pressure causing decreased venous return and a subsequent drop in cardiac output. Cough syncope is a prime example and tends to occur after a fit of vigorous coughing in those with chronic bronchitis. Other situations associated with this type of syncope include weight lifting and trumpeting.

Syncope may result from a primary cardiac disorder, and in such cases accurate diagnosis is crucial, as the risk of sudden death is 24% by 1 year.[6] The most common cause is arrhythmia, particularly complete heart block from interruption of atrioventricular conduction (Stokes-Adams attack). Ventricular tachycardia and fibrillation are also associated with syncope and sudden death. In the case of tachyarrhythmias, the patient may experience palpitations before the bout of syncope. Cardiac outflow obstruction may also result in syncope, which is often triggered by exertion. Potential etiologies may include hypertrophic cardiomyopathy, aortic stenosis, mitral stenosis, pulmonic stenosis, subclavian steal, poor left ventricular compliance, and cardiac tamponade.

Vascular syncope occurs as a result of hypotension, which may be due to hypovolemia or inadequacy of autonomic controls for blood pressure maintenance. Patients typically experience orthostatic hypotension and syncope on standing. In subclavian steal syndrome, there is a proximal blockage of the subclavian artery, and syncope may be precipitated by use of the arm and the subsequent "steal" of blood flow from the vertebrobasilar system.

Areflexic or paralytic syncope occurs due to failure of autonomic hemodynamic reflexes to maintain adequate cerebral perfusion. The clinical presentation is similar to vascular syncope with orthostatic hypotension. Etiologies include neuropathies (e.g., diabetic, tabes dorsalis), central autonomic disorders (e.g., Shy-Drager disorder), medications (e.g., antihypertensives, antidepressants), and structural abnormalities (e.g., paraplegia).

Syncope in children deserves special mention. Breath-holding spells are the primary cause. These occur before the age of 2 years, are always provoked, and are self-limited, usually resolving by 4 years of age. There are two varieties of breath-holding spells: cyanotic and pallid. Cyanotic breath-holding spells are most common and are triggered by anger, pain, or fright. There is always vigorous crying, after which the child becomes cyanotic and holds his or her breath in expiration. The child then becomes limp. After approximately 30 seconds, rigidity and opisthotonic posturing occur, which may be followed by clonic activity if the apnea persists. The episode terminates in a gasp with a subsequent return to normal, although transient drowsiness may occur.

Pallid events are due to transient asystole from excess vagal tone. They occur with sudden fright or pain, particularly with head injury. If crying occurs, it is generally brief, as opposed to cyanotic episodes. Stiffening occurs with upward rolling of the eyes and a few myoclonic jerks, after which the child awakens transiently, only to then fall asleep. Rarely, a true epileptic seizure may be precipitated after 15 seconds of asystole.[6] This may be a result of an underlying epileptic diathesis or lowered seizure threshold.

Breath-holding spells may be confused with atonic or tonic seizures, and the occurrence of a secondary tonic-clonic seizure may add further diagnostic confusion. Consistent precipitation of events by fright, pain, or crying suggests the diagnosis. The EEG is normal, but asystole and typical events may be precipitated by ocular compression in 60–75% of patients with pallid spells, 25% with cyanotic spells, and 7% of healthy patients.[9] However, this procedure is risky and of uncertain value.

Occasionally, patients with epilepsy may present with true or apparent syncope. Rarely, ictal cardiac arrhythmias may occur that may result in secondary syncope.[10] In addition, patients who have chronic temporal lobe epilepsy may develop "temporal lobe syncope," which is a complex partial seizure with the appearance of syncope.[11]

The differentiation of syncope from seizures relies primarily on a detailed history and physical examination. These, combined with an electrocardiogram, have a diagnostic yield of 50% in patients with syncope.[12] In some instances, there may be a family history of similar events. A history of precipitating circumstances, such as standing, urinating, coughing, pain, or the sight of blood, is extremely helpful in supporting the diagnosis of syncope. In some instances, the diagnosis may be confirmed by recreating an episode with the usual provocative circumstances while the patient is closely monitored.

In patients with syncope, the physical examination is usually normal. Vital signs must be checked for evidence of arrhythmias or hypotension, including orthostatic changes. A careful cardiac examination must be performed to look for evidence of murmurs suggestive of valvular disease, as cardiac causes of syncope usually involve obstructive pathology or an arrhythmia.

In terms of laboratory testing, blood tests should be performed to rule out causes of syncope, such as anemia or metabolic derangements. An electrocardiogram with a rhythm strip and a chest x-ray should be performed to rule out cardiopulmonary causes. If heart disease is suspected or syncope is exertional, cardiac testing should be performed, which may include echocardiography, stress testing, Holter monitoring, or intracardiac electrophysiologic testing.[12] Tilt-table testing may confirm the diagnosis in cases of orthostatic or neurocardiogenic syncope and has a diagnostic yield of up to 60%.[12] Testing is performed for 15–30 minutes unless symptoms occur or syncope is produced by decreased cardiac rate or hypotension.

A normal EEG is helpful in excluding epilepsy, but one must keep in mind that a routine interictal EEG is normal in 50% of epilepsy patients.[2] If suspicion for seizures is strong, sleep deprivation may increase yield. Electroencephalographically, diffuse slowing is seen during syncope, followed by attenuation if hypoperfusion persists. This is also the case during convulsive syncope. Neuroimaging is recommended only if a primary neurologic etiology is suspected.

For a more detailed discussion of the treatment of syncope, the reader is referred to an excellent review article.[13] Basically, the treatment of syncope is dependent on its underlying mechanism. In cases of orthostatic syncope, the patient may be instructed to get up slowly, avoid prolonged standing, and increase salt and fluid intake. Pressure stockings may also be helpful. If syncope is neurocardiogenic and related to anxiety or panic, reassurance, behavioral therapy, and antianxiety agents may be effective. Adrenergic agents such as pseudoephedrine may be used in neurocardiogenic syncope, but there is a small risk of seizure precipitation with such drugs. Mineralocorticoids, such as florinef acetate, may be helpful, but the use of hepatic enzyme-inducing antiepileptic drugs (AEDs), such as phenobarbital, may cause a fall in the serum level of such drugs, as well as the level of beta-blocking agents, which may also be effective in neurocardiogenic syncope.

In syncope of cardiac etiology, treatment may involve antiarrhythmic agents, cardiac pacing, or invasive electrophysiologic ablation techniques. Of the antiepileptic medications, on rare occasions carbamazepine may cause arrhythmias and phenytoin may cause a worsening of heart block, both of which are conditions theoretically capable of resulting in syncope. Thus, if seizures and cardiac syncope coexist, one should use these agents with caution.

Cerebrovascular Disease

Cerebrovascular disturbances may at times be confused with seizures owing to the fact that both disorders present with sudden symptoms. In most instances, vascular events can be relatively easily distinguished from seizures, although the occurrence of TIAs or seizures with transient postictal deficits may lead to diagnostic confusion. Most important, in light of the objective of this textbook, is the fact that seizures commonly occur as a consequence of cerebrovascular disease. This section concentrates on the clinical differentiation of vascular events and seizures. For a more detailed discussion of cerebrovascular disease and its relationship to seizures, please refer to Chapter 15.

Of all cerebrovascular events, TIAs are the most likely to be confused with seizures owing to their relative brevity. TIAs last less than 24 hours, with 50% resolving within 30 minutes.[14] Most seizures last for only a minute or two, making the differentiation from TIAs relatively easy, although seizures may be more prolonged, or postictal states may be mistakenly considered a part of the event itself, prolonging the apparent ictal duration. Differentiation of TIAs from seizures can also usually be made based on the nature of the clinical signs and symptoms. Cerebrovascular events are usually associated with "negative" neurologic phenomena, such as weakness, numbness, or blindness, as opposed to "positive" ictal phenomena during seizures, such as clonic motor activity, paraesthesias, or visual hallucinations. However, seizures with negative phenomenology can occur (e.g., focal or generalized atonic seizures), as can transient postictal neurologic deficits (e.g., Todd's paralysis). Alternatively, TIAs may rarely present with positive motor activity (see later).

Cranial bruits may rarely be mistaken for a simple partial seizure arising from the auditory portion of the temporal lobe. In the case of carotid disease, the patient usually perceives the sound diffusely, although it may be localized to the region of the ear on the involved side. It may be most apparent in a quiet environment or with the ear against a pillow. Audible bruits may also arise from arteriovenous malformations or fibromuscular hyperplasia of the internal carotid artery. In all cases, the sounds experienced would be expected to follow the time course of the patient's pulse, allowing differentiation from a seizure.

Vertebrobasilar TIAs are perhaps the most likely cerebrovascular disorder to be confused with epilepsy owing to the fact that they may be associated with a loss of consciousness. This does not occur without the presence of associated symptoms, such as weakness or paraesthesias of any or all extremities, ataxia, unilateral or bilateral visual field defects, vertigo, diplopia, dysphagia, or dysarthria.[15] Less commonly, visual inversion, blindness, deafness, tinnitus, or tremor may occur.[15] Differentiation from seizures may be confounded by symptoms such as vertigo, leading to the impression of a temporal lobe seizure. However, the episode would have the appearance of syncope and would not be associated with true tonic-clonic activity.

Auditory hallucinosis mimicking simple partial sensory seizures may occur with cerebrovascular disease of the pontine tegmentum and midbrain.[16,17] In such patients, the correct diagnosis can be made by the presence of associated neurologic signs implicating the posterior circulation, normal EEG, structural lesions on neuroimaging in the appropriate locations, or documentation of posterior circulation vascular disease.

Cerebrovascular disease of the posterior diencephalon or midbrain may cause Lhermitte's syndrome, consisting of peduncular hallucinosis, which is characterized by vivid, colorful, pleasurable visual hallucinations, often involving moving patterns, people, or animals. These appear to be release hallucinations that possess all the qualities of true visual perceptions. Confusion is possible with simple partial visual seizures arising in the occipital, and possibly temporal, regions. Similar to ictal hallucinations, but quite different from psychotic illness, the patient is aware that the hallucinations are unreal. Because the etiology of peduncular hallucinosis typically involves infarction or intracranial lesions, hallucinations would be expected to be much more prolonged and persistent than those occurring as an ictal manifestation. However, brief episodes have been reported.[18,19] The presence of clinical or ultrasonic evidence of cerebrovascular disease, as well as a normal EEG, would support the diagnosis of peduncular hallucinosis due to a vascular etiology.

Patients with cerebral amyloid angiopathy may at times present with transient neurologic symptoms due to petechial hemorrhages.[20] These episodes involve paraesthesias, numbness, or weakness with a rapid march to contiguous areas. It is presumed that these most likely represent focal seizures, with TIAs being a less likely etiology.[20]

Transient global amnesia is another entity with presumed cerebrovascular etiology, which usually involves the abrupt onset of a single bout of pure short-term memory dysfunction in an older person and lasts for less than 24 hours.[6] Given the gap in memory, episodes may be confused with complex partial seizures. However, there is no associated alteration of awareness or other cognitive processes, as would be expected during such a seizure. Retrograde and anterograde amnesia are seen, with the retrograde component largely resolving by the time the episode resolves, but with permanent loss of memory for events occurring between onset and termination. During the episode, the patient is awake and responsive, but also disoriented, asking the same questions repeatedly. Episodes may at times be precipitated by immersion in cold water, sexual intercourse, severe pain, physical exertion, or emotional stress.[6] Patients typically experience only a single episode, and the prognosis is uniformly good. Interictal epileptiform activity has only rarely been seen on EEG during episodes.[6] On rare occasions, pure ictal amnesia may occur as a result of hippocampal ictal activity and may be mistaken for transient global amnesia,[21] although such episodes would be expected to be much briefer than a bout of transient global amnesia.

Akinetic mutism is a state characterized by poverty of movement and lack of speech. It may be seen in cases of bilateral frontal ischemic strokes or hemorrhage, such as from a ruptured aneurysm in the anterior cerebral distribution. Bithalamic infarction has also resulted in this syndrome.[22] Notably, a case of akinetic mutism due to phenytoin toxicity has been reported.[23] Akinetic mutism may be confused with catatonic psychosis or a state of nonconvulsive status epilepticus (NCSE). In the case of stroke, the patient's clinical state would be expected to remain static, whereas most cases of NCSE, which are partial in nature, show a cyclic pattern of multiple discrete complex partial events with intervening confusion. Notably, a case of episodic, epileptic, akinetic mutism with video-EEG confirmation has been reported.[24] On occasion, generalized "spike-wave stupor" may occur as an expression of a primary generalized absence NCSE with a constant unresponsive state. In such instances, small rhythmic movements involving the face and midline may provide a clue to diagnosis. Definitive exclusion of NCSE is based on performance of an EEG. If this is problematic, consideration can be given to a diagnostic or therapeutic trial of a short-acting benzodiazepine.

In patients with severe carotid occlusive disease, "limb-shaking" TIAs have been reported that may be mistaken for simple partial motor seizures.[25,26] The patient experiences brief, coarse, wavering or trembling movements of the distal arm contralateral to the occluded internal carotid artery due to orthostatic hypoperfusion. At times, the leg may also be affected and, rarely, motor activity may be bilateral when there is more diffuse cerebrovascular disease combined with hypotension.[27] Episodes usually last for seconds to minutes. As opposed to seizures, rhythmic clonic activity and version do not occur. The presence of a carotid bruit or evidence of significant carotid occlusive disease on ultrasonic testing, as well as provocation of the episodes by standing and resolution by sitting or lying down, allows differentiation from a seizure.

As many as 30% of patients with pontine hemorrhagic stroke may experience episodes of flexor spasm that may resemble seizures of a tonic nature.[28] Diagnosis should not be difficult owing to the presence of associated neurologic signs, a normal EEG, and demonstration of pontine hemorrhage on neuroimaging.

In moyamoya disease, patients may experience seizures, but they are even more prone to experience brief TIAs, which usually involve hemiparesis,[29] suggesting the possibility of atonic or inhibitory motor seizures. Paresis may remain unilateral or may alternate sides. Episodes may be triggered by hyperventilation, playing instruments, sucking, or the Valsalva maneuver, all of which decrease cerebral blood flow. The presence of such precipitating factors and alternation of the side involved would support the diagnosis of TIAs.

Nonepileptic drop attacks in the elderly, which may be due to vertebrobasilar ischemia in some, may also be confused with epilepsy, particularly with atonic seizures. There is transient weakness of both legs with a fall, but no alteration in consciousness. On rare occasions, carotid disease may be responsible when associated with contralateral anterior cerebral artery hypoplasia.[30] Anterior spinal artery TIAs may also produce paraparesis associated with radicular pain, areflexia, and a spinal pain and temperature level.[31] Epilepsy patients with atonic seizures predominantly experience Lennox-Gastaut syndrome and typically have an abnormal EEG, usually demonstrating generalized slow spike-wave activity. In addition, other seizure types, such as tonic, myoclonic, atypical absence, and tonic-clonic, would generally be associated.

In determining whether a patient has cerebrovascular disease as opposed to seizures, the physical examination is of prime importance. Vital signs should be assessed for the presence of abnormalities of pulse or blood pressure. The cranium and carotid arteries should be auscultated for the presence of bruits. A cardiac examination should be performed to determine whether there are clicks or murmurs suggestive of valvular disease. A peripheral vascular examination may indicate the presence of diffuse vascular disease.

Neuroimaging studies, including magnetic resonance imaging and possibly magnetic resonance angiography, may document the presence of vascular lesions. In the case of suspected vasculitis, angiography may be indicated. Doppler flow studies help to document the presence of clinically relevant vascular lesions, primarily in the carotid territory. An echocardiogram may be indicated in those with possible valvular disease.

A normal EEG makes the presence of seizures less likely, although it does not rule out this possibility entirely. One must also be aware that vascular abnormalities may be associated with EEG findings, such as focal slowing or even sharp waves, that do not necessarily prove the presence of epilepsy.

A detailed discussion of the treatment of cerebrovascular disease is beyond the scope of this chapter. There are important potential interactions between AEDs and medications used in the treatment of cerebrovascular disease. Many patients with cerebrovascular disease are treated prophylactically with aspirin or other antiplatelet agents. Aspirin can interact with AEDs via displacement from albumin binding sites and can cause an elevation in the free level of phenytoin and valproate.

Other patients, particularly those with embolic disease due to atrial fibrillation, are treated with coumarins. These agents also have the potential for protein binding interactions and may cause an elevation of phenytoin levels. Similarly, valproate may lead to an elevation in free warfarin levels. Alternatively, owing to hepatic enzyme induction, phenytoin, carbamazepine, and phenobarbital cause a lowering of coumarin levels. As a result of such interactions, cotherapy with these agents must be monitored closely with coagulation studies.

It should also be realized that patients with seizures who are treated with anticoagulants for cerebrovascular disease may be at much greater risk for complications such as subdural hematomas. As a result, in some patients, uncontrolled epilepsy with major motor seizures may represent a relative contraindication to long-term anticoagulation.

Migraine

Migraine is a common hereditary disorder that is related to epilepsy in several ways. Often, the two disorders coexist. In some cases, migraine attacks may culminate in a seizure, or a migraine syndrome may later evolve into epilepsy. Phenomena experienced during several types of migraine may easily lead to a misdiagnosis of epilepsy, particularly if headache is not associated (migraine equivalent). When visual in nature, migrainous phenomena may suggest the possibility of occipital lobe epilepsy. Seizures may also be followed by a migrainous postictal headache. This section highlights the clinical differentiation of migraines and epilepsy. For a more detailed discussion of migraine, as well as its interface with epilepsy, please see Chapter 13.

Classic migraine has many neurologic manifestations that occur during the initial aura phase, which typically lasts for 20–30 minutes, much longer than most seizures. These may include visual abnormalities, diplopia, numbness, weakness, aphasia, confusion, or loss of consciousness. Visual loss is the most common transient neurologic deficit associated with migraines, but visual field defects, scintillating scotomata, fortification spectra, or complex visual hallucinations may also occur.[32] Complex hallucinations are generally more suggestive of seizures than migraines. The temporal progression of migrainous phenomena is also generally slower than seizures, occurring over minutes rather than seconds, as is often the case

with seizures. After the aura phase, the patient typically experiences a throbbing headache associated with nausea, vomiting, photophobia, and sonophobia. However, with acephalic migraines (migraine equivalents), there is an absence of headache after the aura, making differentiation from seizures more difficult. In such cases, the slow progression of migraine assists in making the correct diagnosis.

For years, a syndrome primarily seen in children with episodes of abdominal pain, dizziness or vertigo, and intense autonomic output was labeled *abdominal epilepsy*, although this appears to actually be migrainous in nature.[33] Epileptiform activity on EEG in many of these patients supported the theory that it was epileptic in nature.

Confusional migraine may be mistaken for complex partial seizures or a postictal confused state. The patient may demonstrate confusion, disorientation, hyperactivity, impaired responsivity, amnesia, lethargy, and vomiting.[34] The episodes last for several hours and resolve with sleep. Diagnosis is assisted by an absence of automatisms, as would be seen during complex partial seizures, and preceding headache or visual symptoms consistent with migraine. An EEG can be helpful, as it may demonstrate lateralized slowing during a confusional migraine[34] but not epileptiform activity. However, similar findings may be seen during a postictal state.

In hemiplegic migraine, the aura is associated with transient hemiparesis or hemiplegia. This is generally more likely to be confused with a TIA than a seizure, given the duration and negative phenomenology of such events. Inhibitory motor seizures can be considered, although they are generally much briefer. Confusion with a postictal Todd's paralysis might occur, but one would expect a history of a more obvious, initial clinical seizure. Aside from the time course, a very helpful historical feature allowing differentiation from a seizure would be an alternation of the side of hemiplegia during various attacks.

Alternating hemiplegia is a disorder of early childhood related to migraine that presents before 18 months of age.[35] These are attacks of hemiplegia or dystonia, or both, that usually alternate sides, although bilateral and synchronous involvement also occurs. Episodes last for minutes to days, may be precipitated by fatigue or emotion, and resolve after sleep. Nystagmus may occur with these episodes or independently. The dystonic episodes may be confused with tonic or dystonic seizures. However, such seizures are usually very brief, so more prolonged episodes are less likely to be epileptic in nature. In addition, the alternation of sides is uncommon in epilepsy. It should be noted that older patients with this disorder may also develop true tonic-clonic seizures. Patients eventually develop mental deterioration and choreoathetosis, and these associated clinical findings help confirm the diagnosis.

Basilar artery migraine is particularly likely to be confused with epilepsy due to associated loss of consciousness. It is most common in adolescent girls. Attacks are characterized by dysfunction of the posterior circulation and begin with a gradual onset of drowsiness or stupor, possibly preceded by phenomena such as vertigo, visual loss, diplopia, alternating hemimotor or hemisensory symptoms, or ataxia.[36] Afterward, there is a severe occipital headache. The presence of vertigo preceding an alteration in consciousness may lead to a suspicion of temporal lobe epilepsy, and visual phenomena to a suspicion of occipital lobe epilepsy. However, the duration of episodes is more prolonged than most seizures and the loss of consciousness more gradual, and the patient can usually be aroused with stimulation. Diagnostic confusion can also arise from the frequent presence of epileptiform EEG patterns in patients with basilar migraine, although seizures are not associated.[32]

The diagnosis of migraine is based purely on clinical signs and symptoms. Differentiation from seizures may be difficult, but the more prolonged duration of the aura, gradual onset, presence of a subsequent throbbing headache, associated photophobia, improvement with antimigraine medications, and a family history of migraine are particularly helpful in making the diagnosis. Alternation of neurologic symptoms or headache from one side to the other during various episodes also makes migraine much more likely than seizures. Migraines have a propensity to be triggered by factors such as certain foods (e.g., sharp cheese), caffeine withdrawal, alcohol, and sleep deprivation. However, seizures may also be precipitated by such circumstances. Sudden onset, the occurrence of events in sleep, and the presence of other episodes consistent with seizures suggest the diagnosis of epilepsy.

Physical examination in patients with migraine is usually normal. In addition, there are no specific tests to be performed in diagnosing a patient with migraines. However, if headaches are invariably on one side, consideration might be given to performing an imaging study to identify intracranial lesions, such as arteriovenous malformations. EEG is generally not helpful and may lead to diagnostic confusion, as epileptiform EEG abnormalities are not uncommon in patients with migraine,[32] especially basilar migraine. However, an EEG during a clinical episode demonstrating a clearcut ictal electroencephalographic pattern strongly suggests epilepsy. During migraines, lumbar puncture may reveal elevated white blood cell count and protein and opening pressure, and similar findings may be seen during active seizures.[32]

Diagnostic-therapeutic trials of medication often do not allow a differentiation of migraines from seizures. Antiepileptic medications such as carbamazepine, valproate, benzodiazepines, phenobarbital and topiramate may improve both disorders. However, a response to dietary manipulation, nonsteroidal anti-inflammatory drugs, ergots, tricyclics, beta-blockers, or serotonin antagonists favors a migraine diagnosis.[32]

Movement Disorders

Movement disorders and many seizure types are characterized by involuntary movements, and it is not surprising that the two disorders are easily confused with each other. Movement disorders may be mistaken for simple partial motor, myoclonic, tonic, dystonic, or atonic seizures. On occasion, medications used for the treatment of movement disorders may precipitate seizures via a lowering of seizure threshold or alterations in blood levels of antiepileptic medications. Alternatively, the use of virtually all antiepileptic medications may be associated with the appearance of abnormal movements, which may at times be mistaken for seizures and lead to diagnostic confusion.

A full discussion of movement disorders is beyond the scope of this chapter, and the reader is referred to an excellent review.[37] Movement disorders express clinically as either akinesis or abnormal involuntary movements, known as *dyskinesias*. Such movements are of five general types: tremor, chorea, myoclonus, tics, and dystonias. They arise primarily from dysfunction of various portions of the basal ganglia or their connections.

There are several general characteristics of movement disorders that may help to distinguish them from seizures. The movements of movement disorders tend to occur much more persistently than seizures, which generally occur intermittently for only brief periods of time. With few exceptions, movement disorders disappear in sleep, whereas seizures generally become more frequent. With many movement disorders, such as tics, the patient may be able to suppress the movements at least temporarily, which is usually not the case with seizures. In addition, as opposed to most seizures, many movement disorders can be provoked by movement or manipulation. However, epilepsia partialis continua, also termed *focal cortical reflex myoclonus*, may attenuate or be provoked by tactile stimuli.

Tremor is a rhythmic oscillation of a body part around a fixed point. The movement is biphasic and involves alternating agonist and antagonist muscle group action. Tremor may occur primarily or exclusively on sustension or intention, such as in cases of essential or cerebellar tremor. In such instances, there is usually little confusion with simple partial motor seizures, which would be expected to occur regardless of the state of activity, although reflex motor seizures are a possibility. Resting tremor, such as in parkinsonism, is more likely to be confused with seizures. Differentiation of tremor from seizures is based on the greater persistence of tremor, constant association with either rest or active use of the limbs, disappearance of tremor in sleep or with manipulation of the affected limb, a family history of tremor, and, in the case of parkinsonism, associated akinesis and rigidity.

Chorea involves rapid forceful jerky arrhythmic "dancing" movements of the extremities or face that tend to flow to contiguous body parts. Respiratory sounds and grimacing may be associated. Athetosis, which is often seen associated with chorea, consists of slower sinuous writhing movements with rotation about the long axis of extremities and a tendency for extremes of flexion and extension to flow into one another. Differentiation from simple partial motor or tonic seizures is usually not problematic, as the movements in most forms of choreoathetosis occur quite persistently. However, in some instances, choreoathetosis may occur paroxysmally and is then more likely to be confused with epilepsy. In general, choreoathetosis is also more likely to involve multiple areas of the body variably, whereas motor seizures would be expected to be more stereotypical, involving a specific extremity or side of the body.

Paroxysmal dystonic choreoathetosis (PDC; formerly familial paroxysmal choreoathetosis) is an autosomal dominant disorder with incomplete penetrance, which is characterized by dystonic quality choreoathetotic movements lasting minutes to hours, and is precipitated by caffeine, alcohol, strong emotion, cold, and prolonged physical exertion.[38] Any portion of the body may be involved, and there may be prodromal anxiety, weakness, muscle weakness, or paraesthesias, suggesting an epileptic aura. Attacks may be rare, or may occur multiple times per day, suggesting the possibility of seizures, particularly if the episodes are brief. Episodes may be differentiated from seizures by the presence of a family history, purely diurnal episodes, a more prolonged event duration, and a normal EEG.

Choreoathetosis also occurs paroxysmally in paroxysmal kinesigenic choreoathetosis, a familial or sporadic disorder with bouts of dystonia or choreoathetosis, or both, triggered by startle or sudden movement after a period of rest. Reflex tonic or dystonic motor seizures may be suggested. Episodes are brief, lasting seconds to minutes, which makes confusion with seizures more likely. Attacks can occur up to 100 times per day, generally much more than is seen in seizure disorders. As in PDC, somatosensory auras may occur, again suggesting the possibility of a seizure disorder. As opposed to PDC, antiepileptic medications such as carbamazepine are often effective in this disorder.[38] With this in mind, it is not surprising that some researchers have proposed that PDC represents a seizure disorder, possibly basal ganglionic in origin, although there is little evidence to prove this contention.[38]

In hypnogenic paroxysmal dystonia, episodes of diffuse tonic posturing, choreoathetotic movements, or ballismus occur on partial arousal from stage 2 non–rapid eye movement sleep.[39] Episodes typically last for 30–60 seconds and often occur several times per night. Tonic seizures may be suggested, and this entity may also be very difficult to distinguish from frontal epilepsy, because both disorders are characterized by brief attacks with tonic or, occasionally, bizarre posturing, as well as nocturnal clusters. In addition, it is notable that carbamazepine may effectively treat this disorder. The EEG is normal during attacks, as it may also be during frontal seizures. In fact, some patients with brief attacks may actually experience mesial frontal lobe epilepsy.[40]

The main epileptic disorder to be distinguished from forms of paroxysmal choreoathetosis is frontal lobe epilepsy, particularly that which arises from the supplementary motor area, which may present with brief seizures characterized by tonic or dystonic posturing with retention of consciousness and, often, a normal ictal EEG. However, this form of epilepsy is usually most prominent in sleep, whereas the paroxysmal choreoathetoses (except hypnogenic paroxysmal dystonia) are diurnal disorders. In addition, because the paroxysmal dyskinesias commence in childhood, later onset may suggest the possibility of seizures, as would epileptiform activity on EEG, the presence of clonic activity, and tonic as opposed to dystonic or choreoathetotic posturing.

Ballismus usually involves unilateral proximal violent flinging movement of the extremities and is due to pathology in the region of the subthalamic nucleus. Hemiballismus usually can be differentiated from clonic simple partial motor seizures by its greater persistence and the presence of proximal extremity movements, which is unusual for seizures because there is a much greater representation of distal musculature on the motor homunculus. In addition, as opposed to seizures, there is a disappearance of movements in sleep.

Paroxysmal ataxia is a sporadic or familial disorder characterized by bouts lasting minutes to hours that involve an inability to walk, dysarthria, autonomic symptoms, and shaking limbs that might be mistaken for myoclonic or simple partial seizures or side effects related to antiepileptic medications. It may be familial, sporadic, or secondary to diffuse perinatal encephalopathy.[33] It may be differentiated from epilepsy by purely diurnal occurrence, longer duration (if greater than a few minutes), and normal EEG findings. This disorder may respond to treatment with acetazolamide.[33]

Tics are involuntary movements, typically involving the face or neck, that may be clonic (e.g.,

eye blinking, facial grimacing, vocalizations) or dystonic (e.g., eye deviation, blepharospasm, neck movements) in nature. They resemble simple partial motor seizures, and both are brief, repetitive, and stereotyped. A simple tic involves sudden movement in a few related muscle groups rather than in multiple systems of muscles.[38] There is often an antecedent irresistible urge to perform the tic, and it may be suppressed at least temporarily. Tics also worsen with stress and disappear in sleep, as with most movement disorders. These characteristics may allow differentiation from seizures. Tourette's syndrome arises in childhood and is characterized by multiple rapid tics and involuntary vocalizations. Echolalia and coprolalia may be seen, as well as complex stereotypes, obsessive-compulsive disorder, attention deficit hyperactivity disorder, and learning disabilities.

Stereotypical movements and self-stimulatory behavior are very common in the developmentally disabled population and may be mistaken for seizures. Activity may involve head shaking, swaying, rocking, staring, chewing, "hand-washing," tonic postures, and tics. Such behaviors tend to occur for longer and more variable periods of time than seizures and may be at least temporarily halted by distracting or restraining the patient.

Dystonia results in the assumption of a fixed abnormal body posture due to slow sustained stereotyped muscle contractions. Many dystonias are focal in nature and may be confused with focal tonic or clonic seizures. Those most likely to be confused are torticollis, blepharospasm, Meige's syndrome, and hemifacial spasm.

In idiopathic cervical dystonia, there are sudden episodes of dystonic head and neck posturing with face rotation to the opposite side. Duration can be minutes to days. In two-thirds of cases, head twisting is interrupted by jerks, leading to the designation *spasmodic torticollis*.[38] In children, benign paroxysmal torticollis presents within the first few months, and attacks are also associated with ataxia, gastrointestinal (GI) symptoms, and drowsiness.[38] Diagnostic confusion could occur with simple partial motor or focal tonic seizures, but episodes are purely diurnal and generally much longer than seizures, and the patient's EEG is normal. In children, the benign form usually resolves spontaneously within a few years. It may be important to exclude pathology of the posterior fossa or cervical cord, but in such instances the movements are usually sustained.

Blepharospasm is a facial dystonia that initially involves compulsory blinking. This is commonly associated with a feeling of irritation in the eyes. There is usually progression to clonic and later, sustained tonic contractions of the orbicularis oculi, leading to forceful closure of the eyelids, which can lead to functional blindness in many patients. Up to 20% of patients have unilateral involvement at the onset, but the opposite eye becomes involved later in all patients. Blepharospasm is rarely an isolated condition and is often associated with dystonia in other facial, cervical, perioral, and mandibular muscles. Dystonia in the limbs, trunk, and vocal cords may also be associated. Blepharospasm is usually exacerbated by bright light and activity, and the spasms may be transiently alleviated by pulling on an upper eyelid or an eyebrow, pinching the neck, talking, humming, yawning, singing, sleeping, relaxing, reading, concentrating, looking down, and other maneuvers.[41] Episodes may be differentiated from simple partial seizures by an absence of rhythmic clonic activity, disappearance in sleep, characteristic progression over time, and a normal EEG.

Blepharospasm may be combined with oromandibular dystonia in Meige's syndrome, which usually presents in middle age. The disorder is characterized by involuntary contractions of the muscles innervated by the fifth and seventh cranial nerves, producing repetitive, patterned mouth, jaw, and tongue movements. Patients have difficulty chewing, eating, and speaking because of an inability to open or close their jaws, and there is often lingual dystonia, activated by eating, which causes the tongue to push food out of the mouth. Involuntary vocalizations, such as humming, grunting, belching, and gasping, can occur.

Hemifacial spasm is a disorder characterized by involuntary, paroxysmal, tonic or clonic contractions of the muscles innervated by the seventh cranial nerve.[42] Ipsilateral vascular compression of the seventh nerve may be present in the majority of patients.[43] At onset, the patients experience twitches of the upper face and eyelid akin to blepharospasm, but with progression, the movements become more prolonged and dystonic, and involve the lower facial musculature. Contractions are triggered by action, such as smiling, talking, eating, or blinking. As opposed to the majority of movement disorders, hemifacial spasm may persist in sleep, which may make differentiation from simple partial motor seizures more difficult. However, a normal EEG, characteristic progression over time, sparing of pharyngeal, laryngeal, and masticatory muscles, and precipitation by facial motor activity would aid in diagnosis.

Startle disease, or hyperexplexia, is a hereditary disorder commencing in childhood that is characterized in its minor form by an exaggerated startle response to any type of stimulus. In its major form, diffuse stiffness occurs when an infant is handled that may cause apnea and bradycardia. Episodes may be mistaken for tonic seizures and result in falls in ambulatory patients. The episode may terminate with forced flexion of the neck or hips, allowing differentiation from a seizure. Also associated are ataxia, hyper-reflexia, and episodic limb shaking, suggesting a myoclonic or clonic seizure. A normal EEG during episodes helps to differentiate this disorder from startle epilepsy, in which partial or generalized seizures follow a startle, usually due to a sudden sound.[34] In addition, enhanced somatosensory evoked potentials may be seen.[44]

Myoclonus consists of sudden brief, shocklike, involuntary movements caused by muscular contraction (positive myoclonus) or inhibitions (negative myoclonus).[45] It can arise from the cortex, brain stem, or spinal cord. Potential etiologies are numerous, and the reader is referred to an excellent review.[38] Myoclonus can be classified as focal, multifocal, or generalized and may be symmetric or asymmetric. Events may occur at rest, with activity (intention myoclonus), or with stimuli (reflex myoclonus). Myoclonus may be rhythmic, in which case it is usually due to a focal lesion of the spinal cord or brain stem. In such cases, events may be mistaken for tonic-clonic seizures, although there is an absence of a tonic phase and the periods of jerking are briefer. Myoclonus may also be mistaken for myoclonic seizures, as are seen in secondary generalized epilepsies, juvenile myoclonic epilepsy, and progressive myoclonic epilepsies. In these patients, multiple seizure types occur, and an EEG demonstrates generalized spike or polyspike and slow-wave activity.

Benign neonatal myoclonus involves myoclonic jerks occurring in sleep in early infancy. The jerks are bilateral, asynchronous, and asymmetric and migrate among muscle groups.[34] Rhythmic activity may occur but is not prolonged as in seizures. The attacks are usually a few minutes long but may last for hours. The myoclonus is purely nocturnal and the EEG is normal.

Benign myoclonus of early infancy is a disorder characterized by what appear to be tonic-myoclonic seizures involving axial musculature, with or without limb involvement, that may resemble infantile spasm.[9] Clusters of episodes occur, particularly on awakening, a time when infantile spasms and generalized epilepsies also tend to express themselves. However, in this disorder, neurologic examination is normal, as is the EEG, even ictally. The episodes usually begin between 3 and 9 months of age and typically resolve by 2 years of age.[9]

Familial essential myoclonus is usually an autosomal dominant disorder, with the onset of myoclonus in the first or second decade of life. The myoclonus may be rhythmic or arrhythmic and multifocal or generalized, and the disorder is benign and nonprogressive.[46] Activity may be more prominent at rest or on intention.

In children, myoclonus may be associated with opsoclonus, consisting of rapid conjugate multidirectional oscillating eye movements. This association should raise suspicion for a neuroblastoma.[34] Children may also demonstrate myoclonus in the setting of metabolic abnormalities, such as hypoglycemia or biotinidase deficiency.[9]

Hypnagogic myoclonus (sleep starts; hypnic jerks) are single myoclonic jerks affecting the entire body, more prominently in the legs, that occur at sleep onset and are often associated with a perception of falling.[47] In children with mental retardation and spastic diplegia, repetitive hypnic jerks suggesting seizures have been reported.[48] However, the timing of such events usually leaves little confusion as to their nature. Fragmentary myoclonus may be seen during drowsiness or rapid eye movement (REM) sleep and consists of fine jerks of the face or hands.

Focal myoclonus involves a small group of muscles and may occur in an isolated or rhythmic fashion, in which case it may be mistaken for a simple partial motor seizure. However, as opposed to seizures, myoclonus does not demonstrate a motor march, does not occur for a sustained period of time, and is not associated with sensory symptoms. Palatal myoclonus is a rare focal myoclonic disorder consisting of continuous rhythmic synchronous jerks of the soft palate, muscles innervated by other cranial nerves, and, rarely, trunk and limb muscles. The myoclonus is usually rhythmic and unaffected by action, sleep, or distraction. It usually develops secondary to brain stem or cerebellar disease. Patients with palatal myoclonus have objective rhythmic clicking noises, which may be mistaken for simple auditory hallucinations.[49] However, examination of the oropharynx should lead immediately to the appropriate diagnosis.

Cortical myoclonus is frequently multifocal and stimulus sensitive, and involves distal muscles more prominently. Spinal myoclonus is seen in patients with spinal cord injuries and is usually symmetric, rhythmic, and continuous but may be stimulus sensitive, which would help to establish the correct diagnosis.[50] As with palatal myoclonus, movements persist in sleep.

Asterixis, a type of "negative myoclonus," consists of irregular inhibitory lapses of posture affecting various parts of the body independently.[51] These lapses are caused by silent periods appearing in muscles that are tonically active, such as on extension of the arms. When bilateral, asterixis is almost always due to a metabolic encephalopathy. Unilateral asterixis is due to a localized lesion, which may not be clinically evident, in the contralateral cerebral hemisphere. Episodes of asterixis may on occasion be mistaken for atonic seizures, but an EEG does not demonstrate epileptiform activity. However, rhythmic sharp triphasic waves may be seen in the setting of a metabolic encephalopathy.

There are also several movement disorders that occur exclusively in children. Spasmus nutans involves diurnal episodes of head nodding without an alteration in consciousness, commencing in children between 4 and 12 months of age.[9] Later, nystagmus and torticollis are associated. Resolution typically occurs in 1–2 years. In these children, the neurologic exam and the EEG are normal. Confusion might occur with atonic or dystonic frontal seizures, but such patients would generally also have prominent nocturnal seizures and an abnormal EEG. In addition, nystagmus is not associated with such seizures.

Shuddering attacks consist of sudden episodes of rapid 8- to 12-Hz tremors of the head, trunk, arms, and sometimes legs, with the elbows flexed and adducted.[9] Episodes last for only a few seconds, occur multiple times per day, and may be confused with myoclonic events. The neurologic exam and the EEG are normal, and antiepileptic medications do not alter the episodes. A diagnostically helpful finding may be an increased incidence of essential tremor in the family.[9,34] Onset occurs from infancy into early childhood, and resolution usually occurs in late childhood.[9]

In newborns, tremulousness or "jittery" movements may be seen in the setting of drug withdrawal, hypoxic encephalopathy, hypoglycemia, or hypocalcemia. Confusion with clonic or tonic-clonic seizures may occur. However, the EEG is normal, and the movements appear more tremor-like, show marked stimulus sensitivity, and stop with passive limb flexion.[47]

Formal testing is generally much less important than clinical assessment in differentiating seizures and movement disorders. An EEG may help by demonstrating clear-cut epileptiform activity, but a normal EEG does not definitively rule out the possibility of epilepsy, particularly if events are simple partial in nature. In some instances, video-EEG monitoring may be necessary to allow accurate diagnosis of events.

A detailed discussion of the treatment of movement disorders is beyond the scope of this text. It is most important for the clinician to be aware that some drugs used for movement disorders, such as major tranquilizers (e.g., chlorpromazine, haloperidol), may increase the risk of seizures in patients with epilepsy via lowering of the seizure threshold. AEDs may also alter the levels of drugs used for movement disorders. For example, phenytoin may lower the serum level of levodopa and carbamazepine that of haloperidol. Selegiline, used in Parkinson's disease, may inhibit the metabolism of carbamazepine, resulting in potential carbamazepine toxicity.

Movement disorders have been reported with the use of virtually all AEDs, particularly with toxic levels and often in those with baseline neurologic disabilities. Tremor, dyskinesias, and myoclonus are most common. Carbamazepine can cause asterixis and myoclonus and may also provoke tics in those with underlying movement disorders.[52] Valproic acid commonly causes tremor and may also cause dyskinesias and a reversible parkinso-nian syndrome.[53] Tremor is also caused by lamotrigine. Phenytoin is known to cause asterixis, ballismus, and also choreoathetosis,[54] usually with toxic blood levels. Gabapentin has recently been reported to cause myoclonus.[55] Alternatively, several AEDs may actually be helpful in the treatment of certain movement disorders. For example, valproic acid can be very efficacious in the treatment of myoclonus. Gabapentin and topiramate have been reported to be efficacious in the treatment of benign essential tremor.[56,57]

Dizziness and Vertigo

Dizziness is perhaps the most common episodic neurologic complaint, particularly in the elderly, and its meaning often varies from person to person. Thus, it is first crucial to determine the true nature of the complaint. Dizziness generally describes an unpleasant sensation of imbalance, altered spatial orientation, or lightheadedness. Patients with epilepsy may experience various types of ictal dizziness and may also experience dizziness as a side effect of their antiepileptic medications. However, in the majority of cases, dizziness is not related to epilepsy or its treatment. As a result, determining the cause of dizziness in patients with epilepsy can be particularly challenging.

There are four major categories of dizziness that must be distinguished: vertigo, dysequilibrium, presyncope, and psychogenic. Table 1-3 lists the various types of dizziness as well as possible etiologies.

Vertiginous dizziness implies a sense of motion, usually of rotation in space, or alternatively of body tilting. Simple partial seizures of temporoparietal origin may be suggested. Associated signs and symptoms include nystagmus, oscillopsia, imbalance, and autonomic symptoms, such as nausea and vomiting. Vertigo is usually due to abnormalities of the vestibular system or its central nervous system connections. Peripheral causes of vertigo are most common and involve pathology in the semicircular canals, vestibular nerve, or vestibular nuclei. These include cupulolithiasis, middle ear infections, vestibular neuronitis, head trauma, cervical deceleration injuries, cervical spine pathology, and normal aging.[58] Central causes of vertigo include seizures, medication side effects (e.g., antiepileptic medications), vertebrobasilar vascular disease, migraine, neurosyphilis, posterior fossa tumors, vasculitis, and multiple sclerosis.[58]

Benign positional vertigo is the most common vestibular disorder and is usually due to cupulolithiasis of the posterior semicircular canal.[58] It typically arises in the sixth decade of life or later. Vertigo is positional and typically occurs when the head is tilted backward or when turning in bed. A specific, evocative direction of head movement is usually noted by the patient. There is typically a brief delay to the onset of vertigo and nystagmus, and the attacks last less than a minute. With repeated stimulation, habituation occurs. The patient does not experience auditory or other neurologic symptoms, and an EEG is normal. On examination, nystagmus may be elicited by the Hallpike maneuver (Nylen-Barany), although this is often normal.[58]

Vestibular neuronitis involves the acute onset of vertigo, normal hearing, spontaneous nystagmus to the side of the healthy semicircular canal, and decreased caloric response on the affected side.[58] Patients worsen with any movement, as opposed to specific positions. Attacks last for hours to days, much longer than seizures. Akin to Bell's palsy, viruses have been etiologically implicated.[58] Acute labyrinthitis presents in a similar fashion.

Ménière's disease involves a clinical tetrad of vertigo, tinnitus, ear fullness, and progressive hearing loss.[58] Again, the bouts of vertigo are much longer than seizures, lasting hours and recurring every few weeks or months. Associated tinnitus may be mistaken for a simple partial sensory seizure but is more persistent. The disorder is assumed to be due to endolymphatic hydrops.

Acoustic neuromas may cause vertigo, although dysequilibrium is a more common effect. They typically present early with tinnitus and hearing loss. With growth, there is progressive involvement of the fifth and seventh cranial nerves.

Benign paroxysmal vertigo is a migrainous disorder of childhood characterized by bouts of vertigo and ataxia that are associated with secondary fear, generally lasting less than 5 minutes, but at times for hours. Rarely, autonomic phenomena such as vomiting, pallor, and sweating may occur. Nystagmus or torticollis may be associated. The child may cling to his or her parents or may lie still on the floor, suggesting an atonic event or syncope. However, consciousness and responsivity are pre-

Table 1-3. Differential Diagnosis of Dizziness

Character of Dizziness	Examples
Light-headedness (presyncope)	Volume depletion
	Severe anemia
	Orthostatic hypotension
	Aortic stenosis
	Carotid sinus hypersensitivity
	Neurocardiogenic presyncope
	Autonomic neuropathy
	Drugs
	Hypoxia
	Hypoglycemia
	Anxiety
Vertigo	Benign positional vertigo
	Vestibular neuronitis
	Acute labyrinthitis
	Ménière's disease
	Acoustic neuroma
	Ototoxic drugs
	Vertebrobasilar insufficiency
	Multiple sclerosis
	Drugs/alcohol
	Seizure
Dysequilibrium	Impaired vision
	Motor dysfunction
	Sensory dysfunction
	Cerebellar pathology
	Diabetes mellitus
Ill-defined giddiness	Anxiety
	Depression
	Psychosis

served. Onset is usually from 1 to 3 years of age, with typical resolution by 5–8 years.[9] The EEG is normal, but vestibular caloric testing is abnormal in the majority and may help in diagnosis.[9] Frequently, there is a family history of migraine, and most of these children go on to develop migraines.[9]

Dysequilibrium involves a sense of unsteadiness or imbalance when mobile but does not involve the actual perception of movement. If episodic, partial seizures may be suggested. Pathology in such cases may involve the vestibular system but also may be associated with abnormalities in other systems involved in the maintenance of equilibrium, such as the visual, motor, or proprioceptive systems. Those with sensory dysequilibrium perform worse in the dark or with eyes closed, which is not the case in motor dysequilibrium. Patients often improve with minor stabilization, such as the use of a cane. Etiologies include the effects of alcohol or medications; hypotension; lesions of the cerebellum, basal ganglia, or spinal cord; peripheral neuropathies; lesions of dorsal ganglia; hydrocephalus; hypothyroidism; refractive errors; anxiety or panic disorders; hyperventilation syndrome; depression; and conversion.[58] Given these possibilities, neurologic examination is important in deciding on a probable etiology for dysequilibrium.

Presyncope is characterized by lightheaded nonvertiginous dizziness that is commonly associated with weakness, diaphoresis, nausea, pallor, and visual dimming. Recumbency generally relieves the symptoms in most cases. The diagnostic considerations are similar to those discussed in the preceding section, Syncope. The history may provide clues as to the etiology of presyncope. For example, a history of fasting may suggest hypoglycemia. Prolonged standing or a temporal relationship to medications may suggest orthostatic presyncope. Occurrence with pain or fright would suggest a neurocardiogenic mechanism.

Psychogenic dizziness involves a vague giddiness or feeling of dissociation, usually in patients with anxiety. Symptoms are not relieved by recumbency and are usually continuous, with periodic exacerbations and bouts of presyncope induced by hyperventilation. Specific environmental triggers, such as enclosed spaces, may be identified. The diagnosis can be confirmed by having the patient hyperventilate to recreate typical symptoms.

In cases of epilepsy, nonspecific dizziness may occur during epileptic auras, as can true vertigo, which arises from ictal activity in the temporoparietal region. Both types of dizziness may also be seen as side effects of AEDs. In addition, nystagmus may be seen related to seizures or antiepileptic medications. If ictal in nature, dizziness or vertigo would tend to be brief in duration, would occur in any position, would not be triggered or worsened by movements, and would not be associated with other ictal phenomena. If related to medications, duration would be longer and bouts would tend to occur with a similar temporal association to the administration of medications.

The treatment of vertigo in patients with seizures raises some concerns. Most of the drugs used for the symptomatic treatment of vertigo are anti-histamines (e.g., meclizine, trimethobenzamide, dimenhydrinate) or phenothiazines (e.g., promethazine, prochlorperazine), classes of drugs that are known to lower seizure threshold. Thus, these agents should be used with caution in seizure patients experiencing vertigo, although there is usually a low risk when low doses are used.

Sleep Disorders

Of all the various types of disorders discussed in this text, the relationship of epilepsy to sleep and its disorders is perhaps the closest. In both, alterations in consciousness, motor tone, and paroxysmal EEG changes occur. In addition, approximately 60% of patients with epilepsy experience at least some seizures in sleep, with 10–25% having purely nocturnal events.[59] It is also well known that sleep deprivation may precipitate seizures or the appearance of epileptic interictal activity in EEGs. Many sleep disorders present with nocturnal, behavioral paroxysms, suggestive of seizures of various types, and diurnal phenomena of narcolepsy, such as sleep attacks, cataplexy, and automatic behavior, which may also be mistaken for seizures. This section concentrates on the differentiation of sleep disorders and seizures. For a more detailed discussion of sleep disorders, please refer to Chapter 14.

There are several types of sleep disorders, but those most likely to be confused with epilepsy are disorders of hypersomnolence (e.g., narcolepsy, sleep apnea) and parasomnias (e.g., sleep walking, night terrors, REM behavior disorder). Insomnia is the most common sleep problem, but it presents little diagnostic confusion.

Narcolepsy involves the intrusion of various aspects of REM sleep into wakefulness, as well as the disruption of nocturnal sleep. The most common clinical episodes are brief, irresistible sleep attacks (microsleeps), which can occur even when the patient is stimulated by his or her environment. These may last only seconds to minutes, and afterward the patient typically feels refreshed. Also associated are sleep paralysis, vivid hallucinations at sleep-wake transitions (hypnagogic and hypnopompic hallucinations), and cataplexy, involving a loss of tone, but not consciousness, usually precipitated by intense emotion or startle. Periods of automatic behavior can also occur, for which the patient is amnestic. Individuals do not necessarily experience all of these symptoms, but the essential characteristics of the disorder are excessive daytime sleepiness and REM sleep attacks.

Diagnostic confusion with epilepsy can occur, although the presence of multiple typical symptoms of the disorder usually makes the diagnosis clear. Sleep attacks may be mistaken for absence or complex partial seizures, but attacks are characteristically preceded by an irresistible urge to sleep, which is unusual for these seizure types. Observers report the appearance of normal sleep during episodes, as opposed to staring or automatic activity, and the patient can be aroused, which would be less likely were a seizure occurring. In addition, patients are refreshed afterward and are not "postictal." Bouts of automatic behavior with amnesia are more likely to be mistaken for such seizures, but such behavior is more complex and goal directed than ictal or postictal automatisms, typically consisting of normal routines.[59] Cataplectic attacks may be mistaken for atonic seizures, although there is no alteration of awareness, and they are typically precipitated by strong emotion. Hallucinations may be mistaken for simple or complex partial seizures, but this is unlikely given their specific occurrence at sleep-wake transitions and the presence of other features of narcolepsy. Sleep paralysis might be mistaken for inhibitory motor seizures, but the duration is typically much longer than a seizure; it may be terminated by touching the patient and, once again, the timing is characteristic, occurring on awakening.

The diagnosis of narcolepsy is established by demonstrating hypersomnolence (sleep onset of less than 5 minutes) and sleep-onset REM periods (within 15 minutes of sleep onset) on a multiple sleep latency test. In addition, more than 90% of patients with narcolepsy carry the human leukocyte antigens (HLA) HLA-DR2 and HLA-DQw1,[60] and their demonstration may help to confirm the diagnosis.

Sleep apnea is characterized by daytime hypersomnolence due to repeated bouts of nocturnal apnea, which are most commonly due to upper airway obstruction. The patient may experience sleep attacks during the day that are typically not refreshing, as opposed to the sleep attacks of narcolepsy. As with narcolepsy, patients may perform automatic behavior for which they have no recall, which may be mistaken for complex partial seizures. Differentiation from epilepsy is based on clinical characteristics of episodes similar to those described for narcolepsy. A history of obesity, snoring, and headaches on awakening suggests the possibility of sleep apnea. Hypersomnolence may be noted on a routine EEG, and the diagnosis is confirmed with overnight polysomnography.

Somnambulism (sleep walking) occurs primarily in children and occurs within the first 2 hours of sleep, during slow-wave sleep.[59] Episodes last up to 30 minutes and may be confused with complex partial seizures or poriomania, a postictal automatism of aimless wandering. In fact, some sleep-walking attacks may actually be epileptic in nature.[61] Semipurposeful, moderately complex behavior is seen, with the patient arising and walking around, at times even outside. Patients have a glassy stare and may mumble, but communication with them is difficult or impossible. They may perform activities such as eating, carrying objects, or rearranging furniture. Frenzied behavior and wielding of weapons can occur and may result in injury. Amnesia for the event is typical, and patients may awaken in bed or in other rooms, unaware of how they have gotten there. Somnambulism can be differentiated from seizures by the fact that a single bout of somnambulism occurs during the night, usually early in the night when slow-wave sleep occurs, whereas seizures may occur several times in a single night at various times. The automatisms of somnambulism also tend to be more complex than the simple, often oroalimentary automatisms of complex partial seizures. In addition, somnambulists can more easily be led back to bed than epilepsy patients, who are in a confused postictal state. There is also often a family history of somnambulism. Electroencephalographically, somnambulist attacks arise out of slow-wave sleep and demonstrate unreactive monomorphic theta range activity.[59] Although complex partial seizures are frequently associated with a theta range ictal discharge, there is typically a gradual slowing of ictal activity into the delta frequency range before termination, as well as a postictal delta range slowing postictally.

Night terrors (pavor nocturnus) also occur primarily in young children and, as with somnambulism, episodes occur out of slow-wave sleep within the first few hours of the night. A family history of parasomnias is common. The attacks involve abrupt arousal from sleep with unresponsiveness and inconsolable screaming and crying for up to 10 minutes, followed by amnesia for the event.[59] Intense sympathetic outflow is associated with tachycardia, tachypnea, diaphoresis, piloerection, and mydriasis.[59] As opposed to nightmares, patients do not recall a frightening dream, although they may recall sensations of choking or suffocation at the onset. Confusion with complex partial seizures can occur, particularly with seizures arising from the frontal lobe, which can be associated with intense affective vocalizations. However, such frontal seizures are typically only 20–30 seconds in duration and usually occur multiple times per night at various times, whereas night terrors occur as a single event during the early portion of the night. Notably, there are rare cases of patients diagnosed with night terrors that were proven to be epileptic in nature.[62]

Confusional arousal, or sleep drunkenness, most commonly occurs with incomplete arousals during the first 2 to 3 hours of sleep, although they may occur with morning arousals as well. There is mental confusion, relative unresponsiveness to environmental stimuli, and difficulty in fully awakening the patient.[63] Relatively complex and inappropriate automatic behavior occurs, such as uttering unintelligible speech or attempting to speak to a lamp when the phone has rung.[63] Aggression can occur toward the person attempting to awaken the patient, and this, combined with gait instability, leads to the name *sleep drunkenness*. There is amnesia for the episode and no recalled associated dreaming. Episodes are differentiated from complex partial seizures by their specific precipitation by arousal.

REM behavior disorder is an entity involving periods of REM sleep that occur without the usual associated muscular atonia, resulting in patients' "acting out" their dreams. The episodes occur primarily in middle-aged to older men. The episodes typically occur late in the sleep cycle, when there is greatest REM density, and involve sudden apparent arousal with unresponsiveness, but immediate aggressive or defensive behavior, including punching, kicking, or running. Injuries to self or bed partners are common. Amnesia for their behavior is typical, although patients recall vivid dreams in which they are attacked.

Episodes of REM behavior disorder may be confused with rage attacks or frontal lobe complex partial seizures, particularly those arising from the orbitofrontal cortex. However, episodes of REM behavior disorder arise out of REM sleep, the sleep stage least likely to be associated with clinical seizures. They tend to occur late in the sleep cycle, whereas seizures may occur at various times during the night. Patients recall threatening nightmares associated with the episodes, which is unusual for seizures. The complex motor activity displayed is more violent and goal directed than the automatisms seen with most seizures, although frontal lobe complex partial seizures may have bizarre complex motor automatisms (e.g., thrashing, kicking, punching, cursing, spitting) and commonly occur in sleep.[3] However, such seizures would generally not be expected to arise from REM sleep. Violence may also occur during the postictal phase of more typical complex partial seizures, although this is much less goal directed and typically occurs only when attempts are made to restrain the patient.

Nocturnal anxiety attacks may raise a suspicion for complex partial seizures. These are related to nightmares and occur as arousals from REM sleep, usually late in the sleep cycle, when REM density is highest.[59] Patients recall the frightening dream before arousal and then are awake and fearful without the unresponsiveness, automatic behavior, or postictal state of seizures, parasomnias, or REM behavior disorder.

Two sleep-related neuromuscular disorders occur in older adults, often manifest together, and may result in insomnia and daytime sleepiness: restless legs syndrome and periodic limb movements in sleep (PLMS). Restless legs syndrome is characterized by unpleasant leg sensations at rest described as "itching," "tingling," "pulling," or "crawling." There is a very strong presleep urge to move or stimulate the legs to eliminate these feelings, which results in insomnia. The majority of patients with restless legs syndrome also have PLMS.

PLMS occurs in light sleep, may result in arousals and daytime sleepiness, and may be mistaken for simple partial motor seizures. Episodes involve dorsiflexion of the foot and great toe, with flexion at the knee; last 1–2 seconds; and recur approximately every 30 seconds over the course of minutes to hours.[59] In some cases, the arms may also be involved. Patients may not be aware of the movements, although bed partners complain of kicking movements.[64] PLMS may be associated with EEG arousal, K complexes, or no change in the EEG. Periods of sleep apnea may be associated.[65] Diagnosis is established by performing a polysomnographic study.

Hypnagogic and fragmentary myoclonus may be mistaken for simple partial motor or myoclonic seizures and were previously discussed in the section Movement Disorders. In that section, paroxysmal nocturnal dystonia was also discussed.

Sleep bruxism and enuresis may occasionally lead to concern about possible nocturnal seizures. Sleep bruxism is characterized by repeated rhythmic grinding or clenching of the teeth during all stages of sleep, with each bout lasting for a few seconds.[59] It is most common in children and adolescents and is often related to anxiety or depression.[59] Morning jaw pain may be present, and temporomandibular joint syndrome can be associated. Dental damage may occur, as well as ulceration and ridging of the buccal mucosa opposite the molars, but tongue biting, as might be seen with a seizure, is unusual.

Nocturnal enuresis is characterized by recurrent involuntary urination during sleep after toilet training has been achieved, usually after the age of 5 years. Differentiation from seizures is based on an absence of associated postictal signs or symptoms (e.g., tongue biting, diffuse muscle soreness, lethargy), a normal EEG, and a family history of enuresis.

Another childhood parasomnia that may raise suspicion for nocturnal tonic-clonic seizures is jactatio capitis nocturna. This disorder is most common in association with static encephalopathy or stress and consists of a rhythmic rocking of the head or entire body in light sleep, which lasts for 5–15 minutes.[59] It may be differentiated from seizures by the typical presentation and an ability to terminate the movements with arousal of the child.

The assessment of sleep disorders and their differentiation from seizures relies first on a detailed sleep history from the patient and observers. In many instances, this alone provides the correct diagnosis or at least allows a general differentiation of sleep disorders from seizures. The presence of a normal EEG, particularly during sleep, also makes the diagnosis of a seizure disorder much less likely.

Formal diagnostic testing for most sleep disorders usually first involves an overnight polysomnogram with measurement of EEG, eye movements, electromyography of chin and tibialis anterior muscles, respiratory effort and flow, oxygenation via pulse oximetry, and cardiac rhythm. In the case of narcolepsy, diagnosis is obtained with a multiple sleep latency test that involves three to six trials of sleep given every 2 hours. The latency to sleep onset is measured, and narcolepsy is suggested by the demonstration of sleep-onset REM periods (within 15 minutes) or sleep latency of 5 minutes or less, or both. However, sleep-onset REM periods may be seen with sleep deprivation or suppression of natural REM by medications, such as antidepressants. For this reason, a polysomnogram may be indicated before performing a multiple sleep latency test.

There are several treatment issues to be considered in patients who have sleep disorders and seizures. In patients with epilepsy, the use of antiepileptic medications may cause alterations in sleep patterns. In patients with coexistent epilepsy and sleep apnea, seizure control is improved with correction of the apnea.[66] In narcolepsy, stimulants such as dextroamphetamine, methylphenidate, and pemoline that are used to treat hypersomnolence, as well as tricyclic agents used for cataplexy, may cause a lowering of the seizure threshold. Alternatively, some AEDs, such as benzodiazepines or gabapentin, may be useful in sleep disorders such as restless legs syndrome.[67]

Endocrine and Metabolic Disorders

There are a number of ways in which endocrine and metabolic disorders may interact with and be mistaken for seizures. Metabolic changes, either primary or secondary to an endocrine disturbance, may precipitate seizures directly or lower seizure threshold and hormonal changes, such as those associated with menses, may alter seizure susceptibility. There are several endocrine and metabolic disorders that present with paroxysmal episodes to suggest seizures. This section places an emphasis on phenomenology and differentiation from seizures. Further information regarding these disorders can be found in Chapters 3 and 10.

In many instances, patients with endocrine or metabolic disorders present with other symptoms characteristic of these disorders, making the diagnosis of paroxysms clearer. In addition, the characteristics of the episodes, such as timing of occurrence, may provide further clues. For example, occurrence at a fixed time relative to meals or intake of oral hypoglycemics may suggest a disorder of glucose homeostasis.

Abnormalities of glucose regulation are the endocrine disturbances most commonly confused with epilepsy, and they are also capable of producing physiologic seizures. Hypoglycemia generally causes clinical symptoms at serum levels below 45 mg/dl,[68] with lethargy, confusion, and behavioral changes suggesting complex partial seizures. Focal weakness may occur, suggesting an inhibitory simple partial motor seizure or a vascular event. In addition, physiologic seizures may occur, generally tonic-clonic in nature, which may lead to further diagnostic confusion. Associated anxiety, palpitations, tachycardia, hyperventilation, sweating, blurry vision, nausea or vomiting, and tremor may suggest an anxiety disorder or a simple partial autonomic seizure. The duration of symptoms is typically longer than that of a seizure, and one may also note a specific timing of events in relationship to the consumption of food, fasting, or the administration of hypoglycemic medications. The diagnosis is made with documentation of a low blood glucose or correction of symptoms with the administration of glucose, or both.

Nonketotic hyperglycemia presents with symptoms that are gradual and progressive in onset, unlike seizures.[68] Altered consciousness can occur, suggesting the possibility of a complex partial event. Abnormal movements, such as asterixis and paroxysmal choreoathetosis, occur in up to 6% of cases, presenting possible confusion with primary movement disorders, as well as myoclonic or simple partial motor seizures.[68] Focal seizures may be precipitated, including epilepsia partialis continua, which may be resistant to antiepileptic medications.[68] Diagnosis is based on the gradual onset of symptoms and documentation of hyperglycemia.

Hypoparathyroidism with hypocalcemia may present with paraesthesias and, when severe, tetany with painful tonic muscular contractions (carpo-

pedal spasm) that increase gradually and symmetrically.[68] Associated symptoms include irritability, depression, psychosis, and focal or generalized tonic-clonic seizures.[68] There may be a similarity to tonic seizures, but episodes are longer and more gradual in onset than seizures. Tapping the parotid region may induce unilateral facial contraction (Chvostek's sign), and serum calcium level is low.

Symptoms of hyponatremia are dependent on the degree of hyponatremia and the rate of fall. Confusion and stupor may occur at sodium levels of 120 mEq/liter or less,[68] suggesting complex partial seizures or NCSE given the more prolonged duration of symptoms, but the EEG would not be expected to demonstrate epileptiform activity. Seizures and coma may occur with lower levels.[68] The AED carbamazepine is notable for causing the syndrome of inappropriate secretion of antidiuretic hormone with associated hyponatremia.

Both hyper- and hypothyroidism are associated with encephalopathies and choreoathetotic movements that may mimic seizures.[68] In addition, seizures, usually tonic-clonic in nature, have been reported in both conditions.[68] Diagnosis is established by the presence of associated signs and symptoms of these disorders, as well as documentation of abnormal thyroid function tests. Periodic paralysis may sometimes be associated with thyroid disease and may present the impression of inhibitory motor seizures. However, as opposed to seizures, in this disorder, weakness progresses over minutes to an hour, symptoms last for less than an hour to several days, and facial and respiratory muscles are usually spared. There is often an association with rest after exercise and, during attacks, the potassium level is found to be either depressed or elevated.

Pheochromocytomas and other paragangliomas produce symptoms via the secretion of excess catecholamines. Symptoms include headache, visual changes, pallor, sweating, malaise, and hypertension.[68] Anxiety, dizziness, palpitations, dyspnea, paraesthesias, flushing, and epigastric or chest discomfort may cause confusion with panic disorder or simple partial autonomic seizures. However, there is no relationship to emotional stress, as might be the case in panic disorder. Tremor may be mistaken for myoclonic or simple partial motor seizures. Syncope and convulsions have been reported, which can lead to further diagnostic confusion. The episodes typically last for less than 20 minutes, which is brief, but still longer than most seizures. Historically, episodes may be found to be triggered by movements that displace the abdominal contents.[68] Diagnosis is via the demonstration of elevated catecholamine levels in the blood or elevated urinary metabolites of catecholamines.

Carcinoid syndrome is due to carcinoid tumor secretion of serotonin. Clinical episodes consist of flushing with erythema (limited to the face, neck and upper trunk), a sensation of warmth, GI hypermotility (at times with diarrhea and abdominal cramps), and occasional palpitations and dizziness.[68] On occasion, syncope can occur. The presence of a warm sensation and GI symptoms may be mistaken for a simple partial autonomic seizure with origin in the temporal lobe. Diagnosis is made by the demonstration of elevated serotonin metabolites in the urine.

Mastocytosis presents with symptoms very similar to the carcinoid syndrome—vasodilatation and flushing, tachycardia, abdominal cramps, and occasional hypotension and nausea or vomiting.[68] These symptoms are then followed by lethargy and prostration. Again, symptoms may be mistaken for a temporal lobe simple partial autonomic seizure, but the duration of paroxysms is longer than most seizures, and the EEG is normal.

The symptoms of acute intermittent porphyria may sometimes be mistaken for seizures, and this disorder is also capable of producing focal and generalized seizures.[69] In addition, it is important to be aware that hepatically metabolized drugs, such as phenobarbital and phenytoin, may precipitate or worsen an attack of this disorder. For this reason, newer AEDs without significant hepatic metabolism, such as gabapentin, may be advantageous.[70] Autonomic symptoms, such as abdominal pain, tachycardia, and diaphoresis may raise suspicion for an autonomic temporal lobe seizure. Aside from seizures, cerebral symptoms can include headaches, aphasia, apraxia, homonymous hemianopsia, and psychosis.[69] Delirium with confusion, paranoia, and hallucinations or a catatonic state may occur, suggesting complex partial seizures or NCSE. The correct diagnosis may be established by the presence of a nonepileptiform EEG, documentation of elevated urinary porphobilinogen and δ-aminolevulinic acid during attacks, and associ-ated neurologic findings, such as flaccid paralysis with areflexia.

In treating patients with seizures and endocrine or metabolic disorders, it is important to be aware of potential drug effects and interactions. Hormones and AEDs can have reciprocal effects via hepatic enzyme induction. For example, enzyme-inducing AEDs lead to a hypermetabolism of thyroid hormones, with phenytoin and carbamazepine causing 60% and 74% decreases in total T4, respectively.[71] However, these AEDs displace T3 and T4 from binding proteins, resulting in normal free levels of these hormones.[71] When abnormalities are found, a thyroid-stimulating hormone level should be checked to confirm the euthyroid state of the patient.[71] Enzyme-inducing AEDs also cause an increase in hepatic synthesis of sex hormone–binding globulin and also increase the metabolism of hormones, including contraceptives, leading to an increase in the required dosage. Phenytoin and carbamazepine may directly block the synthesis of testosterone[72] and may also elevate estradiol levels.[73] Menstrual disorders are also seen with AEDs, such as carbamazepine and valproic acid, and correlate with sex hormone changes.[74] In women, exposure to valproic acid has been associated with hyperandrogenism, polycystic ovarian disease, obesity, and menstrual irregularities.[75] Conversely, steroid hormones may also cause increased metabolism of AEDs, resulting in lower serum levels of drugs such as phenobarbital or phenytoin.

Toxic Disorders

Toxic substances may cause many neurologic effects, but they are most likely to be confused with seizures when they cause a clinical picture of delirium, which may also be seen in the setting of metabolic, infectious, and structural disease. Delirium is an acute organic mental syndrome characterized by a reduced level of consciousness, global cognitive impairment, attentional abnormalities, increased or decreased psychomotor activity, and a disordered sleep-wake cycle.[76] Patients are disoriented and may experience visual and auditory illusions and hallucinations. They may be agitated or apathetic. The clinical presentation may be confused with complex partial seizures or a postictal state, although most cases of delirium can be differentiated from seizures by their much longer duration.

Alcohol use and withdrawal may cause seizures, as well as several clinical states that may be confused with seizures. The effects of acute intoxication are usually clinically obvious, and diagnosis can be confirmed with a blood alcohol level.

Pathologic intoxication may be seen with even small amounts of alcohol and may consist of inappropriate behavior or even outbursts of rage and aggression followed by sleep and then partial or total amnesia for the event. Confusion can occur with complex partial seizures or postictal agitation, but there would be an absence of an unresponsive phase and automatisms, and the antecedent consumption of alcohol would suggest the diagnosis. Alcoholic blackouts involve a period of amnesia for events occurring during severe intoxication, although the patient's state of consciousness is not severely altered. There may be confusion with complex partial seizures, but observers' reports of the patient's relatively normal behavior during the episodes, as well as the history of alcohol consumption, should make the diagnosis apparent.

Wernicke's encephalopathy is a result of thiamine deficiency and presents as an acute or subacute confusional state with disorientation, inattention, memory impairment, and drowsiness, suggesting complex partial seizures or a postictal state. The diagnosis is suggested by a history of alcohol intake, as well as associated abducens or conjugate gaze palsies.[77]

Alcohol withdrawal is associated with a state of central nervous system excitation with initial tremulousness. Within 12–24 hours of abstinence, alcoholic hallucinosis can occur, which is characterized by primarily visual hallucinations without a clouded sensorium that might be mistaken for simple partial occipital or temporal lobe seizures. However, as opposed to seizures, such hallucinations would tend to be less stereotypical and more illusory in nature, involving the misperception of environmental stimuli. Visual hallucinations in this setting tend to involve animate objects. Auditory hallucinosis also may occur at this time and may involve elementary sounds, such as buzzing, or may be musical in nature.[78] Vocal hallucinations usually also occur, are perceived as real and objective in origin, and may be threatening and disturbing to the patient.[78] They may react emotionally to

auditory or visual hallucinations as if they represent an actual threat. Conversely, ictal hallucinations are usually perceived as unreal by patients.

Twenty-four to forty-eight hours after alcohol abstinence, a state of delirium tremens may develop, characterized by delirium, agitation, insomnia, and auditory or visual illusions and hallucinations.[78] Complex partial seizures might be suggested. Notably, in this state hallucinations may be provoked by suggestion,[78] which would be very unusual for seizures. Autonomic hyperactivity is also seen, with tachycardia, hyperthermia, and diaphoresis. Seizures may be excluded by the typical combination of mental and physical symptoms, a nonepileptiform EEG, and a history of alcohol abstinence.

There are many drugs of abuse that may cause delirium, suggesting the possibility of complex partial seizures, particularly when illusions or hallucinations are associated. Examples include the hallucinogens lysergic acid diethylamide, phencyclidine, methylenedioxymethamphetamine (ecstasy), mescaline, and psilocybin. However, with the exception of short-acting agents, such as dimethyltryptamine, the duration of the drug's effects is much longer than would be expected for a seizure. NCSE might be considered, but there would be an absence of automatisms, and an EEG would not be expected to demonstrate epileptiform activity.

Tetanus may occur in local and generalized forms, and it is the latter that may be mistaken for seizures. Early symptoms include rigidity of the masseters and facial muscles, with straightening of the upper lip (risus sardonicus). Rigidity of axial muscles follows, and then of the limbs, with relative sparing of distal segments. Paroxysmal, violent contractions of the involved muscles (reflex spasms) appear repetitively in severe cases in response to voluntary movement and even to slight external and internal stimuli.[79] As a result, patients are kept in darkened rooms with little external stimuli. The clinical impression can be one of tonic or tonic-clonic seizures, but retention of consciousness and stimulus sensitivity, as well as a normal EEG, would suggest otherwise. Generalized spasms as well as laryngospasm contribute to ventilatory insufficiency and asphyxia, which may result in alteration of consciousness and true convulsive seizures. Autonomic instability, with a hypersympathetic state, may complicate severe cases. The symptoms worsen for 10–14 days after onset, and recovery usually begins after a month.

Poisoning with strychnine may be fatal and results in an excitatory state owing to competition with the inhibitory neurotransmitter glycine.[80] There is initial excitement and irritability followed by generalized rigidity with trismus, opisthotonus and extension of the limbs, although the arms can be flexed. Muscular fasciculations are seen, as well as hyper-reflexia. The patient may then experience tonic or clonic "seizures," which are generated at the spinal level and may be triggered by stimuli. This phase may last for a few to 30 minutes and may be clinically mistaken for tonic, clonic, or tonic-clonic seizures. However, at this stage, patients have a clear sensorium during the events and no postictal state, helping to differentiate these events from cortical seizures.[81] This period may then be followed by true generalized tonic-clonic seizures. The clinical course may be complicated by respiratory failure, acidosis, and rhabdomyolysis. Treatment involves supportive care, as well as a darkened room with minimal stimulation, as is done in cases of tetanus, and possible neuromuscular blockade.[81] If necessary, AEDs are used for associated seizures.

Poisoning with camphor may occur as a suicidal gesture or accidentally in young children, as it is a constituent of mothballs. Patients experience headache, warmth, blurry vision, vertigo, and abdominal pain. At this stage, a simple partial temporal seizure may be suspected. After minutes to hours, delirium and confusion occur and, rarely, excitement with hallucinations and aggressivity,[82] potentially raising suspicion for a complex partial seizure or postictal state. There may then be twitching of buccal and oral mucosa, as well as rigidity with trismus, which may be followed by a loss of consciousness,[82] suggesting seizure generalization. This phase may then be followed by actual tonic-clonic seizures, which may be repetitive.[82] Death may occur from respiratory or circulatory collapse. This syndrome can be differentiated from seizures by the presence of a nonepileptiform EEG, progression over a much longer time course than seizures, and a camphor smell to the breath and urine. However, the occurrence of true generalized convulsions may lead to diagnostic confusion.

Table 1-4. Psychiatric Disorders Misdiagnosed as Epilepsy

Panic disorder
Post-traumatic stress disorder
Impulse control disorder
Dissociative disorder
Psychotic disorders
Seizurelike episodes:
Unconscious—conversion
Somatoform disorder (with conversion)
Conscious—malingering
Factitious disorder

Psychiatric Disorders

Many symptoms of psychiatric disorders occur paroxysmally and may also be seen as part of an epileptic aura, as well as during ictal or postictal phases. As a result, it is not uncommon for psychiatric symptoms to be misdiagnosed as epileptic in nature. Alternatively, ictal symptoms may at times be misinterpreted as an expression of a primary psychiatric disorder, particularly because patients with epilepsy have a higher rate of psychopathology than the general population.[83] In patients with epilepsy who have such symptoms, it is important to determine whether there is a temporal association to seizures, as proper treatment in this case requires primarily seizure control as opposed to the use of psychotropic medications. Differentiation of epileptic and psychiatric symptoms can be particularly challenging because cortical regions generating such phenomena lie deep within the limbic system and, as a result, one may not even rely on ictal EEG recordings. As a result, differentiation once again rests on the clinical history.

Table 1-4 contains a list of psychiatric disorders with episodic symptoms that may be misdiagnosed as epilepsy. The primary symptoms of these disorders involve hallucinations, panic or anxiety, aggression or rage, dissociation or amnesia, or seizurelike episodes. As discussed previously, nonepileptic paroxysmal behavioral events suspected of being seizures are termed NESs. Patients with seizurelike episodes are distinguished from other NES patients with psychological symptoms by the belief and intentional attempt (conscious or unconscious) to make others believe that the episodes represent epileptic seizures. Such classic "pseudoseizures" are most commonly conversion symptoms, attributable to pure conversion disorder or somatization disorder with conversion seizures as a symptom and are formally classified as *conversion NESs*. NESs that are not conversion reactions but are paroxysmal behavioral features of other psychiatric syndromes are referred to as *nonconversion NESs*.

Primary psychiatric disorders can most reliably be differentiated from epilepsy by the same diagnostic principles previously discussed. Epileptic paroxysms are brief, stereotypical, and less likely to be related to environmental stimuli than are primary psychiatric symptoms. Additionally, in patients with primary psychiatric disorders, there is usually no history of other phenomena suggestive of seizures. The routine EEG cannot be relied on completely to exclude seizures as a cause of episodic psychiatric symptoms, because epileptiform activity in such cases may not be seen due to its location in deep limbic structures, such as the amygdala. Yield may be increased in such cases by the use of sphenoidal electrodes. Alternatively, the presence of epileptiform activity, particularly in the anterior temporal region, must make the clinician even more diligent in performing a detailed clinical history to determine the true nature of the patient's symptoms. In such instances, caution must be exercised in attributing a patient's symptoms to epilepsy, as epileptiform EEG abnormalities are found with higher frequency in patients with psychiatric disorders, and as many as 10% of healthy patients also demonstrate such abnormalities.[4]

Hallucinatory phenomena in multiple sensory modalities may occur as part of psychotic disorders, such as schizophrenia or psychotic depression. In general, hallucinations associated with psychiatric disorders are most commonly auditory, more prolonged and variable in content than ictal hallucinations, and often self referential and persecutory in nature. Ictal auditory hallucinations tend to be more elementary in nature (e.g., buzzing, humming), brief, and stereotypical, and there may be a past history of such symptoms that precede a more obvious clinical seizure. Visual hallucinations are more common as ictal phenomena and, again, are stereotypical in nature. They typically have a translucent ghostlike appearance. As opposed to the case with psychoses, reality testing is maintained, and the ictal hallucinations are perceived as unreal by the patient.[84] Hallucinations may also occur during a postictal psychosis and, in this setting, are more prolonged, variable, and likely to be confused with a primary psychiatric disorder. Such postictal psychoses typically occur 24–48 hours after a cluster of seizures and have prominent mood symptoms with paranoid delusions and hallucinations.[85] There is a similarity to psychotic depression, but the temporal association with seizures is the key to diagnosis. Amygdaloid seizures may be associated with the ictal sensation of someone standing behind the contralateral shoulder, leading to the misdiagnosis of a paranoid disorder. The ictal nature of this phenomenon is suggested by its brevity, as well as the presence of consistent lateralization of the sensation.

Symptoms of anxiety disorders, including panic and post-traumatic stress disorders, may be confused with simple partial seizures of an autonomic nature, which usually have their onset in the amygdala or insular cortex. Ictal fear arises from the amygdala and is the most common ictal emotion.[84] It must be differentiated from reactive fear secondary to the experience of some other preictal symptom. Symptoms shared with anxiety or panic attacks include tachycardia, piloerection, sweating, flushing, hyperventilation, paraesthesias, and nausea. These symptoms may also be mistaken for a cardiac disorder or pheochromocytoma. At times, confusion, derealization, depersonalization, and amnesia can be associated with panic, leading to the impression of a complex partial seizure. Focal neurologic symptoms, such as hemisensory numbness, blindness, vertigo, and visual distortions, can sometimes be seen with panic, and attacks may occur out of sleep, all suggesting the possibility of a seizure.[86] Anxiety or panic attacks differ from seizures in having a much greater likelihood of being triggered by environmental stressors, such as large crowds or other phobic stimuli. In addition, when ictal in nature, the panic tends to be maximal at onset with a total duration of only a few minutes, whereas "functional" panic attacks develop maximal intensity within 5–10 minutes and have a total duration of 15–20 minutes. Patients with hyperventilation syndrome may have overlap with anxiety or panic disorders, which may cause cerebral vasoconstriction on the basis of hypocarbia, which results in ischemia leading to dizziness, dysequilibrium, confusion, and states such as depersonalization. Perioral and digital paraesthesias are usually present, and carpopedal spasms may occur, suggesting the possibility of a tonic seizure. Patients often also complain of dyspnea, palpitations, and chest discomfort. A diagnosis can be made by having the patient recreate typical symptoms through hyperventilation, and bouts can be terminated via rebreathing into a paper bag.

There are several psychiatric disorders that are characterized by bouts of rage or aggression, or both, that may be confused with epilepsy. Ictal aggression is extremely rare, occurs unprovoked, and usually consists of poorly organized acts, rather than a series of intentional acts, such as obtaining and using a weapon against someone.[87] Most commonly, aggression in epilepsy occurs only during the immediate postictal period in a state of confusion and only when attempts are made to restrain the patient. Such aggression is, again, generally unorganized and simple, such as pushing or shoving. Directed, organized acts of aggression are unusual in epilepsy. However, of note, there has been a report of delayed postictal aggression of a more organized and directed manner that is stereotypical and follows a time course similar to postictal psychosis, with an approximately 24-hour period of postictal lucidity before onset.[88]

In young children, temper tantrums may at times be mistaken for complex partial seizures, although there is usually a clear association with frustration, the duration is much longer than a seizure, and the episode may be terminated by distraction or eliminating the cause of frustration. Intermittent explosive disorder (previously episodic dyscontrol syndrome) occurs in older children and adults, and the episodes are often called *rage attacks*. These episodes occur unprovoked or are triggered by even relatively minor frustration or other environmental stressors and involve directed and undirected aggression against people or inanimate objects. Unlike seizures, the duration of episodes varies from minute to hours. Recall of the episode may be absent or patchy, leading to confusion with complex partial seizures. Patients may feel remorse after the episode, as such behavior may be out of character for the patient's usual per-

sonality. Differentiation from seizures may be made based on the presence of a triggering stimulus, the occurrence of directed aggression, an ability to modify behavior with distraction, and a lack of stereotypy in the nature and duration of episodes. An increased incidence of temporal lobe spikes has been reported in such patients,[89] although an epileptic etiology is far from established.

Dissociative disorders are characterized by an alteration in the normally integrative functions of identity, memory, or consciousness, and they may be confused with simple partial psychic or complex partial seizures. When disruption of identity occurs, the disorder is either dissociative fugue or dissociative identity disorder (formerly multiple personality disorder). In dissociative fugue, there is travel away from one's home with an inability to recall one's past, often with confusion about personal identity. Episodes can last hours to months and are often related to severely traumatic life events. Poriomania (fugue with wandering) may occur in patients with epilepsy, but as opposed to patients with dissociative fugue, such patients would be expected to demonstrate a clouding of consciousness. In dissociative identity disorder, there are multiple well-organized personalities that interchange and the patient experiences gaps in time or fugues that suggest the possibility of complex partial seizures. A history of childhood abuse is not uncommon. This disorder has been reported in association with complex partial seizures,[90] but an analysis of patients with only dissociative identity disorder did not disclose an increased incidence of EEG epileptiform abnormalities.[91] Depersonalization disorder involves episodes of unreality (derealization) and detachment from oneself (depersonalization). Out of body experiences (autoscopy) may occur. All of these phenomena may occur during temporal lobe seizures.[92] Dissociative disorders can usually be differentiated from epilepsy based on an absence of altered consciousness or episodes involving automatisms, a much more prolonged duration of episodes, an abrupt resolution of amnesia, a loss of personal identity without altered sensorium, and a resolution of symptoms to suggestion, hypnosis, or Amytal interview.[86]

Seizurelike nonepileptic psychogenic seizures (pseudoseizures) most commonly represent a conversion symptom, which is related to subconscious

Table 1-5. Differentiating Nonepileptic from Physiologic Seizures.

Nonepileptic	Physiologic
Nonstereotypical phenomena	Stereotypical
Duration variable	Duration stereotypical; usually 1–2 mins
Clonic activity, often intermittent and of fixed frequency; absence of facial clonic activity	Clonic activity demonstrates gradual slowing
Incontinence rare but possible	Frequent incontinence
Tongue biting on anterior tip	Tongue biting posterolaterally
Injury occurs, but not burns	Injury frequent, including burns
Postictal state often absent	Postictal state usually present

psychological conflict (conversion NES). Although the occurrence of events is often related to environmental stress, such a relationship is usually denied by the patient and is more common in those with physiologic seizures. They are a common problem and may be seen in 10–40% of medically refractory epilepsy patients evaluated in comprehensive epilepsy centers.[93] They may also be seen in the context of somatization disorder, in which case they represent only one of a multitude of physical maladies. NESs are also seen in the setting of factitious disorder (e.g., Munchausen syndrome) or malingering, in which case there is a conscious intent to create the impression of an epileptic seizure for secondary gain. This section concentrates on the clinical differentiation of epileptic and nonepileptic psychogenic seizures. A more in-depth discussion of this topic can be found in Chapter 19.

The clinical diagnosis of conversion NES might at first seem easy, but clinical features of physiologic and psychogenic seizures may be very similar. As a result, continuous video-EEG monitoring to capture events is usually required. Conversion NESs may take any form but most commonly resemble either complex partial or tonic-clonic seizures. Patients with tonic-clonic type events may be more likely to have been the victims of sexual abuse.[94]

Many studies have examined ictal clinical features differentiating such episodes, and the results are mixed. Table 1-5 lists clinical signs that may be helpful in differentiating physiologic seizures from conversion NESs. Stereotypy applies to all possible seizures, but the other clinical features mentioned pertain to episodes of a generalized tonic-clonic nature. An apparent generalized tonic-clonic seizure without facial involvement is

a very useful clue, highly suggestive of conversion NES.[95] Significant injury can occur during conversion NES and may indicate an increased risk of suicide.[96] However, only patients with physiologic seizures have burns.[96]

Frontal complex partial seizures are particularly likely to be confused with conversion NES, as they can be extremely bizarre, with screaming, cursing, thrashing, boxing, or bicycling movements.[3] The ictal EEG can be normal in 25% of such seizures, so one cannot rely on the EEG.[3] As a result, the most reliable indication of physiologic seizures is the presence of stereotypy—identical duration and phenomenology from event to event. Video-EEG analysis is usually required to perform such an analysis.

Another means of proving that a seizure is nonepileptic in nature is by producing typical episodes with methods that should not cause a physiologic event, such as with photic stimulation in a patient without photosensitive epilepsy. Suggestive testing with placebo, such as alcohol pads on the carotid arteries or saline injection, can be extremely helpful in establishing the diagnosis of NES. In such instances, it must be verified with the patient and habitual observers that the event produced is the same as spontaneous episodes, as some patients may be extremely suggestible or may produce an event to please the physician. Although ethically controversial, one must weigh the costs and risks of continued misdiagnosed seizures to the patient, family, and society. For example, overtreatment of pseudo–status epilepticus is associated with significant morbidity and mortality.[97]

Postictal elevation of serum prolactin has been used to differentiate conversion NES from physiologic seizures, but with a classification accuracy of only 72%.[98] With such testing, false-negatives may occur with seizures that are not generalized in nature. In addition, prolactin has been reported to be elevated after NES and may also be elevated by neuroleptics.[99]

Most AEDs are capable of producing psychiatric symptoms, more commonly with polytherapy and high serum levels. For example, it is well known that phenobarbital and primidone may cause depression, although this may also occur with most other AEDs. The stimulant AEDs felbamate and lamotrigine may cause the appearance or exacerbation of anxiety. Psychosis may occur with the use of ethosuximide, carbamazepine, zonisamide, and vigabatrin.

Many AEDs have demonstrated usefulness in psychiatric disorders. For example, carbamazepine, valproate, gabapentin, lamotrigine, and topiramate have shown efficacy in bipolar disorder. Lamotrigine appears to have antidepressant effects.[100] Carbamazepine, valproate, and gabapentin have demonstrated efficacy in intermittent explosive disorder. Benzodiazepines and gabapentin may also be useful in anxiety disorders.[101] As a result of such psychotropic effects of AEDs, the choice of an AED in patients with epilepsy and coexistent psychiatric disorders may be governed by the desire to treat both disorders. Similarly, certain AEDs may be avoided to prevent the exacerbation of a pre-existing psychiatric disorder. For example, phenobarbital should generally be avoided in those with depressive symptoms and stimulant AEDs avoided in those with anxiety or panic.

Alternatively, some psychotropic medications may cause the occurrence or exacerbation of seizures, which may cloud the diagnostic picture. For example, major tranquilizers such as chlorpromazine or haloperidol, as well as antidepressants such as buspirone and bupropion, may lower the seizure threshold. The antipsychotic clozapine is quite notable in this regard, with an incidence of seizures of 1.3%.[102] Withdrawal of agents such as benzodiazepines, used in epilepsy and anxiety disorders, may also precipitate seizures.

It is also important to be aware of potential interactions between AEDs and psychotropic medications, which may occur via protein-binding interactions or hepatic enzyme induction. Such problems are more common with earlier and gener-

ally highly protein-bound or hepatically active, or both, AEDs, such as phenobarbital, phenytoin, carbamazepine, and valproate. For example, phenothiazines elevate levels of phenytoin or valproate. Fluoxetine, fluvoxamine, paroxetine, and sertraline elevate levels of phenytoin and carbamazepine.[103] Phenobarbital, phenytoin, and carbamazepine lower levels of tricyclic antidepressants, mirtazapine, and olanzapine.[103]

Miscellaneous Disorders

Disorders of the eye or visual pathways, such as macular degeneration, may result in hallucinosis with even, complex visual phenomena.[104] Symptoms likely represent "release hallucinations" as a result of sensory deprivation. Confusion with simple partial occipital or temporal seizures may occur. Historically, the hallucinations are more prominent with diminished sensory input (e.g., darkness), are more persistent and prolonged than ictal hallucinations, and also transiently disappear with retinal refixation and the associated increase in sensory input.

Sandifer's syndrome involves esophageal reflux and in infancy triggers attacks of generalized stiffening, usually with head deviation to the side, which may be associated with apnea.[9] The episodes may be mistaken for tonic or dystonic frontal seizures. Confusion with seizures is enhanced by decreased responsiveness, although the child is awake. Patients have a normal EEG and often have a history of frequent vomiting. In addition, episodes may be found to occur predominantly when eating or in the supine position.

Infantile masturbation is rarely suspected and may lead to the impression of complex partial or tonic-clonic seizures or a postictal state, as children may demonstrate tonic posturing, rhythmic activity, sympathetic outflow, and a dazed appearance without obvious genital stimulation. Episodes can be differentiated from seizures by their voluntary nature and the ability to terminate episodes, which may cause the child to seem resentful.[47]

Particularly in children, daydreaming or inattentiveness may be mistaken for an absence or complex partial seizure. Such episodes can be differentiated from seizures by termination with stimuli, such as calling the patient's name. In addition, there is no evidence of a postictal state. The EEG is normal, even with prolonged hyperventilation, which would generally be expected to precipitate an absence attack. In addition, in patients with attention deficit and hyperactivity disorder, one expects an associated history of hyperactivity.

After an incubation period of 1–2 months, rabies presents with nonspecific prodromal symptoms and often with paresthesiae of the bitten area.[105] Approximately 80% of patients then develop a "furious" or encephalitic form of the disease with episodes of excitement, terror, hallucinations, confusion, and aggressive behavior separated by lucid intervals, suggesting the possibility of complex partial seizures, delirium tremens, or drug intoxication.[105] Hydrophobia develops in 50% of patients, and fever and autonomic signs, such as hypersalivation, tachycardia, and sweating, may be present.[105] Seizures occur in some patients, adding to diagnostic confusion. Paralysis and coma develop within a few days.

Flumazenil-responsive recurring stupor is a disorder due to elevation of endozepine-4, an endogenous ligand for benzodiazepine recognition sites on γ-aminobutyric acid A receptors in the nervous system.[106] The bouts of stupor last for hours to days and are characterized by initial drowsiness, staggering, and behavioral changes.[106] This is followed by deep sleep and then a return to normal with postictal amnesia. The clinical presentation can suggest a state of complex partial status epilepticus. However, the EEG during these episodes demonstrates unreactive, 14- to 16-Hz fast activity as opposed to ictal activity. EEG changes and stupor are reversible with the administration of flumazenil, a benzodiazepine antagonist.[106]

Patients with multiple sclerosis may experience brief paroxysmal bouts involving brain stem or spinal dysfunction that may be characterized by, among other symptoms, tonic spasms, which may be unilateral and associated with the experience of pain and heat contralateral.[107] The episodes typically last for seconds to a few minutes and occur multiple times per day, either arising spontaneously or triggered by movement, sensory stimuli, or hyperventilation. Episodes usually resolve spontaneously over the course of weeks or months. Confusion with focal or generalized tonic seizures is possible, but the correct diagnosis is established by their occurrence in patients with known multiple sclerosis, a normal EEG, and the ictal occurrence of crossed sensory symptoms or other symptoms of brain stem dysfunction, such as diplopia or dysarthria.

In patients with brain stem lesions, bouts of tonic posturing lasting 1–10 minutes occur, during which there is opisthotonic posturing with extension of the legs and flexion (decorticate) or extension (decerebrate) of the arms.[45] There may be associated shivering, suggesting a tonic-clonic event. Events are differentiated from seizures by precipitation with noxious stimuli and an absence of ictal EEG activity during events.

Summary

Epilepsy is a disorder with numerous clinical manifestations. There is also a multitude of nonepileptic paroxysmal disorders that can present with very similar manifestations. Unfortunately, the EEG, an invaluable standard tool for the diagnosis and classification of epilepsy, often cannot be relied on to distinguish epileptic and nonepileptic disorders. As a result, diagnosis is primarily clinical, and the neurologist must be equipped with a sound knowledge of various seizure types, as well as the clinical manifestations of the numerous disorders contained within their differential diagnoses.

References

1. Day SC, Cook EF, Funkenstein H, Goldman L. Evaluation and outcome of emergency room patients with transient loss of consciousness. Am J Med 1982;73:15–23.
2. Salinsky M, Kanter R, Dashieff RM. Effectiveness of multiple EEGs in supporting the diagnosis of epilepsy: an operational curve. Epilepsia 1987;28:331–334.
3. Quesney LF. Seizures of Frontal Lobe Origin. In B Meldrum, TA Pedley (eds), Recent Advances in Epilepsy. Edinburgh, UK: Churchill Livingstone, 1986;81–110.
4. Zivin L, Ajmone-Marsan C. Incidence and prognostic significance of "epileptiform" activity in the EEG of nonepileptic subjects. Brain 1968;91:751–778.
5. Savage DD, Corwin L, McGee DL, et al. Epidemiologic features of isolated syncope. The Framingham study. Stroke 1985;16:626–629.
6. Krumholz A. Syncope. In RS Fisher (ed), Imitators of Epilepsy. New York: Demos, 1994;91–107.

7. Taylor B, Green MS. Evaluating and managing syncope. Clin Rev 2000;10:55–64,71–72.

8. Bandinelli G, Cencetti S, Bacalli S, Lagi A. Disease-related syncope. Analysis of a community-based hospital registry. J Intern Med 2000;247:513–516.

9. Ritter FJ, Kotagal P. Non-Epileptic Seizures in Children. In JR Gates, AJ Rowan (eds), Non-Epileptic Seizures (2nded). Boston: Butterworth–Heinemann, 2000;95–110.

10. Devinsky O, Price BH, Cohen SI. Cardiac manifestations of complex partial seizures. Am J Med 1986;80:195–202.

11. Gambardella A, Reutens DC, Andermann F, et al. Late-onset drop attacks in temporal lobe epilepsy: a reevaluation of the concept of temporal lobe syncope. Neurology 1994;44:1074–1078

12. Linzer M, Yang EH, Estes NA 3rd, et al. Diagnosing syncope. Part 1: value of history, physical examination, and electrocardiography. Clinical efficacy assessment project of the American College of Physicians. Ann Intern Med 1997;126:989–996.

13. Kapoor WN. Workup and management of patients with syncope. Med Clin North Am 1995;79:1153–1170.

14. Scheinberg P. Transient ischemic attacks: an update. J Neurol Sci 1991;101:133–140.

15. Feldmann E, Wilterdink JL. The symptoms of transient cerebral ischemic attacks. Semin Neurol 1991;11:135–145.

16. Cambier J, Decroix JP, Masson C. Allucinose auditive dans les lésions du tronc cérébral. Rev Neurol 1987;143:255–262.

17. Cascino GD, Adams RD. Brain stem auditory hallucinosis. Neurology 1986;36:1042–1047.

18. Williams D, Wilson TG. The diagnosis of the major and minor syndromes of basilar insufficiency. Brain 1962;85:741–743.

19. Wenzel C, Pearlstein L. Peduncular hallucinosis as a transient ischemic attack. J Am Osteopath Assoc 1993;93:129–130.

20. Greenberg SM, Vonsattel JP, Stakes JW, et al. The clinical spectrum of cerebral amyloid angiopathy: presentations without lobar hemorrhage. Neurology 1993;43:2073–2079.

21. Rowan AJ, Rosenbaum DH. Ictal amnesia and fugue states. Adv Neurol 1991;55:357–367

22. Van Domburg PH, ten Donkelaar HJ, Notermans SL. Akinetic mutism with bithalamic infarction. Neurophysiological correlates. J Neurol Sci 1996;139:58–65.

23. Tutuncuoglu S, Kantar M, Tekgul H, Candan C. Akinetic mutism due to diphenylhydantoin toxicity. Turk J Pediatr 1997;39:403–407.

24. Aylett SE, Cross JH, Taylor DC, et al. Epileptic akinetic mutism following temporal lobe lobectomy for Rasmussen's syndrome. Eur Child Adolesc Psychiatry 1996;5:222–225.

25. Fisch BJ, Tatemichi TK, Prohovnik I, et al. Transient ischemic attacks resembling simple partial motor seizures. Neurology 1988;38[Suppl 1]:S264.

26. Yanagihara T, Piepgras DG, Klass DW. Repetitive involuntary movement associated with episodic cerebral ischemia. Ann Neurol 1985;18:244–250.

27. Wada Y, Kita Y, Yamamoto T. Orthostatic hypotension with repeated bilateral limb shaking and metamorphopsia. A case of hemodynamic transient ischemic attacks. Rinsho Shinkeigaku 2000;40:582–585.

28. Dinsdale HB. Spontaneous hemorrhage in the posterior fossa. Arch Neurol 1964;10:98–115.

29. Fukuyama Y, Umezu R. Clinical and cerebral angiographic evolutions of idiopathic progressive occlusive disease of the circle of Willis ('moyamoya' disease) in children. Brain Dev 1985;7:21–37.

30. Ho RT, Harrison MJ, Earl CJ. Transient paraparesis—a manifestation of ischemic episodes in the anterior cerebral artery territory. J Neurol Neurosurg Psychiatry 1983;46:786.

31. Bromfield EB. Somatosensory, special sensory, and autonomic phenomena in seizures. Semin Neurol 1991;11:91–99.

32. Fisher RS, Buchholz D. Migraine and Epilepsy. In RS Fisher (ed), Imitators of Epilepsy. New York: Demos, 1994;125–144.

33. Andermann F. Non-Epileptic Paroxysmal Neurologic Events. In JR Gates, AJ Rowan (eds), Non-Epileptic Seizures (2nd ed). Boston: Butterworth–Heinemann, 2000;51–69.

34. Pellock JM. The Differential Diagnosis of Epilepsy: Nonepileptic Paroxysmal Disorders. In E Wyllie (ed), The Treatment of Epilepsy: Principles and Practice (2nd ed). Baltimore: Williams & Wilkins, 1996;681–689.

35. Bourgeois M, Aicardi J, Goutieres F. Acute hemiplegia in childhood. J Pediatr 1993;122:673–679.

36. Golden GS, French JH. Basilar artery migraine in young children. Pediatrics 1975;56:722–726.

37. Watts RL, Keller WC. Movement Disorders. Neurologic Principles and Practice. New York: McGraw-Hill, 1997.

38. Fisher RS, Blum D. Movement Disorders That Imitate Epilepsy. In RS Fisher (ed), Imitators of Epilepsy. New York: Demos, 1994;165–198.

39. Lugaresi E, Cirignotta F, Montagna P. Nocturnal paroxysmal dystonia. J Neurol Neurosurg Psychiatry 1986;49:375–380.

40. Tinuper P, Cerullo A, Cirignotta F, et al. Nocturnal paroxysmal dystonia with short lasting attacks. Three cases with evidence for an epileptic frontal lobe origin of seizures. Epilepsia 1990;31:549–556.

41. Jankovic J, Fahn S. Dystonic Disorders. In J Jankovic, E Tolosa (eds), Parkinson's Disease and Movement Disorders (3rd ed). Baltimore: Williams & Wilkins, 1998;513–551.

42. Wang A, Jankovic J. Hemifacial spasm: clinical correlates and treatments. Muscle Nerve 1998;21:1740–1747.

43. Adler CH, Zimmerman RA, Savino PJ, et al. Hemifacial spasm: evaluation by magnetic resonance imaging and magnetic resonance tomographic angiography. Ann Neurol 1992;32:502–506.
44. Markand ON, Garg BP, Weaver DD. Familial startle disease (hyperexplexia). Electrophysiologic studies. Arch Neurol 1984;41:71–74.
45. Schmidt D, Lempert T. Differential Diagnoses in Adults. In M Dam, L Gram (eds), Comprehensive Epileptology. New York: Raven Press, 1991;449–471.
46. Bressman S, Fahn S. Essential myoclonus. Adv Neurol 1986;43:287–294.
47. Pranzatelli MR, Pedley TA. Differential Diagnoses in Children. In M Dam, L Gram (eds), Comprehensive Epileptology. New York: Raven Press, 1990;423–447.
48. Fusco L, Pachatz C, Cusmai R, Vigevano F. Repetitive sleep starts in neurologically impaired children: an unusual non-epileptic manifestation in otherwise epileptic subjects. Epileptic Disord 1999;1:63–67.
49. Deuschl G, Mischke G, Schenck E, et al. Symptomatic and essential rhythmic palatal myoclonus. Brain 1990;113:1645–1672.
50. Davis SM, Murray NM, Diengdoh JV, et al. Stimulus-sensitive spinal myoclonus. J Neurol Neurosurg Psychiatry 1981;44:884–888.
51. Young RR, Shahani BT. Asterixis: one type of negative myoclonus. Adv Neurol 1986;43:137–156.
52. Kurlan R, Kersun J, Behr J, et al. Carbamazepine-induced tics. Clin Neuropharm 1989;12:298–302.
53. Armon C, Shin C, Miller P, et al. Reversible parkinsonism and cognitive impairment with chronic valproate use. Neurology 1996;47:626–635.
54. Harrison MB, Lyons GR, Landow ER. Phenytoin and dyskinesias: a report of two cases and review of the literature. Mov Disord 1993;8:19–27.
55. Asconape J, Diedrich A, DellaBadia J. Myoclonus associated with the use of gabapentin. Epilepsia 2000;41:479–481.
56. Galvez-Jimenez N, Hargreave M. Topiramate and essential tremor. Ann Neurol 2000;47:837–838.
57. Gironell A, Kulisevsky J, Barbanoj M, et al. A randomized placebo-controlled comparative trial of gabapentin and propranolol in essential tremor. Arch Neurol 1999;56:475–480.
58. Fisher RS. Dizziness and Vertigo as Imitators of Epilepsy. In RS Fisher (ed), Imitators of Epilepsy. New York: Demos, 1994;235–253.
59. Labar DR. Sleep disorders and epilepsy: differential diagnosis. Semin Neurol 1991;11:128–134.
60. Aldrich MS. Narcolepsy. Neurology 1992;42[Suppl 6]:34–43.
61. Plazzi G, Tinuper P, Montagna P, et al. Epileptic nocturnal wanderings. Sleep 1995;18:749–756.
62. Lombroso CT. Pavor nocturnus of proven epileptic origin. Epilepsia 2000;41:1221–1226.
63. Broughton R. Sleep disorders: disorders of arousal? Science 1968;159:1070–1078.
64. Montplaisir J, Godbout R. Restless Legs Syndrome and Periodic Movements During Sleep. In MH Kryger, T Roth, WC Dement (eds), Principles and Practice of Sleep Medicine. Philadelphia: Saunders, 1989;402–409.
65. Coccagna G. Restless Legs Syndrome/Periodic Leg Movements in Sleep. In MJ Thorpy (ed), Handbook of Sleep Disorders. New York: Marcel Dekker Inc, 1990;457–478.
66. Devinsky O, Ehrenberg B, Barthlen GM, et al. Epilepsy and sleep apnea syndrome. Neurology 1994;44:2060–2064.
67. Adler CH. Treatment of restless legs syndrome with gabapentin. Clin Neuropharmacol 1997;20:148–151.
68. Bouloux PM, Kaplan P. Endocrine Imitators of Epilepsy. In RS Fisher (ed), Imitators of Epilepsy. New York: Demos, 1994;199–214.
69. Glaser GH, Pincus JH. Neurologic Complications of Internal Disease. In AB Baker, LH Baker (eds), Clinical Neurology (vol 4). Philadelphia: Harper & Row, 1987;1–57.
70. Zadra M, Grandi R, Erli LC, et al. Treatment of seizures in acute intermittent porphyria: safety and efficacy of gabapentin. Seizure 1998;7:415–416.
71. Surks MI, DeFesi CR. Normal serum free thyroid hormone concentrations in patients treated with phenytoin or carbamazepine. A paradox resolved. JAMA 1996;275:1495–1498.
72. Kuhn-Velten WN, Herzog AG, Muller MR. Acute effects of anticonvulsant drugs on gonadotropin-stimulated and precursor-supported androgen production in the rat testis. Eur J Pharmacol 1990;181:151–155.
73. Herzog AG, Levesque LA, Drislane FW, et al. Phenytoin-induced elevation of serum estradiol and reproductive dysfunction in men with epilepsy. Epilepsia 1989;32:550–553.
74. Waisburg H, Alvarez N. Carbamazepine in the treatment of epilepsy in people with intellectual disability. J Intellect Disabil Res 1998;42[Suppl 1]:36–40.
75. Vainionpaa LK, Rattya J, Kinp M, et al. Valproate-induced hyperandrogenism during pubertal maturation in girls with epilepsy. Ann Neurol 1999;45:444–450.
76. Kaplan PW, Schulz P. Delirium and Epilepsy. In RS Fisher (ed), Imitators of Epilepsy. New York: Demos, 1994;215–234.
77. Caine D, Halliday GM, Kril JJ, Harper CG. Operational criteria for the classification of chronic alcoholics: identification of Wernicke's encephalopathy. J Neurol Neurosurg Psychiatry 1997;62:51–60.
78. Victor M. Neurologic Disorders Due to Alcoholism and Malnutrition. In AB Baker, LH Baker (eds), Clinical Neurology (vol 4). Philadelphia: Harper & Row, 1987;1–94.
79. Bleck TP, Brauner JS. Tetanus. In WM Scheld, RJ Whitley, DT Durack (eds), Infections of the Central Nervous System (2nd ed). Philadelphia: Raven Press, 1997;629–653.

80. Palatnick W, Meatherall R, Sitar D, Tenenbein M. Toxicokinetics of acute strychnine poisoning. J Toxicol Clin Toxicol 1997;35:617 620.

81. Smith BA. Strychnine poisoning. J Emerg Med 1990;8:321–325.

82. Goetz CG, Klawans HL, Cohen MM. Neurotoxic Agents. In AB Baker, RJ Joynt (eds), Clinical Neurology (vol 2). Philadelphia: Harper & Row, 1987;1–84.

83. Smith DB, Craft BR, Collins J, et al. Behavioral characteristics of epilepsy patients compared with normal controls. Epilepsia 1986;27:760–768.

84. Gloor P, Olivier A, Quesney LF, et al. The role of the limbic system in experiential phenomena of temporal lobe epilepsy. Ann Neurol 1982;12:129–144.

85. Szabo CA, Lancman M, Tagno S. Postictal psychosis: a review. Neuropsychiatry Neuropsychol Behav Neurol 1996;9:258–264.

86. Stonnington CM. Psychiatric Imitators of Epilepsy. In RS Fisher (ed), Imitators of Epilepsy. New York: Demos, 1994;255–281.

87. Fenwick P. Aggression and Epilepsy. In O Devinsky, WH Theodore (eds), Epilepsy and Behavior. New York: Wiley, 1991;85–96.

88. Gerard ME, Spitz MC, Towbin JA, Shantz D. Subacute postictal aggression. Neurology 1998;50:384–388.

89. Bach-y-Rita P, Lion JR, Climent CE, Ervin FR. Episodic dyscontrol: a study of 130 violent patients. Am J Psychiat 1971;127:1473–1478.

90. Benson DF, Miller BL, Signer SF. Dual personality associated with epilepsy. Arch Neurol 1986;43:471–474.

91. Devinsky O, Putnam F, Grafman J, et al. Dissociative states and epilepsy. Neurology 1989;39:835–840.

92. Devinsky O, Luciano D. Psychic phenomena in partial seizures. Semin Neurol 1991;11:100–109.

93. Gates JR, Luciano D, Devinsky O. The Classification and Treatment of Nonepileptic Events. In O Devinsky, WA Theodore (eds), Epilepsy and Behavior. New York: Wiley-Liss, 1991;251–263.

94. Luciano D, Barkan M, Devinsky O, Alper K. Abuse history and ictal semiology of nonepileptic psychogenic seizures. Epilepsia 1995;36:161.

95. Kanner AM, Morris HH, Luders H, et al. Supplementary motor seizures mimicking pseudoseizures: some clinical differences. Neurology 1990;40:1404–1407.

96. Peguero E, Abou-Khalil B, Fakhoury T, Mathews G. Self-injury and incontinence in psychogenic seizures. Epilepsia 1995;36:586–591.

97. Alper K. Nonepileptic Seizures. In O Devinsky (ed), Neurologic Clinics. Epilepsy 2: Special Issues. Philadelphia: Saunders, 1994;153 173.

98. Laxer KD, Mullooly JP, Howell B. Prolactin changes after seizures classified by EEG monitoring. Neurology 1985;35:31–35.

99. Alving J. Serum prolactin levels are elevated also after pseudo-epileptic seizures. Seizure 1998;7:85–89.

100. Maltese TM. Adjunctive lamotrigine treatment for major depression. Am J Psychiatry 1999;156:1833.

101. Brannon N, Labbate L, Huber M. Gabapentin treatment for posttraumatic stress disorder. Can J Psychiatry 2000;45:84.

102. Pacia S, Devinsky O. Clozapine-related seizures: experience with 5,629 patients. Neurology 1994;44:2247–2249.

103. Luciano D, Alper K. Psychiatric Aspects of Seizures and Epilepsy. In A Stoudemire, BS Fogel, DB Greenberg (eds), Psychiatric Care of the Medical Patient (2nd ed). Oxford: Oxford University Press, 2000;635–651.

104. Lalla D, Primeau F. Complex visual hallucinations in macular degeneration. Can J Psychiatry 1993;38:584–586.

105. Warrell DA. The clinical picture of rabies in man. Trans R Soc Trop Med Hyg 1976;70:188–195.

106. Lugaresi E, Montagna P, Tinuper P, et al. Endozepine stupor. Recurring stupor linked to endozepine-4 accumulation. Brain 1998;121:127–133.

107. Osterman PO, Westerberg CE. Paroxysmal attacks in multiple sclerosis. Brain 1975;98:189–202.

Section B

Medical Conditions and Epilepsy

Chapter 2

Cardiac Disorders

Jane Boggs

When cardiac or central nervous systems (CNSs) interact with diseases of one system, the function of both systems is usually affected. Neurocardiology, the study of heart and brain interactions in both health and disease, is a subspecialty of neurologists and cardiologists. Although regulation of the heart via the autonomic nervous system usually maintains cardiovascular homeostasis, neurologic dysfunction disrupts the balance of these two vital systems. Isolated seizures can transiently influence cardiac function. Epilepsy can result in progressive neurologic dysfunction and, rarely, serious cardiac dysfunction if not managed appropriately. Some epilepsy treatments may have potential cardiac complications, adding another level of complexity to patient management. Also, many cardiovascular symptoms can imitate seizures, and extensive evaluation of both systems may be necessary for diagnosis. This chapter addresses cardiovascular disease and treatments that precipitate seizures and epilepsy, as well as the cardiovascular complications of epilepsy and its management.

Etiologies

Structural cardiac disease and arrhythmias can precipitate seizures. Impaired or turbulent cardiac output can impair poor cerebral perfusion either globally or in areas of vascular compromise. Embolic and hemorrhagic strokes that compress or injure the cerebral cortex cause seizures more commonly than subcortical thrombotic strokes or lacu-

nas. However, ischemia or infarction of any etiology can cause seizures. The Rotterdam study determined that a history of stroke, or risk factors for stroke, was associated with an increased lifetime risk for epilepsy.[1] Also, cardiovascular compromise with diffuse cerebral hypoperfusion can result in epileptogenic injury to watershed areas of the cerebral cortex or to areas sensitive to hypoxia, such as the hippocampus. Such effects can result from cardiac arrest and subsequent resuscitation, congestive heart failure, cardiomyopathy, and cardiogenic shock. Congenital cardiac anomalies and conduction defects can have significant hemodynamic effects that can lower seizure threshold, or they may be primarily associated with congenital CNS abnormalities that cause seizures. Cardiac interventions, surgery, and medications can also lower seizure threshold.

Conversely, epilepsy and its treatments may be associated with cardiac complications, as discussed subsequently in the section Cardiac Complications of Epilepsy.

Frequency and Phenomenology

Atherosclerotic cardiovascular disease (ASCVD) is associated with an increased risk for thromboembolic strokes due to atheromata and calcific lesions and hemorrhagic strokes due to reperfusion and therapy, including thrombolysis and anticoagulation. Strokes more commonly complicate large, acute myocardial infarctions (MIs) of the anterior and apical wall rather than those of the inferior wall.[2] The highest risk of embolization is in the first 4 months after acute MI, especially in the first week.[3]

Myocardial Infarction

Although uncommon, in the setting of acute MI, seizures can occur as complications of lobar cerebral hemorrhages with thrombolytic therapy. Rarely, thrombolysis precipitates seizures without evidence of hemorrhage on neuroimaging.[4] Cocaine, other CNS stimulants, and intravenous drug use may result in both MI and seizures, with or without identifiable cerebrovascular involvement. Other systemic vasculitides, such as giant cell arteritis and systemic lupus erythematosus, can also result in seizures and infarctions of both cardiac and cerebral vascular beds.

Left ventricular hypertrophy in the setting of hypertension is associated with increased risk for seizures. A population-based case control study from Rochester, Minnesota, found that severe uncontrolled hypertension increased the risk for seizure.[5] Hypertensive patients who were treated with diuretics did not have an increased risk. Dilated cardiomyopathy is associated more with cerebral complications than with hypertrophic cardiomyopathy, probably owing to the association with atrial fibrillation (AF).[6]

Valvular Disease

Cerebral thromboembolism is also a major complication of native mitral valvular disease. Mitral stenosis is the most common valvular disease precipitating cerebral thromboembolism, which may be the presenting manifestation of this valvular disease in more than 10% of patients.[7] The Framingham study estimated up to an 18-fold increased risk of thromboembolism if AF occurred with mitral disease.[8] Mitral regurgitation is less likely to result in embolic events, although concomitant mitral stenosis increases the risk of complications from mitral regurgitations.[9] Mitral valve prolapse (MVP), often asymptomatic, occurs in 5–7% of the adult population and therefore is commonly cited as a cause for many medical disorders, including

epilepsy and stroke.[10] Some patients with MVP and no other risk factors have recurrent cerebral ischemic events, suggesting a possible causal relationship.[11] Because of the vague association between stroke risk and MVP, the need for antiplatelet prophylaxis remains controversial in asymptomatic MVP. Mitral annular calcification predicts a doubled risk of embolic stroke, which is independent from other ASCVD risk factors of age, gender, systolic blood pressure, diabetes mellitus, and cigarette smoking. AF occurs more commonly in the presence of mitral annular calcification, but the risk of stroke also appears independent of AF.[12] Aortic stenosis and insufficiency can result in diffuse cerebral hypoperfusion but are unusual causes of clinically symptomatic cerebral ischemic events unless associated with another source of emboli (e.g., mitral valve disease, AF, endocarditis). Anticoagulation is recommended for all patients with mechanical valves and for higher-risk patients with bioprosthetic valves, which increase the risk of stroke and subsequent seizures. Balloon valvuloplasty is used as an alternative treatment in patients for whom surgery is inappropriate. Despite systemic heparinization during the procedure, embolization from release of calcific material results in embolic strokes in approximately 1% of cases.[13] Seizures can result from exuberant dosing of lidocaine during such procedures.[14]

Infective endocarditis can precipitate seizures in up to 11% of patients, due to embolization of septic material, formation of cerebral abscess, or rupture of mycotic aneurysms.[15] Neurologic complications more commonly occur from involvement of left-sided valvular disease, especially the mitral valve. Prosthetic valves are associated with larger and less adherent vegetations, which are especially prone to embolization. Focal seizures usually result from localized infarction, hemorrhage, or abscess, whereas generalized seizures are more likely due to associated metabolic factors, hypoxia, or medications. Beta-lactam (e.g., penicillin and imipenem) and quinolone (e.g., levofloxacin and ciprofloxacin) antibiotics are especially associated with seizures. Infections by highly virulent organisms, such as *Staphylococcus aureus*, increase the likelihood of neurologic events. Signs of cerebral embolization are the presenting symptoms in up to 23% of patients with endocarditis[16] and occur soon after initiation of antibiotic therapy in up to 30%.[15] Patients with prosthetic valve endocarditis do not have a greater cerebral risk over those with native valve disease. Cerebral hemorrhage, however, is more likely in anticoagulated patients who have infective endocarditis, as the intraluminal arterial walls undergo inflammatory destruction, increasing the chance of hemorrhage.

Congenital Heart Disease

Congenital heart disease may result in seizures through neurovascular events caused by cyanotic right-to-left shunts. Transposition of the great arteries and tetralogy of Fallot account for 90% of such neurologic complications, owing to associated hypoxia, polycythemia, clotting factor deficiencies, and thrombocytopenia. Children younger than 4 years of age are at higher risk of anemic and thromboembolic complications of cyanotic heart disease, with autopsy series documenting up to 19% incidence of cerebrovascular events.[17] A series of patients with suspected congenital heart disease underwent electroencephalogram (EEG) and neurologic examination before cardiac catheterization. Even in those with normal neurologic examinations, a high proportion of EEG abnormalities was found, suggesting subclinical neurologic involvement in both cyanotic and acyanotic congenital heart disease.[18] Seizures were the second most common neurologic complication after hypothermic cardiopulmonary bypass surgery in young infants, occurring in 15% of patients. Seventy percent of these were focal seizures.[19] Seizures after repair of cyanotic disease also occur frequently. In a study from Boston Children's Hospital, the incidence of electrographic seizures after correction of transposition of the great arteries was 20%, but only 6% had clinically apparent seizures. Seizures were associated with longer duration of deep hypothermic circulatory arrest and diagnosis of ventricular septal defects.[20]

Congenital heart disease with left-to-right shunts may also cause neurologic injuries associated with seizures. Silent atrial septal defects, including patent foramen ovale, may go unrecognized until adulthood, when they are often detected by investigation of the cause of stroke in young

adults. Routine transthoracic echocardiography fails to identify up to 75% of patent foramen ovale defects, resulting in an underestimate of this congenital defect in series not using more sensitive echocardiographic procedures, such as transesophageal echocardiography with contrast.[21]

Brain abscesses can occur when hypoxic blood bypasses the lungs via a right-to-left shunt, especially with abnormal cardiac structure allowing embolization. Rare under 2 years of age, brain abscesses occur in 2% of cyanotic congenital heart disease patients, with a peak incidence between 4 and 7 years of age.[22]

Congenital heart disease also occurs in syndromes of multiple congenital abnormalities, further predisposing them to seizures. Such multisystem genetic conditions include Down's syndrome,[23] Kallmann's syndrome,[24] and tuberous sclerosis.[25] Congenital heart diseases in autopsy series are associated with a 68% incidence of cerebral malformations.[26] Infants with severe cardiac and neurologic anomalies may not survive childhood, and those who have successful surgical repair commonly experience serious arrhythmias and may require antiarrhythmics and anticoagulants. These arrhythmias can precipitate convulsive syncope and occasionally recurrent seizures if permanent CNS structural damage results (e.g., stroke). Coarctation of the aorta may be associated with intracranial aneurysms, although subarachnoid hemorrhage due to aneurysmal rupture is rare in pediatric patients, and early repair further minimizes risk of cerebrovascular complications.[27]

Arrhythmias

Both atrial and ventricular arrhythmias can produce transient neurologic symptoms by disrupting cerebral perfusion. However, ventricular arrhythmias rarely cause seizures. Although nonvalvular AF confers a five- to sevenfold increased risk of stroke, without evidence of infarction arrhythmia-induced convulsive syncope can be difficult to distinguish clinically from seizure. Multivariate analysis has found an overall higher risk for embolic strokes in nonvalvular AF patients who also have hypertension, are older than 75 years of age, and have had a previous transient ischemic attack and diabetes mellitus.[28] In the Copenhagen Stroke

Table 2-1. Potential Drug Interactions between Aspirin or Warfarin with Antiepileptic Drugs

Antiepileptic Drug	Antiplatelet/Anticoagulant	Potential Clinical Effect
Phenytoin (PHT)	Warfarin	Increases international normalized ratio (INR)
	Aspirin	Increases free PHT
Carbamazepine	Warfarin	Decreases INR
Phenobarbital	Warfarin	Decreases INR
Primidone	Warfarin	Decreases INR
Valproic acid (VPA)	Warfarin	Slight decrease in INR
	Aspirin	Increases free VPA

Study, 4.2% of patients had seizures within 2 weeks of embolic stroke.[29] Early seizures were associated with worse stroke severity at presentation but predicted better clinical outcome, suggesting that they may be characteristic of strokes with a large reversible ischemic penumbra. Current recommendations by the Third Consensus Conference on antithrombotic therapy strongly suggest chronic warfarin therapy (international normalized ratio, 2–3) for all patients with AF, except those younger than 60 years old with no associated cardiac disease.[30] For these and patients in whom warfarin is contraindicated, 325 mg of aspirin daily should be used. Antiepileptic drugs (AEDs) with potential interactions with warfarin or aspirin should be avoided, not only to optimize seizure prophylaxis, but also to minimize stroke risk. Valproic acid can produce a serum-level-dependent thrombocytopenia and may result in abnormal platelet function by inhibiting the second phase of platelet aggregation. These effects are reversible with decreasing dose. The clinical risk of bleeding diatheses is minimal but may be more significant in patients with other risks of hemorrhage. Such risks include the therapeutic use of agents, such as aspirin or warfarin. Potentially clinically important interactions of these drugs with AEDs are listed in Table 2-1.

Sick-sinus syndrome, especially bradycardia-tachycardia types, is also a risk for cerebral embolism. These arrhythmias may result in misdiagnosis of epilepsy, especially in children. Long Q-T syndromes are rare congenital channelopathies that produce episodic ventricular arrhythmias with resultant seizures, syncope, and potentially sudden death. Romano-Ward syndrome is characterized by prolonged Q-T interval and autosomal-dominant inheritance, with six identifiable genetic variants (LQT1–6). Jervell and Lange-Nielsen syndrome has marked prolongation of the Q-T interval and sensorineural deafness and is much rarer. Three long Q-T syndrome genes have been identified: SCN5A on 3p21-24, HERG on 7q35-36, and KVLQT1 on 11p15.5, and genetic tests have been developed and are available.[31] Mutations of various cardiac voltage-dependent sodium channels and potassium-current mechanisms occur, although some cases are sporadic.[32] Clinically, there is an imbalance in sympathetic influences on the heart, and symptoms often appear with exercise or stress. Although EEGs may be abnormal, measurement of the corrected Q-T interval obtained in one EEG channel can document the cardiac abnormality.[33]

Cardiac Complications of Epilepsy

Case reports document cardiac arrhythmias recorded during and after seizures. Bradyarrhythmias may occur with temporal lobe foci,[34] termed the *ictal bradycardia syndrome*.[35] The majority of observed arrhythmias are clinically benign, such as premature atrial and ventricular contractions and beat-to-beat variations in R-R intervals.[36] Photic stimulation, however, can trigger either benign sinus tachycardia or clinically significant bradycardia with sinus arrest requiring cardiopulmonary resuscitation.[37] The most common rhythm seen intraictally is sinus tachycardia, which is a normal stress-induced sympathetic response and sometimes is mistakenly categorized as an arrhythmia.[38] The failure to develop sinus tachycardia with a prolonged seizure suggests cardiovascular dysfunction or incompetence of the autonomic response to seizures. Arrhythmias are less common than repolarization and conduction abnormalities.[39,40] Such functional cardiac electrical changes may impart instability to ventricular function and lower the threshold for ventricular fibrillation and tachycardia. In the Greater Richmond Metropolitan Area Status Epilepticus study, acute fatal cardiac decompensation was most typically associated with ventricular tachyarrhythmias.[41] These patients did not usually have increased premature ventricular contractions before death, indicating a latent cardiac arrhythmogenicity, possibly induced by prolonged effects of seizures on their hearts. Similar potential myocardial damage may be induced by long-standing refractory epilepsy, which has been suggested as a risk factor for sudden unexpected death in epilepsy.[42]

Sudden Unexpected Death in Epilepsy

Although there are differences of opinion of the specific definition of sudden unexpected death in epilepsy, there is general agreement that "definite" cases require autopsy confirmation that no anatomic or toxicologic cause of death can be identified. The exact incidence is unclear, owing to the low rate of autopsies, but is estimated to be 0.35–1.00 per 1,000 patients per year.[42,43] The incidence is estimated to be at least 24 times higher than the rate of sudden death in the general population without epilepsy. Higher incidences are found in refractory seizure patients and appear independent of the type of treatment. Proposed mechanisms of sudden unexpected death in epilepsy include fatal cardiac arrhythmia,[44] microscopic myocardial damage from seizure-induced catecholamine effects, neurogenic pulmonary edema, and central apnea.[45]

Assessment

The initial assessment of any patient with a seizure should ideally include a complete medical history, a review of systems, and a family history. The medical history should inquire about cardiac conditions, previous cardiac testing, and medications. Inquiry about palpitations, dyspnea, chest pressure, or "heaviness" can help identify ASCVD or valvular disease as a cause of seizure. The question of whether seizures are episodes of convulsive syncope rather than manifestations of epilepsy can often be resolved by appropriately directed questions and cardiac testing. Awareness as postural tone is lost during a blackout and hemodynamic symptoms such as blurring vision and light-headedness are helpful signs of syncope, although they can be experienced in seizures. Exercise-induced loss of consciousness frequently suggests cardiac, instead of neurologic, etiology of symptoms. Risk factors of prior ASCVD events, smoking, diabetes mellitus, hypertension, cholesterol levels, and family history of ASCVD events at a young age need to be reviewed carefully. Medications, doses, and timing, relative to onset of symptoms, of all medications may reveal precipitating factors for either cardiac or neurologic events. A complete list of cardiac medications is also necessary to allow appropriate selection of AEDs.

The physical examination screening should include respiratory rate and routine and orthostatic blood pressure with heart rate. Auscultation for cardiac murmurs, carotid bruits, and extrapulmonary sounds should be performed; evidence of hypertension, including funduscopic vascular changes, cardiac enlargement, jugular venous distension, and peripheral edema, should be noted. If no recent laboratory evaluations are available, electrolytes and a complete blood count, including platelets and coagulation parameters, should be obtained. Patients with suspected acute cardiac symptoms should have creatine phosphokinase and troponin as well as an electrocardiogram (ECG). Children and known cardiac patients with new-onset syncope or seizures should routinely have an ECG.

Evaluation by EEG should always include at least one reliably recorded ECG channel. As in bedside telemetry, this channel is typically useful only for assessing conduction intervals and rhythm. Any suspected ischemic changes should be confirmed by performing a 12-lead ECG. For patients with possible syncope or seizure, video-EEG with an ECG channel may be necessary to document the nature of the typical clinical event.

Convulsive syncope may be clinically difficult to distinguish from generalized convulsive seizures,

Table 2-2. Acute Seizure Medications and Cardiac Effects

Medication	Potential Cardiac Effects	Electrocardiogram Monitoring Recommended
Phenobarbital (IV)*	Hypotension, arrhythmia	Yes
Phenytoin (IV)*	Hypotension, arrhythmia	Yes
Fosphenytoin		
(IV)	Minimal	Yes
(IM)	Minimal	No
Depacon	Minimal	No
Valium* (IV)	Hypotension	No
(PR)	Minimal	No
Ativan*	Hypotension	No
Versed	Hypotension	No
Paraldehyde	Hypotension	No

*Contains propylene glycol.

although a history of exertion, micturition, or cough immediately preceding the event should argue against epilepsy. Focal symptoms associated with the event or stereotypical semiology argue against syncope and may support a diagnosis of partial seizures, and simultaneous recording of clinical and EEG data is confirmatory in many cases. In the Framingham study, more than 3% of patients had at least one syncopal episode. Cardiac causes can be identified in between 8% and 39% of patients.[46] The major cardiac causes of syncope include mechanical cardiac disease, cardiac arrhythmias, bradyarrhythmias, ventricular tachyarrhythmias, and neurocardiogenic (vasovagal) syncope. In patients studied with induced ventricular tachyarrhythmias, two-thirds had generalized tonic contraction of axial muscles, sometimes followed by irregular jerking of the extremities.[47]

Managing Cardiac Disease

Cardiac medications at therapeutic doses rarely increase the risk for seizures. The group I antiarrhythmics are the most common culprits.[48] Case reports of seizures related to digoxin, verapamil, beta-blockers, mexiletine, tocainide, disopyramide, ergonovine, sympathomimetics, and lidocaine may result from therapeutic and excessive use.[49] Nonspecific medications used to treat cardiac conditions (e.g., antibiotics

for endocarditis and immunosuppressants for cardiac transplantation) can also lower seizure threshold. All medications used to treat cardiac disease should be evaluated for their potential to interact adversely with highly protein bound and liver-metabolized AEDs.

Diagnostic cardiac catheterization has a low risk of cerebral complications (0.2%); the largest proportion of embolic and hemodynamic events occurs in the posterior circulation and is not associated with seizures.[50] Percutaneous transluminal coronary angioplasty has a similar low rate of cerebral complication, although events are more commonly in the anterior and middle cerebral circulation.[51]

In patients with cardiac disease and epilepsy, treatments for both must be cautiously balanced to avoid provoking adverse events. In cardiac patients for whom surgery is contemplated, management of pre-existing epilepsy must take into consideration the duration of anesthesia, type of anesthesia, and time *non per os*. Patients should be advised to take their usual AEDs with a sip of water, even when *non per os* for surgery. In many cases, the use of benzodiazepine or barbiturates intraoperatively may help in acute seizure prophylaxis but may also contribute to subsequent withdrawal seizures. In cardiac surgery with patients who unexpectedly develop seizures, acute treatment with agents least likely to affect cardiac function is imperative. The parenteral AEDs with the safest cardiovascular profile are fosphenytoin and sodium valproate, although benzodiazepines can be used temporarily. If enteral agents can be administered, AEDs such as gabapentin, tiagabine, valproic acid, and levetiracetam have good cardiac safety profiles and achieve steady states rapidly compared to other AEDs. For patients with chronic, stable cardiac conditions, AEDs should be selected with a low potential for interactions with cardiac medication. Usually, this implies avoiding AEDs that are highly protein-bound (i.e., phenytoin and valproic acid) and potent cytochrome P450 inducers (i.e., carbamazepine, phenytoin, phenobarbital, and their derivatives). Implantation of the vagal nerve stimulator (VNS) can be more anatomically complex, although not contraindicated, in patients with implanted defibrillators and pacemakers.

Some AEDs can cause cardiovascular side effects, rendering management of patients with coexisting cardiac disease difficult. The most common cardiovascular complications of AEDs are hypotension and arrhythmia, especially with rapid infusions of some parenteral agents. Symptomatic heart block has been described with voltage-dependent, sodium channel–blocking AEDs, especially carbamazepine.[52] Agents with more complex, multiple mechanisms of action, such as lamotrigine, have not clearly been associated with cardiac conduction abnormalities.[53] Calcium channel blockers, conversely, have been investigated as potential AEDs.[54,55]

Parenteral AEDs may also be associated with hemodynamic instability due to propylene glycol, which is used to solubilize phenobarbital, phenytoin, and some benzodiazepines. Parenteral phenytoin also has proarrhythmic effects when administered rapidly in large doses. Although parenteral administration and overdose should be monitored by ECG telemetry, oral phenytoin doses of up to 75 μg/ml do not usually require telemetry management.[56] Some previous formulations of phenobarbital contained ethanol rather than propylene glycol, with less tendency for hypotension; these formulations are no longer available. VNS has rarely been associated with bradycardia or asystole on initiation of programming.[57] Little information of the potential for risk of VNS in patients with pre-existing bradycardia or conduction delays has been accumulated, although VNS can have minimal effects on heart rhythm or heart period variability.[58]

The ketogenic diet has been associated not only with abnormal lipid profiles, but also prolongation of the Q-T interval and dilated cardiomyopathy.[59] Adrenocorticotropic hormone may result in hypertension and, ultimately, even hypertrophic cardiomyopathy.[60] Electrical stimulation of the insular region causes lateralized cardiac chronotropic effects before surgical resection.[61] Table 2-2 lists potential cardiac effects of acute seizure treatments. Familiarity with the cardiac effects of AEDs is essential in optimally managing patients with epilepsy.

Summary

Cardiac disease and seizures are common medical conditions with significant morbidity and mortality. Sudden death is associated with epilepsy, as well as ASCVD, leading to speculations of the neurocardiac effects of seizures. Patients who have seizures and heart disease warrant careful attention to the interactions of medications, diagnostic studies, and disease. As knowledge of cardiovascular disease and epilepsy rapidly expands, the neurologist must remain abreast of their important interface.

References

1. Li X, Breteler MM, de Bruyne MC, et al. Vascular determinants of epilepsy: the Rotterdam Study. Epilepsia 1997;38:1216.
2. Komrad MS, Coffey CE, Coffey KS, et al. Myocardial infarction and stroke. Neurology 1984;34:1403.
3. Weinrich DJ, Burke JF, Pauletto FJ. Left ventricular thrombi complicating acute myocardial infarction. Long term follow up with serial echocardiography. Ann Intern Med 1984;100:789–794.
4. Caramelli P, Mutarelli EG, Caramelli B, et al. Neurological complications after thrombolytic treatment for acute myocardial infarction: emphasis on unprecedented manifestations. Acta Neurol Scand 1999;85:331–333.
5. Hesdorffer DC, Hauser WA, Annegers JF, Rocca WA. Severe uncontrolled hypertension and adult-onset seizures: a case-control study in Rochester, Minnesota. Epilepsia 1996;37:736–741.
6. Russell JW, Biller J, Hajduczok ZD, et al. Ischemic cerebrovascular complications and risk factors in idiopathic subaortic stenosis. Stroke 1991;22:1143.
7. Chesebro JH, Adams PC, Fuster V. Antithrombotic therapy in patients with valvular heart disease and prosthetic heart valves. J Am Coll Cardiol 1986;8:41B.
8. Wolf PA, Dawber TR, Thomas HE Jr, et al. Epidemiologic assessment of chronic atrial fibrillation and risk of stroke: the Framingham study. Neurology 1978;28:973.
9. Neilson GH, Galea EG, Hossack KF. Thromboembolic complications of mitral valve disease. Aust N Z J Med 1978;8:372.
10. Boughner DR, Barnett NJ. The enigma of risk of stroke in mitral valve prolapse. Stroke 1985;16:175.
11. Barnett HJ, Boughner DR, Taylor DW, et al. Further evidence relating mitral-valve prolapse to cerebral ischemic events. N Engl J Med 1980;302:139.
12. Benjamin EJ, Plehn JF, D'Agostino RB, et al. Mitral annular calcification and the risk of stroke in an elderly cohort. N Engl J Med 1992;327:374–379.
13. McKay RG. The Mansfield Scientific Aortic Valvuloplasty Registry: overview of acute hemodynamic results and procedural complications. J Am Coll Cardiol 1991;17:485.
14. Ryan CA, Robertson M, Coe JY. Seizures due to lidocaine toxicity in a child during cardiac catheterization. Pediatr Cardiol 1993;14:116–118.

15. Salgado AV, Furlan AJ, Keys TF, et al. Neurologic complications of endocarditis: a 12-year experience. Neurology 1989;39:173.

16. Harrison MJ, Hampton JR. Neurological presentation of bacterial endocarditis. BMJ 1967;2:148.

17. Berthrong M, Sabiston DC. Cerebral lesions in congenital heart disease Bull Johns Hopkins Hosp 1951;89:384.

18. John K, Bachman DS, Cooper RF, et al. Electroencephalographic abnormalities in children with congenital heart disease. Arch Neurol 1985;42:794–796.

19. Miller G, Eggli KD, Contant C, et al. Postoperative neurologic complications after open heart surgery on young infants. Arch Pediatr Adolesc Med 1995;149:764–768.

20. Helmers SL, Wypij D, Constantinou JE, et al. Perioperative seizures in infants undergoing repair of complex congenital cardiac defects. Electroencephalogr Clin Neurophysiol 1997;102:27–36.

21. Belkin RN, Pollack BD, Ruggiero ML, et al. Comparison of transesophageal and transthoracic echocardiography with contrast and color flow Doppler in the detection of patent foramen ovale. Am Heart J 1994;128:520–525.

22. Fischbein CA, Rosenthal A, Fischer EG, et al. Risk factors of brain abscess in patients with congenital heart disease Am J Cardiol 1974;34:97.

23. Stafstrom CE, Patxot OF, Gilmore HE, Wisniewski KE. Seizures in children with Down syndrome: etiology, characteristics, and outcome. Dev Med Child Neurol 1991;33:191–200.

24. Moorman JR, Crain B, Osborne D. Kallman's syndrome with associated cardiovascular and intracranial anomalies. Am J Med 1984;77:369.

25. Quek SC, Yip W, Quek ST, et al: Cardiac manifestations in tuberous sclerosis: a 10-year review. J Paediatr Child Health 1998;34:282–287.

26. Jones M. Anomalies of the brain and congenital heart disease: a study of 52 necropsy cases. Pediatr Pathol 1991;11:721.

27. Shearer WT, Rutman JY, Weinberg WA, et al. Coarctation of the aorta and cerebrovascular accident: a proposal for early corrective surgery. J Pediatr 1970;77:1004.

28. Morley J, Marinchak R, Rials SJ, Kowey P. Atrial fibrillation, anticoagulation, and stroke. Am J Cardiol 1996;77:38A–44A.

29. Reith J, Jorgensen HS, Nakayama H, et al. Seizures in acute stroke: predictors and prognostic significance. The Copenhagen Stroke Study. Stroke 1997;28:1585–1589.

30. Laupacis A, Albers G, Dunn M, Feinberg W. Antithrombotic therapy in atrial fibrillation. Chest 1992; 102[Suppl]:426S.

31. Wang Q, Chen Q, Li H, Towbin JA. Molecular genetics of long QT syndrome from genes to patients. Curr Opin Cardiol 1997;12:310–320.

32. Chiang CE, Roden DM. The long QT syndromes: genetic basis and clinical implications. J Am Coll Cardiol 2000;36:1–12.

33. Gospe SM, Choy M. Hereditary long Q-T syndrome presenting as epilepsy: electroencephalography laboratory diagnosis. Ann Neurol 1989;25:514–516.

34. Devinsky O, Pacia S, Tatambhotla G. Bradycardia and asystole induced by partial seizures: a case report and literature review. Neurology 1997;48:1712–1714.

35. Reeves A, Nollet KE, Lass DW, et al. The ictal bradycardia syndrome. Epilepsia 1996;37:983–987.

36. Blumhardt LD, Smith PE, Owen L. Electrocardiographic accompaniments of temporal lobe epileptic seizures. Lancet 1986;1:1051.

37. Ossentjuk E, Elink Sterk CJ, Storm van Leeuwen W. Flicker-induced cardiac arrest in a patient with epilepsy. Electroencephalogr Clin Neurophysiol 1966;20:257.

38. Erickson TC. Cardiac activity during epileptic seizures Arch Neurol Psychiatry 1939;41:511.

39. Boggs JG, Painter JA, DeLorenzo RJ. Analysis of electrocardiographic changes in status epilepticus. Epilepsy Res 1993;14:87–94.

40. Keilson MJ, Hauser A, Magrill JP, et al. ECG abnormalities in patients with epilepsy. Neurology 1987;37:1624.

41. Boggs JG, Marmarou A, Agnew JP, et al. Hemodynamic monitoring at the time of death in status epilepticus. Epilepsy Res 1998;31:199–209.

42. Ficker DM. Sudden unexplained death and injury in epilepsy. Epilepsia 2000;41[Suppl 2]:S7–S12.

43. Walczak TS, Hauser WA, Leppik IE, et al. Incidence and risk factors for sudden unexpected death in epilepsy: a prospective cohort study. Neurology 1998;50[Suppl 4]:443–444.

44. Lathers CM, Schraeder PL, Boggs JG. Sudden Unexpected Death and Autonomic Dysfunction. In J Engel Jr, TA Pedley (eds), Epilepsy: a Comprehensive Textbook. Philadelphia: Lippincott–Raven, 1997;1943–1955.

45. Johnston SC, Siedenberg R, Min J, et al. Central apnea and acute cardiac ischemia in a sheep model of epileptic sudden death. Ann Neurol 1997;42:588–594.

46. Kapoor WN. Diagnostic evaluation of syncope. Am J Med 1991;90:91–94.

47. Aminoff MJ, Schienman MM, Griffin JC, et al. Electrocerebral accompaniments of syncope associated with malignant ventricular arrhythmias. Ann Intern Med 1988;108:791–795.

48. Wijdicks EF, Sharborough FW. New-onset seizures in critically-ill patients. Neurology 1993;43:1042–1044.

49. Zaccara G, Muscas GC, Messori A. Clinical features, pathogenesis, and management of drug-induced seizures. Drug Saf 1990;5:109–151.

50. Keilson GR, Schwaartz WJ, Recht LD. The preponderance of posterior circulatory events is independent

of the route of cardiac catheterization. Stroke 1992;23:1358.

51. Galbreath C, Salgado ED, Furlan AJ, Hollman J. Central nervous system complications of percutaneous transluminal angioplasty. Stroke 1986;17:616.

52. Takyanagi K, Hisauchi I, Watanabe J, et al. Carbamazepine-induced sinus node dysfunction and atrioventricular block in elderly women. Jpn Heart J 1998;39:469–479.

53. Steinhoff BJ, Stodiek SR, Tiecks FP, et al. Cardiac side effects and ECG changes with lamotrigine? A clinical study. Schweiz Arch Neurol Psychiatr 1994;145:8–12.

54. Meyer FB, Cascino GD, Whisnant JP, et al. Nimodipine as an add-on therapy for intractable epilepsy. Mayo Clin Proc 1995;70:623–627.

55. Pledger GW, Sackellares JC, Treiman DM, et al. Flunarizine for treatment of partial seizures: results of a concentration-controlled trial. Neurology 1994;44:1830–1836.

56. Evers ML, Izhar A, Aquil A. Cardiac monitoring after phenytoin overdose. Heart Lung 1997;26:325–328.

57. Asconape JJ, Moore DD, Zipes DP, et al. Bradycardia and asystole with the use of vagus nerve stimulation for the treatment of epilepsy: a rare complication of intraoperative device testing. Epilepsia 1999;40:1452–1454.

58. Setty AB, Vaughn BV, Quint SR, et al. Heart period variability during vagal nerve stimulation. Seizure 1998;7:213–217.

59. Best TH, Franz DN, Gilbert DL, et al. Cardiac complications in pediatric patients on the ketogenic diet. Neurology 2000;54:2328–2330.

60. Starc TJ, Bierman FZ, Pavlakis SG, et al. Cardiac size and function during ACTH-induced systolic systemic hypertension in infants. Am J Cardiol 1993;73:57–64.

61. Oppenheimer SM, Gelb A, Girvin JP, et al. Cardiovascular effects of human insular cortex stimulation. Neurology 1992;42:1727–1732.

Chapter 3

Renal Disorders

Thomas R. Browne

The neurologist usually is asked to consult with patients with renal disease and seizures for two reasons: (1) seizures associated with renal insufficiency or dialysis, or both, and (2) management of antiepileptic drug (AED) therapy in patients with renal disease, alone or in combination with hemodialysis. Thus, this chapter covers three areas: (1) diagnosis and management of seizures associated with renal insufficiency or dialysis, or both; (2) effects of renal insufficiency and hemodialysis on drug pharmacokinetics; and (3) effects of renal insufficiency and hemodialysis on the pharmacokinetics of specific AEDs. For reviews of the many facets of renal disease and the many neurologic complications of renal disease, see Brenner[1] and Denker.[2]

Seizures Associated with Renal Insufficiency or Hemodialysis, or Both

Seizures are associated with four conditions occurring with renal insufficiency: uremic encephalopathy, dialysis disequilibrium syndrome, aluminum encephalopathy in infants and children, and dialysis encephalopathy syndrome. These four conditions have been comprehensively reviewed by Gobbi et al.,[3] and the author used this review in preparing this section.

Uremic Encephalopathy

Diagnosis

Uremia is a systemic intoxication due to renal insufficiency, resulting in disturbances in tubular and endo-crine functions of the kidney, production of toxic metabolites, changes in volume and electrolyte composition of the body fluids, and an excess or deficiency of various hormones.[3,4] Seizures may be due to hypertension, electrolyte imbalance, aluminum toxicity, drug toxicity, or infection.[3] Also, uremia may lead to seizures owing to elevation of intracellular sodium, accumulation of toxic metabolites, and inhibition of γ-aminobutyric acid responses.[3]

Uremic encephalopathy is characterized by an alteration in mental status, hypoxia, seizures, movement disorders, nystagmus, and ataxia.[3] Similar symptoms and signs occur in acute and chronic renal insufficiency, and their severity correlates with the severity of renal insufficiency.[3]

Early movement disorders include muscle cramps, tremor, and asterixis.[3] In more severe uremia, muscle fasciculations and myoclonus may appear.[3] The combination of asterixis and myoclonus may be severe and has been termed *uremic twitching*.[3,5] Chorea and athetosis may occur. These abnormal movements are sometimes confused with seizures. The electroencephalogram (EEG) is helpful in distinguishing movement disorders from seizures, because paroxysmal activity is not recorded during abnormal movements.

Seizures occur in approximately one-third of patients with uremic encephalopathy.[3] The seizures are usually tonic-clonic or myoclonic, but partial motor seizures may occur.[3,5] In acute renal failure, seizures usually occur within the first 15 days.[5] In chronic renal failure, seizures usually occur late in the disease and may be a preterminal event.[3,6]

Table 3-1. Risk of Drug Removal by Hemodialysis

Low:	Intermediate:
Carbamazepine	Lamotrigine
Clonazepam	Valproate
Phenytoin	
Tiagabine	
High:	**Undetermined:**
Ethosuximide	Felbamate
Gabapentin	Oxcarbazepine
Levetiracetam	Primidone
Phenobarbital	Zonisamide
Topiramate	

The EEG background in uremic encephalopathy demonstrates bilateral, frontal-predominant, slow activity, which may include diphasic and triphasic waves.[3] Photomyoclonic and photoconvulsive responses to photic stimulation may occur.[3]

When seizures occur in the context of renal insufficiency, it is necessary to exclude complications other than uremia as the cause of the seizures. The other conditions to exclude are electrolyte imbalance (e.g., water intoxication, hypocalcemia, hyponatremia, hypomagnesemia), aluminum encephalopathy, drug intoxication, hypertensive encephalopathy, intracranial hemorrhage, and subdural hematoma.[3] Also, Wernicke's encephalopathy can occur in dialysis. Thiamine is a water-soluble vitamin removed by dialysis. Tests to be performed include bone and plasma aluminum concentrations, plasma and urinary electrolyte concentrations, osmolality, volume, and antidiuretic hormone level.[3] The record should be reviewed for administration of drugs that may cause seizures, and drug plasma concentration of drugs that may cause seizures should be determined if possible. Hypertensive encephalopathy, intracranial hemorrhage, and subdural hematoma can be diagnosed by imaging studies.

Management

Definitive management of uremic encephalopathy requires dialysis or renal transplant. Seizures are managed with the standard AEDs for tonic-clonic and partial seizures. If dialysis is to be undertaken, a drug with a low risk for removal by dialysis should be selected (see section Hemodialysis; Table 3-1). In

practice, phenytoin is often selected because it is effective for tonic-clonic and partial seizures and can be given intravenously in loading doses to maintain a desired plasma concentration (e.g., after hemodialysis), using procedures described in the section Hemodialysis, and relatively little phenytoin is removed by hemodialysis (see section Phenytoin). Free, rather than total, phenytoin plasma concentration should be monitored in renal insufficiency, because the free fraction increases and the total concentration decreases in renal insufficiency (see section Phenytoin). The effects of renal insufficiency and hemodialysis on phenytoin and other AEDs are discussed in the sections Seizures Associated with Renal Insufficiency or Hemodialysis, or Both and Effects of Renal Insufficiency and Hemodialysis on Drug Pharmacokinetics. Clonazepam is effective for the myoclonus of uremia.[7]

Dialysis Disequilibrium Syndrome

Diagnosis

Dialysis disequilibrium syndrome usually occurs during the patient's first few dialysis sessions.[3] The symptoms of the syndrome include irritability, restlessness, headache, nausea, emesis, hypertension, blurred vision, seizures, muscular twitching, fasciculations, asterixis, and confusion.[3] When delirium appears, it may last for several days.[3] Deaths from cerebral edema and herniation have been reported in the past but are rare with newer dialysis techniques.[3]

The mechanism of dialysis disequilibrium syndrome is that urea is more rapidly cleared from the plasma than the brain.[8] After dialysis, water enters the brain following an osmotic gradient. This results in an increase in brain extracellular water and brain edema.[8,9] Decrease in intracellular pH and generation of osmolar molecules may contribute to cerebral edema.[3,10,11]

The EEG between dialysis sessions may show background slowing.[12,13] During dialysis, increased slow activity, bursts of bilaterally symmetric slow waves, and increased photic sensitivity may be seen.[12,13] The EEG can determine whether abnormal movements are due to seizures or movement disorder by the presence or absence of paroxysmal activity.

The presence of other disorders that can cause seizures in renal insufficiency needs to be excluded. See Uremic Encephalopathy, Diagnosis, for a list of disorders and diagnostic tests. In addition, lowered serum concentration of ionized calcium (due to abrupt increase in plasma pH) and nonketotic hyperosmolar coma in nondiabetic patients (due to increased plasma glucose concentration in repeated peritoneal dialysis) need to be considered.[3,14,15]

Management

Dialysis must be discontinued until the seizure and vital signs have been stabilized. AED therapy may help reduce seizures. A drug not removed by dialysis should be selected (see section Hemodialysis and Table 3-1). Most often, phenytoin is selected for the reasons listed in Uremic Encephalopathy, Management, following the guidelines given in that section. Therapy begins with a loading dose of intravenous phenytoin of 15–20 mg/kg. Additional intravenous loading doses of phenytoin may be administered, if necessary, after dialysis, following the guidelines given in the section Hemodialysis. Hypocalcemic seizures may be controlled with calcium gluconate.[3]

Aluminum Encephalopathy Syndrome

Diagnosis

Aluminum encephalopathy syndrome is a progressive encephalopathy of infants and children (occasionally adults) with chronic renal insufficiency who have taken aluminum containing products such as phosphate binders for several years.[3,16–18] Such patients have an elevated brain-aluminum concentration.[17,19] In renal insufficiency, aluminum absorption is increased by secondary hypoparathyroidism, and aluminum excretion is reduced.[3] Aluminum is stored in bones and other tissues.[17] Aluminum encephalopathy occasionally is seen in patients with normal renal function who are receiving large amounts of aluminum, such as aluminum bladder irrigation.[20,21] There is speculation that aluminum intoxication may play a role in Alzheimer's disease, based on the morphologic

and immunologic similarities of the two conditions.[22]

The clinical features of aluminum encephalopathy are motor disturbances (e.g., dysmetria, tremor, hypotonia, myoclonus), seizures, speech disturbances, and, ultimately, a vegetative state.[3] The seizures usually are tonic-clonic but may be simple or complex partial.[23]

The EEG in aluminum encephalopathy syndrome has a characteristic pattern of a slow background with superimposed bursts of high-amplitude slow waves and sharp waves and complexes of spikes and slow waves.[6,23] Imaging studies show cortical atrophy.

The diagnosis of aluminum encephalopathy syndrome is suggested by the presence of typical symptoms in a child with chronic renal disease who has been taking aluminum-containing products.[3] The diagnosis is confirmed by elevated plasma and bone aluminum concentrations and by typical EEG and imaging findings.[3] Aluminum encephalopathy syndrome must be differentiated from uremic encephalopathy and electrolyte imbalances, such as acute hypercalcemia and severe phosphate depletion.[3]

Management

Aluminum-containing products must be eliminated from the diet of the child with chronic renal insufficiency. Aluminum chelation with deferoxamine is indicated in advanced cases.[3,21] Infant diets should consist of low-phosphate formulas with calcium carbonate added.[3] Calcium citrate and aluminum-containing antacids should be avoided.[3] Benzodiazepines, such as clonazepam and diazepam, are effective in controlling the myoclonus. Phenytoin usually is used for the tonic-clonic seizures, for reasons discussed in the section Uremic Encephalopathy, Management.

Dialysis Encephalopathy Syndrome (Dialysis Dementia)

Diagnosis

Dialysis encephalopathy syndrome (also called *dialysis dementia*) occurs in patients on chronic hemodialysis. Some cases are due to aluminum toxicity from aluminum in the dialysis bath,[19] and the incidence of the disease has decreased with the use of aluminum-free water.[7]

Presenting symptoms consist of dysarthria, apraxia, and slurred speech with stuttering and hesitation.[3,24] Within months, myoclonus, asterixis, movement dyspraxias, seizures, memory loss, personality changes, and frank psychosis develop.[3,16,24]

The disease usually progresses to apneic spells and death within 1–15 months from sepsis or suicide.[3,16,19,24] However, in some patients, the disease is transient, and others have a variable course lasting several years.[24]

The EEG shows changes similar to those in aluminum encephalopathy syndrome.[13] The bursts of sharp and slow activity and the clinical symptoms sometimes are suppressed by oral or intravenous diazepam early in the disease.[25] Epileptic and non-epileptic movements can be distinguished by combined EEG and electromyography recordings.

Symptoms similar to dialysis dementia can be caused by acute hypercalcemia[26] and severe hypophosphatemia,[27] which can occur during hemodialysis. Pyridoxine is removed during hemodialysis, and this can lead to drug-resistant seizures.[3,28]

Management

Aluminum-containing phosphate binders and infant formulas should be removed from the diets of those patients on chronic hemodialysis. Aluminum chelation with deferoxamine may lead to dramatic improvement, even in advanced cases.[3,21] Pyridoxine supplementation must be given when pyridoxine deficiency is present.[27] Control of secondary hyperthyroidism, iron deficiency anemia, and hyperphosphatemia reduces aluminum absorption by the gastrointestinal tract.[3] The concentration of aluminum in the dialysate should be monitored periodically.[3]

Benzodiazepines such as clonazepam and diazepam are effective in controlling the myoclonus. Benzodiazepines may temporarily control the bursts of sharp and slow activity on the EEG and may temporarily reduce the clinical symptoms of dialysis encephalopathy syndrome.[25] Phenytoin usually is used for tonic-clonic seizures, for reasons discussed in the section Uremic Encephalopathy, Management.

Effects of Renal Insufficiency and Hemodialysis on Drug Pharmacokinetics

This section reviews the normal physiology of renal clearance of drugs and the effects of renal impairment and hemodialysis on drug steady-state plasma concentration. These topics have been exhaustively reviewed by Matzke and Millikin,[29] and the author used this review in preparing this section.

Physiology of Renal Clearance of Drugs

Principles of Renal Clearance

Drugs may be eliminated entirely by renal excretion, by hepatic or other nonrenal routes, or by both renal and nonrenal routes. The proportion of a drug excreted by the renal route determines the importance of renal disease on the drug's elimination.[30,31]

Renal excretion of drugs and their metabolites is determined by three processes: glomerular filtration, tubular secretion, and passive tubular resorption. Filtration is determined primarily by glomerular filtration (measured clinically as creatinine clearance) and plasma-protein binding. Only non–protein-bound (free) drugs in the plasma can pass through the glomerular filter. This has important implications that are discussed later.

Some drugs are actively transported from the plasma to the urine by two independent carrier systems. One carrier system transports organic acids, such as acetazolamide and glucuronide drug metabolites. The other carrier system transports organic bases, such as cimetidine. In practice, the only AED with significant tubular secretion is acetazolamide (80% excretion via acidic secretion system).[32] A small portion (probably not clinically important) of gabapentin is excreted via the basic secretion system, as evidenced by the inhibition of renal clearance of gabapentin by co-administration of cimetadine.[33] Otherwise, renal tubular secretion is not an important mechanism for clearance of unchanged AEDs.

Lipid-soluble (nonionized) molecules pass through biological membranes by simple diffusion, whereas water-soluble (ionized) molecules do not. Resorption of water in renal tubules creates a concentration gradient that facilitates back diffusion of lipid-soluble drugs from the glomerular filtrate into the plasma. Thus, water-soluble drugs (e.g., gabapentin, levetiracetam) are excreted in the urine. Lipid-soluble drugs (e.g., carbamazepine, phenytoin) are not excreted via the urine.

The renal elimination of ionizable drugs with pK_a values within the range of urinary pH (5–8) can be increased or decreased by altering urine pH. Such alterations in pH will alter the proportions of the drug that are ionized (water soluble, excreted in urine) and nonionized (lipid soluble, resorbed into plasma). For example, alkalinization of the urine increases the rate of elimination of phenobarbital (weak acid, pK_a = 7.3) in the case of phenobarbital overdose.[34]

In summary, the renal clearance of AEDs is determined by protein binding, glomerular filtration rate, and the drug's water solubility. Water-soluble (ionized) drugs are excreted via the urine, whereas lipid-soluble (nonionized) drugs are not. Most drug metabolites (e.g., epoxides, glucuronides) are more water soluble than the parent drug and are excreted in the urine.

Factors Determining Steady-State Drug Plasma Concentration

The mean steady-state plasma concentration of a drug during chronic oral dosing is

$$\bar{C}_{ss} = \frac{F \times (D/t)}{Cl_R + Cl_H + Cl_O} \quad (1)$$

where F = fraction of drug absorbed, D = dose, t = dosing interval, Cl_R = renal clearance, Cl_H = hepatic clearance and Cl_O = clearance via other routes. For drugs having no renal tubular secretion (all AEDs except acetazolamide), renal clearance can be defined as

$$Cl_R = GFR = \frac{C_{ur} \times Q_{ur}}{C_p} \quad (2)$$

where GFR = glomerular filtration rate, C_{ur} = concentration of drug in urine, C_p = concentration of drug in plasma, and Q_{ur} = urine flow rate.

The hepatic clearance of a drug by a hepatic enzyme system is

$$Cl_H = \frac{Q_H \times f \times (V_{max}/K_M)}{Q_H + f \times (V_{max}/K_M)} \quad (3)$$

where Q_H = hepatic blood flow rate, f = free (non–protein-bound) fraction of drug on plasma, V_{max} = the maximum velocity of the enzyme, and K_M = the Michaelis-Menten constant of the enzyme.

Combining equations 1, 2, and 3 yields

$$-C = \frac{F \times (D/t)}{\dfrac{(C_{ur} \times Q_{ur})}{C_p} + \dfrac{[QH \times f \times (V_{max}/K_M)]}{QH + f \times (V_{max} \times K_M)}} \quad (4)$$

Equation 4 is admittedly cumbersome and complex and need not be memorized. However, equation 4 provides a useful checklist of all of the factors that may influence drug plasma concentration. Most of the factors listed in equation 4 can be affected by renal impairment, as discussed in the next section.

Effects of Renal Impairment and Hemodialysis on Drug Steady-State Plasma Concentration

Renal impairment can alter the fraction of drug dose absorbed, protein binding, renal drug clearance, and hepatic drug clearance. These changes can alter drug steady-state plasma concentration (see equations 1 and 4).

Effect of Renal Impairment on Fraction of Drug Absorbed (F)

There are reports that renal disease may reduce oral absorption, owing to alteration of gastric pH; edema of the gastrointestinal tract due to irritant properties of waste products, such as urea; and administration of antacids.[29] However, bioavailability studies typically compare area under the plasma concentration (AUC) versus time of drug given for healthy persons and renally impaired patients. AUC is determined by the fraction of drug absorbed, drug clearance, and drug protein binding. Because the latter two factors can be affected by renal impairment, simple measurements of AUC for determination of F may be invalidated, owing to alterations in drug clearance or protein binding, or both.[29] The use of techniques that correct for changes in clearance and protein binding has produced variable results when applied to studies of F in patients with renal impairment.[29]

Effect of Renal Impairment on Drug Protein Binding

The plasma protein binding of acidic drugs (e.g., phenytoin, valproic acid) is markedly reduced in patients with severe renal impairment.[35] The effects of lesser degrees of renal impairment have not been studied as extensively. The proposed mechanisms for reduced protein binding in renal insufficiency include decreased plasma albumin concentration, accumulation of endogenous binding inhibitors, and competition for binding sites by metabolites of the administered parent drug.[29,35,36]

For drugs cleared principally by hepatic enzymes, equation 4 can be simplified to

$$\bar{C}_{ss} \cong \frac{1}{f} \qquad (5)$$

Thus, total (protein bound and nonbound) mean steady-state plasma concentration decreases when the free fraction of drug increases in situations, such as renal insufficiency.

The mean steady-state free or non–protein-bound concentration of a drug (C_{ssF}) can be expressed as

$$\bar{C}_{ssF} = \bar{C}_{ss} \times f \qquad (6)$$

Combining equations 5 and 6 yields

$$\bar{C}_{ssF} \cong \frac{1}{f} \times \bar{C}_{ss} \times f \qquad (7)$$

Note this important relationship: *For drugs metabolized by hepatic enzymes, changes in protein binding affect the total steady-state plasma concentration, but the free drug plasma concentration remains constant.*

For example, in the presence of renal insufficiency, the total plasma concentration of a protein-bound drug cleared by the liver, such as phenytoin, decreases owing to an increase in the free fraction of the drug, but the free concentration of phenytoin remains unchanged.[37] Seizure patients with renal insufficiency may receive excessive (toxic) dosing rates of phenytoin, if the total phenytoin plasma concentration is the basis for selecting dosing rate.

Another example of the effects of changes in protein binding on free and total drug plasma concentration is the interaction of valproate with phenytoin. Both drugs are highly protein-bound. When valproate is added to phenytoin, the free fraction of phenytoin increases, owing to the displacement of phenytoin from protein-binding sites by valproate. The total phenytoin plasma concentration decreases, but the free phenytoin plasma concentration remains constant.[38] This can lead to excessive (toxic) dosing rates of phenytoin, if the phenytoin dosing rate is based on total phenytoin plasma concentration.

Effect of Renal Impairment on Drug Metabolism

Renal impairment decreases excretion of drugs eliminated by renal clearance (see next section). Certain drugs (no AEDs), such as acetaminophen, are metabolized by the kidney, and this metabolism is reduced in renal failure.[29] There is animal and human evidence that the nonrenal clearance of certain drugs is decreased by 20–80% in the presence of renal insufficiency.[29]

Metabolic enzyme systems that may be affected by renal impairment are hydroxylation, *O*-demethylation, *N*-demethylation, glucuronidation, deacetylation, and sulfoxidation.[29] The mechanism of these metabolic changes may be the accumulation of inhibitors or toxins or the collateral effects of the disease causing renal insufficiency.

Hydroxylation, demethylation, and glucuronidation are results of the metabolism of some AEDs. This raises the possibility of a decrease in nonrenal clearance of some AEDs in renal failure. This possibility has not been studied extensively.

Effect of Renal Impairment on Drug Excretion

The total clearance of a drug is the sum of renal clearance (CL_R) plus hepatic clearance (CL_H) plus other routes of clearance (e.g., sweat).

$$CL_T = CL_R + CL_H + CL_O \qquad (8)$$

Renal clearance can be defined as

$$CL_R = CL_F + \frac{R_S - R_R}{C_p} \qquad (9)$$

where CL_F = clearance via filtration, R_S = the rate of renal tubular secretion, R_R = the rate of renal tubular resorption, and C_p = drug plasma concentration. The effect of renal disease on drug clearance thus depends on the relative contribution of renal clearance to total clearance, drug filtration, tubular secretion rate, tubular resorption rate, and drug plasma concentration.

For some drugs (e.g., gabapentin, levetiracetam), renal clearance accounts for most or all of total clearance.[39] For other drugs (e.g., phenytoin, carbamazepine), renal clearance accounts for little of total clearance.

The rate of filtration of a drug (R_f) depends on GFR, drug plasma concentration, and free fraction of the drug in plasma.

$$R_f = GFR \times C_p \times f \qquad (10)$$

In renal impairment, the GFR decreases, and the free fraction of drug in plasma may increase (see section Effect of Renal Impairment on Drug Protein Binding). Renal tubular secretion does not occur with the commonly used AEDs.

Tubular resorption is dependent on lipid solubility and the ability to cross biological membranes. Lipid-soluble drugs readily cross the renal tubule and are resorbed. For example, phenytoin is highly lipid soluble, and almost no phenytoin is cleared by the kidney.[40]

Thus, there can be no general statement about how renal impairment affects total drug clearance. The effect of renal impairment in total drug clearance depends on the combined effects of the factors listed previously in this section. In the section Effects on Renal Impairment and Hemodialysis on the Pharmacokinetics of Specific Antiepileptic Drugs, the effects of renal impairment on specific AEDs are presented.

Drug Dosing Rate Adjustments in Renal Insufficiency

Changes in renal clearance are correlated with changes in creatinine clearance (CL_{CR}) by a constant q, which is different for each drug.

$$CL_R = q \times CL_{CR} \qquad (11)$$

Total drug clearance (CL_T) is the sum of renal clearance (CL_R) plus nonrenal clearance (CL_N).

$$CL_T = CL_R + CL_N \qquad (12)$$

Steady-state mean drug plasma concentration (C_{ss}) is equal to dosing rate (D) divided by total clearance.

$$\overline{C}_{ss} = \frac{D}{CL_T} \qquad (13)$$

Rearranging this equation leads to

$$D = \overline{C}_{ss} \times CL_T \qquad (14)$$

Thus, the simplest approach to adjusting dosing rate in renal insufficiency is to empirically determine q for a drug, measure creatinine clearance for

an individual, select a desired plasma concentration, and calculate dose from the given equations.

Although simple, this first approach fails to account for differences in age and weight and for changes in volume of distribution, bioavailability, and nonrenal clearance that may occur in renal insufficiency. Roland and Tozer[41] have described a more complete method for dosage adjustment in renal failure, using the volume of distribution of an unbound drug in healthy subjects and in renal insufficiency, the fraction of the drug absorbed in healthy subjects and in renal insufficiency, the ratio of the individual patient's creatinine clearance to normal creatinine clearance, the fraction of the unchanged drug eliminated renally in healthy persons, age, and weight.

Other, more complex, methods of adjusting dosing regimen in renal failure have been reported. These are reviewed by Matzke and Millikin.[29]

All available methods for computing dosing regimens in renal insufficiency have errors. The actual plasma drug concentration obtained with the calculated dosing rate may vary considerably from the desired plasma concentration. Monitoring of the patient and the drug plasma concentration is necessary. The dosing rate may need to be modified from the calculated dosing rate.

Hemodialysis

AEDs are cleared from the circulation by hemodialysis, principally by diffusion from the blood into the dialysate through the filter membrane. The drug moves from the blood (high concentration) to the dialysate (low concentration) via a concentration gradient. There are many factors that determine the rate of clearance of a drug via hemodialysis.[29]

Molecular Size. Drugs must pass through pores of a specified size during hemodialysis. Molecules larger than 500 atomic mass units usually do not pass through hemodialysis filters. In practice, the AEDs have atomic masses of less than 500, and molecular size is not an issue for the dialysis of AEDs.

Water Solubility. Drugs that are water soluble readily cross dialysis membranes, whereas drugs that are not readily water soluble do not. Many central nervous system drugs (e.g., carbamazepine, phenytoin, tricyclics) are lipid-soluble compounds (i.e., not readily water soluble), because lipid solubility permits passage across the blood-brain barrier. This is discussed further in the following sections.

Protein Binding.   Only non–protein-bound drugs can cross dialysis membranes. Drugs that are highly protein bound (e.g., phenytoin, valproate) are difficult to remove from the systemic circulation by hemodialysis.

Volume of Distribution.   Drugs that remain mainly in the blood are more readily removed than are drugs that are distributed extensively into tissues.

Dialysis Conditions.   Filter characteristics (there are many types of filters), filter size, blood flow rate, and dialysis flow rate all effect the hemodialysis clearance of a drug.

Peritoneal Dialysis.   The principles applicable to hemodialysis are also applicable to peritoneal dialysis.

Conclusion.   There is no simple equation to predict the amount of an AED that is lost during dialysis. Drugs that are water soluble and not highly protein bound and that have a small volume of distribution are readily removed by hemodialysis. Drugs with high lipid solubility (i.e., low water solubility), high protein binding, and high volume of distribution are difficult to remove by hemodialysis. See Table 3-1 for a listing of risk of drug removal by hemodialysis.

Note that even low-risk drugs will have some removal during dialysis.

Correction for Drug Loss during Hemodialysis. The plasma concentration of a drug that has been partially removed during dialysis can be restored to the desired plasma concentration using the following equation and a loading dose (*LD*) of drug:

$$LD = C_{change} \times VD \qquad (15)$$

where C_{change} = desired change in plasma concentration and VD = volume of distribution.

For example, let us suppose it is desired to increase phenytoin plasma concentration by 5 mg/ liter (5μg/ml). Then the loading dose equals 5.0

mg/liter × 0.7 liter/kg (phenytoin volume of distribution) or 3.5 mg/kg.

For gabapentin, levetiracetam, and topiramate, a standard replacement dose is recommended after hemodialysis. See the next section for details.

Effects on Renal Impairment and Hemodialysis on the Pharmacokinetics of Specific Antiepileptic Drugs

Carbamazepine (Tegretol)

The absorption and clearance of carbamazepine do not appear to be influenced by renal impairment.[42] However, carbamazepine has a significant antidiuretic effect and may promote fluid retention.

Carbamazepine is poorly soluble in water and is 80% protein bound. As expected, hemodialysis has little effect on carbamazepine plasma concentration.[43]

Clonazepam (Klonopin)

The effects of renal insufficiency on clonazepam have not been studied.[44] Clonazepam is poorly soluble in water, is 85% protein bound, has a large volume of distribution, and is cleared almost exclusively by the liver. It is unlikely that renal insufficiency alters clonazepam clearance or that hemodialysis has much effect on clonazepam plasma concentration.

Ethosuximide (Zarontin)

There are no studies on the effect of renal insufficiency on ethosuximide pharmacokinetics.[45] Approximately 80% of ethosuximide is cleared via the liver and 20% via the kidney.[45] Therefore, it is unlikely that renal insufficiency greatly alters ethosuximide clearance.

Ethosuximide is water soluble, is not bound to plasma proteins, and has a small volume of distribution. As expected, large amounts of ethosuximide are removed during hemodialysis and peritoneal dialysis.[45,46] One study reported that approximately 50% of the ethosuximide stored in the body can be removed during a 6-hour dialysis session.[46]

Felbamate (Felbatol)

Approximately 50% of felbamate is cleared via the renal route.[47] Reduced felbamate clearance and lengthened felbamate elimination half-life are associated with diminishing renal function.[47] Felbamate is poorly soluble in water, has low plasma protein binding, and has a low volume of distribution. This combination of characteristics does not clearly predict the effect of hemodialysis on felbamate plasma concentration. There are no reports of the effect of hemodialysis on felbamate plasma concentration.[48] Caution should be used when performing hemodialysis on a patient taking felbamate.

Fosphenytoin (Cerebyx)

Fosphenytoin is the water-soluble disodium phosphate ester of phenytoin. Despite its water solubility, less than 5% of fosphenytoin is excreted via direct renal clearance in healthy subjects.[40] This presumably is due to rapid conversion of fosphenytoin to phenytoin (see section Phenytoin). The rate of conversion of fosphenytoin to phenytoin may be greater in persons with renal insufficiency than in healthy subjects, owing to decreased protein binding of fosphenytoin in renal insufficiency.[49]

The extent of removal of fosphenytoin by hemodialysis is unknown.[50] The water solubility of fosphenytoin would suggest that it is subject to removal during hemodialysis. The rapid conversion of fosphenytoin to phenytoin (not removed by hemodialysis; see section Phenytoin) would suggest that little fosphenytoin would be removed during hemodialysis. It may be prudent to use injectable sodium phenytoin, rather than fosphenytoin, for administration of phenytoin during dialysis.

Gabapentin (Neurontin)

Gabapentin is cleared almost entirely by glomerular filtration. Gabapentin clearance decreases in proportion to a decrease in creatinine clearance in patients with renal insufficiency.[51] Table 3-2 lists the decreases in gabapentin dosing rate as a function of decreased creatinine clearance.

Gabapentin is water soluble, has low protein binding, and has a low volume of distribution.

Table 3-2. Gabapentin Dosing in Renal Impairment

Creatinine Clearance (ml/min)	Total Daily Dose (mg/day)	Dose Regimen (mg)
>60	1,200	400 t.i.d.
30–60	600	300 b.i.d.
15–30	300	300 q.d.
<15	150	300 q.o.d.

Large amounts of gabapentin are lost during hemodialysis.[52] The sponsor recommends a loading dose of 200–300 mg of gabapentin after every 4 hours of hemodialysis.[51,53]

Lamotrigine (Lamictal)

Only approximately 10% of lamotrigine is cleared by the kidney. Nevertheless, the elimination half-life of lamotrigine is increased by approximately 50% in patients with renal insufficiency.[54] The dose of lamotrigine may need to be reduced in patients with renal insufficiency.[54,55]

Lamotrigine is poorly soluble in water, is approximately 50% bound to plasma proteins, and has a modest volume of distribution. In a study of six subjects on hemodialysis, an average of 20% (range, 5.6–35.1%) of lamotrigine present in the body was eliminated during a 4-hour hemodialysis session.[54]

Levetiracetam (Keppra)

Approximately two-thirds of administered levetiracetam is cleared by the kidney via glomerular filtration.[55] Clearance of levetiracetam decreases in proportion to a decrease in creatinine clearance in patients with renal insufficiency.[56] Table 3-3 lists the dosing of levetiracetam as a function of creatinine clearance.

Levetiracetam is water soluble, has low protein binding, and has a low volume of distribution.[55] Approximately 50% of the body pool of levetiracetam is removed during a 4-hour hemodialysis session.[56] The sponsor recommends a supplemental dose of 250–500 mg of levetiracetam after dialysis.[57]

Table 3-3. Levetiracetam Dosing in Renal Impairment

Creatinine Clearance (ml/min)	Dosage (mg)	Frequency
>80	500–1,500	Every 12 hrs
50–80	500–1,000	Every 12 hrs
30–50	250–750	Every 12 hrs
<30	250–500	Every 12 hrs

Oxcarbazepine (Trileptal)

After oral administration, oxcarbazepine is rapidly converted to its active monohydroxy metabolite (MHD). Most of the antiepileptic activity of oxcarbazepine is provided by MHD. Approximately 25% of MHD is cleared via the kidney.[58] There is a linear correlation between decreased creatine clearance and decreased MHD clearance.[58] The sponsor recommends that, in persons with creatine clearance, values less than 30 ml per minute oxcarbazepine be initiated at one-half the usual starting dose (300 mg/day). The dose then should be increased to achieve the desired clinical response.[58]

There are no clinical studies of the effects of hemodialysis on MHD plasma concentration.[50] Oxcarbazepine is poorly soluble in water and has 40% protein binding and a low volume of distribution. Given this profile, it is difficult to predict the extent of drug removal by hemodialysis. Plasma concentration determinations of MHD usually are not readily available for dosage adjustments after dialysis. Patients on oxcarbazepine and hemodialysis should be followed closely.

Phenobarbital

Approximately 25% of an administered dose of phenobarbital is cleared by the kidney as an unchanged drug. It is often necessary to lower phenobarbital dosage in patients with renal insufficiency, but there are no clear guidelines for this dosage adjustment.[59] Patients with renal insufficiency taking phenobarbital should have their dosage adjusted as dictated by phenobarbital plasma concentration determinations.

Phenobarbital is sparingly soluble in water, is approximately 50% protein bound, and has a modest volume of distribution. Significant amounts of the drug are lost during dialysis. Supplemental phenobarbital, after dialysis, is often required for both hemodialysis and peritoneal dialysis.[59,60] However, there are no clear guidelines as to how much supplemental drug is required. The postdialysis, phenobarbital loading dose requirement should be determined by obtaining a postdialysis, phenobarbital plasma concentration determination and using equation 16 with an assumed volume of distribution of 0.7 liter/kg.

Phenytoin (Dilantin)

Less than 5% of phenytoin is cleared by renal clearance.[40] Nevertheless, renal impairment has significant effects on phenytoin pharmacokinetics.

Because of decreased protein binding in renal failure, the following occur: (1) decreased total phenytoin–plasma concentration, (2) no change in the free phenytoin concentration because hepatic metabolism is unchanged (see section Effects of Renal Impairment of Drug Protein Binding), and (3) an increase in the free fraction of phenytoin.[61] These changes can lead to overdosing of phenytoin if the dosing rate is based on total phenytoin–plasma concentration. Monitoring of free phenytoin–plasma concentration is preferred to the monitoring of total phenytoin–plasma concentration in patients with renal insufficiency. Monitoring of total phenytoin–plasma concentration may lead to overdosage and toxicity.

Phenytoin is poorly soluble in water, is 90% protein bound, and has a modest volume of distribution. As predicted, little phenytoin is lost in hemodialysis (2–4%),[62] peritoneal dialysis,[63] or continuous, ambulatory peritoneal dialysis.[64] In a patient undergoing plasmapheresis, 10% of total phenytoin was removed with each treatment.[65]

Primidone (Mysoline)

Little has been published on the effects of renal impairment on primidone pharmacokinetics. In adults on primidone monotherapy, approximately

60% of primidone is cleared via the kidney.[66] In adults on polytherapy and in children, approximately 40% of primidone is cleared via the kidney.[66] Also, 5–10% of an administered dose of primidone is excreted as phenobarbital via the kidney.[66] These observations suggest the dose of primidone probably should be reduced in patients with renal impairment. The amount of this reduction should be based on a determination of the plasma concentrations of primidone and phenobarbital.

Primidone is poorly soluble in water, is 0–20% protein bound, and has a modest volume of distribution.[66] Significant amounts of primidone and its metabolites (phenobarbital and phenylethylmalonamide) are lost during dialysis.[67,68] Plasma concentrations of primidone and phenobarbital should be checked after hemodialysis and an additional loading given, if needed, following the procedure given in the section Hemodialysis.

Tiagabine (Gabitril)

Tiagabine is cleared almost entirely by the liver. The pharmacokinetics of total and unbound tiagabine are similar in subjects with normal renal function and in subjects with mild, moderate, and severe renal impairment.[69] The pharmacokinetics of total and unbound tiagabine were not altered by hemodialysis in a study of subjects with chronic renal failure.[69]

Topiramate (Topamax)

Approximately 85% of an administered dose of topiramate is excreted as the unchanged drug in the urine in monotherapy. In combination therapy, the proportion of topiramate cleared by the kidney decreases owing to hepatic enzyme induction. The clearance of topiramate is decreased by 42% in patients with moderate renal impairment (creatinine clearance, 30–69 ml/minute/1.73 m^2) and by 54% in severely impaired subjects (creatinine clearance less than 30 ml/minute/1.73 m^2).[70] The sponsor recommends reducing the dosing rate of topiramate in patients with moderate or severe renal impairment.

Topiramate is water soluble and weakly protein bound. Significant amounts of topiramate are cleared during hemodialysis.[70] The plasma concen-

tration of topiramate may fall below the minimum concentration to maintain antiepileptic effect.[70] Thus, a supplemental dose of topiramate may be required *before* dialysis. There are no guidelines for determining the size of the supplemental dose. The volume of distribution for topiramate has not been determined. Thus, equation 16 cannot be used to compute a loading dose. The elimination half-life of topiramate is 21 hours in healthy subjects, and the clearance of topiramate is decreased by 50% in severe renal impairment.[70] These data suggest the elimination half-life of topiramate is 36 hours in patients with severe renal insufficiency. Thus, a supplemental dose equal to the dose administered over 36 hours would supply one-half of the drug needed to produce a peak plasma concentration.

Valproate (Depakene, Depakote)

Valproate is eliminated almost entirely by hepatic metabolism (>96%), and renal disease has little effect on valproate metabolism.[71] However, valproate is 85–95% protein bound, and renal disease significantly affects valproate protein binding.[71,72] In renal disease, the total valproate–plasma concentration falls, but the free valproate level remains unchanged. This change is principally owing to decreased protein binding. See the section Effect of Renal Impairment on Drug Protein Binding for a detailed discussion of this phenomenon. Allosteric changes in protein binding[73] and endogenous toxic products, displacing valproate from protein binding sites,[74] may also contribute to decreased protein binding.

Valproate is poorly soluble in water, is highly protein bond, and has a small volume of distribution. Less than 20% of valproate is removed by hemodialysis[75] or peritoneal dialysis.[76]

Zonisamide (Zonegran)

Significant amounts of zonisamide are cleared by both the renal and hepatic routes.[77] The clearance of zonisamide has been shown to decrease with decreasing creatinine clearance.[78] In patients with severe renal impairment (creatinine clearance less than 20 ml/minute), mean plasma concentration of zonisamide increased by 35%.[78] The sponsor provides no specific guidelines for reduction of zonisamide dosing rate in renal insufficiency and recommends frequent monitoring of such patients.

Zonisamide is moderately soluble in water, is 40% protein bound, and has a moderate volume of distribution. There are no clinical studies of the effects of hemodialysis on zonisamide plasma concentration.[50] The pharmacokinetics of zonisamide suggest that there is some loss of the drug with hemodialysis.

References

1. Brenner BM (ed). The Kidney (6th ed). Philadelphia: Saunders, 2000.
2. Denker BM, Chertow GM, Owen WF. Hemodialysis. In BM Brenner (ed), The Kidney (6th ed). Philadelphia: Saunders, 2000;2373–2453.
3. Gobbi G, Bertani G, Pini A. Electrolyte, Sporadic, Metabolic, and Endocrine Disorders. In J Engel, TA Pedley (eds), Epilepsy: a Comprehensive Textbook. Philadelphia: Lippincott–Raven, 1998;2605–2627.
4. Bergstrom J. Uremia is an intoxication. Kidney Int 1985;28[Suppl 17]:52–54.
5. DeDeyn PP, Saxena VK, Abts H, et al. Clinical and pathophysiological aspects of neurological complications of renal failure. Acta Neurolog Belg 1992;92:191–206.
6. Raskin NA, Fishman RA. Neurologic disorders in renal failure (part I). N Engl J Med 1976;294:143–148.
7. Aicardi J. Diseases of the Nervous System in Children (Clinics in developmental medicine; No 115/118). London: MacKeith Press, 1992;1241–1278.
8. Arieff AI. Dialysis disequilibrium syndrome: current concepts on pathogenesis and prevention. Kidney Int 1994;45:629–635.
9. Galous JP, Trouard T, Gmitro AS, et al. Hemodialysis increases apparent diffusion coefficient of brain water in nephrectomized rats measured by isotopic diffusion-weighted magnetic imaging. J Clin Invest 1996;98:750–755.
10. Arieff AI, Guisado R, Massry SG, Lazarowitz VC. Central nervous system pH in uremia and effects of hemodialysis. J Clin Invest 1976;58:306–311.
11. Silver SM, Sterns RH, Halperin ML. Brain swelling after dialysis: old urea or new osmoles? Am J Kidney Dis 1996;28:1–13.
12. Kennedy AC. Dialysis disequilibrium syndrome. Electroencephalogr Clin Neurophysiol 1970;29:213–220.
13. Saunders MG, Westmoreland BF. The EEG in Evaluation of Disorders Affecting the Brain Diffusely. In DW Klass, DD Daly (eds), Current Practice of Clinical Electroencephalography. New York: Raven Press, 1979;343–379.
14. Boyer J, Gill GN, Epstein FH. Hypoglycemia and hyperosmolality complicating dialysis. Ann Intern Med 1967;67:568–572.
15. Waking KG. The pathophysiology of dialysis disequilibrium syndrome. Mayo Clinic Proc 1969;44:406–429.
16. Pillion G, Loirat C, Blum C, et al. Aluminum encephalopathy: a potential risk of aluminum gels in children with chronic renal failure. Int J Pediatr Nephrol 1981;2:29–32.
17. Reusche E, Koch V, Friedrich HJ, et al. Correlation of drug-related aluminum intake and dialysis treatment with deposition of argyrophilie aluminum containing inclusions in CNS and other systems of patients with dialysis associated encephalopathy. Clin Neuropathol 1996;15:342–347.
18. Russo LS, Beale G, Sandroni S, Ballinger WE. Aluminum intoxication in undialysed adults with chronic renal failure. J Neurol Neurosurg Psychiatry 1992;55:697–700.
19. Alfrey AC, LeGendre GR, Kachney MD. The dialysis encephalopathy syndrome: possible aluminum intoxication. N Engl J Med 1976:294:184–188.
20. Hoang-Xuan K, Perrotte P, Dubas F, et al. Myoclonic encephalopathy after aluminum exposure. Lancet 1996;347:910–911.
21. Nakamura H, Rose PG, Blumer JL, et al. Acute encephalopathy due to aluminum toxicity successfully treated by intravenous deferoxamine and hemodialysis. J Clin Pharmacol 2000;40:296–300.
22. Huang Y. Herman MM, Liu J, et al. Neurofibrillary lesions in experimental aluminum-induced encephalopathy and Alzheimer's disease share immunoreactivity for amyloid precursor proteins beta, alpha l-antichymotrypsin and ubiquitin-protein conjugates. Brain Res 1997;771:213–220.
23. Anghes JR, Schreader MT. EEG in dialysis encephalopathy. Neurology 1980;30:148–154.
24. Lederman RJ, Henry CE. Progressive dialysis dementia. Ann Neurol 1978;4:199–204.
25. Nadel AM, Wilson WP. Dialysis encephalopathy possible seizure disorder. Neurology 1976;26:1130–1134.
26. Rivera-Vasquez AB, Nuriega-Sanchez A, Ramirez-Gonzales R, et al. Acute hypercalcemia in hemodialysis patients: distinction from dialysis dementia. Nephron 1980;25:243–246.
27. Pierides AM, Ward MK, Kerr DN. Hemodialysis encephalopathy: possible role of phosphate depletion. Lancet 1976;1:1234–1235.
28. Joshioka T, Itaki K, Kasai N. Uncontrollable convulsions responsive to pyridoxal phosphate in a uremic child. Int J Pediatr Nephrol 1984;5:221–222.
29. Matzke GR, Millikin SP. Influence of Renal Function and Dialysis on Drug Disposition. In WE Evans, JJ Schentag, WJ Jusko (eds), Applied Pharmacokinetics:

principles of therapeutic drug monitoring (3rd ed). Vancouver, WA: Applied Therapeutics, 1992;1–49.

30. Levy RH, Thummel KE, Unadkat JD. Drug Absorption, Distribution, and Elimination. In RH Levy, RH Mattson, BS Meldrum (eds), Antiepileptic Drugs (4th ed). New York: Raven Press, 1995;13–30.

31. Perucca ER, Richens A. Biotransformation. In RH Levy, RH Mattson, BS Meldrum (eds), Antiepileptic Drugs (4th ed). New York: Raven Press, 1995;31–50.

32. Ramsay RE, DeToledo J. Acetazolamide. In J Engel, TA Pedley (eds), Epilepsy: a Comprehensive Textbook. Philadelphia: Lippincott–Raven, 1998;1455–1462.

33. Richens A. Clinical Pharmacokinetics of Gabapentin. In D Chadwick (ed), New Trends in Epilepsy Management: the Role of Gabapentin. London: Royal Society of Medicine Services, 1993;41–46.

34. Dodson WE, Rust RS. Phenobarbital: Absorption, Distribution, and Excretion. In RH Levy, RH Mattson, BS Meldrum (eds), Antiepileptic Drugs (4th ed). New York: Raven Press, 1995;379–397.

35. Reidenberg M, Drayer DE. Alteration of drug-protein binding in renal disease. Clin Pharmacokinet 1984;9:18–26.

36. Matzke GR, Flaherty FJ. Drug Dosing in Renal Failure. In LY Young, MA Koda-Kimble (eds), Applied therapeutics : the clinical use of drugs (4th ed). Vancouver, WA: Applied Therapeutics, 1988;571–586.

37. Blum MR, Rigelman S, Becker CE. Altered protein binding of diphenylhydantoin in uremic plasma. N Engl J Med 1972;286:109–112.

38. Mattson RH, Cramer JA, Williamson PD, et al. Valproic acid in epilepsy: clinical and pharmacologic effects. Ann Neurol 1978;3:20–25.

39. Vollmer KO, Von Hodenberg A, Kolle EV. Pharmacokinetics and metabolism of gabapentin in rat, dog, and man. Arzneimittelforschung 1986;36:830–839.

40. Browne TR, Szabo GK, McEntaget E, et al. Bioavailability studies of drugs with non-linear pharmacokinetics: II. Absolute bioavailability of intravenous phenytoin prodrug at therapeutic phenytoin serum concentration determined by double stable isotope technique. J Clin Pharmacol 1993;33:89–94.

41. Rowland M, Tozer TN. Clinical Pharmacokinetics: Concepts and Applications (2nd ed). Philadelphia: Lea & Febiger, 1989;238–254.

42. Morselli PL. Carbamazepine: Absorption, Distribution, and Excretion. In RH Levy, RH Mattson, BS Meldrum (eds), Antiepileptic Drugs (4th ed). New York: Raven Press, 1995;515–528.

43. Kandrotas RF, Oles KS, Gal P, Love JM. Carbamazepine clearance in hemodialysis and hemoperfusion. DICP 1989;23:137–140.

44. Clonazepam package insert. Basel, Switzerland: Roche Laboratories, Inc., 2000.

45. Bialer M, Xiaodoug S, Pesucca E. Ethosuximide Absorption, Distribution, and Excretion. In RH Levy,

RH Mattson, BS Meldrum (eds), Antiepileptic Drugs (4th ed). New York: Raven Press, 1995;659–666.

46. Marbury TC, Lee CC, Perchalski RJ. Hemodialysis clearance of ethosuximide in patients with chronic renal failure. Am J Hosp Pharm 1981;30:1757–1760.

47. Perhatch JL, Shumaker RC. Felbamate: Absorption, Distribution, and Excretion. In RH Levy, RH Mattson, BS Meldrum (eds), Antiepileptic Drugs (4th ed). New York: Raven Press, 1995;807–813.

48. Felbamate [package insert]. Cranbury, NJ: Wallace Laboratories, 2000.

49. Aweeka FT, Gottwald MD, Gambertoglio JG, et al. Pharmacokinetics of fosphenytoin in patients with hepatic or renal disease. Epilepsia 1999;40:777–782.

50. Pub Med Search. July 22, 2000.

51. Blum RA, Comstock TJ, Sica DA, et al. Pharmacokinetics of gabapentin in subjects with various degrees of renal function. Clin Pharmacol Ther 1994;56:154–159.

52. Wong MO, Elson MA, Keane WF, et al. Disposition of gabapentin in anuric subjects on hemodialysis. J Clin Pharmacol 1995;35:622–626.

53. Gabapentin [package insert]. New York: Pfizer, Inc., 2000.

54. Fillastre JP, Tabaret AM, Fialaire A, et al. Pharmacokinetics of lamotrigine in patients with renal impairment: in hemodialysis. Drugs Exp Clin Res 1993;19:25–32.

55. Lamotrigine [package insert]. Research Triangle Park, NC: Glaxo Wellcome, Inc., 2000.

56. Patsalos PN. Pharmacokinetic profile of levetiracetam: toward ideal characteristics. Pharmacol Ther 2000;85:87–88.

57. Levetiracetam [package insert]. Smyrna, GA: UCB Pharma Inc., 2000.

58. Oxcarbazepine package insert. East Hanover, NJ: Novartis Pharmaceuticals Co., 2000.

59. Rainter MJ, Gaus LM. Phenobarbital: Clinical Use. In RH Levy, RH Mattson, BS Meldrum (eds), Antiepileptic Drugs (4th ed). New York: Raven Press, 1995;401–408.

60. Porto I, John EG, Heilliczer J. Removal of phenobarbital during continuous cycling peritoneal dialysis in a child. Pharmacotherapy 1997;17:432–435.

61. Browne TR. Phenytoin and Other Hydantoins. In J Engel, TA Pedley (eds), Epilepsy: a Comprehensive Textbook. Philadelphia: Lippincott–Raven, 1998;1557–1580.

62. Martin E, Gambertoglio JG, Adler DS, et al. Removal of phenytoin by hemodialysis in uremic patients. JAMA 1977;238:1750–1753.

63. Czajlia PA, Anderson WA, Christoph RA, et al. A pharmacokinetic evaluation of peritoneal dialysis for phenytoin. J Clin Pharmacol 1980;20:565–569.

64. Hays DP, Primack WA, Abrams IF. Phenytoin clearance by continuous ambulatory peritoneal dialysis. Drug Intell Clin Pharm 1985;19:429–431.

65. Liu E, Rubenstein M. Phenytoin removal by plasmapheresis in thrombotic thrombocytopenic purpura. Clin Pharmacol Ther 1982;31:782–785.

66. Cloyd JC, Leppik IE. Primidone: Absorption, Distribution, and Excretion. In RH Levy, RH Mattson, BS Meldrum (eds), Antiepileptic Drugs (4th ed). New York: Raven Press, 1995;459–466.

67. Lee CS, Marbury TC, Perchalski RT, et al. Pharmacokinetics of primidone elimination by anuric patients. J Clin Pharmacol 1982;22:301–308.

68. Streete JM, Berry DJ, Jones JA, et al. Clearance of phenylethylmalonamide during hemodialysis of a patient with renal failure. Ther Drug Monit 1980;12:281–283.

69. Cato A, Gustauson LE, Oian J, et al. Effect of renal impairment on the pharmacokinetics and tolerability of tiagabine. Epilepsia 1998;39:43–47.

70. Topiramate [package insert]. Raritan, NJ: Ortho-McNeil Pharmaceutical, Inc., 2000.

71. Levy RH, Shen DD. Valproic Acid: Absorption, Distribution, and Excretion. In RH Levy, RH Mattson, BS Meldrum (eds), Antiepileptic Drugs (4th ed). New York: Raven Press, 1995;605–620.

72. Bruni J, Wang LH, Marbury TC, et al. Protein binding of valproic acid in uremia patients. Neurology 1980;30:557–559.

73. Scheyer RD, Mattson RH. Valproic Acid: Interactions with Other Drugs. In RH Levy, RH Mattson, BS Meldrum (eds), Antiepileptic Drugs (4th ed). New York: Raven Press, 1995;621–632.

74. Perracca E, Gatti G, Frigo GM, et al. Sodium valproate in epileptic patients. Br J Pharmacol 1978;5:495–499.

75. Marbury TC, Lee CS, Brunni J, Wilder BJ. Hemodialysis of valproic acid in uremic patients. Dral Transpl 1980;9:961–964.

76. Orr JM, Farrell K, Abbott FJ, et al. The effects of peritoneal dialysis on the single dose and steady state pharmacokinetics of valproic acid in a uremic epileptic child. Eur J Clin Pharmacol 1983;24:387–390.

77. Leppik IE. Zonisamide. Epilepsia 1999;40[Suppl 5]:S23–S29.

78. Zonisamide [package insert]. Dublin, Ireland: Elan Pharma, 2000.

Chapter 4

Gastrointestinal and Hepatic Disease

William R. Garnett

Patients with epilepsy often have other diseases. Because such patients are typically excluded from premarketing, antiepileptic drug (AED) trials, these studies lend little insight into the effects of concurrent disease on AED pharmacokinetics and pharmacodynamics. When such testing is performed in the face of comorbid conditions, such as liver impairment, studies are usually conducted in only mild to moderate disease, and the drug is given only as a single dose or in multiple doses for a short time period, thereby limiting understanding of pharmacokinetics. Nevertheless, clinical experience and select studies clearly indicate that gastrointestinal (GI) or liver disease produces unique considerations in the administration of AEDs. This chapter summarizes our understanding of the potential for GI and hepatic diseases to alter the pharmacokinetics and pharmacodynamics of AEDs.

Liver Disease

The liver is the major body site for xenobiotic (i.e., a chemical not normally present in biological systems, such as environmental pollutants and drugs) metabolism, and it determines the disposition of many drugs. The liver has a dual blood supply, receiving blood from the hepatic artery and the portal veins. After transcoursing through the liver, blood returns to the systemic circulation via the hepatic vein and into the vena cava. The *extraction ratio* is a measure of the efficiency of the liver in removing a drug from hepatic inflow. High-extraction drugs are absorbed from the gut and delivered to the liver, where they may be metabolized before reaching the systemic circulation. This is known as *first-pass metabolism*. Drugs with a high extraction ratio and significant first-pass metabolism have a low oral bioavailability—that is, much of the administered drug does not reach the systemic circulation. An extraction ratio of one would indicate that all of the drug is metabolized before it can reach the systemic circulation. The portion of drug reaching the systemic circulation does return to the liver for metabolism. The metabolism of high-extraction drugs is affected by liver blood flow and by the functional ability of liver enzymes. A decrease in liver blood flow decreases the first-pass metabolism and increases bioavailability, making more drug available to the systemic circulation. Low-extraction drugs reach the systemic circulation and are brought back to the liver for metabolism. An extraction ratio of zero would indicate that none of the drug is metabolized by the liver. The metabolism of low-extraction drugs is minimally affected by liver blood flow but is extensively affected by the functional capacity of hepatocytes. It is important to remember that the hepatic extraction ratio is a measure of the efficiency of the extraction, rather than the extent of the extraction. Hepatic metabolic enzymes are diverse and are classified as phase I (nonsynthetic or functionalization metabolism, which includes oxidation, reduction, and hydrolysis reactions) and phase II (synthetic or conjugation metabolism, which involves glucuronidation, methylation, and acetylation reactions). There are multiple forms of cytochrome P-450 involved in phase I metabolism, and there may be genetic polymorphic distribution of these enzymes. Therefore, some individuals may be inherently fast or slow metabolizers. It has become critical to know which of the isoenzymes of cytochrome is involved in a specific drug's metabolism and whether there is genetic polymorphism for metabolism. Drug-metabolizing enzymes may also be induced or inhibited. When enzymes are induced, drugs are metabolized more quickly, which increases the clearance, shortens the half-life, and decreases the bioavailability. Conversely, when drug-metabolizing enzymes are inhibited, drugs are metabolized more slowly, which decreases the clearance, increases the half-life, and increases the bioavailability. The capacity for the liver to metabolize drugs depends on hepatic blood flow and liver enzyme activity.[1]

The liver produces albumin and alpha glycoprotein, to which some drugs are extensively bound. An alteration in the ability of the liver to synthesize proteins decreases the amount of bound drug and increases the drug's free fraction that binds at receptor sites, exerting its pharmacologic activity. Liver disease may also alter the binding characteristics of plasma proteins in a manner similar to that encountered with renal disease, and therefore, even if plasma proteins are normal, there may also be a decrease in plasma protein binding. By altering the binding characteristics, the percent bound will be changed. An increase in free fraction also makes more of the drug available for metabolism, which increases clearance if the hepatocytes are functioning. If the hepatocytes are not functioning, there is an increase in the free drug concentration.[1,2]

Several patient factors alter the liver's ability to metabolize drugs. For example, the presystemic clearance of high-extraction drugs, (e.g., propranolol) is significantly reduced, and bioavailability significantly increased when administered within 3 hours after eating. Other influencing factors include age, gender, race, pregnancy, hormones, circadian variability, and concurrently administered medications. Drugs have the ability to induce and inhibit the enzymes responsible for drug metabolism. Drug interactions may occur when new drugs are added or if a concurrent drug is discontinued. Concurrent drug administration may also change protein binding.[1,2]

Liver disease causes multiple pathophysiologic changes that influence drug disposition. Decreased hepatic blood flow, extrahepatic and intrahepatic blood shunting, and loss of hepatocytes alter the ability to metabolize drugs. This increases the bioavailability of administered medications, effectively increasing the dose. Decreased protein synthesis decreases the percentage of drug bound to plasma proteins and increases the amount of "free" or unbound drug. The increase in free fraction makes more of the drug available to the receptor site and more of the drug available for metabolism, thereby increasing its clearance. Increased clearance does not occur if hepatocytes are not capable of drug metabolism. An increase in free fraction and a decrease in hepatocyte function result in an increase in free drug concentration. Liver diseases that alter drug disposition include chronic liver disease (e.g., cirrhosis), acute hepatitis, drug-induced hepatotoxicity, cholestasis, and hepatic infiltrative or neoplastic disease.[1–3]

In renal disease, the creatinine clearance expresses the degree of remaining function. There is no comparable measure of residual liver function. Endogenous biochemical markers, such as aspartate aminotransferase, alanine aminotransferase, bilirubin, and international normalized ratio, are qualitative but not quantitative for liver function. Clearance tests of exogenous markers such as aminopyrine, indocyanine green, and lorazepam have not proved to be clinically useful. The Child-Pugh classification of liver disease can be used clinically to indicate mild (type A), moderate (type B), or severe (type C) disease, but this does not predict drug metabolism.[1,2]

With the exception of gabapentin and levetiracetam, all AEDs have some liver metabolism. Also, phenytoin and valproic acid are highly (>90%) bound to albumin, and carbamazepine is extensively bound to albumin and alpha glycoprotein. Liver disease patients with concurrent renal disease may experience further changes in the protein binding of drugs, because patients with renal failure retain a high-molecular-weight protein that displaces drugs (e.g., phenytoin) and also may have a low albumin. Therefore, there is a significant potential for liver disease to alter the pharmacokinetics of AEDs. Liver disease may alter the pharmacodynamics of AEDs. For example, some patients with chronic liver disease (e.g., alcoholic cirrhosis) may have chronic mild to moderate encephalopathy. This could make these patients more sensitive to the central nervous system (CNS) side effects of AEDs.[1-3]

Gastrointestinal Disease

Orally administered medications must dissolve and go into solution in the GI tract before absorption across the gut wall into circulating blood. These processes are dependent on lipid solubility, concentration of nonionized molecules, gastric blood flow, gastric emptying time, gut pH, administration of meals, meal content, bowel length, and other factors.[4] GI diseases that alter these factors may therefore affect drug absorption and disposition. However, it is difficult to perform prospective trials in patients with acute GI disease. For example, it would be hard to study the pharmacokinetics and pharmacodynamics of a drug in a patient with diarrhea secondary to influenza. Patients with chronic GI diseases may have confounding factors that make pharmacokinetic and pharmacodynamic evaluation difficult. In addition to the GI tract's role in absorption, the GI tract also contributes to drug metabolism. For example, alcohol dehydrogenase and CYP3A4 are two enzymes that contribute to xenobiotic metabolism and are found in the gut.

Specific Antiepileptic Drugs

Phenobarbital

Pharmacokinetics

Phenobarbital is well absorbed from a variety of oral formulations, with peak concentrations reached in 2–12 hours. The bulk of phenobarbital is absorbed from the small intestine, where the unionized fraction is smaller but intraluminal dwell time is longer. Phenobarbital disseminates into all body tissues but is only 40–50% plasma protein bound. Phenobarbital is eliminated by a first-order process and has a low extraction ratio. In the liver, phenobarbital is parahydroxylated and, subsequently, conjugated to glucuronic acid. The extent of glucuronide formation of phenobarbital varies widely. Approximately 60–80% of the drug is metabolized by the liver, but alkalinization of the urine increases the amount of phenobarbital excreted unchanged by the kidney.[5,6]

Effect of Liver Disease

Although a significant amount of phenobarbital is excreted unchanged in the urine, the clearance of phenobarbital is altered in patients with liver disease. In cirrhotic patients, the half-life of phenobarbital is 130 ± 15 hours compared to 86 ± 3 hours in healthy controls. However, the half-life of only one dose of phenobarbital is not altered in patients with acute hepatitis. Patients with cirrhosis have a decreased ability to form the parahydroxy metabolite of phenobarbital.[7] It is unlikely that there are any clinically relevant changes in the protein binding of phenobarbital in patients with liver disease.

Effect of Gastrointestinal Disease

The presence of food and neutralizing agents or the occurrence of rapid gastric emptying slows phenobarbital absorption.[6] Therefore, GI disease may alter the absorption of phenobarbital.

Phenytoin

Pharmacokinetics

Very little of an orally administered dose of phenytoin is absorbed from the stomach, because phenytoin is poorly soluble at a low pH. Absorption increases when the drug passes into the duodenum and continues at a slower rate in the jejunum and ileum. Absorption from the colon is poor. The oral absorption of phenytoin is somewhat irregular and prolonged, and it is not first order. The extent of phenytoin's absorption is dependent on the rate at which it can enter the bloodstream. There is a maximal amount of GI fluid in which the drug can be dissolved. At higher doses, some of the drug is left undissolved, resulting in prolonged or decreased absorption. The lack of linearity has been shown in animals, where the percent absorbed is inversely related to the concentration or dose. Phenytoin is highly (>90%) protein bound and is extensively metabolized by the liver. Less than 5% of the drug is excreted unchanged in the liver. Phenytoin exhibits nonlinear (e.g., Michaelis-Menten) pharmacokinetics, indicating that the metabolism saturates at doses given clinically. Isoforms of the CYP2C subfamily are responsible for the metabolism of phenytoin. Fosphenytoin is a diphosphate ester of phenytoin that is very water soluble, making it a convenient intravenous dose form. The molecular weight of fosphenytoin is 1.5 times that of phenytoin. However, the commercial product is labeled in terms of phenytoin equivalents. Fosphenytoin should be dosed on the basis of phenytoin equivalents. It is rapidly converted systemically to phenytoin.[8-10]

Effect of Liver Disease

Changes in hepatic blood flow do not alter phenytoin clearance, because it is a low-extraction drug.[10] However, the loss of functional hepatocytes decreases phenytoin metabolism. Phenytoin accumulates as hepatic dysfunction increases.[11] As a result of decreased albumin production, hepatic disease is associated with decreased protein-binding capacity for phenytoin. Furthermore, bilirubin may compete for binding sites of the albumin molecule, further increasing the unbound concentration.[12-17] The effect of liver diseases on fosphenytoin was evaluated in four patients with liver dysfunction, four patients with renal dysfunction, and four control subjects. There was no difference in the time to peak fosphenytoin concentrations, but the time to achieve peak plasma concentrations of phenytoin was faster in the patient with liver and renal impairment because of decreased protein binding of fosphenytoin and phenytoin.[18]

Effect of Gastrointestinal Disease

The absorption of phenytoin is pH dependent and is maximal in the duodenum.[9] It is likely that diseases that alter gut pH and decrease duodenal dwell time alter the absorption of phenytoin. Nasogastric feedings, which increase GI transit, decrease the absorption of phenytoin. The mechanism of this interaction remains unclear but may result from the binding of phenytoin to proteins in the feeding or from decreased time in the duodenum, where absorption is optimal.

Ethosuximide

Pharmacokinetics

Absorption of ethosuximide is more complete and is faster from the syrup than the capsule-dose form. Ethosuximide is extensively distributed throughout the body but is not bound to plasma proteins. There is no first-pass metabolism, but the drug is extensively metabolized in the liver to inactive metabolites.[19] CYP3A4 is the main isoenzyme involved in the metabolism of ethosuximide, although CYP2E also has an important role, and CYP2B may be involved.[20,21]

Effect of Liver Disease

Because of extensive liver metabolism, significant impairment of liver function may decrease the clearance of ethosuximide.

Effect of Gastrointestinal Disease

The effects of GI disease on ethosuximide are unknown.

Carbamazepine

Pharmacokinetics

The absorption of carbamazepine from immediate release tablets is slow, erratic, and unpredictable. Absorption does not follow a simple first-order process. Absorption occurs faster from the syrup-dose form than from immediate-release tablets. A controlled-release dose form and a sustained-release dose form administered every 12 hours are bioequivalent to immediate-release tablets administered every 6 hours. Carbamazepine is 75–85% bound to plasma proteins, including albumin and alpha glycoprotein. The free fraction has been reported to be inversely related to the concentration of alpha glycoprotein concentration. Carbamazepine is extensively metabolized primarily by CYP3A4 to an active metabolite that is further metabolized. Carbamazepine induces its own metabolism.[22,23]

Effect of Liver Disease

Carbamazepine is a low-extraction drug but is extensively metabolized by the liver. Therefore, it is expected that the metabolism of carbamazepine is sensitive to decreased hepatic function but not to changes in hepatic blood flow. A reduction in protein binding can occur in patients with liver disease.[24]

Effect of Gastrointestinal Disease

The effect of GI disease has not been studied in patients receiving carbamazepine. However, because carbamazepine is poorly water soluble and the immediate-release tablet results in erratic and prolonged absorption, it is likely that GI disease alters carbamazepine absorption. The absorption of the new ostomotic-release oral system (controlled-release preparation) of carbamazepine can be affected by GI diseases that alter GI transit. In healthy volunteers, Wilding demonstrated significant variability in GI transit time of the ostomotic-release oral system formulation that resulted in variability in carbamazepine absorption.[25] Absorption variability from immediate-release tablets is also likely, because the absorption is slow, erratic, and prolonged. Absorption from the suspension and the sustained-dose forms is unknown.

Valproic Acid

Pharmacokinetics

Valproic acid has excellent bioavailability and is absorbed through the intestine with no site specificity. The rate of absorption depends on the dose form. Absorption is faster from the syrup and the gelatin capsule. The enteric-coated formulation was developed to minimize GI irritation. The coating does not dissolve in the acid medium of the stomach, resulting in delayed absorption with trough levels occurring 4–6

hours after dose administration. Recently, a controlled-release dose form was introduced for once-a-day dosing.

Valproic acid is highly (>90%) bound to albumin, but the bound percentage decreases as the concentration increases. Whereas the unbound concentration is between 7% and 9% at total concentrations below 75 μg/ml, the unbound concentration increases to 15% at total concentrations of approximately 100 μg/ml and 30% at total concentrations above 150 μg/ml. The changes in free fraction result in a change in clearance. Valproic acid is metabolized by a variety of conjugation and oxidative processes. There are multiple metabolites of valproic acid. These metabolites may contribute to both the efficacy and the toxicity of valproic acid. Evidence supporting the contribution of the metabolites of valproic acid to the desired pharmacologic effects includes the observations that the pharmacologic effects of valproic acid do not correlate well with the steady-state concentrations of the parent drug and that the time course of the pharmacologic effects differs from the pharmacokinetics of the drug—that is, the full effects of the drug are not seen until some time after steady state is achieved and persist for some time after the drug is discontinued. However, although some of the metabolites are active, some authors have argued that they are present only in low plasma and brain concentrations and that they may not contribute much to the efficacy of valproic acid. Also, the metabolites of valproic acid may contribute to the rare, but potentially fatal, hepatotoxicity.[26] Valproic acid is a low-extraction drug, and its clearance is independent of hepatic blood flow.[26,27]

Effect of Liver Disease

The protein binding of valproic acid is decreased in alcoholic cirrhosis and viral hepatitis. The elimination half-life is increased, although there is no change in total clearance, because clearance of the unbound drug is reduced. The result is an increase in unbound drug, with no change in the total drug concentration.[28] Liver disease alters the profile of valproic acid metabolites, but it is not possible to distinguish between benign and life-threatening hepatic adverse reactions based on the profile of the valproic acid metabolites.[29] Valproic acid may cause hepato-toxicity, especially in young children with polytherapy or inborn errors of metabolism. Two retrospective reviews demonstrated that the risks of fatal hepatotoxicity associated with valproic acid are highest in children younger than 2 years of age who are taking multiple medications. For example, the risk of fatal hepatotoxicity was 1 in 500 patients who were younger than 2 years of age and on polytherapy and 1 in 7,000 patients who were younger than 2 years of age on mono-therapy. In patients older than 2 years of age on polytherapy, the risk was 1 in 12,000, and in patients older than age 2 years on monotherapy, the risk was 1 in 45,000. In these reports, no patient over age 10 years developed fatal hepato-toxicity with valproic acid. However, case reports have associated valproic acid with fatal hepatotoxicity in adults. The hepatotoxicity may be the result of a metabolite that is normally not present or present in low concentrations. This is suggested by the fact that the children who received multiple AEDs had severe epilepsy associated with mental retardation, neurologic deficits, congenital anomalies, and other develop-mental delays. These factors, as well as the co-medication, may alter the metabolism of valproic acid.[26,29] Animal studies indicate the mechanism of valproic acid–induced hepatotoxicity is differ-ent from its mechanism for antiepileptic activity. The use of *L*-carnitine supplementation in the treat-ment and prophylaxis of valproic acid–induced liver disease remains controversial. However, a recent consensus panel recommended *L*-car-nitine supplementation in patients with certain secondary carnitine deficiency syndromes, symptomatic valproic acid–associated hyperam-monemia, multiple risk factors for valproic acid toxicity or renal associated syndrome, infants and young children taking valproic acid, patients with epilepsy using the ketogenic diet who have hypocarnitinemia, patients receiving dialy-sis, and premature infants who are receiv-ing total parenteral nutrition.

Effect of Gastrointestinal Disease

Changes in gastric pH could change the dissolu-tion of the enteric coating of valproic acid. Because the absorption of valproic acid is not site specific, it is difficult to predict the effect of GI disease.

Felbamate

Pharmacokinetics

Felbamate is well absorbed after oral adminis-tration, with bioavailability exceeding 90%. Felbamate is not extensively bound to plasma proteins, is approximately 40–50% eliminated via hepatic metabolism, and is approximately 50–60% excreted unchanged in the urine. Felbamate is a low-extraction drug and is metabolized mainly by hydroxylation and conjugation.[30,31]

Effect of Liver Disease

Because felbamate is not extensively protein bound, the free fraction is not significantly changed in liver disease. The effect of liver dis-ease on the metabolism of felbamate is unknown. The mixture of renal and hepatic elimination may minimize the effect of liver disease. Patients with impairment of both renal and liver function would be expected to have a reduced clearance of felbamate.

When felbamate was approved initially by the U.S. Food and Drug Administration, it was believed to be extremely well tolerated. How-ever, after 100,000 patient exposures, the use of felbamate was associated with the occurrence of aplastic anemia and hepatotoxicity. These side effects are potentially fatal. Hepatotoxicity occurs less often than aplastic anemia, and the incidence is believed to be comparable to that of valproic acid. The patients developing hepato-toxicity were predominantly female, were equally divided among adult and pediatric patients, and had a broad range of time to presentation after starting felbamate therapy. The role of concomi-tant therapy with other drugs that may cause liver disease is unclear. A reactive metabolite, atropaldehyde, may be responsible for the hepa-totoxicity. Human leukocyte antigen studies may identify high-risk patients. Although felbamate is still available, the approval of other AEDs has relegated felbamate to deep-reserve status. It is unlikely that it would be used without careful consideration for patients with liver disease. Felbamate may be considered for patients who have failed other therapies. It is also useful in treating the Lennox-Gastaut syndrome. If patients are started on felbamate, they should be closely monitored for any signs of bone marrow suppression, such as easy bruising, sore throat, or infections, and for the prodromal symptoms of liver disease, such as lethargy, dark urine, and jaundice.

Effect of Gastrointestinal Disease

The effect of GI disease on the pharmacokinetics of felbamate is unknown.

Gabapentin

Pharmacokinetics

Gabapentin is rapidly absorbed, reaching a peak in 2–4 hours. It binds to a leucine–amino acid protein in the gut and is actively absorbed. The bioavailability of gabapentin decreases with an increase in dose. It is not metabolized, is not bound to plasma proteins, and is excreted unchanged in the urine.[32]

Effect of Liver Disease

Liver disease should not affect gabapentin, because it is not hepatically metabolized and is not protein bound.

Effect of Gastrointestinal Disease

It is unknown whether GI disease affects the leucine-amino protein that is responsible for the active absorption of gabapentin.

Lamotrigine

Pharmacokinetics

Lamotrigine is rapidly absorbed, reaching peak concentrations in 1–3 hours. It is well absorbed and has an oral bioavailability of 98%. The pro-

tein binding of lamotrigine is only 55%. It is metabolized by glucuronide conjugation, and less than 1% is excreted renally.[33–35]

Effect of Liver Disease

There is one report describing the metabolism of lamotrigine in seven subjects with Gilbert's syndrome (a benign deficiency in the enzyme bilirubin uridine diphosphate glucuronyl transferase). Although clearance was reduced and half-life was prolonged, these effects were considered clinically insignificant.[36] Because lamotrigine is extensively metabolized, loss of hepatocyte function may decrease clearance. However, phase I metabolism is generally affected more by loss of hepatocyte function than is phase II. Protein binding of lamotrigine would not be expected to be significantly altered by liver disease.

Effect of Gastrointestinal Disease

The effect of GI disease on the pharmacokinetics of lamotrigine is unknown.

Topiramate

Pharmacokinetics

The absorption of topiramate is rapid and nearly complete. Topiramate is poorly bound (9–17%) to plasma proteins. There is both renal and hepatic elimination of topiramate. In the absence of enzyme induction, greater than 80% of a single radiolabeled dose of topiramate is excreted unchanged in the urine.[37]

Effect of Liver Disease

The effect of liver impairment on the metabolism of topiramate was evaluated in patients with moderate to severe hepatic impairment, as defined by Child-Pugh.[1] When compared to healthy subjects, the plasma clearance was reduced by 26% and the half-life prolonged by 36%, both clinically insignificant.[38] However, in selected patients, these changes may be clinically significant. Liver disease would not be expected to cause significant changes in the protein binding of topiramate.

Because the protein binding of topiramate is only 9–17% and the alteration in metabolism by liver disease is not clinically significant, there does not need to be any dosage adjustment of topiramate in patients with liver disease.

Tiagabine

Pharmacokinetics

There is rapid and nearly complete absorption of tiagabine, with peak concentrations achieved in 30–90 minutes. Tiagabine is 96% bound to albumin and alpha glycoprotein and is extensively metabolized by the hepatic CYP3A4 isoenzyme.[39]

Effect of Liver Disease

The pharmacokinetics of tiagabine were evaluated in four subjects with mild liver impairment and three subjects with moderate hepatic impairment who were compared to matched controls. The maximal drug concentration (C_{max}), minimal drug concentration (C_{min}), area under the curve, and elimination half-lives were all higher in the patients with liver impairment. The free fractions were also increased in the hepatically impaired subjects. It was recommended that the dose or the dosing interval, or both, of tiagabine be reduced in patients with liver impairment.[40]

Effect of Gastrointestinal Disease

The effect of GI disease on the pharmacokinetics of tiagabine is unknown.

Levetiracetam

Pharmacokinetics

Levetiracetam is absorbed rapidly and almost completely. Protein binding is less than 10% with leve-

tiracetam. Sixty-six percent of levetiracetam is excreted renally as the unchanged drug. The remaining drug undergoes metabolism by hydrolysis of the acetamide group and is not cytochrome P-450 dependent.[41]

Effect of Liver Disease

The clearance of levetiracetam is reported to be unaffected by liver disease.

Effect of Gastrointestinal Disease

The effect of GI disease on levetiracetam is unknown.

Oxcarbazepine

Pharmacokinetics

More than 96% of an orally administered dose of oxcarbazepine is absorbed. Oxcarbazepine is rapidly converted to a monohydrate derivative that is the active component by cytosol arylketone reductase. The monohydroxy metabolite (MHD) is further metabolized by glucuronide conjugation. There is no evidence of autoinduction. However, the metabolism of oxcarbazepine to an inactive metabolite may be induced. Approximately 60% of oxcarbazepine and 40% of MHD are bound to plasma proteins.[42,43]

Effect of Liver Disease

Oxcarbazepine is only approximately 60% protein bound and is rapidly converted to its active metabolite, MHD, by nonliver enzymes. Therefore, it is unlikely that liver disease alters the pharmacokinetics of the parent drug. The active metabolite does undergo metabolism to an inactive metabolite by glucuronide conjugation. Phase II metabolism is less likely to be affected by liver disease than phase I pathways (e.g., CYP). Therefore, it is unlikely that liver disease affects the pharmacokinetics of oxcarbazepine or its active metabolite, MHD. Therefore, dosage adjustments of oxcarbazepine for patients with liver impairment are unlikely.

Effect of Gastrointestinal Disease

The effect of GI disease on oxcarbazepine is unknown.

Zonisamide

Pharmacokinetics

Zonisamide is rapidly and completely absorbed, reaching peak concentrations in 2–6 hours. Zonisamide is approximately 70% metabolized by the liver, with reduction by CYP3A4 accounting for approximately 50% and *N*-acetylation accounting for 20% of the metabolism. There are no active metabolites. Other drugs that induce or inhibit CYP3A4 may increase or decrease the clearance of zonisamide, but zonisamide does not alter the concentrations of other AEDs or induce its own metabolism. Zonisamide has a long half-life, around 63 hours in an uninduced patient and around 27–38 hours in an induced patient. The half-life would be expected to be greater than 63 hours in a patient taking enzyme-inhibiting drugs. Approximately 30% of a dose of zonisamide is excreted unchanged in the urine. Zonisamide is only approximately 40% protein bound.[44–46]

Effect of Liver Disease

The pharmacokinetics of zonisamide have not been formally evaluated in patients with liver dysfunction. However, because the drug is approximately 70% metabolized by reduction and acetylation, it is anticipated that the metabolism of zonisamide would be reduced in patients with liver dysfunction. Drugs like zonisamide with long half-lives require longer intervals between dosage adjustments to achieve a steady state. Rapid titration of zonisamide has resulted

in an increase in CNS side effects. Because the half-life of zonisamide is likely to be prolonged in patients with liver dysfunction, there should be a longer interval between dosage adjustments. Patients should be carefully evaluated clinically.

Effect of Gastrointestinal Disease

The effect of GI disease on zonisamide is unknown.

Summary

AEDs are given to patients with concurrent medical conditions, although they are not routinely studied in patients with concurrent disease. Patients with GI or liver disease are predisposed to alteration in the pharmacokinetics of many AEDs. Although the effect of GI disease is poorly studied, it is known that diseases that alter GI transit have the potential to alter absorption. The effect of gut metabolism is unknown. The acute and intermittent nature of many GI disorders makes it difficult to anticipate or titrate AED dosage changes. Clinicians should obtain a careful history from the patient if there are changes in seizure activity or drug concentrations to determine whether these changes are temporarily related to a GI disease.

The liver is the primary site for the metabolism of many drugs. Factors that favor an altered elimination in liver disease are high extraction ratio, significant metabolism by the liver, and high protein binding. The currently available AEDs are low-extraction drugs and are less likely to be affected by alterations in liver blood flow. However, the metabolism of low-extraction drugs is altered by decreased hepatocyte function, and low-extraction drugs can have a decreased clearance, increased half-life, and increased bioavailability in patients with liver disease. With the exception of gabapentin, most AEDs have some liver metabolism, even if the liver is not the primary means of elimination, as in the case of topiramate and levetiracetam. Therefore, liver disease has the potential to alter the elimination of most AEDs. In addition, those AEDs that are highly protein bound (e.g., phenytoin, carbamazepine, valproic acid, and tiagabine) may have alterations in the percent of free or unbound fraction in patients with liver disease, because there is a decreased production of plasma proteins or an alteration in the binding sites. The increase in the free fraction increases clearance if the hepatocytes are functional, causing the total concentration to decrease. Therefore, it is better to monitor the unbound concentration of highly protein-bound AEDs in patients with liver disease. The pharmacodynamic effects of liver disease on AEDs are completely unknown. However, because some patients with chronic liver disease have mild encephalopathy, it is possible that they are more sensitive to the CNS side effects of AEDs. Because there is no endogenous or exogenous marker of liver function, it is not possible to quantify the amount of liver function that is remaining or lost in a patient with acute or chronic liver disease. Therefore, when giving AEDs to patients with liver disease, clinicians should anticipate initiating a maintenance therapy with lower doses and making dose adjustments at longer intervals. A lower dose or a decreased frequency of dosing should be anticipated.

The adverse reactions of AEDs may include hepatic and GI side effects. The AED effects on the liver range from elevation of liver enzymes to hepatic disease. Elevations of liver enzymes are much more common than liver disease. For example, up to 50% of patients taking AEDs have an elevation of gamma-glutamyl transferase.[47] In a study of 786 patients taking carbamazepine, 14% had an aspartate aminotransferase that was two to three times normal, and 9% had an increase in bilirubin, but all were asymptomatic for liver disease.[48] Valproic acid may be associated with a dose-dependent increase in serum glutamic-oxaloacetic transaminase,[49] and as many as 50% of patients taking valproic acid develop hyperammonemia.[50,51] The increase in ammonia associated with valproic acid is seen more often in patients taking other AEDs and is usually seen without associated liver enzyme abnormalities or liver disease. However, serious hepatotoxicity caused by aromatic AEDs, such as carbamazepine, phenytoin, and phenobarbital, is very rare, with an incidence of less than one case in 3,000 exposures. The hepatotoxicity associated with the aromatic AEDs usually begins within 2–8 weeks after the initiation of therapy and presents with a rash, fever, and internal organ involvement. The hepatotoxicity may be a part of an AED hypersensitivity syndrome.[52,53] The hepatotoxicity associated with valproic acid and felbamate appears to be different histopathologically from that associated with the aromatic AEDs. Therefore, mild to moderate elevations of liver enzymes are common with AEDs, but true hepatotoxicity is rare. Elevation of liver enzymes is a poor predictor of impending liver toxicity. Patients should be carefully monitored clinically. Other GI symptoms that may result from AED use include nausea, vomiting, and indigestion. These are usually seen in the early stages of dosage titration and may be ameliorated by slowing the titration. GI symptoms associated with valproic acid may be reduced by using the enteric-coated dose form. The use of valproic acid has been associated with pancreatitis.[54,55]

Both GI and liver diseases have the potential to alter the pharmacokinetics and pharmacodynamics of AEDs. Because it is not possible to quantify liver function, it is not possible to calculate a dosage adjustment for patients with liver impairment. Some GI diseases (e.g., constipation or diarrhea) may be episodic and transitory, making it difficult to prospectively evaluate or assess how to alter drug dosing. Also, AEDs are associated with side effects affecting the liver and GI tract. Therefore, clinicians should carefully monitor their patients who have GI or liver disease to ensure that the therapeutic outcomes are achieved—that the patient achieves optimal seizure control with minimal side effects.

References

1. Brouwer KL, Dukes GE, Powell JR. Influence of Liver Function on Drug Disposition. In WE Evans, JJ Schentag, WJ Jusko (eds), Applied Pharmacokinetics:

Principles of Therapeutic Drug Monitoring (3rd ed). Vancouver, WA: Applied Therapeutics Inc, 1992;1–59.

2. Rodighiero V. Effects of liver disease on pharmacokinetics. An update. Clin Pharmacokinet 1999;37:399–431.

3. Boggs J, Waterhouse E, DeLorenzo RJ. The Use of Antiepileptic Medications in Renal and Liver Disease. In E Wyllie (ed), The Treatment of Epilepsy: Principles and Practice (2nd ed). Baltimore: Williams & Wilkins, 1996;753–762.

4. Rowland M, Tozer TN. Absorption. In M Rowland, TN Tozer (eds), Clinical Pharmacokinetics: Concepts and Applications (2nd ed). Philadelphia: Lea & Febiger, 1989;113–130.

5. Anderson GD, Levy RH. Phenobarbital: Chemistry and Biotransformation. In RH Levy, RH Mattson, BS Meldrum (eds), Antiepileptic Drugs (4th ed). New York: Raven Press, 1995;371–377.

6. Dodson WE, Rust RS Jr. Phenobarbital: Absorption, Distribution, and Excretion. In RH Levy, RH Mattson, BS Meldrum (eds), Antiepileptic Drugs (4th ed). New York: Raven Press, 1995;379–387.

7. Alvin J, McHorse T, Hoyumpa A, et al. The effect of liver disease in man on the disposition of phenobarbital. J Pharmacol Exp Ther 1975;192:224–235.

8. Browne TR, LeDuc B. Phenytoin: Chemistry and Biotransformation. In RH Levy, RH Mattson, BS Meldrum (eds), Antiepileptic Drugs (4th ed). New York: Raven Press, 1995;283–300.

9. Treiman DM, Woodbury DM. Phenytoin: Absorption, Distribution, and Excretion. In RH Levy, RH Mattson, BS Meldrum (eds), Antiepileptic Drugs (4th ed). New York: Raven Press, 1995;301–314.

10. Tozer TN, Winter ME. Phenytoin. In WE Evans, JJ Schentag, WJ Jusko (eds), Applied Pharmacokinetics: Principles of Therapeutic Drug Monitoring (3rd ed). Vancouver, WA: Applied Therapeutics Inc, 1992;1–44.

11. Kutt H, Winters W, Scherman R, McDowell R. Diphenylhydantoin and phenobarbital toxicity. The role of liver disease. Arch Neurol 1964;11:649–656.

12. Hooper WD, Bochner F, Endre MJ, Tyrer JH. Plasma protein binding of diphenylhydantoin. Effects of sex hormones, renal and hepatic disease. Clin Pharmacol Ther 1974;15:276–282.

13. Olsen GD, Bennett WM, Porter GA. Morphine and phenytoin binding to plasma proteins in renal and hepatic failure. Clin Pharmacol Ther 1975;17:677–684.

14. Reidenberg MN, Affrime M. Influence of disease on binding of drugs to plasma proteins. Ann N Y Acad Sci 1973;226:115–126.

15. Blaschke TF, Meffin PJ, Melmon KL, Rowland M. Influence of acute viral hepatitis on phenytoin kinetics and protein binding. Clin Pharmacol Ther 1975;17:685–691.

16. Lunde PK, Rane A, Yaffe SJ, et al. Plasma protein binding of diphenylhydantoin in man. Interaction with other drugs and the effect of temperature and plasma dilution. Clin Pharmacol Ther 1970;11:846–855.

17. Rane A, Lunde PK, Jalling B, et al. Plasma protein binding of diphenylhydantoin in normal and hyperbilirubinemic infants. J Pediatr 1971;78:877–882.

18. Aweeka FT, Gottwald MD, Gambertoglio JG, et al. Pharmacokinetics of fosphenytoin in patients with hepatic and renal disease. Epilepsia 1999;40:777–782.

19. Garnett WR. Ethosuximide. In WJ Taylor, MH Caviness (eds), A Textbook for the Clinical Application of Therapeutic Drug Monitoring. Irving, TX: Abbott Laboratories, Diagnostics Division, 1986;225–235.

20. Pisani F, Bialer M. Ethosuximide: Chemistry and Biotransformation. In RH Levy, RH Mattson, BS Meldrum (eds), Antiepileptic Drugs (4th ed). New York: Raven Press, 1995;655–658.

21. Mialer M, Xiaodong S, Perucca E. Ethosuximide: Absorption, Distribution, and Excretion. In RH Levy, RH Mattson, BS Meldrum (eds), Antiepileptic Drugs (4th ed). New York: Raven Press, 1995;659–665.

22. Faigle JW, Feldmann KF. Carbamazepine: Chemistry and Biotransformation. In RH Levy, RH Mattson, BS Meldrum (eds), Antiepileptic Drugs (4th ed). New York: Raven Press, 1995;499–513.

23. Morselli PL. Carbamazepine: Absorption, Distribution, and Excretion. In RH Levy, RH Mattson, BS Meldrum (eds), Antiepileptic Drugs (4th ed). New York: Raven Press, 1995;515–528.

24. Hooper WD, Dubetz DK, Bochner F, et al. Plasma protein binding of carbamazepine. Clin Pharmacol Ther 1975;17:433–440.

25. Wilding IR, Davis SS, Hardy JG, et al. Relationship between systemic drug absorption and GI transit after the simultaneous oral administration of carbamazepine as a controlled-release system and as a suspension of 15N-labelled drug to healthy volunteers. Br J Clin Pharmacol 1991;32:573–579.

26. Baillie TA, Sheffels PR. Valproic Acid: Chemistry and Biotransformation. In RH Levy, RH Mattson, BS Meldrum (eds), Antiepileptic Drugs (4th ed). New York: Raven Press, 1995;589–604.

27. Levy RH, Shen DD. Valproic Acid: Absorption, Distribution, and Excretion. In RH Levy, RH Mattson, BS Meldrum (eds), Antiepileptic Drugs (4th ed). New York: Raven Press, 1995;605–619.

28. Klotz U, Rapp T, Mueller WA. Disposition of valproic acid in patients with liver disease. Eur J Clin Pharmacol 1978;13:55–60.

29. Siemes H, Nau H, Schulze K, et al. Valproate (VPA) metabolites in various clinical conditions of probable VPA-associated hepatotoxicity. Epilepsia 1993;34:332–346.

30. Kucharczk N. Felbamate: Chemistry and Biotransformation. In RH Levy, RH Mattson, BS Meldrum (eds), Antiepileptic Drugs (4th ed). New York: Raven Press, 1995;799–806.

31. Perhach JL, Shumaker RC. Felbamate: Absorption, Distribution, and Excretion. In RH Levy, RH Matt-

son, BS Meldrum (eds), Antiepileptic Drugs (4th ed). New York: Raven Press, 1995;807–812.

32. McLean MJ. Gabapentin: Chemistry, Absorption, Distribution, and Excretion. In RH Levy, RH Mattson, BS Meldrum (eds), Antiepileptic Drugs (4th ed). New York: Raven Press, 1995;843–849.

33. Garnett WR. Lamotrigine: pharmacokinetics. J Child Neurol 1997;12[Suppl 1]:S10–S15.

34. Dickins M, Sawyer DA, Morley TJ, Parsons DN. Lamotrigine: Chemistry and Biotransformation. In RH Levy, RH Mattson, BS Meldrum (eds), Antiepileptic Drugs (4th ed). New York: Raven Press, 1995;871–875.

35. Parsons DN, Dickins M, Morley TJ. Lamotrigine: Absorption, Distribution, and Excretion. In RH Levy, RH Mattson, BS Meldrum (eds), Antiepileptic Drugs (4th ed). New York: Raven Press, 1995;877–881.

36. Posner J, Cohen AF, Land G, Peck AW. The pharmacokinetics of lamotrigine (BW 430C) in healthy subjects with unconjugated hyperbilirubinemia (Gilbert's syndrome). Br J Clin Pharmacol 1989:28:117–120.

37. Garnett WR. Clinical pharmacology of topiramate: a review. Epilepsia 2000;41[Suppl 1]:S61–S65.

38. Doose DR, Walker SA, Venkataramanan R, et al. Topiramate pharmacokinetics in subjects with liver impairment. J Pharm Res 1994;11[Suppl]:S446.

39. Gustavson LE, Mengesl HB. Pharmacokinetics of tiagabine, a gamma-aminobutyric acid-uptake inhibitor, in healthy subjects after single and multiple doses. Epilepsia 1995;36:605–611.

40. Lau AH, Gustavson LE, Sperelakis R, et al. Pharmacokinetics and safety of tiagabine in subjects with various degrees of hepatic function. Epilepsia 1997;38:445–451.

41. Patsalow PN. Pharmacokinetic profile of levetiracetam: toward ideal characteristics. Pharmacol Ther 2000;85:77–85.

42. Tecoma ES. Oxcarbazepine. Epilepsia 1999;40[Suppl 5]:S37–S46.

43. Dam M, Ostergaard LH. Oxcarbazepine. In RH Levy, RH Mattson, BS Meldrum (eds), Antiepileptic Drugs (4th ed). New York: Raven Press, 1995;987–995.

44. Leppik IE. Zonisamide. Epilepsia 1999;40[Suppl 5]:S23–S29.

45. Kochak GM, Page JG, Buchanan RA, et al. Steady-state pharmacokinetics of zonisamide, an antiepileptic agent for treatment of refractory complex partial seizures. J Clin Pharmacol 1998;38:166–171.

46. Seino M, Naruto S, Ito T, Miyazaki H. Zonisamide. In RH Levy, RH Mattson, BS Meldrum (eds), Antiepileptic Drugs (4th ed). New York: Raven Press, 1995;1011–1023.

47. Krauss G, Crone N. Non-CNS side effects of antiepileptic drugs. Medscape (http://www.medscape.com/Medscape/Neurology/TreatmentUpdate/2000/tu02/public/toc-tu02.html).

48. Camfield C, Camfield P, Smith E, Tibbles JA. Asymptomatic children with epilepsy: little benefit from screening for anticonvulsant-induced liver, blood, or renal damage. Neurology 1986;36:838–841.

49. Haidukewych D, John G. Chronic valproic acid and coantiepileptic drug therapy and incidence of increases in serum liver enzymes. Ther Drug Monit 1986;8:407–410.

50. Kugoh T, Yamamoto M, Hosokawa K. Blood ammonia level during valproic acid therapy. Jpn J Psychiatry Neurol 1986;40:663–668.

51. Zaccara G, Paganini M, Campostrini R, et al. Effect of associated antiepileptic treatment on valproate-induced hyperammonemia. Ther Drug Monit 1985;7:185–190.

52. Schlienger RG, Shear NH. Antiepileptic drug hypersensitivity syndrome. Epilepsia 1998;39:S3–S7.

53. Knowles SR, Shapiro LE, Shear NH. Anticonvulsant hypersensitivity syndrome: incidence, prevention and management. Drug Saf 1999;21:489–501.

54. Asconape JJ, Penry JK, Dreifuss FE, et al. Valproate-associated pancreatitis. Epilepsia 1993;34:177–183.

55. Binek J, Hany A, Heer M. Valproic acid–induced pancreatitis. Case report and review of the literature. J Clin Gastroenterol 1991;13:690–693.

Chapter 5

Transplantation and Seizures

E. Cruz-Martinez and Robin L. Gilmore

Increasingly available and widespread organ transplantation has led to newly recognized disorders of the central nervous system (CNS) and new manifestations of old disorders. Seizures occur in 6–36% of transplant patients.[1] Patients anticipating or having undergone transplantation may have seizures that are difficult to manage for several reasons: (1) metabolic stressors, (2) pre-existing diseases, and (3) prior therapies. Any of these factors can affect the CNS. For instance, bone marrow transplant (BMT) patients may have had L-asparaginase for treatment of acute lymphocytic leukemia. Because L-asparaginase is associated with cerebral hemorrhage and infarction, an asparaginase-treated patient may have ischemic seizures, especially when metabolically stressed. The immunosuppressive drugs used to treat patients, especially cyclosporine, may in themselves be associated with seizures[2] or be affected by the drugs used to treat seizures.[3] Other traditional immunosuppressive or immunomodulating agents commonly used for transplantation include busulfan, methylprednisolone, prednisone, azathioprine, and cyclophosphamide. Newer agents include tacrolimus, mycophenolate, and daclizumab. Some of these have also been implicated in seizures in transplantation patients.[4–8] High-dose methylprednisolone given concurrently with cyclosporine seems to precipitate seizures, especially in patients with underlying metabolic disturbances.[4] Although azathioprine is not commonly associated with seizures, it has been associated with intracranial hypertension leading to generalized seizures. Foscarnet, used in treatment of cytomegalovirus hepatitis after BMT,[9] has been associated with seizures.[10]

Immunosuppression increases the risk for opportunistic CNS infection, which may manifest with seizures as a presenting feature of an intercurrent clinical problem during treatment. For instance, imipenem, commonly used in bacterial infections, has been associated with seizures.[11]

Transplant patients undergo procedures in intensive care units and operating rooms that require sedatives, anesthetics, and narcotics with many side effects. Many drugs used in anesthesia and the intensive care unit may cause seizures as a toxic side effect. Although enumeration of each drug is outside the scope of this chapter, we review a common syndrome known as the *central anticholinergic syndrome* (CAS).[12] It is associated with blockage of the central cholinergic neurotransmission and presents with symptoms identical to the central symptoms of atropine intoxication, including seizures. Additionally, agitation, hallucinations, disorientation, stupor, coma, and respiratory depression may occur. Such disturbances may be induced by opiates, ketamine, etomidate, propofol, nitrous oxide, and halogenated inhalation anesthetics as well as by histamine 2 (H_2)–blocking agents, such as cimetidine. Although there is an individual predisposition for CAS, it is unpredictable from laboratory findings or other signs. Postanesthetic CAS can be prevented by administration of physostigmine during the anesthesia procedure. There are some common denominators to all transplantation patients. However, each type of organ transplantation carries its own unique features and peculiarities. The following sections address these specific issues.

Kidney Transplantation

The kidney is the most frequently transplanted organ. The most common underlying diseases leading to kidney transplantations are glomerulonephritis, diabetes, and hypertensive renal disease, all of which produce uremia, which in turn may be associated with neurologic dysfunction and seizures.

As in all metabolic encephalopathies, a change in mental status is the hallmark of uremic encephalopathy. An unusual feature of uremic encephalopathy is simultaneous neural depression (obtundation) and neural excitation (twitching, myoclonus, generalized seizures). Seizures occur in one-third of uremic patients.[13] The reasons for this are diverse.

Uremic amaurosis, a condition that presents with blindness, is associated with focal and persistent seizures. Gross et al. described a syndrome of encephalopathy associated with acute rejection of renal allograft.[14] The clinical picture consisted of headaches, altered mental status, and seizures without focal neurologic deficits, fever, weight gain, renal failure, and graft tenderness.

The treatment of renal failure also may lead to *dialysis disequilibrium*. This syndrome is characterized by headache, nausea, and irritability that may progress to seizures, coma, and death, which is caused by the entry of free water into the brain, leading to edema. Dialysis dementia, caused by the toxic effects of aluminum, is now rare. Renal transplant recipients may develop cerebrovascular disease, infections by opportunistic organisms, or malignant neoplasms, particularly primary lymphoma of the brain. Antibiotic-associated adverse reactions in patients with renal insufficiency are other common conditions in which uremic patients have seizures.[15]

Patients may have focal motor or generalized seizures or myoclonus. Decreased protein binding of drugs in uremia results in an increased free fraction of highly protein-bound drugs in serum (and therefore in the CNS), which can be neurotoxic (e.g., cephalosporins). This may lead to lowered seizure threshold and increased seizure susceptibility. This may be further enhanced by the altered blood-brain barrier in uremia that leads to increased CNS concentrations of drugs.

Phenytoin is a frequently used antiepileptic drug (AED) for nontransplanted uremic patients. Because uremic patients have plasma protein-binding abnormalities and phenytoin is moderately protein bound, the drug is managed somewhat differently than in nonuremic patients. In nonuremic patients, 10% of phenytoin is not protein bound, whereas in uremic patients, as much as 75% is not protein bound. Thus, it is necessary to use free phenytoin levels instead of total phenytoin levels.[8] Therapeutic free phenytoin levels are between 1 and 2 µg/ml.[16]

The patient undergoing hemodialysis represents a special challenge, because one can expect a decrease in AED concentration when the drug is dialyzable. Plasma protein binding of a drug determines how effectively it can be dialyzed. Drugs, such as gabapentin and levetiracetam, with less than 10% plasma protein binding and topiramate, approximately 15% plasma protein bound, are dialyzed. This leads to reduced serum concentration and the possibility of increased seizure frequency. Dosage adjustments may be necessary. The AEDs with a high degree of protein binding are removed less by dialysis, because the drug-protein complex is too large to cross the dialysis membrane. The more protein bound a drug, the less dialyzable it is. Hence, the concentration of a drug, such as phenobarbital (40–60% bound), lamotrigine (55% bound), and zonisamide (40% bound), decreases during dialysis more than that of valproic acid, which is more highly protein bound (approximately 95%). One way to avoid "losing" the drug in these circumstances is to dialyze against a dialysate containing the drug, but this is a cumbersome solution. If the patient has more frequent seizures around the time of dialysis, it may be useful to use a highly protein-bound drug, such as valproic acid, which is not dialyzed completely. If drugs with low protein binding, such as gabapentin, are used, supplemental doses may be needed.

Drugs excreted by the kidney, such as gabapentin, levetiracetam, and topiramate, have prolonged half-lives when the patient is not undergoing hemodialysis. The clinician needs to adjust dosages and drug schedule timing (Table 5-1).

The immunosuppressant agents that make organ transplantation possible are usually metabolized via hepatic pathways. The use of phenytoin in patients treated with cyclosporin can be difficult. Phenytoin may decrease the plasma concentration of cyclosporin by enzyme induction.[17] It may also decrease cyclosporin levels by reducing absorption.[18] Other AEDs that induce the hepatic enzyme system CYP450, such as carbamazepine[3] and phe-

Table 5-1. Antiepileptic Drugs in Transplantation Patients

Antiepileptic Drug (protein bound %)	Renal	Hepatic	Bone Marrow	Heart	Comment
Phenytoin (80–90)	Use free phenytoin levels	Use free phenytoin levels		Use free phenytoin levels	Monitor cyclosporin level Steroid metabolism altered
Carbamazepine (65–80)	Hyponatremia		Leukopenia anemia Avoid during engraftment	Hyponatremia	Monitor cyclosporin level Steroid metabolism altered
Phenobarbital (40–60)	Sedating	Sedating	Useful during engraftment		Monitor cyclosporin level Steroid metabolism altered
Valproate (~95)	Useful during hemodialysis because little is removed	Avoid during hepatic failure	Avoid during engraftment Thrombocytopenia at high concentrations		Severe hepatotoxicity or pancreatitis are rare Avoid in patients <2 yrs of age
Gabapentin (3)	300 mg q.o.d. for severe renal failure 300 mg after ~4 hrs hemodialysis				
Lamotrigine (55)	$T_{1/2}$ ~48 hrs during severe renal failure $T_{1/2}$ ~12 hrs during hemodialysis	$T_{1/2}$ ~110 hrs during severe hepatic failure			Serious rashes: ~3/1,000 in adults ~1/100 in children
Topiramate (~15)	Clearance reduced ~50% in renal failure Need to adjust dose during hemodialysis				Kidney stone: ~1% incidence
Levetiracetam (<10)	Reduce dose during renal failure Supplemental dose after hemodialysis				
Zonisamide (~40)	Avoid in renal failure	Not studied in hepatic failure	Avoid during engraftment		A sulfonamide Kidney stone: ~4% incidence
Oxcarbazepine (MHD is ~40)	Hyponatremia	Liver converts to active MHD Not studied in severe failure	Avoid during engraftment	Hyponatremia	Both an inhibitor and inducer of P-450 Monitor cyclosporin level

MHD = monohydroxy derivative (active metabolite); $T_{1/2}$ = terminal half-life.

nobarbital, may also decrease the plasma concentration of cyclosporin. We highly recommended that cyclosporin levels be monitored when these AEDs are used.

Liver Transplantation

Hepatic Encephalopathy

Hepatic encephalopathy may result from a variety of liver disorders, including hepatitis, Wilson's disease, acquired hepatocerebral degeneration, alcoholic hepatitis, and cirrhosis. Hepatic encephalopathy is classified into stages: in stage I, encephalopathy is incipient; in stage II, the mental status deteriorates and asterixis develops; and in stage III, focal or generalized seizures may occur, and the incidence of seizures varies widely. Hypoglycemia may complicate liver failure and may be responsible for some seizures. Hyperammonemia is associated with seizures and may contribute to the encephalopathy of primary hyperammonemic disorders. Treatments that reduce ammonia also ameliorate the encephalopathy.[19] Treatment should be directed at the underlying etiology of the hepatic failure. The cornerstone of treatment is the reduction of gastrointestinal protein and lactulose. Lactulose increases ammonia elimination. Treatment with chronic AEDs is usually not necessary, unless there is a known predisposition to seizures (e.g., from previous cerebral injury). Because sedating AEDs may precipitate coma, they are generally avoided. Phenytoin is probably a reasonable choice when chronic AED treatment is necessary. Valproate should be avoided in hepatic failure. The AEDs excreted by the kidney are particularly useful in this setting.

Three to thirty-six percent[20–23] of patients who undergo liver transplantation develop seizures. The majority of these seizures are single episodes. If recurrent, these seizures are usually easily controlled with AEDs. Seizures after liver transplantation in patients were thought to herald a catastrophic course. Recently, this has been questioned: Wijdicks et al. reported that 4% of their large series of patients had seizures. However, in only 1% of 630 patients was it an agonal event.[22] In most patients, the seizures were associated with toxic levels of immunosuppressant drugs or with opportunistic infections. Thus, the majority of patients with seizures after liver transplantation

have an unremarkable course. The patients of Wijdicks et al. were usually treated with phenytoin. Phenytoin was discontinued after approximately 3 months without seizure recurrence.

Recurrent partial seizures occurring immediately after liver transplantation are most likely the result of focal cerebral infarction.[24] The use of cyclosporin may be correlated with seizures and other neurologic complications.[25] Cyclosporin toxicity may be enhanced by hypocholesterolemia[26] and hypomagnesemia.[27] Hypocholesterolemia may be associated with an increased intracellular transport of cyclosporin. Cyclosporin may cause renal wasting of magnesium, therefore magnesium levels should be checked at regular intervals in cyclosporin treated patients.[28] Phenobarbital has been commonly used in the past. However, with the advent of effective AEDs not metabolized by the liver, such as zonisamide, topiramate, and levetiracetam, chronic oral phenobarbital may be used less. Topiramate is not extensively metabolized and is primarily excreted unchanged in the urine. Zonisamide has not been studied in hepatic failure. If possible, it is best to avoid the use of chronic benzodiazepines, barbiturates, and valproate in liver transplantation patients with chronic seizures.

Other factors associated with seizures during cyclosporin use include hypertension, fluid retention, high-dose steroids, leukoencephalopathy and graft function, and age.[29–34] No clear relationship between neurologic toxicity and blood cyclosporin levels has been established.

Tacrolimus (FK506), an immunomodulator, has also been implicated as a cause of seizures, particularly when toxic blood levels occur.[35,36] When abrupt increases in drug level by 100% occur, patients can develop occipitoparietal white matter lesions on computed tomography (CT) or magnetic resonance imaging,[37] persistent confusional state, tremor, or seizures.[22]

Hypocholesterolemia exacerbates cyclosporin toxicity; this may be due to up-regulation of low-density lipoprotein receptors that increase the intracellular transport of cyclosporin.[29]

Lung Transplantation

Lung transplantation has become a viable treatment modality for patients with end-stage pulmonary disease. CNS complications include seizures.[38,39] A high incidence of seizures in young cystic fibrosis lung transplant recipients was first reported by Vaughn et al.[38] Age dependence is also noted in BMT and heart transplant recipients. The risk of seizures is greatest in the early course after surgery, a relationship that has also been seen in heart and liver transplant and BMT recipients. Double lung transplant recipients are more likely to have seizures than are single lung transplant recipients. Most patients in the series of Vaughn et al. had partial-onset seizures. This contrasts with other types of transplant series.[8,30,31,40] However, earlier series may have included secondarily generalized seizures.

Most seizures associated with lung transplantation occur during organ rejection.[38] Focal breakdown of the blood-brain barrier, similar to that in strokes and postulated in graft-versus-host disease, is a possible mechanism. Lung transplant recipients with cystic fibrosis have an elevated incidence of seizures.[39] Strokes, cyclosporin toxicity, and electrolyte abnormalities commonly occur in these patients.[39,41] The outcome of these complications is usually favorable, with long-term AED therapy needed only in a very small portion of cases.

Seizures are frequent after lung transplantation in pediatric patients; the most common etiologies are cyclosporin toxicity and hypoxia, followed by strokes and metabolic derangement.[42] Seizures occur early in the postoperative course. The electroencephalogram in the majority of these patients shows generalized slowing consistent with diffuse encephalopathy. Imaging studies often show changes consistent with cyclosporin toxicity—that is, reversible low-attenuation white matter changes on CT and hyperintense signals in the cortex or white matter of the cerebral hemispheres. These changes of T2 signal intensity suggest a microvascular injury.[43–45] The seizures are most often self-limited.

Heart Transplantation

The reasons for needing a heart transplant may be classified into ischemic heart disease and idiopathic cardiomyopathy. In the former, cerebrovascular disease may be much more common than in other transplant patients, and, subsequently, the incidence of cerebral infarct–related seizures may be higher.

During transplantation, patients are on bypass pumps for several hours and are vulnerable to significant hypoperfusion and hypoxia.[46,47] Grigg et al. reported seizures in 15% of consecutive orthotopic heart transplant recipients.[48] All of these

patients were treated with cyclosporin. Postoperative focal cerebral ischemic infarctions were noted in two-thirds of patients.[48] Ischemic injury experienced during surgery increases the incidence of postoperative seizures.[49]

Bone Marrow Transplantation

The incidence of seizures among 800 BMT patients treated with cyclosporin is 5.5%.[50] Seizures occurred in more than 10% of BMT recipients in Patchell et al.'s study.[51] In the latter series, patients were not treated with AEDs, but seizures did not recur. Seizures are usually generalized, mostly associated with metabolic derangements, and sometimes associated with the drugs used to "condition" the bone marrow (e.g., busulfan).[52,53]

Patients undergoing BMT may have significant thrombocytopenia secondary to the condition for which they are being treated or from the conditioning regimen before the transplant procedure. Thrombocytopenia makes them more susceptible to cerebral hemorrhage and associated seizures.

Infarction with subsequent seizures may result from venous thrombosis due to the fluid dynamic alteration that occurs in patients with extremely high white blood cell count or due to embolization from nonbacterial thrombotic endocarditis.[54] Occasionally, BMT patients may have had L-asparaginase for the treatment of acute lymphocytic leukemia. Because L-asparaginase is associated with cerebral hemorrhage and infarction, an asparaginase-treated patient may have ischemic seizures.

Pancreas Transplantation

Pancreatic transplants are not as common as other transplants and are usually performed in patients with type I diabetes who have extensive end-organ damage.[55] Most pancreas transplantation procedures are performed together with renal transplantation. Because most patients have end-stage renal disease from diabetes, they also may experience the same seizure rate postoperatively.

Diagnostic Approach to Transplantation Patients with Seizures

Seizures may occur in transplantation pre-, peri-, or postoperatively. The physician should consider the seizure as a symptom of CNS dysfunction. The first step should be to identify the process responsible for the seizure as a partial versus generalized one. A careful history and physical examination are invaluable. Metabolic disturbances are a common course of seizures in all the transplantation patients, so they should always be sought and corrected. Infections may occur in afebrile patients. Infections may be systemic or may specifically involve the CNS. A detailed investigation for infections, including cerebrospinal fluid analysis, is imperative even when metabolic abnormalities are present, because the latter do not exclude the possibility of the former. A normal cerebrospinal fluid does not exclude infection.

Cranial imaging studies are useful in identifying a structural lesion. Magnetic resonance imaging identifies more abnormalities than CT.[56] Although cranial imaging studies may not demonstrate a new or treatable lesion as an etiology for the seizures, such studies should be obtained when any type of seizure occurs in these patients.[8] There are exceptions to this rule, of course, such as when seizures occur as a preterminal or terminal event or after marked hypoxia. Thus, the decision to obtain a cranial imaging study should be individualized.

The electroencephalogram is still very useful in assessing patients. It provides information about background rhythms, is a qualitative marker of encephalopathy, and helps characterize epileptiform discharges with regard to focal or generalized distribution, leading to clarification of seizure etiology.

Treatment of Seizures

Acute Management

As with any seizure, attention should be directed to determine its cause or precipitant. The acute management of the prolonged seizure in the transplantation patient is somewhat different than for acute seizures in other medical conditions. One wishes to use AEDs that are least likely to induce the enzyme system responsible for metabolizing immunosuppressant drugs. It is paramount to prevent cardiorespiratory compromise of the patient. If the convulsive seizures last more than 3 minutes, recur frequently, or the patient develops status epilepticus, then a parenteral AED should be used. The use of the benzodiazepines, such as diazepam and lorazepam, is preferred.[8] In principle, the AED used acutely should be the least likely to induce the hepatic enzyme system responsible for the metabolism of cyclosporin, methylprednisolone, prednisone, and tacrolimus. However, the rigid adherence to this principle would exclude the two most effective, longer-acting parenteral AEDs available: fosphenytoin and phenobarbital. Sometimes compromises are necessary. Fosphenytoin should be considered over parenteral phenytoin, because it can be infused at a higher rate and it lacks direct vascular injury that has been associated with intravenous phenytoin.

There have been recent reports about parenteral valproate, mostly in patients with nonconvulsive status epilepticus.[57,58] However, it is not recommended as a first-line drug in the treatment of status epilepticus, nonconvulsive or convulsive. Rapid infusion (greater than 20 mg/minute) of valproate may lead to increased adverse effects. More important, its efficacy for convulsive status epilepticus is unknown.

Chronic Management

The chronic management of seizures is determined after etiology has been ascertained and a decision regarding the need for long-term therapy has been made. The choice of AED is determined by consideration of several factors, including the type of transplant.

Allograft survival in patients treated with AEDs is an important issue. Renal allograft survival is decreased in patients treated with phenytoin or phenobarbital and steroids.[59,60] Hence, discontinuing AEDs has been actively advocated.[60] The half-lives of prednisolone[61] and probably cyclosporine are decreased when phenobarbital, phenytoin, and carbamazepine are used. Thus, in patients other than hepatic transplantation patients and BMT patients during engraftment, valproate is a reasonable antiepileptic choice. For liver transplant patients or those in hepatic failure, gabapentin or levetiracetam may be a more appropriate choice. When phenytoin, phenobarbital, or carbamazepine is used, the medical team caring for the patient should increase the dosages of immunosuppressive drugs to ensure therapeutic immunosuppressant drug levels.

During BMT engraftment, phenytoin and valproate should be avoided. Carbamazepine is relatively contraindicated in BMT patients, both during and after engraftment, as the major serious side effect is hematologic toxicity. Although oxcarbazepine is chemically related to carbamazepine, oxcarbazepine has much less potential for hematologic toxicity risks. During the 2- to 6-week period of engraftment, reasonable choices include phenobarbital, gabapentin, and levetiracetam.

The recent introduction of several new AEDs has proven beneficial. Gabapentin, lamotrigine, topiramate, zonisamide, levetiracetam, and oxcarbazepine are new oral antiepileptics that have negligible hepatic CYP450 enzyme-inducing activity and fewer systemic or neurologic side effects compared to older AEDs. Lamotrigine and oxcarbazepine are approved for monotherapy in adults with partial seizures. The others are indicated as adjunctive therapy. Selection of AEDs can be complex in transplantation patients. It requires careful evaluation of the patient's general medical condition and consideration of potential adverse effects of individual drugs.

References

1. Patchell RA. Neurological complications of organ transplantation. Ann Neurol 1994;36:688–703.
2. Polson RJ, Powell-Jackson PR, Williams R. Convulsions associated with cyclosporin A in transplant recipients. BMJ (Clin Res Ed) 1985;290:1003.
3. Soto Alvarez J, Sacristan Del Castillo JA, Alsar Ortiz MJ. Effect of carbamazepine on cyclosporin blood level. Nephron 1991;58:235–236
4. el Dahr S, Chevalier RL, Gomez RA, Campbell FG. Seizures and blindness following intravenous pulse methylprednisolone in a renal transplant patient. Int J Pediatr Nephrol 1987;8:87–90.
5. Ghany AM, Tusschka PJ, McGhee RB Jr, et al. Cyclosporine-associated seizures in bone marrow transplant recipients given busulfan and cyclophosphamide preparative therapy. Transplantation 1991;52:310–315.
6. Cilio MR, Danhaive O, Gadisseux JF, et al. Unusual cyclosporin related neurological complications in recipients of liver transplants. Arch Dis Child 1993;68:405–407.
7. Seifeldin RA, Lawrence KR, Rahamtulla AF, Monaco AP. Generalized seizures associated with the use of morumonab-CD3 in two patients after kidney transplantation. Ann Pharmacother 1997;31:586–589.
8. Gilmore RL. Seizures and antiepileptic drug use in transplant patients. Neurol Clin 1988;6:279–296.
9. Zomas A, Mehta J, Powles R, et al. Unusual infections following allogeneic bone marrow transplantation for chronic lymphocytic leukemia. Bone Marrow Transplant 1994;14:799–803.
10. Lor E, Liu YQ. Neurologic sequelae associated with foscarnet therapy. Ann Pharmacother 1994;28:1035–1037.
11. Calandra G, Lydick E, Carrigan J, et al. Factors predisposing to seizures in seriously ill, infected patients receiving antibiotics: experience with imipenem/cilastatin. Am J Med 1988;84;911–918.
12. Schneck HJ, Rupreht J. Central anticholinergic syndrome (CAS) in anesthesia and intensive care. Acta Anaesthesiol Belg 1989;40:219–228.
13. Plum F, Posner JB. Diagnosis of stupor and coma (3rd ed). Philadelphia: FA Davis Co, 1980.
14. Gross ML, Pearson RM, Kennedy J, et al. Rejection encephalopathy. Lancet 1982;2:1217.
15. Manian FA, Stone WJ, Alford RH. Adverse antibiotic effects associated with renal insufficiency. Rev Infect Dis 1990;12:236–249.
16. DeMonaco HJ, Lawless LM. Variability of phenytoin protein binding in epileptic patients. Arch Neurol 1983;40:481–482.
17. Keown PA, Laupacis A, Carruthers G, et al. Interaction between phenytoin and cyclosporine following organ transplantation. Transplantation 1984;38:304–306.
18. Rowland M, Gupta SK. Cyclosporin-phenytoin interaction: re-evaluation using metabolite data. Br J Clin Pharmacol 1987;24:29–34.
19. Rothstein JD, Herlong HF. Neurologic manifestations of hepatic disease. Neurol Clin 1989;7:563–578.
20. Estol CJ, Brenner RP, Martinez AJ. Seizures after liver transplantation: a clinicopathologic study. Neurology 1989;39:1297–1301.
21. Wijdicks EF, Wiesner RH, Krom RA. Neurotoxicity in liver transplant recipients with cyclosporine immunosuppression. Neurology 1995;45:1962–1964.
22. Wijdicks EF, Plevak DJ, Wiesner RH, Steers JL. Causes and outcome of seizures in liver transplant recipients. Neurology 1996;47:1523–1525.
23. Bronster DJ, Emre S, Boccagni P, et al. Central nervous system complications in liver transplant recipients—incidence, timing, and long-term follow-up. Clin Transplant 2000;14:1–7.
24. Starzl TE, Schneck SA, Mazzoni G, et al. Acute neurological complications after liver transplantation with particular reference to intraoperative cerebral air embolus. Ann Surg 1978;187:236–240.
25. Adams HP, Ponsford S, Gunson B, et al. Neurological complications following liver transplantation. Lancet 1987;1:949–951.
26. Cooper DK, Novitzky D, Davis L, et al. Does central nervous system toxicity occur in transplant patients with hypocholesterolemia receiving cyclosporine? J Heart Transplant 1989;8:221–224.
27. Thompson CB, June CH, Sullivan KM, et al. Association between cyclosporin neurotoxicity and hypomagnesaemia. Lancet 1984;2:1116–1120.
28. Vogt DP, Lederman RJ, Carey WD, Broughan TA.

Neurologic complications of liver transplantation. Transplantation 1988;45:1057–1061.

29. de Groen PC, Aksamit AJ, Rakela J, et al. Central nervous system toxicity after liver transplantation. The role of cyclosporine and cholesterol. N Engl J Med 1987;317:861–866.

30. Allen RD, Hunnisett AG, Morris PJ. Cyclosporin and magnesium. Lancet 1985;1:1283–1284.

31. Durrant S, Chipping PM, Palmer S, Gordon-Smith EC. Cyclosporin A, methylprednisolone, and convulsions. Lancet 1982;2:829–830.

32. Nordal KP, Talseth T, Dahl E. Aluminum overload: a predisposing condition for epileptic seizures in renal transplant patients treated with cyclosporin? Lancet 1985;2:153–154.

33. Wszolek ZK, Steg RE. Seizures after liver transplantation. Liver Transpl Surg 1995;1:334–339.

34. Menegaux F, Keeffe EB, Andrews BT, et al. Neurological complications of liver transplantation in adult versus pediatric patients. Transplantation 1994;58:447–450.

35. Mueller AR, Platz KP, Bechstein WO, et al. Neurotoxicity after orthotopic liver transplantation. A comparison between cyclosporine and FK506. Transplantation 1994;58:155–170.

36. Wijdicks EF, Wiesner RH, Dahlke LJ, Krom RA. FK 506-induced neurotoxicity in liver transplantation. Ann Neurol 1994;35:498–501.

37. Jarosz JM, Howlett DC, Cox TC, Bingham JB. Cyclosporine-related reversible leukoencephalopathy: MRI. Neuroradiology 1997;39:711–715.

38. Vaughn BV, Ali II, Oliver KN, et al. Seizures in lung transplant recipients. Epilepsia 1996;37:1175–1179.

39. Goldstein LS, Haug MT III, Perl J, et al. Central nervous system complications after lung transplantation. J Heart Lung Transplant 1998;17:185–191.

40. Boogaerts MA, Zachee P, Verwilghen RL. Cyclosporine, methylprednisolone and convulsions. Lancet 1982;2:1216–1217.

41. Graver B, Lee SH. Worldwide transplant center directory. Lung transplants. Clin Transpl 1989;580–582.

42. Wong M, Mallory GB Jr, Goldstein J, et al. Neurologic complications of pediatric lung transplantation. Neurology 1999;53:1542–1549.

43. Scheinman SJ, Reinitz ER, Petro G, et al. Cyclosporin central neurotoxicity following renal transplant. Transplantation 1990;49:215–216.

44. Truwit CL, Denaro CP, Lake JR, Demarco T. MR imaging of reversible cyclosporine A-induced neurotoxicity. Am J Neuroradiol 1991;12:651–659.

45. Pace MT, Slovis TL, Kelly JK, Abelle SD. Cyclosporine A toxicity: MRI appearance of the brain. Pediatr Radiol 1995:25:180–183.

46. Hotson JR, Pedley TA. The neurological complications of cardiac transplantation. Brain 1976;99:673–694.

47. Eidelman BH, Obrist WD, Wagner WR, et al. Cerebrovascular complications associated with the use of artificial circulatory support services. Neurol Clin 1993;11:463–474.

48. Grigg MM, Constanzo-Nordin MR, Celesia GG, et al. Cyclosporine-induced seizures following cardiac transplantation: fact or fiction? Epilepsia 1987;28:626.

49. Sila CA. Spectrum of neurologic events following cardiac transplantation. Stroke 1989;20:1586–1589.

50. O'Sullivan DP. Convulsions associated with cyclosporin A. BMJ 1985;290:858.

51. Patchell RA, White CL III, Clark AW, et al. Neurologic complications of bone marrow transplantation. Neurology 1985;35:300–306.

52. Marcus RE, Goldman JM. Convulsions due to high-dose busulfan. Lancet 1984;2:1463.

53. Murphy CP, Harden EA, Thompson JM. Generalized seizures secondary to high-dose busulfan therapy. Ann Pharmacother 1992;26:30–31.

54. Patchell RW, White CL III, Clark AW, et al. Nonbacterial thrombotic endocarditis in bone marrow transplant patients. Cancer 1985;55:631–635.

55. Morel P, Goetz FC, Moudry-Munns K, et al. Long-term glucose control in patients with pancreatic transplants. Ann Intern Med 1991;115:694–699.

56. Bleck TP. Management approaches to prolonged seizures and status epilepticus. Epilepsia 1999;40[Suppl 1]:S59–S63; discussion S64–S66.

57. Chez MG, Hammer MS, Lkoeffel M, et al. Clinical experience of three pediatric and one adult case of spike-and-wave status epilepticus treated with injectable valproic acid. J Child Neurol 1999;14:239–242.

58. Kaplan PW. Intravenous valproate treatment of generalized nonconvulsive status epilepticus. Clin Electroencephalogr 1999;30:1–4.

59. McEnery PT, Stempel DA. Commentary: anticonvulsant therapy and renal allograft survival. J Pediatr 1976;88:138–139.

60. Wassner SJ, Malekzadeh MH, Pennisi AJ, et al. Allograft survival in patients receiving anticonvulsant medications. Clin Nephrol 1977;8:293–297.

61. Gambertoglio JG, Holford NH, Kapusnik JE, et al. Disposition of total and unbound prednisolone in renal transplant patients receiving anticonvulsant. Kidney Int 1984;25:119–123.

Chapter 6

Infectious States

Martin Adam Goldstein and Cynthia L. Harden

Alien they seemed to be
No mortal eye could see
The intimate welding of their later history
Or sign that they were bent by paths coincident
On being twin halves of one august event

—Hardy

Importance and Types of Comorbidity

Comorbid seizure and infection represent a subdivision of the larger phenomenon of infection and central nervous system (CNS) dysfunction. Four major potential temporal permutations exist:

1. A patient with an acute infection can have a seizure.
2. A patient with epilepsy can develop an acute infection.
3. Epilepsy can follow an acute infection as a neurologic sequela.
4. Epilepsy can develop during a chronic infection.

As with all illness comorbidities in medicine, three possible causal relationships can exist between seizure and infection:

1. An infectious state can be a causative factor in the development of a seizure disorder (infections are among the most common causes of seizures).
2. A seizure disorder can be a causative factor in the development of an infectious state.

3. An infectious state and a seizure disorder can occur coincidentally but independently, without any causal connection existing between their origins, yet, nevertheless, carry possible interactions in their natural histories and managements.

Regardless of temporal sequence and the potential causality existing between components of the comorbid dyad, it is important to maintain the perspective of comorbidity significance for three fundamental reasons: diagnosis, management, and prognosis.

Diagnosis

Attending to the concept of comorbidity can facilitate elucidation of the etiologic pathogenesis of either or both disorders. For example, functioning via a limited number of final common pathways (e.g., fever, metabolic derangement, inflammatory reaction, cerebrovascular disruption, and mass effect), almost any infection can potentially be complicated by a seizure. However, certain infections and certain loci of infection are more likely to be associated with seizure expression. Conversely, consideration of seizure semiology can aid determination of infection type and locus. A seizure can be the initial presentation of an infectious state, providing a crucial overt clinical manifestation of a previously covert infection or heralding the progression of a known infection now impacting the CNS.

Table 6-1. Anticonvulsant and Antimicrobial Cytochrome P-450 Effects

Cytochrome P-450 Isoenzyme	Antimicrobial			Anticonvulsant		
	Substrate	Inducer	Inhibitor	Substrate	Inducer	Inhibitor
1A2	Ritonavir	Rifampin Ritonavir	Ciprofloxacin Clarithromycin Erythromycin Isoniazid Ketoconazole Levofloxacin Ritonavir	Diazepam	Carbamazepine Phenobarbital Phenytoin Primidone	
2A6	Ritonavir		Ritonavir		Phenobarbital	
2B6					Phenobarbital Phenytoin Primidone	
2C		Rifampin	Isoniazid Ketoconazole		Carbamazepine Phenobarbital Phenytoin Primidone	
2C8		Rifampin		Carbamazepine Diazepam	Carbamazepine Phenobarbital Phenytoin Primidone	
2C9	Dapsone Metronidazole Ritonavir	Fluconazole Rifampin	Chloramphenicol Isoniazid Ketoconazole Metronidazole Ritonavir Sulfamethox- azole- trimethoprim Sulfonamides	Phenytoin	Carbamazepine Phenobarbital Phenytoin	Valproic acid
2C18		Rifampin			Carbamazepine Phenobarbital Phenytoin	
2C19	Pentamidine Ritonavir	Rifampin	Fluconazole Isoniazid Ketoconazole Ritonavir	Phenobarbital Phenytoin Topiramate Valproate	Carbamazepine Phenobarbital Phenytoin	Felbamate Oxcarbazepine Topiramate
2D6		Chloroquine Quinidine Ritonavir		Tiagabine	Valproate	
2E1	Dapsone Isoniazid Ritonavir	Isoniazid	Ritonavir			
3A3/4	Clarithromycin Clindamycin Dapsone Erythromycin Indinavir Itraconazole Ketoconazole Miconazole	Griseofulvin Nafcillin Rifabutin		Carbamazepine Clonazepam Diazepam Tiagabine	Carbamazepine Oxcarbazepine Phenobarbital Phenytoin Primidone	

Table 6-1. *Continued*

Cytochrome P-450 Isoenzyme	Antimicrobial			Anticonvulsant		
	Substrate	Inducer	Inhibitor	Substrate	Inducer	Inhibitor
	Nelfinavir Quinidine Rifampin Ritonavir Saquinavir					
3A5-7	Quinidine	Rifampin	Clotrimazole Ketoconazole Metronidazole		Phenobarbital Phenytoin Primidone	

Source: Data from CF Lacy, LL Armstrong, MP Goldman. Drug Information Handbook. Hudson, OH: Lexi-Comp, 2000;1092–1100; P Hantson, F Leonard, JM Maloteaux, P Mahieu. How epileptogenic are the recent antibiotics? Acta Clin Belg 1999;54:80–87.

Management

Comorbid seizure and infection mandate implementation of a multisystemic management approach, as the likelihood that other systems (e.g., respiratory, cardiovascular, renal, or metabolic) can become clinically impacted, either by the disease processes or by their contemporaneous management, increases. For example, a seizure occurring within the context of infection means that the special circumstances of the CNS (e.g., its physical encasement), its immunologic sequestration, and the implications of its involvement (i.e., interpreting a seizure as signifier of a "CNS-at-risk" event) now must be incorporated within the overall management strategy. Speed of intervention becomes even more crucial, and potential interactions among interventions (e.g., adverse drug interactions between simultaneous anticonvulsant and antimicrobial treatment; Tables 6-1 and 6-2) must be considered diligently.

CNS damage with potentially long-lasting neurologic sequelae.

In general, choice of antiseizure treatment is not influenced by infection type, per se, but by how the infection disturbs seizure-generating CNS circuitry. Hence, throughout this chapter, especially when considering seizure complications of an acute infectious process, emphasis is placed on infection pathophysiology, because the potential diagnostic value of the seizure can best be appreciated and, subsequently, used for planning seizure management by understanding how a seizure's expression is a logical by-product of the infectious process. Non–seizure-related clinical manifestations are given to facilitate infectious syndrome recognition when a patient's presenting sign is seizure. Infection management guidelines are also provided, because even the clinician solely concerned with the epileptic clinical component needs to be aware of concomitant infection treatment.

Prognosis

The development of one disorder within the context of the other can significantly impact the subsequent morbidity of the initial disease process, yielding important prognostic implications. For example, development of pneumonia secondary to seizure-related aspiration can significantly affect overall outcome. Alternatively, seizure onset during comorbid infection can indicate

Locus of Infection

As elsewhere in neurology, "Where is the problem?" is a fundamental organizing question in the management of comorbid seizure and infection. Because diagnosis and management often depend on the pathogenic focus (e.g., it is conceptually useful to consider bacterial pathogens that can cause meningitis separately from the bacteria that cause epidural abscesses), it is useful to explicitly

Table 6-2. Major Antimicrobial-Anticonvulsant Interactions

Antimicrobial	Anticonvulsant	Antimicrobial Effect	Anticonvulsant Effect
Itraconazole	Carbamazepine	None	↓ level
	Phenytoin	↓ level	↑ level
Fluconazole	Phenytoin	↓ level	↑ level
Ketoconazole	Phenytoin	↓ level	↑ level
Chloramphenicol	Phenytoin	None	↑ toxicity
Clindamycin	Diazepam	None	↑ effect
Doxycycline	Phenobarbital	↓ absorption, ↓ serum terminal half-life	↑ level
Ciprofloxacin	Phenytoin	None	↑ or ↓
Isoniazid	Carbamazepine	None	↑ level
	Phenytoin	None	↑ level
Erythromycin	Carbamazepine	None	↑ level, toxicity
	Phenytoin	None	↑ level
	Valproate	None	↑ level
Clarithromycin	Carbamazepine	None	↑ level, toxicity
	Phenytoin	None	↑ level
	Valproate	None	↑ level
Mefloquine	Valproate	None	↓ level
Metronidazole	Phenobarbital	↓ level	
	Phenytoin	↓ level	
Pentamidine	Valproate	↑ risk of pancreatitis	None
Nelfinavir	Carbamazepine	↓ level	↑ level
	Clonazepam	↓ level	↑ level
	Phenobarbital	↓ level	↑ level
	Phenytoin	↓ level	↑ level
Ritonavir	Carbamazepine	↓ level	↑ level
	Clonazepam	↓ level	↑ level
	Phenobarbital	↓ level	↑ level
	Phenytoin	↓ level	↑ level
Saquinavir	Carbamazepine	↓ level	↑ level
	Clonazepam	↓ level	↑ level
	Phenobarbital	↓ level	↑ level
	Phenytoin	↓ level	↑ level
Rifamycins	Phenytoin	None	↓ level
Sulfonamides	Phenytoin	None	↑ level
Sulfamethoxazole-trimethoprim	Phenytoin	None	↑ level
Zalcitabine (ddC)	Valproate	↑ risk of pancreatitis	None

↓ = decreased; ↑ = increased.
Source: Data from P Hantson, F Leonard, JM Maloteaux, P Mahieu. How epileptogenic are the recent antibiotics? Acta Clin Belg 1999;54:80–87; DN Gilbert, RC Moellering, MA Sande. Guide to Antimicrobial Therapy. Hyde Park, VT: Antimicrobial Therapy, 2000;129–133.

review the biological "topography" of infection relative to the nervous system. Infection can be localized to the following areas:

1. Non-CNS systemic (e.g., bacteremia, viremia, and fungemia)
2. Para-CNS (e.g., epidural abscess)
3. Cerebrospinal fluid (CSF) (e.g., meningitides)
4. Parenchymal CNS (e.g., encephalitides, intra-parenchymal abscess)

A summary of the major CNS infection syndromes that can be complicated by seizures is given in Table 6-3.

Table 6-3. Central Nervous System (CNS) Infection Syndromes That Can Be Complicated by Seizures

CNS Infection Syndrome	Onset	Duration	Systemic Features
Acute meningitis (e.g., bacterial, viral, fungal)	Sudden	Days	Present
Subacute or chronic meningitis (e.g., tuberculous, cryptococcal, syphilitic)	Gradual	Weeks to years	Variable
Acute encephalitis (e.g., arbovirus, rickettsia, toxoplasmosis)	Sudden	Days to weeks	Usually
Chronic encephalitis (e.g., subacute sclerosing panencephalitis, human immunodeficiency virus, Lyme disease, syphilis)	Gradual	Months to years	Variable
Focal mass infections (e.g., abscess, cysticercosis)	Crescendo	Days to months	Variable
Encephalopathy secondary to extra–central nervous system or systemic infection (e.g., infective endocarditis, malaria)	Variable	Days to months	Present
Postinfectious/immunization syndromes (postvaccine encephalomyelitis)	Variable	Days to years	Absent
Slow viral syndromes (e.g., Creutzfeldt-Jakob disease)	Very gradual	Months to years	Absent

Source: Adapted from DT Durack, RJ Whitley, WM Scheld. Approach to the patient with central nervous system infection. In WM Scheld, RJ Whitley, DT Durack (eds), Infections of the Central Nervous System. Philadelphia: Lippincott–Raven, 1997;3.

Epilepsy as a Consequence of a Comorbid Infectious State

A seizure can arise as an acute, subacute, or long-term consequence of an infectious state. Furthermore, a seizure complication of an infection can consist of a single seizure or can go on to become a chronic epilepsy. When and what type of epileptic complication arises from an infection depend on the nature of the infectious illness, its duration, and the type and extent of damage that the infection does to the CNS. Although quantitative seizure risk data in the context of infection would be extremely useful, there are few detailed quantitative studies. One reason for this is that retrospective analysis of seizure risk factors is complicated by the interdependence of the manifold multisystemic and iatrogenic events typically impacting patients during their course of illness.

To get a general idea of the impact of direct CNS infection in particular on seizure genesis, a retrospective study of survivors of encephalitis or meningitis between 1935 and 1981 was conducted to assess the risk of unprovoked seizures after CNS infection.[5] The 20-year risk of developing unprovoked seizures was 6.8%, and the ratio of observed to expected cases of unprovoked seizures was 6.9. The increased incidence of unprovoked seizures was highest during the first 5 years after CNS infection but remained elevated over the next 15 years of follow-up. Type of CNS infection and seizure occurrence during the acute phase of CNS infection greatly influenced the risk of subsequent unprovoked seizures. The 20-year risk of developing unprovoked seizures was 22% for patients with viral encephalitis and acute-context seizures, 10% for patients with viral encephalitis without acute-context seizures, 13% for patients with bacterial meningitis and acute-context seizures, and 2.4% for patients with bacterial meningitis without acute-context seizures. The 20-year risk of 2.1% for patients with aseptic meningitis was not increased over the general population seizure incidence.

Bacterial Infections

An overview of the most clinically relevant bacterial pathogens is given in Table 6-4.

Bacterial Infections in General

A number of studies have investigated the epileptic complication effect of having any type or severity of bacterial infection. Iavanainen et al. found that increased serum levels of various bacterial antibodies were more common in patients with recent seizures than in healthy control subjects (17 of 29 vs. 2 of 31;

Table 6-4. Taxonomic Classification of Neurologically Relevant Bacterial Pathogens

Aerobic gram-positive cocci
  Streptococcus pneumoniae
  Streptococcus agalactiae (group B)
  Enterococcus
Aerobic gram-positive rods
  Listeria monocytogenes
Aerobic gram-positive cocci
  Neisseria meningitidis
Aerobic gram-negative rods
  Escherichia coli
  Haemophilus influenzae (type b)
  Legionella pneumophila
  Salmonella
  Pseudomonas aeruginosa
Anaerobic gram-positive cocci
  Peptostreptococcus
Anaerobic-gram positive rods
  Actinomyces
  Propionibacterium
  Clostridium botulinum, Clostridium tetani, Clostridium perfringens
Anaerobic gram-negative rods
  Bacteroides fragilis
Spirochetes
  Borrelia burgdorferi (Lyme disease)
  Treponema pallidum (syphilis)
Intracellular
  Rickettsia (Rocky Mountain spotted fever)

Table 6-5. Seizure Risk Index for Adult Intensive Care Unit Patients with Gram-Negative Infections

Factor	Risk Index Weight
Before admission	
Prior seizure history	2
Central nervous system (CNS) tumor history	4
Concurrent factors (within 1 mo)	
Acute stroke (ischemic or hemorrhagic)	3
CNS surgery	3
CNS infection	3
While in intensive care unit	
Coma or anoxic encephalopathy	1
Renal impairment (serum creatinine >1.6 mg/dl)	2
Acute hypotensive episode	1

Source: Adapted from HA Guess, LJ Resseguie, LJ Melton, et al. Factors predictive of seizures among intensive care unit patients with gram negative infections. Epilepsia 1990;31:567–573.

$p <.001$).[6] In most of these cases, no infections were recognized clinically or bacteriologically. The mechanistic significance of higher antibody titers in epileptics is unclear (e.g., whether seizure production was related to the bacterial infection or a nonspecific immune response). Besides bolstering long-standing theories regarding the epileptogenic effect of infection in general, these results also suggest that epileptic seizures can be triggered by bacterial infections even when no clinically apparent infection is recognized.

In a study investigating an animal model for the study of the neurotoxicity of bacterial products, pentylenetetrazol (PTZ), a convulsant drug, was injected into mice.[7] Increased seizure induction sensitivity to PTZ was used as an indicator of neurotoxicity. Preinjection of sonicates of *Shigella dysenteriae* or *Escherichia coli* enhanced seizure response to PTZ, as indicated by a higher mean convulsion score, and increased the number of mice responding to PTZ and

the induction of seizures in animals pretreated with a subepileptic dose of PTZ.

In one of the few studies attemping to formulate a quantitative means of predicting seizure risk in the context of serious acute infection, Guess et al. reviewed records of intensive care unit patients with gram-negative infections to develop a predictive score of clinical risk for seizure occurrence.[8] Based on this review, they were able to develop an inventory of clinical risk factors with individual seizure risk weights (derived from regression coefficients determined by the frequency with which each clinical condition was associated with seizure occurrence in retrospective chart review), as exemplified in Table 6-5.

A seizure risk index greater than or equal to 3 was considered suggestive of relatively high seizure risk, whereas a risk factor index less than or equal to 2 was considered low seizure risk. To evaluate the predictive value of this scoring system, the authors applied it to a separate population of seriously ill inpatients with similar gram-negative infections. Seizure risk index scores and actual seizure occurrences were then compared; whereas positive predictive values were low (26%), negative predictive values were high ($\geq$97%). Thus, this index better identifies patients at low risk for sei-

Table 6-6. Relative Species Etiology Incidences of Bacterial Meningitis

Organism	Neonates	Children	Adults
Haemophilus influenzae	+	++++	+
Neisseria meningitidis	+	+++	+++
Streptococcus pneumoniae	+	++	++++
Listeria species	++	+	+
Group B Streptococci	++++	+	+
Gram-negative bacilli (E. coli)	++++	+	++
Staphylococci	+	+	++

+ = infrequent; ++ = occasional; +++ = common; ++++ = most common.
Source: Adapted from KL Roos, AR Tunkel, WM Scheld. Acute bacterial meningitis in children and adults. In WM Scheld, RJ Whitley, DT Durack (eds), Infections of the Central Nervous System. Philadelphia: Lippincott–Raven, 1997;336–401.

Table 6-7. Neurologic Symptoms and Signs of Bacterial Meningitis by Age Group

Age Group	Neurologic Manifestations
Child	Consciousness level change
	Headache
	Irritability
	Photophobia
	Nuchal rigidity
	Seizures
	Focal neurologic deficits
Adult	Headache
	Consciousness level change
	Photophobia
	Nuchal rigidity
	Seizures
	Focal neurologic deficits
Elderly	Consciousness level change
	Headache
	Nuchal rigidity
	Seizures, including non–convulsive status epilepticus

Source: Adapted from KL Roos, AR Tunkel, WM Scheld. Acute bacterial meningitis in children and adults. In WM Scheld, RJ Whitley, DT Durack (eds), Infections of the Central Nervous System. Philadelphia: Lippincott–Raven, 1997;336–401.

zures than it predicts seizure occurrence in individual patients.

In a study of seizure complications of bacterial sepsis–related encephalopathy, approximately 40% of cases manifested seizures.[9] Although systemic sepsis may cause seizures by disturbing cortical function (e.g., synaptic transmission, cerebral energy production) via diffuse toxic or metabolic mechanisms, other potential autopsy-revealed etiologies included bacterial intraparenchymal invasion with microabscess formation, cortical proliferation of astrocytes and microglia, microinfarcts, multiple small white-matter hemorrhages, and central pontine myelinolysis.

Bacterial Meningitis

Epidemiology

Approximately 25,000 cases of bacterial meningitis occur annually in the United States, with approximately 70% of all cases occurring in children younger than 5 years old.[10] The relative frequency with which each bacterial species causes meningitis is age related, as summarized in Table 6-6.

In a large review (n = 493) of adult bacterial meningitis cases managed at Massachusetts General Hospital from 1962 to 1988, 40% of cases were nosocomial, of which 33% were caused by gram-negative bacilli. In the 60% of cases that were community acquired, the most common pathogens were *Streptococcus pneumoniae* (37%), *Neisseria meningitidis* (13%), and *Listeria monocytogenes* (10%).[11]

Diagnosis of Bacterial Meningitis

Table 6-7 summarizes the common neurologic manifestations of bacterial meningitis by age group.

Laboratory Diagnosis

Cerebrospinal Fluid Analysis. The decision to perform a lumbar puncture (LP) is based on clinical presentation (i.e., meningitic signs). When the clinical threshold for LP has been reached, LP performance requires confirmation that a focal intracranial mass lesion (e.g., tumor, abscess, epidural abscess, subdural empyema [SDE]) causing increased intracranial pressure, which might predispose to brain herniation after LP, does not exist. This is especially relevant when the clinical presentation includes a

Table 6-8. Characteristic Cerebrospinal Fluid Profile of Bacterial Meningitis

Opening pressure	>180 cm H_2O
Glucose	<40 mg/dl
Cerebrospinal fluid: serum to glucose ratio	<0.31
Protein	>50 mg/dl
Red blood cell	Usually 0
White blood cell	>10 to <10,000/mm^2 (neutrophil predominance)
Gram's stain	Positive in >70% cases
Culture	Species-specific positive in 70–90% of untreated cases

Source: Adapted from KL Roos, AR Tunkel, WM Scheld. Acute bacterial meningitis in children and adults. In WM Scheld, RJ Whitley, DT Durack (eds), Infections of the Central Nervous System. Philadelphia: Lippincott–Raven, 1997;336–401; F Plum, JB Posner. Infectious and Inflammatory Disorders of the Nervous System. In TE Andreoli, CC Carpenter, F Plum, et al. (eds), Cecil Essentials of Medicine. Philadelphia: Saunders, 1990;806–816.

seizure, particularly a seizure of focal onset. If history and neurologic examination (e.g., papilledema) suggest existence of such a mass lesion, then LP must be delayed until neuroimaging is performed. If such neuroimaging imposes a significant treatment delay, then antimicrobial therapy must be started empirically. Table 6-8 summarizes the typical CSF profile of bacterial meningitis.

Other diagnostics serve only as adjuncts to CSF analysis in the diagnosis of acute bacterial meningitis; however, they can provide useful information about neurologic and systemic complications, including seizure occurrence.

Serologic Culture. Because bacterial entry into CSF is usually via a hematogenous route, blood cultures can be positive in up to 75% of cases of *untreated* meningitis.[10, 12]

Neuroimaging. During acute bacterial meningitis, computed tomography (CT) can be normal or can demonstrate meningeal or ependymal enhancement, or both, and cortical sulci or basal cistern, or both, widening secondary to purulent exudate accumulation or bacterial meningitic complications (e.g., subdural effusion or empyema and diffuse cerebral edema), or both. Development of a seizure (or focal neurologic signs) during meningitis is an additional indication for CT, besides the initial pre-LP screen-

ing CT. Magnetic resonance imaging (MRI) is generally more useful than CT; subdural effusions and empyemas, cortical infarctions, and extent of leptomeningeal enhancement are better imaged by MRI.

Electroencephalography. A full range of electroencephalogram (EEG) abnormalities can be seen in the context of acute bacterial meningitis, from nonspecific slowing to status epilepticus. A corresponding variety of EEG findings can occur as part of the neurologic sequelae of bacterial meningitis. Both situations are described in further detail in the following discussion.

Epileptic Complications of Bacterial Meningoencephalitides

Seizures occur in approximately 25% of children with bacterial meningitis and in more than 30% of adults with pneumococcal meningitis in the first few days of illness. Generalized convulsive seizures may occur as part of the presentation of bacterial meningitis, along with the classic triad of fever, headache, and stiff neck. Of bacterial pathogens, seizures are most often associated with *Haemophilus influenzae*.[13]

Generalized seizures and a depressed level of consciousness can occur as a consequence of inflammation and bacterial toxin accumulation in the subpial space early in the course of infection. As the meningeal infectious process progresses, meningeal veins can become thrombosed, producing focal neurologic deficits including focal seizures.[13]

In the large meningitis case review performed at Massachusetts General Hospital, which was discussed previously, seizures occurred in 23% of patients with community-acquired meningitis, and risk factors for death among those patients with single episodes of community-acquired meningitis included seizure occurrence within 24 hours of presentation.[11]

Patients with bacterial meningitis who have been taking oral antibiotics can present with seizure as the sole initial sign or symptom; hence, all patients taking antibiotics who develop a seizure require an LP to exclude meningitis. Rosenberg et al. reviewed the records of 187 patients with bacterial meningitis. Seizures were a presenting manifestation in 13%, and 28% of these patients had been taking antibiotics before diagnosis. Twenty-five percent of pretreated patients had no signs or symptoms other than seizure, whereas all patients without pretreatment had additional findings (p <.01). Patients with seizures had a poorer outcome than those without seizures.[14]

Listeria represents an important cause of meningitis and meningoencephalitis, frequently complicated by seizures. In a large (n = 820) retrospective case review of CNS listeriosis (excluding pregnancy), compared to patients with acute meningitis secondary to other bacteria, patients with *Listeria* had a significantly lower incidence of meningeal signs. Further, CSF profile was significantly less likely to have a high white blood cell (WBC) count or elevated protein concentration, and Gram's stains were negative in two-thirds of CNS listeriosis cases. However, 25% of cases developed seizures. Mortality was 26% overall and was higher among patients with seizures.[15]

Of Rickettsial diseases, only Rocky Mountain spotted fever has significant epileptic comorbidity, with almost 10% of cases manifesting seizure as an acute illness component. *Rickettsia rickettsii* is transmitted via a number of different tick species. Treatment of infection is by tetracycline or doxycycline. After successful management of acute illness, CNS abnormalities, including EEG abnormalities, can persist in up to 50% of patients.[16]

Cerebral ischemia is a common complication of bacterial meningitis. Increased cerebral blood flow velocity (CBFV) in intracranial arteries, probably secondary to vasospasm, is a known finding in cerebral ischemia. In a prospective study of intracranial CBFVs via transcranial Doppler sonography in patients with bacterial meningitis, *seizures were more frequent (43% vs. 7%) in patients with CBFV greater than 210 cm per second.* Thus, because transcranial Doppler sonography is an easily applicable, noninvasive technique for revealing vascular changes, even in severely ill patients, and because data suggest a greater seizure complication risk with increased CBFV, transcranial Doppler sonography could potentially be used to identify high-risk patients who could benefit from seizure prophylaxis.[17]

Treatment

Complicated factors involving etiologic bacterial species, blood-brain barrier penetration, antibacterial activity within purulent CSF, drug metabolism, potential drug interactions, and host defense status affect antibiotic choice. However, general guidelines are well developed and summarized in Table 6-9.

Table 6-9. Antibacterial Management of Bacterial Meningitis

Organism	Antibiotic
Streptococcus pneumoniae	
Penicillin-sensitive	Penicillin G or ampicillin
Partial penicillin-sensitive	Third generation cephalosporin
Penicillin-resistant	Vancomycin + third generation cephalosporin
Neisseria meningitidis	Penicillin G or ampicillin
Haemophilus influenzae	
Beta-lactamase negative	Ampicillin
Beta-lactamase positive	Third generation cephalosporin
Enterobacteriaceae	Third generation cephalosporin
Pseudomonas aeruginosa	Ceftazidime
Listeria monocytogenes	Penicillin G or ampicillin
Staphylococcus aureus	
Methicillin-sensitive	Nafcillin or oxacillin
Methicillin-resistant	Vancomycin
Staphylococcus epidermidis	Vancomycin

Source: Adapted from KL Roos, AR Tunkel, WM Scheld. Acute bacterial meningitis in children and adults. In WM Scheld, RJ Whitley, DT Durack (eds), Infections of the Central Nervous System. Philadelphia: Lippincott–Raven, 1997;336–401.

Epileptic Complications of Pediatric Bacterial Meningitis

Neonatal bacterial meningitis is associated with significant neurologic sequelae. In a retrospective study of infants with culture-proven neonatal meningitis, a review of EEGs obtained during the acute phase of infection demonstrated that degree of background abnormality proved to be an accurate predictor of outcome. Infants who had normal or mildly abnormal backgrounds had normal outcomes, whereas those with markedly abnormal EEGs died or manifested severe neurologic sequelae at follow-up. When EEG was considered in the context of presence or absence of clinical seizures and level of consciousness, an accurate prediction of neurologic outcome was obtained in 93% of cases. Although EEG patterns were generally nonspecific, some abnormalities (i.e., positive rolandic sharp waves, persistent hemispheric or focal voltage attenuation) suggested more specific pathology (e.g., deep white matter necrosis, large-vessel infarction and abscess, respectively). Thus, besides being valuable for recognition of subtle and subclinical seizures, EEG proved valuable for predicting long-term prognosis of infants with neonatal bacterial meningitis.[18]

Inoue et al. studied seizures occurring in the acute phase of aseptic and bacterial meningitis in children. Of the study sample with aseptic meningitis, approximately 5% had seizures; 80% of these developed seizures within 24 hours of initial symptom onset (fever in 60%), and 60% had repeated seizures on the first day. Of the study sample with bacterial meningitis, approximately 17% had a seizure, which in all cases occurred on the second day of illness. Abnormal head CT was found in all bacterial meningitis cases of patients who seized. The authors inferred that seizures occurring in the acute phase of aseptic meningitis tend to reflect transient cortical dysfunction secondary to nonstructural (e.g., metabolic) mechanisms (e.g., fever or syndrome of inappropriate secretion of antidiuretic hormone), whereas seizures complicating bacterial meningitis tend to be associated with structural factors.[19]

To study risk factors for adverse outcomes from pediatric bacterial meningitis, Grimwood et al. prospectively studied 166 cases for 5–9 years with neurologic, neuropsychologic, audiologic, and behavioral assessments. Statistical analysis revealed that seizures complicating the acute episode were associated with an adverse outcome.[20] Baraff at al. performed a meta-analysis of pediatric bacterial meningitis reports to determine neurologic sequelae frequencies in children 2 months to 19 years of age. Of approximately 1,600 children with acute bacterial meningitis evaluated for at least one sequela after hospital discharge, 4.2% had epilepsy as a likely consequence of having had childhood bacterial meningitis.[21]

In what turned out to be a study of a long-term complication of childhood bacterial meningitis and febrile seizure, Cascino et al. performed a prospective investigation of neuroimaging and temporal lobe pathology in 13 patients with facial asymmetry and intractable partial epilepsy of temporal lobe origin. All patients had a history of childhood bacterial meningitis or febrile seizure. Facial weakness occurred primarily during emotional expression (i.e., spontaneous smiling). Temporal lobe of seizure origin, demonstrated by ictal EEG recording, was always contralateral to the side of facial weakness. Hippocampal atrophy

was present in all epileptic temporal lobes as measured by MRI volume studies. Thus, facial asymmetry and partial epilepsy associated with mesial temporal sclerosis can occur as long-term sequelae of childhood bacterial meningitis.[22]

Spirochetal Infections

Syphilis

Primary syphilis occurs within days of infection via direct inoculation of *Treponema pallidum* at cutaneous or mucous membrane sites and is manifested by a syphilitic ulcer, the chancre. Without treatment, the chancre heals over 3–6 weeks, after which most patients progress to the secondary stage, in which systemic spirochetemia is marked primarily by flulike symptoms. Untreated, secondary syphilis also resolves over weeks to months. After a variable-length clinically silent latency period ranging from months to years, approximately one-third of patients with untreated latent syphilis go on to develop tertiary disease, which can present as cardiovascular syphilis, gummatous syphilis, or neurosyphilis, or a combination of these. Neurosyphilis can be subdivided into several syndromes occurring at different points in the natural history of untreated syphilis; it is useful to categorize these, as shown in Table 6-10, for the purpose of conceptualizing syphilitic seizure occurrence.

As shown, seizures can occur in all clinically expressed stages of neurosyphilis. In syphilitic meningitis, given the nonfocal stimulus of diffuse meningeal inflammation, seizures tend to be generalized. General paresis (dementia paralytica) also tends to be a nonlocalizing syndrome, and complicating seizures tend to be generalized. In contrast, gummatous neurosyphilis presents with signs and symptoms secondary to mass lesions at gummata sites; therefore, partial seizures with localizing quality are often seen.

Diagnosis of CNS syphilitic involvement involves consideration of a constellation of lab tests within the context of careful history taking and physical examination. Well-known serologic screening tests include VDRL and rapid plasma reagent; fluorescent treponemal antibody absorption enhances diagnostic specificity after positive screening test results (although fluorescent treponemal antibody absorp-

Table 6-10. Clinical Classification of Neurosyphilis

Central Nervous System (CNS) Syphilitic Stage	Pathology	Manifestations	Peak Incidence	Neuroimaging
Asymptomatic CNS involvement	Abnormal cerebrospinal fluid ($\uparrow$ protein, white blood cell >5, + VDRL)	Asymptomatic	Anytime	$\pm$ Meningeal enhancement
Syphilitic meningitis (luetic meningitis)	Aseptic meningitis (cerebrospinal fluid profile as above)	$\uparrow$ Intracranial pressure, cranial nerve palsies, seizures	1–2 yrs postinfection	Meningeal enhancement
Meningovascular syphilis				
Cerebrovascular	Endarteritis, $\pm$ infarcts	Sudden-onset focal-cerebral symptoms, seizures	5–7 yrs postinfection	Infarcts (cortical, subcortical)
Spinal	Endarteritis, meningeal inflammation, myelomalacia	Paresthesias, weakness, atrophy, sensory loss	5–7 yrs postinfection	N/A
Parenchymatous neurosyphilis				
Paretic	Meningoencephalitis	Neuropsychiatric symptoms, seizures	10–20 yrs postinfection	Optic atrophy
Tabetic	Leptomeningitis; degeneration of posterior roots, dorsal funiculi, brain stem	Pain, paresthesias, ataxia, Argyll-Robertson pupil, $\downarrow$ deep tendon reflexes, $\downarrow$ proprioception	10–20 yrs postinfection	N/A
Gummatous neurosyphilis	Gummata formation	Signs 2^0 gummata mass effects, seizures	Anytime	Mass lesions

N/A = not available; $\uparrow$ = increased; $\downarrow$ = decreased; $\pm$ = with or without.
Source: Adapted from LP Rowland. Spirochete Infections: Neurosyphilis. In: LP Rowland (ed), Merritt's Textbook of Neurology. Baltimore: Williams & Wilkins, 1995;200–212.

tion has low specificity of disease activity, remaining positive long after successful treatment). Diagnosis of neurosyphilis requires positive serology and reactive CSF–VDRL. CSF pleocytosis is the best measure of disease activity; in an untreated patient, there should be 5 or more WBC/mm^3. CSF protein is usually elevated, and CSF glucose can be mildly decreased. Also, nonspecifically, CSF gamma globulin can be increased, and oligoclonal bands can be present.

Treatment in all of these stages is of course directed at the underlying spirochete, as summarized in Table 6-11.

Anticonvulsant treatment should only be initiated after seizure expression; that is, there is no role for prophylaxis. When needed, routine application of antiepileptic drug principles applies. Seizure-producing gummas responding too slowly to penicillin can be treated with steroids.[23]

Lyme Disease

Lyme disease is a worldwide tick-transmitted spirochetosis with endemic foci throughout North America, Europe, and Asia. *Borrelia burgdorferi* is the etiologic bacterium; the vector is a tick of the genus *Ixodes*. Lyme disease is now the most common vector-borne illness in the United States. Seasonal pattern of tick activity determines seasonal pattern of illness onset; symptoms typically begin in late spring or summer. Because ticks prefer for-

Table 6-11. Antibiotic Treatment of Syphilis

Stage	Treatment
Primary, secondary, or early latent	PCN G 2–4 million U i.m. (PCN-allergic: doxycycline, tetracycline)
Late latent or unknown duration	PCN G 2–4 million U i.m. q.wk. × 3 wks (PCN-allergic: doxycycline, tetracycline)
Tertiary disease, except neurosyphilis	PCN G 2–4 million U i.m. q.wk. × 3 wks (PCN-allergic: doxycycline, tetracycline)
Neurosyphilis	PCN G 2–4 million U i.v. q4h. × 14 days PCN G 2–4 million U i.m. q.d. + probenecid 500 mg q.i.d. × 14 days (PCN-allergic: no alternative)

PCN = penicillin.
Source: Adapted from LP Rowland. Spirochete Infections: Neurosyphilis. In: LP Rowland (ed), Merritt's Textbook of Neurology. Baltimore: Williams & Wilkins, 1995;200–212; EW Hook. Syphilis. In WM Scheld, RJ Whitley, DT Durack (eds), Infections of the Central Nervous System. Philadelphia: Lippincott–Raven, 1997;669–684.

Table 6-12. Clinical Stages of Lyme Disease

Stage	Clinical Abnormality
Early localized	*Erythema migrans* (EM)
	Regional lymphadenopathy
	Mild systemic symptoms
Early disseminated	Multiple secondary EM
	Severe systemic symptoms
	Generalized lymphadenopathy
	Migratory musculoskeletal pain
	Acute arthritis
	Myocarditis
	Pericarditis
	Polyneuritis
	Meningitis
	Early neurologic abnormalities (see Table 6-11)
Late disseminated	Chronic arthritis
	Late neurologic abnormalities (see Table 6-11)

Source: Adapted from L Reik. Lyme Disease. In WM Scheld, RJ Whitley, DT Durack (eds), Infections of the Central Nervous System. Philadelphia: Lippincott–Raven, 1997;685–718; DW Rahn, MW Felz. Lyme disease update. Postgraduate Medicine 1998;103:51–70.

est underbrush, illness is more common in such areas.

Lyme disease begins locally and spreads systemically. Skin, heart, joints, and nervous system are the organ systems most often involved. Illness typically evolves in sequential stages, as outlined in Table 6-12.

Early Localized Infection

Illness begins days to 1 month after tick bite. A red macule or papule arises at tick bite site, which expands centrifugally to form an annular erythematous lesion. *B. burgdorferi* proliferation and the host's immune reaction eventually produce the characteristic skin lesion erythema migrans (EM) in approximately 80% of U.S. cases (40% in Europe). EM is the best clinical marker for Lyme disease.

Early Disseminated Infection

Within days to weeks, *B. burgdorferi* spreads hematogenously. The organism also probably enters the CNS at this time (*B. burgdorferi* DNA, outer

surface protein antigens, and the organism itself have been recovered from CSF as early as 18 days after inoculation). One to two months postinfection, *B. burgdorferi* localizes and becomes sequestered in certain tissues, including the CNS. The CNS is involved in up to 20% of untreated North American patients (50% in European populations). Meningitis, typically lymphocytic, is the most common neuropathologic abnormality in early disseminated Lyme disease. Systemic symptoms can be present, but EM, fever, and lymphadenopathy are usually gone by the time neurologic complications develop. *In fact, neurologic deficits, including seizure, can occur without antecedent EM and can constitute initial disease manifestation.* Multiple neurologic signs have been reported to be associated with early CNS Lyme disease, as outlined in Table 6-13.

Neurologic abnormalities of late Lyme disease usually develop a year or more after illness onset. Although vague neuropsychiatric deficits (e.g., somnolence, emotional lability, depression, impaired memory, and behavioral symptoms) are most common, the best-defined late CNS abnormality is progressive *Borrelia* encephalomyelitis.[27] Seizures can

Table 6-13. Central Nervous System (CNS) Syndromes Associated with Lyme Disease

Early CNS Abnormalities	Late CNS Abnormalities
Acute aseptic meningitis	Progressive
Acute purulent meningitis	encephalomyelitis
Chronic lymphocytic meningitis	Focal encephalitis
Recurrent meningitis	Cerebral vasculitis
Acute meningoencephalitis	Stroke
Acute focal encephalitis	Multi-infarct dementia
Encephalomyelitis	Leukoencephalitis
Leukoencephalitis	Brain stem
Acute cerebellar ataxia	encephalitis
Acute parkinsonian syndrome	Late encephalopathy
Acute transverse myelitis	Cerebellar ataxia
Subacute myelitis	Transverse myelitis
Cognitive deficits	Progressive spastic
Affective disturbance	para- or
Seizures	quadriparesis
	Cognitive deficits
	Affective disturbance
	Seizures

Source: Adapted from L Reik. Lyme Disease. In WM Scheld, RJ Whitley, DT Durack (eds), Infections of the Central Nervous System. Philadelphia: Lippincott–Raven, 1997;685–718.

occur in 7% of these cases.[25] Focal motor, partial complex, and generalized convulsions can all occur.

Lyme disease should be suspected in any patient with chronic lymphocytic meningitis or mild meningoencephalitis with associated cranial neuritis or radiculitis. Lab tests include serologic assays like

Table 6-14. Cerebrospinal Fluid Analysis in Lyme Disease Encephalomeningitis

Opening Pressure	Normal
White blood cell; % lymphocytes	>100; >90
Glucose	Normal
Protein	Mild to moderate ↑
Oligoclonal bands	Present
B. burgdorferi antibody	Positive

↑ = increase.
Source: Adapted from L Reik. Lyme Disease. In WM Scheld, RJ Whitley, DT Durack (eds), Infections of the Central Nervous System. Philadelphia: Lippincott–Raven, 1997;685–718; JR Miller. Spirochete Infections: Lyme Disease. In LP Rowland (ed), Merritt's Textbook of Neurology. Baltimore: Williams & Wilkins, 1995;209–211.

Table 6-15. Diagnostic Criteria for Central Nervous System Lyme Disease

Definite neuroborreliosis	Compatible neurologic abnormality plus one of the following: History of *Erythema migrans* Presence of acrodermatitis chronica atrophicans or lymphocytoma Serum and CSF immunoreactivity or CSF reactivity alone against *B. burgdorferi* by enzyme-linked immunoassay or Western blot Serum immunoreactivity to *B. burgdorferi* and non-neurologic organ system Lyme involvement Seroconversion or fourfold rise in antibody titer between acute and convalescent sera
Probable neuroborreliosis	Compatible neurologic abnormality and serum immunoreactivity to *B. burgdorferi*
Possible neuroborreliosis	Compatible neurologic abnormality and history of tick bite or travel or residence in endemic area

Source: Adapted from L Reik. Lyme Disease. In WM Scheld, RJ Whitley, DT Durack (eds), Infections of the Central Nervous System. Philadelphia: Lippincott–Raven, 1997;685–718.

immunofluorescent assay and enzyme-linked immunoassay tests for anti–*B. burgdorferi* antibodies. Specific anti–*B. burgdorferi* antibody also appears in CSF, where it can be detected even when serum antibody tests are negative (to establish whether these antibodies are synthesized intrathecally, serum and CSF antibody levels should be measured simultaneously).[28] CSF profile and diagnostic criteria set for Lyme neuroborreliosis are outlined in Tables 6-14 and 6-15, respectively.

EEG in most patients with late Lyme disease cortical dysfunction (and many patients without) demonstrates nonspecific generalized slowing, focal slowing, or increases in sharp wave activity, or a combination of these.[13] MRI abnormalities can include multifocal white-matter abnormalities, infarct patterns, periventricular and subinsular encephalomalacia, and pontine and medullary atrophy.[25,27]

Treatment regimens for Lyme disease are outlined in Table 6-16. Comorbid seizures are treated via routine antiepileptic management principles.

Table 6-16. Antibiotic Treatment of Lyme Disease

Lyme Disease Stage	Treatment Options
Erythema migrans and systemic symptoms	
Adults	Amoxicillin 500 mg p.o. + probenecid 500 mg t.i.d. × 2–4 wks
	Doxycycline 100 mg b.i.d. × 2–4 wks
	Cefuroxime 500 mg b.i.d. × 2–4 wks
Children	Amoxicillin 25–50 mg/kg/day × 2–4 wks
	Erythromycin 30 mg/kg/day × 2–4 wks
	Cefuroxime 250 mg b.i.d. × 2–4 wks
Early neurologic involvement	
Facial palsy alone	Oral antibiotics, same treatment as above
All others	
Adults	Ceftriaxone 2 g/day i.v. × 2–4 wks
	Cefotaxime 2 g i.v. t.i.d. × 2–4 wks
	Penicillin G 20 million U/day i.v. × 10–14 days
	Doxycycline 100 mg p.o. b.i.d. × 2–4 wks
Children	Ceftriaxone 75–100 mg/kg i.v. × 2–4 wks
	Penicillin G 300,000 U/kg/day i.v. × 10–14 days
Late neurologic involvement	
Adults	Penicillin, ceftriaxone, or cefotaxime i.v., same treatment as for early involvement
	Doxycycline 100–200 mg p.o. b.i.d. × 30 days
Children	Penicillin or ceftriaxone i.v., same treatment as for early involvement

Source: Adapted from L Reik. Lyme Disease. In WM Scheld, RJ Whitley, DT Durack (eds), Infections of the Central Nervous System. Philadelphia: Lippincott–Raven, 1997;685–718; DW Rahn, MW Felz. Lyme disease update. Postgraduate Medicine 1998;103:51–70; JR Miller. Spirochete Infections: Lyme Disease. In LP Rowland (ed), Merritt's Textbook of Neurology. Baltimore: Williams & Wilkins, 1995;209–211.

Seizure Complications of Bacterial Endocarditis

Neurologic complications occur in approximately 30% of all patients with bacterial endocarditis, and seizures are not uncommon complications. In one series of 218 patients with endocarditis, 39% had a neurologic complication and 58% of these died (in contrast, mortality was only 20% among endocarditis patients without neurologic complications). Of neurologic complications, cerebral embolism is the most frequent and clinically significant and is particularly common in patients with mitral valve infection and with endocarditis due to virulent organisms (e.g., *Staphylococcus aureus* and enteric gram-negative bacilli). Emboli are important not only for their direct morbidity via cerebral infarction, but also because of their role as epileptogenic foci in the form of mycotic aneurysms and brain abscesses. Focal seizures are more commonly associated with acute emboli.[29] Generalized seizures are of diverse etiologies, with systemic (e.g., metabolic) and iatrogenic seizures (e.g., drug induced) being most frequent.[30]

Seizure Complications of Antibacterial Treatment

Most antibiotics are CNS-safe, and neurotoxicity associated with antibiotic administration is infrequent.[31] However, anecdotal reports of seizures complicating antibiotic use exist, and some antibiotics are more frequently reported to be associated with seizures. The exact incidence of seizures complicating antibiotic use is not known. Interpretation of empiric studies and meta-analyses of seizure complications of antibiotic use is complicated by the fact that patients given antibiotics often have other seizure risk factors, making causal attribution of seizure to antibiotic administration difficult. For example, background seizure rate in seriously ill patients likely to receive intravenous antibiotics could be as high as 4%.[32] Beta-lactams are the antibiotic class most commonly associated with adverse CNS events.

Penicillins

The neurotoxicity of penicillin was first reported in 1945 by Johnson and Walker, who observed myoclonic twitching after intravenous administration. Further reports appeared in the 1960s of a penicillin-related syndrome involving serially appearing hyper-reflexia, myoclonic jerks, and sometimes seizures. Semisynthetic penicillins have also been implicated[33]; for example, oxacillin and dicloxacillin induce epileptogenic changes in rabbits.[34]

Epileptogenic characteristics of beta-lactams, like their antimicrobial and antigenic properties, are structure dependent. The beta-lactam ring is a key feature of penicillin epileptogenesis; convulsant properties are abolished after incubation with penicillinase.[35,36] However, ring substitution can influence convulsant activity. For example, substitution of a benzylic hydrogen with an amino group (e.g., as in ampicillin and amoxicillin) reduces epileptogenic potential. Drugs characterized by the presence of a ureido group (e.g., piperacillin) demonstrate epileptogenesis lower than that of penicillin.

Cephalosporins

Cephalosporins differ from penicillins in having a six-membered thiazolide moiety fused to the beta-lactam ring. Different substitutions at different sites can affect epileptogenesis.[37] Accordingly, compounds with similar substituent profiles—ceftriaxone, cefotetan, ceftazidime, and cefepime (heterocyclic ring at position 3 and a heteroaromatic nucleus at position 7 of 7-aminocephalosporanic acid)—show similar evidence of epileptogenesis but less than that of penicillin. Compounds having one heterocyclic ring at position 7, such as cefuroxime and cefixime, show no epileptic activity. In contrast, two other similarly substituted cephalosporins, cefazolin and cefmetazole, have greater epileptogenic activity (in fact, marked similarity to the proconvulsant drug PTZ).[31]

Similar epileptiform electrographic changes to those induced by penicillin have been observed after infusion of high doses of cefazolin.[38,39] However, actual reports of cefazolin-related seizures are unusual.[40] Incidence of CNS adverse events observed during third-generation cephalosporin therapy remains below 1%.[41–44] Clinical experience with fourth-generation cephalosporins (e.g., cefepime) is still limited; however, no significant seizure associations have been reported (only three cases of seizures were reported in a large survey [n >2,000] of patients treated with cefepime, and these were found unrelated to antibiotic administration).[45]

Monobactams

Aztreonam possesses greater convulsant properties than some cephalosporins, but much less than penicillin and cefazolin.[46,47] In a series of 22 bacterial meningitis patients treated with aztreonam, seizures occurred in the acute phase in six cases but were considered more likely related to underlying disease than aztreonam.[48]

Carbapenems

Seizure incidence of imipenem or cilastatin use was first reported by the manufacturer to be 0.4%. Although phase I and II trials did not reveal significant seizure potential, phase III clinical trials and subsequent postmarketing surveys demonstrated that imipenem or cilastatin can be associated with seizures.[49–52] A maximal incidence of 33% was found in a small series of 21 children with bacterial meningitis.[31] Calandra et al. reviewed more than 1,700 patients treated with imipenem or cilastatin to determine carbapenem seizure risk.[32] Patients were moderately to severely ill, with multiple organ system dysfunction, many of whom had independently-associated seizure risks. Three percent of patients had seizures, but in only 0.9% were seizures judged to be possibly, probably, or definitely related to imipenem or cilastatin. A seizure incidence of 2–3% was noted among patients treated with other antibiotics. Average time of seizure onset was 7 days after imipenem or cilastatin initiation. As with other beta-lactam antibiotics, CNS disorders (including premorbid epilepsy) and renal insufficiency were independent risk factors for seizure occurrence. Imipenem dosage in excess of recommended guidelines, especially in patients with renal insufficiency, was also a seizure risk factor. As is usually the case with such retrospective analyses, high background seizure incidence in the severely ill patient population in which these antibiotics are used makes precise seizure etiology attribution difficult.[32]

There is an apparent increase in the proconvulsive activity of imipenem in combination with cilastatin. This could merely be due to elevated imipenem levels in the presence of cilastatin (via cilastatin's inhibition of renal tubular secretion of imipenem). Alternatively, cilastatin might increase CSF levels of imipenem by inhibiting CSF elimination. Cilastatin alone can induce seizures but at doses much higher than those used clinically. De Sarro et al. were able to demonstrate that excitatory amino acid antagonists could counteract seizures induced by imipenem, suggesting an involvement of excitatory amino acids in the genesis of seizures.[53]

In a study of 5,000 patients treated with meropenem, seizure incidence was only 0.08%.[54] Comparison data indicated that seizures occurred no more frequently during treatment with meropenem than during treatment with other beta-lactam antibiotics.[55]

Using the mouse PTZ model, Day et al. found that pretreatment with meropenem did not enhance PTZ-induced seizures, whereas pretreatment with imipenem or cilastatin increased the convulsive activity of PTZ.[56]

Fluoroquinolones

Overall incidence of CNS adverse reactions, including seizure, is less than 1%.[57,58] Isolated case reports note the occurrence of seizures with norfloxacin and ciprofloxacin[59–61]; however, underlying neurologic diseases, renal insufficiency, or concomitant drug use, or a combination of these, known to lower epileptic threshold was almost always present.

Proconvulsant effects of quinolones have been attributed to direct pharmacodynamic effects as well as pharmacokinetic and dynamic interactions with co-administered drugs. Direct pharmacodynamic proconvulsant mechanisms of quinolones may relate to γ-aminobutyric acid (GABA)–like substituents which act as GABA-receptor antagonists.[62] Pharmacokinetic and pharmacodynamic interactions between quinolones and other drugs are best described for concomitant theophylline and nonsteroidal anti-inflammatory drug (NSAID) use.

Several fluoroquinolones potentially interact with theophylline. Vancutsem et al. investigated the influence of fluoroquinolones (ciprofloxacin, norfloxacin) on seizure parameters in amygdaloid-kindled rats and found no change in seizure activity when these antimicrobials were administered alone.[63] However, fluoroquinolone administration concurrent with a nonseizure modulating dose of theophylline resulted in increased seizure activity. Epileptogenic-pharmacodynamic interaction may include centrally mediated mechanisms.[63]

Theophylline, a methylxanthine, is metabolized by several cytochrome P-450 pathway isozymes. Some quinolones exert an inhibitory effect on the cytochrome P-450 system, thereby reducing theophylline clearance with a consequent increase in theophylline blood levels.[64] Meta-analysis of quinolone-theophylline interactions revealed that enoxacin may be the strongest inhibitor of theophylline metabolism.[31]

NSAIDs can also enhance fluoroquinolone toxicity. Certain NSAID metabolites (e.g., biphenylacetic acid) can increase the antagonistic potency of certain quinolones on $GABA_A$ receptors.[65–67]

In sum, although seizures are a relatively unusual complication of antibiotic use, clinical and experimental studies suggest certain risk. For the clinician, seizure risk can be minimized by maintaining cognizance of well-defined predisposing conditions[68,69]:

Age: Age-related changes in drug metabolism, renal clearance, or blood-brain barrier permeability, or a combination of these, may enhance antibiotic seizure risk.

Pre-existing CNS disease: includes epilepsy, intracranial mass, and meningitis.

Renal insufficiency: Excess dosage relative to renal function and body weight seems to be the most common factor explaining antibiotic-related convulsions.

Concomitant use of proconvulsant drugs: Pharmacokinetic or pharmacodynamic, or both, drug interactions increasing *antibiotic epileptogenesis*.

For managing antibiotic-related seizure complications, benzodiazepines and barbiturates should be considered for first-line therapy.[31]

Seizure Complications of Mycobacterial Infections

General Principles

Virtually all mycobacterial infections of the CNS are caused by *Mycobacterium tuberculosis*. Infection begins with inhalation of infectious particles; hematogenous dissemination occurs soon thereafter. The reticuloendothelial system is the main target of organism deposition; the brain and meninges, not part of that system, receive relatively few mycobacteria. T-cell–mediated immunity reaction is induced within 4 weeks after infection. A tubercle forms at the site of immune response to mycobacterium, consisting of macrophages and lymphocytes surrounding a necrotic caseous center. Subsequent illness course is a function of host immunologic capacity and poorly defined genetic factors. At best, small caseous foci are completely eliminated, leaving no residua of infection except positive tuberculin skin test. Less efficient host response results in larger caseous foci which harbor viable mycobacteria with the potential to cause reactivated disease if the host's immune status lessens. In the context of impaired host immunity, primary tubercles continue to grow, the caseous center liquefies, organisms proliferate, and the tubercle ruptures, discharging organisms and their antigenically potent products into surrounding tissues. When these events occur within the brain and meninges, tuberculous (TB) meningitis results. Specific CNS syndromes are a function of the original location of the infecting tubercle. Foci located on brain surface or ependyma can rupture into subarachnoid space or the ventricular system to cause meningitis. Foci deep within brain parenchyma can enlarge to form tuberculomas or, more rarely, TB abscesses.[70]

Tuberculous Meningitis

TB meningitis is correctly characterized as a meningoencephalitis, as it affects not only meninges, but also brain parenchyma and vasculature. The primary pathologic event is formation of thick TB exudate within subarachnoid space, most prominently at the base of the brain.[70] Accompanying this exudate is inflammation affecting adjacent blood vessels. Ischemic cerebral infarction, resulting from

Table 6-17. Clinical Staging of Tuberculous Meningitis

Stage	Neurologic Syndrome
I (early)	Nonspecific (e.g., generalized malaise)
II (intermediate)	Lethargy
	Meningismus
	Moderate focal neurologic deficits (e.g., cranial nerve palsies)
III (advanced)	Seizures
	Severe neurologic deficits (e.g., paresis)
	Stupor or coma

Source: Adapted from MB Bader. Role of ciprofloxacin in fatal seizures. Chest 1992;101:883–884.

vascular occlusion, is a common sequela most often found in the distribution of the middle cerebral artery (reflecting presence of TB exudate within sylvian fissure) and striate arteries as they penetrate the base of the brain.[70] Another characteristic feature of TB meningitis is hydrocephalus secondary to CSF dynamic disturbance. Clinical staging of TB meningitis is outlined in Table 6-17.

Seizures are a presenting complaint in 10–20% of children, and more than 50% can develop seizures during their initial hospitalization.[71] Seizures are generally more frequent in younger children.[70] For adults, seizures are the initial presenting manifestation in 10–15% of CNS TB cases.[70]

Diagnosis of CNS tuberculosis begins with the usual investigations required for diagnosing TB: purified protein derivative delayed-hypersensitivity test, chest x-ray, and sputum acid-fast bacillus. Utility of the tuberculin test in diagnosis of acute TB is controversial, and its use in diagnosing TB meningitis is of similarly questionable value. Up to 60% of patients with TB meningitis do not react to purified protein derivative testing.[72,73]

Opening pressure at initial LP is elevated in approximately 50% of patients. Moderate CSF glucose reduction, protein elevation, and moderate pleocytosis are characteristic. Differentials can be variable: Although initially both neutrophils and lymphocytes can be seen, this usually converts to a predominantly lymphocytic profile over several weeks. The concentration of mycobacteria causing meningitis can be small; consequently, acid-fast bacteria are difficult to isolate on CSF acid-fast bacillus stain. Although culture

Table 6-18. Therapeutic Options for
Tuberculous Meningitis

Low probability of drug resistance:
  A. Isoniazid 300 mg q.d. × 6 mos
     Rifampin 600 mg q.d. × 6 mos
     Pyrazinamide 15–30 mg/kg q.d. × 2 mos
  B. Isoniazid 300 mg q.d. × 9–18 mos
     Rifampin 600 mg q.d. × 9–18 mos
     Pyrazinamide 15–30 mg/kg q.d. × 9–18 mos
  C. Isoniazid 300 mg q.d. × 1 mo, then 900 mg b.i.w. × 8 mos
     Rifampin 600 mg q.d. × 1 mo, then 600 mg b.i.w. × 8
        mos
High probability of drug resistance:
  A. Isoniazid 300 mg q.d. × 9–18 mos
     Rifampin 600 mg q.d. × 9–18 mos
     Pyrazinamide 15–30 mg/kg q.d. × 9–18 mos
     Streptomycin 1 g q.d. × 2 mos
  B. Individual case sensitivity–determined regimen

Source: Adapted from A Zuger, FD Lowy. Tuberculosis. In
WM Scheld, RJ Whitley, DT Durack (eds), Infections of the
Central Nervous System. Philadelphia: Lippincott–Raven,
1997;417–443.

is the diagnostic gold standard for TB meningitis, it is insensitive.

Although there are no pathognomonic radiologic changes, some are sufficiently characteristic to raise clinical suspicion. Noncontrast CT can reveal hydrocephalus and hypodensities (consistent with TB exudate or infarcts, or both). Contrast CT can demonstrate meningeal enhancement, frequently surrounding basal cisterns, sylvian fissure, and brain stem. On MRI, involved cranial nerves appear as thickened structures entrapped in enhancing basilar TB exudate.

Principles guiding treatment of TB meningitis are similar to those for other forms of TB, with the added requirement that antimycobacterial agents must penetrate the blood-brain barrier; therapy is outlined in Table 6-18.

Use of steroids in TB meningitis is controversial. Symptomatic amelioration, including seizure control, spinal block prophylaxis, and reported mortality reduction in children are the prime benefits that must be balanced against the risks of systemic steroid complication, steroid withdrawal, and reports of worsening of long-term neurologic outcome. Most authorities now advocate steroid use in TB meningitis only in the context of extreme neurologic compromise, elevated intracranial pres-

sure, impending herniation, or impending spinal block.

Other Central Nervous System Tuberculous Infections

Initial pathogenesis of CNS tuberculoma is identical to that of TB meningitis. However, instead of rupturing into subarachnoid space, tubercles continue to grow, walled off from brain parenchyma and meninges by a dense fibrous capsule. Grossly, lesions are well-circumscribed masses whose size varies from subcentimeter up to several centimeters; lesion number can range from one to several, localized to any brain region. Occasionally, tuberculomas develop during or after treatment for TB meningitis. Clinical sequelae of CNS tuberculomas are those of single or multiple intracranial mass lesions, primarily seizures and correlates of increased intracranial pressure. Seizure semiology can strongly suggest lesion location. Neuroimaging, especially MRI, is diagnostically indispensable, although biopsy remains the gold standard. Intracranial tuberculoma without evidence of systemic TB is relatively rare and difficult to diagnose, remaining clinically quiescent for a long duration; a seizure can be an important sentinel event in such cases. Tseng et al. reported a patient without any history of TB presenting with focal left-hand seizures; neuroimaging revealed a leptomeningeal lesion in the left frontoparietal region. Subsequent histopathologic analysis of a biopsy sample was consistent with tuberculoma.[74] Tosomeen et al. report a similarly seizure-presenting case of multiple intracranial tubeculomas.[75]

If the caseous core of a tuberculoma liquefies, a TB abscess results. These patients tend to be clinically worse overall than those with correspondingly sized tuberculoma. Again, focal seizures can be an important initial clinical manifestation.[76]

As with other forms of TB, CNS TB incidence is greatly increased in human immunodeficiency virus (HIV)–infected patients.[77] In fact, in some HIV populations, TB meningitis is the most common CNS infection. Strangely, in a study of clinical course difference between cerebral tuberculoma in patients with and without HIV infection, cerebral tuberculoma in HIV-negative patients was more likely to be characterized by seizures.[78]

Antituberculous Treatment-Related Epilepsy Considerations

In the 10–15% of patients who are genetically slow acetylators of isoniazid (INH), significant accumulation of concomitantly administered phenytoin can occur secondary to INH inhibition of 2C9 and 2C19 cytochrome P-450 isoenzyme systems, of which phenytoin is a substrate (Table 6-19).[79] INH has also been reported to markedly increase carbamazepine levels, although mechanism of interaction is less clear.[80]

Seizures are a well-documented complication of INH overdose. In a review of INH poisoning in New York City, Sullivan et al. reviewed 41 cases of patients hospitalized for toxic INH exposure.[81] More than half (53.6%) had seizures. INH toxicity should be considered when young patients present with intractable seizures and otherwise negative etiologic workups. Pyridoxine is the antidote.

Epileptic Complications of Mycoplasmal Infection

The majority of CNS complications of mycoplasmal infection result from *Mycoplasma pneumoniae*. Neurologic complications of *M. pneumoniae* can begin days to weeks after onset of respiratory symptomatology and are varied in type and severity.[82] Seizures can complicate mycoplasmal meningitis and meningoencephalitis. Caceres et al. reported a case of a 10 year-old patient presenting with focal onset and rapid secondary generalization seizure intractable to high-dose multiple anticonvulsants, and, ultimately, requiring a phenobarbital drip. Continuous EEG monitoring demonstrated persistent epileptiform discharges. CSF analysis and brain biopsy studies were unrevealing, but mycoplasma pneumonia titers showed elevated immunoglobulin G (IgG) and immunoglobulin M. High-dose methylprednisolone resulted in marked EEG and rapid clinical improvement. Thus, *M. pneumoniae* CNS infection should be considered in the differential diagnosis of seizure and encephalopathy of unclear etiology.[83]

Table 6-19. Treatment Options for *Mycoplasma pneumoniae* Infection

Adults:
Erythromycin 0.5 g p.o. q6h × 14 days
Tetracycline 0.25–0.50 g p.o. q6h × 14 days
Clarithromycin 0.25 g p.o. q12h × 7–14 days
Azithromycin 0.5 g p.o. × 1 day, then 0.25 g p.o. q.d. × 5 days
Children:
<9 yrs old: erythromycin 30–50 mg/kg p.o. q6h × 14 days
>9 yrs old: erythromycin 30 mg/kg p.o. q6h × 14 days, or tetracycline 30–50 mg/kg p.o. q6h × 14 days
>25 kg: same as adult

Source: Adapted from WA Clyde. Mycoplasmal Diseases. In WM Scheld, RJ Whitley, DT Durack (eds), Infections of the Central Nervous System. Philadelphia: Lippincott–Raven, 1997;603–612.

CSF analysis in mycoplasmal meningitis reveals normal or slightly elevated protein, normal or slightly decreased glucose, and WBC counts averaging 80, with polymorphonuclear leukocytes averaging 25%. Organism isolation is difficult. Antimicrobial treatment for CNS mycoplasmal infection, outlined in Table 6-19, is not well developed beyond standard non-CNS mycoplasmal infection. Anticonvulsant management is routine.

Seizure Complications of Viral Infection

A summary of the principal viral CNS syndromes is given in Table 6-20.

Viral Encephalitis

Viral encephalitis is caused by viral infection of brain parenchyma, producing neuronal and glial degeneration, inflammatory infiltration, edema, and tissue necrosis. Viral encephalitis occurs worldwide, with a higher incidence in tropical regions. Between 1,000 and 2,000 cases per year in the United States are reported by the Centers for Disease Control and Prevention (CDC).[86] Focal or generalized seizures are among the common presenting signs and symptoms of viral encephalitis (along with fever, headache, stiff neck, delirium, and stupor or coma).

Table 6-20. Viral Central Nervous System Syndromes with Potential Seizure Complications

Virus	Central Nervous System Syndrome	Geographic Distribution	Route/Vector	Frequency
DNA viruses:				
Herpes viruses				
Herpes simplex virus 1	Encephalitis Meningitis	Worldwide	Human contact, fluids	+++
Herpes simplex virus 2	Encephalitis (neonates) Meningitis	Worldwide	Human contact	+
Varicella-zoster virus	Encephalitis Meningitis	Worldwide	Human respiratory, contact	++
Cytomegalovirus	Encephalitis	Worldwide	Human contact, fluids	++
Epstein-Barr virus	Encephalitis Meningitis	Worldwide	Human saliva	+
Human herpesvirus 6	Encephalitis Febrile seizures	Worldwide	Human contact	Unknown
Adenoviridae				
Adenovirus	Encephalitis Meningitis	Worldwide	Human respiratory	+
Papovavirus				
Jamestown Canyon virus	Progressive multifocal leukoencephalopathy	Worldwide	Unknown	+
RNA viruses:				
Upper respiratory viruses				
Influenza	Encephalitis	Worldwide	Human respiratory	+
Exanthematous viruses				
Measles	Encephalitis Subacute sclerosing panencephalitis	Worldwide	Human respiratory	++
Mumps	Encephalitis Meningitis	Worldwide	Human respiratory	+++
Rhabdoviridae				
Rabies	Encephalitis	Worldwide	Animal bite	+++
Picornaviridae (enterovirus)				
Echovirus	Meningoencephalitis	Worldwide	Fecal-oral	+++
Coxsackie	Meningoencephalitis	Worldwide	Fecal-oral	+++
Polio	Meningitis	Worldwide	Fecal-oral	Rare where vaccinated
Arboviruses				
Bunyaviridae				
California encephalitis virus	Encephalitis Meningitis	North America	Mosquito	+++
Alphavirus				
Eastern equine encephalitis	Encephalitis Meningitis	United States, Caribbean, South America	Mosquito	+
Western equine encephalitis	Encephalitis Meningitis	Western/central United States, South America	Mosquito	++
Flaviviridae				
Japanese encephalitis	Encephalitis Meningitis	China, southeast Asia, India	Mosquito	++++
St. Louis encephalitis	Encephalitis Meningitis	United States, Caribbean, South America	Mosquito	+++

Virus	Central Nervous System Syndrome	Geographic Distribution	Route/Vector	Frequency
West Nile encephalitis	Encephalitis Meningitis	Middle East, Africa, United States (New York City)	Mosquito	++
Retroviruses				
Human immunodeficiency virus 1	Encephalitis	Worldwide	Human blood, semen	++
Lymphocytic choriomeningitis virus	Encephalitis Meningitis	Worldwide	Rodent	+

+ = infrequent; ++ = occasional; +++ = common; ++++ = very common.
Source: Data from MJ Aminoff, DA Greenberg, RP Simon. Clinical Neurology. Stamford, CT: Appleton & Lange, 1996;29–30; KA Cassady, RJ Whitley. Pathogenesis and Pathophysiology of Viral Infections of the Central Nervous System. In WM Scheld, RJ Whitley, DT Durack (eds), Infections of the Central Nervous System. Philadelphia: Lippincott–Raven, 1997;7–22.

Investigators fail to identify an etiologic agent in up to 75% of presumed viral CNS infection cases.[85] Indeed, the confusing term *aseptic meningitis* is a testament to the historic difficulty of definitively isolating an etiologic agent in presumed viral meningitides. Amplification of viral nucleic acids from CSF, as done by the polymerase chain reaction (PCR) for example, has considerably improved diagnosis of several acute, subacute, and chronic viral CNS infections. PCR has become the method of choice for rapid noninvasive diagnosis of herpes simplex virus (HSV) encephalitis; other herpes viruses which can now be reliably diagnosed include cytomegalovirus (CMV), varicella-zoster virus (VZV), Epstein-Barr virus (EBV), and human herpesvirus 6 (HHV-6). In acquired immunodeficiency syndrome (AIDS), PCR can help differentiate lesions due to HIV itself or to opportunistic infections such as progressive multifocal leukoencephalopathy (PML) caused by Jamestown Canyon virus or CMV-related complications.[87]

Herpes Encephalitis

Epidemiology

HSV causes the most common form of sporadic potentially fatal encephalitis in children older than 6 months and adults worldwide. In the United States, herpes simplex encephalitis (HSE) may account for up to 20% of all encephalitis cases.[88]

HSE occurs in all age groups, strikes without gender or seasonal predilection, and has an annual incidence of 1 per 250,000 to 500,000.[89] CNS HSV infection is divided into two groups: neonatal HSV infection, caused by HSV-2, and HSE, which occurs in children outside the neonatal period and adults and is caused by HSV-1.

Pathophysiology

Approximately half of neonatal HSV cases have CNS involvement, either as part of disseminated infection or as encephalitis alone. Neonatal HSV infection is usually contracted by vertical transmission from infected mother to neonate, mainly via fetal intrapartum contact with genital HSV infection (85% of cases).[13] Congenital infection rarely occurs; remaining infections are due to postpartum virus exposure. Newborns with disseminated disease present within 1 week; when neonatal encephalitis occurs alone, it presents at an average age of 2 weeks. The slightly older age at presentation in the group with isolated encephalitis and the observation that this group usually does not develop skin lesions suggest a different pathogenesis from the cutaneous or disseminated forms of the disease.[90] Access of HSV to CNS in neonatal encephalitis is thought to occur via intraneuronal routes. Brain disease is initially localized to one or both temporal lobes and then may progress to involve all brain regions.[88]

HSE in older children and adults is caused by both primary and recurrent HSV infection. Approximately two-thirds of cases are caused by virus reactivation. The route of access of the virus to CNS in primary infections is under exploration but has been documented to occur after tooth pulp inoculation via the trigeminal nerve[91] and by olfactory bulb involvement.[92] Such infection paths are consistent with temporal and orbitofrontal localization of resulting encephalitis.

Pathology

HSE is characterized by intense meningitis and destructive changes in brain parenchyma. Inflammation with accompanying necrosis and hemorrhage occur, often maximally involving frontal and temporal lobes. Temporal brain regions are most involved quantitatively in autopsy studies.[88]

HSV-1 strains vary widely with regard to their neurovirulence and epileptogenesis. Stroop and Schaefer used clonally related strains (gram-positive cocci [+GC] and gram-negative cocci [–GC]) of HSV-1 to determine the pathophysiologic basis of neurovirulence in a rabbit model. After intranasal inoculation, +GC infection was nearly uniformly fatal, whereas –GC infection was asymptomatic. The +GC infected animals developed EEG abnormalities that preceded severe motor seizures, and +GC antigens were found in the first cortical layer of animals that developed seizures. These results suggest that the ability of HSV-1 to induce electrophysiologic brain abnormalities is associated with its ability to replicate within specific brain centers.[93]

Clinical Manifestations

HSE presents as a focal encephalitis. Neurologic signs found early in disease course (e.g., aphasia, confusion, behavioral changes) can progress to a fulminant illness characterized by recurrent focal or generalized seizures, coma, and death.[88] Hemiparesis is evident at the time of presentation in approximately one-third of cases.[90]

Partial seizures that can secondarily generalize are frequent in HSE, occurring in up to 40% of cases.[13] Abnormal brain electrophysiology without clinical seizure expression is even more common, occurring in most patients.[13] Pathophysiology of epileptogenesis is unclear and the subject of competing theories, including: (1) dysfunction of GABA-ergic neurons; (2) dysfunction of excitatory neurons; (3) deranged acetylcholine (ACh) retention within nerve terminals, resulting in potential excitatory-neurotransmitter release and seizure-focus triggering; (4) suboptimal ACh uptake by malfunctioning infected presynaptic and postsynaptic terminals, resulting in relative excess of ACh and consequent pathologic discharge; (5) deficiency of excitatory-neurotransmitter degradatory enzymes (e.g., acetylcholinesterase); and (6) more general mechanisms by which an infected neuron incurs disturbed homeostasis with predisposition to inappropriate discharge.[88]

The possibility that HSE underlies a variety of epileptic syndromes is being investigated, including epilepsy associated with chronic encephalitides. For example, Jay et al. reported two patients presenting with intractable seizures who eventually had HSV-1 detected.[94] In one patient, an intrauterine infection was suspected as the underlying basis for the seizure disorder and extensive cerebral calcification and gliosis. The other patient underwent temporal lobectomy for medically refractory seizures at age 3 years, and pathologic examination revealed chronic encephalitis. Although immunohistochemical, ultrastructural, and culture studies were negative for viral pathogens, PCR revealed HSV-1 deoxyribonucleic acid sequence in both cases.[94] In another report, Jay et al. detected HSV-1 in the brains of three patients who presented with intractable seizures.[95] All three patients had a previous history of HSV-1 encephalitis and went on to develop a medically refractory seizure disorder necessitating surgical intervention. Pathologic examination revealed chronic encephalitis in all three cases. Although immunohistochemical and ultrastructural studies were negative for viral pathogens, PCR analysis revealed HSV-1 genome. These cases exemplify chronic encephalitis associated with a seizure disorder in which a definitive viral etiology was documented by PCR, demonstrating persistence of viral genome in brain parenchyma long after the initial episode of treated herpes encephalitis.

Diagnosis

Routine blood tests reveal peripheral leukocytosis. LP demonstrates elevated pressure. CSF studies show normal or mildly decreased glucose, mildly elevated protein, and pleocytosis of 10–1,000 cells/mm³, usually with lymphocytic or mixed lymphocytic and neutrophilic predominance.[88] Red blood cells and xanthochromia are frequently seen, although their presence or absence is not diagnostic.[96] Virus is rarely recovered from CSF, and detection of HSV antibodies in CSF is not sensitive or specific enough to make a treatment decision.[88,96] PCR has become the mainstay of noninvasive diagnosis, although the isolation of HSV from the brain biopsy specimen remains the diagnostic gold standard.

CT can demonstrate temporal hypodensity and contrast enhancement but is often normal during the first week of disease. MRI can reveal temporal lobe pathology, including loss of gray-white differentiation, edema, and hemorrhagic components, during the first week of disease.[88,96]

HSE produces dramatic EEG changes that, although not pathognomonic, are highly sugges-tive (80% of biopsy-proven cases).[88,96] EEG patterns include focal slowing, spiking, and paroxysmal lateralizing epileptiform discharges (Figure 6-1).[13] Focal-temporal or lateralized polymorphic delta activity is the earliest change. Diffuse slowing soon follows, with a persistence of temporal predominance. Pseudoperiodic complexes, present on serial EEGs in two-thirds of biopsy-proven cases, appear over temporal regions early in the disease course, usually within 1 month of disease onset.[13] Morphologically, complexes are sharp waves or sharply contoured slow waves and repeat at 1–5 second intervals. Pseudoperiodic complexes can be high amplitude and therefore obviously present but also may be low amplitude and subtle. Bilaterally independent complexes can occur, with a predominance concordant with the severity of the involved side. If bilateral, complexes can be synchronous or asynchronous, with a time-locked relationship between lateralized discharges.[13,88,96]

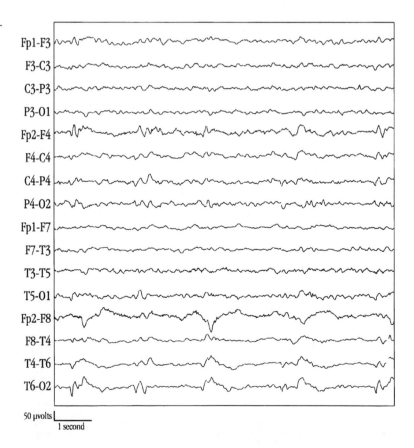

Figure 6-1. Pseudoperiodic lateralized epileptiform discharges in a patient with herpes encephalitis.

Neonatal HSE also produces these complexes, which in the neonate population are often multifocal and shift from side to side. Seizure patterns can evolve from pseudoperiodic complexes. Over time, complexes become less frequent and disappear, leaving low-amplitude polymorphic slowing in their place.[13]

Treatment

Acyclovir is the drug of choice. Recommended dose is 10 mg/kg every 8 hours for 10–14 days.[88] Seizures should be managed routinely with anticonvulsants as needed. Seizure relapse rate is approximately 5–10%.[13]

Prognosis

The majority of HSE cases have long-term neurologic sequelae. Outcome is more favorable in patients who are younger than 30 years old, have been ill for fewer than 4 days, and have little impairment of consciousness at the start of treatment. Mortality rate is 15% at 3 months, and fewer than 40% of patients survive with minimal or no neurologic sequelae, even with acyclovir treatment.[13,88,96]

The association of seizures with HSE morbidity and mortality has been studied via animal models. In another study using rabbits, different strains of HSV-1 were injected to induce focal HSE (subsequent histopathologic analysis confirmed infection focality). Virus strains resulting in greater than 70% mortality produced seizures, and all animals that seized became moribund or died. In contrast, a virus strain resulting in 20% mortality produced no seizures. Administration of daily phenobarbital reduced mortality significantly in animals given epileptogenic virus strains. Although only animal studies, these results emphasize the clinical significance, and specifically the negative prognostic potential, of comorbid seizures complicating infection and underscore the importance of seizure control within infectious states.[97]

Herpes Simplex Virus 2 Meningoencephalitis in an Adult

Cornford and McCormick report a case of an adult man with a chronic genital herpes simplex infection who developed partial-complex temporal lobe seizures of insidious onset, with EEG and MRI evidence of a unilateral temporal-lobe destructive process. Escalating number and severity of daily seizures led to temporal lobectomy. Histologic study revealed active, low-level viral infection in the resected hippocampus and temporal lobe cortex, with immunohistochemical evidence for infection by HSV-2. In situ hybridization confirmed viral presence. Although anticonvulsant-resistant seizure episodes began to recur after surgery, addition of acyclovir resulted in substantial seizure reduction.[98]

Epstein-Barr Virus Infection

Most primary EBV infections of children are asymptomatic. In adolescents and young adults, the usual syndrome associated with primary infection is infectious mononucleosis (35–75% of infections). Potential neurologic complications of EBV infection include encephalitis, meningitis, meningoencephalitis, and cerebellitis. Seizures can complicate acute infection, and even status epilepticus has been reported; most adult patients recover completely.[99]

In children, EBV encephalitis was previously considered a self-limited illness, usually with few or no sequelae. However, a review of pediatric EBV encephalitis or meningoencephalitis cases revealed that acute neurologic manifestations were diverse, including 36% of patients with seizures. Classic findings of infectious mononucleosis were noted infrequently. Sixty-four percent had abnormal EEGs in the acute setting, and of these 43% had persistent abnormalities on follow-up. Thus, although classic signs, symptoms, and lab findings in childhood infectious mononucleosis may be absent in EBV encephalitis, neurologic sequelae including seizures occur in a substantial number of patients.[100]

Human Herpesvirus 6 Encephalitis

HHV-6 has been associated with CNS dysfunction, such as febrile seizures, encephalitis, meningitis, and possibly multiple sclerosis. These manifestations have been reported in both immunocompetent and immunocompromised patients.[101] HHV-6 infection is nearly universal in infancy or early childhood. Convulsive episodes tend to occur during the pre-eruptive stage of exanthem subitum[102] but can appear late and be recurrent.

Controversy exists regarding the causality between HHV-6 infection and febrile seizures. A prospective study of pediatric emergency room (ER) presentation patients revealed HHV-6 infections, accounting for 20% of ER visits for febrile illnesses among children 6–12 months old (no primary HHV-6 infection was found among infants and young children with acute nonfebrile illness or among control subjects without any illness). Of these patients with acute febrile illness and documented HHV-6 infection, 13% had seizures. Furthermore, HHV-6 infection was associated with one-third of all febrile seizures in children up to 2 years old.[103]

In another study, Barone et al. prospectively evaluated febrile convulsions in 42 children to investigate the association between acute HHV-6 infection and first-time febrile convulsions. Twenty-one percent of these had primary HHV-6 infection documented by viral culture or serologic studies, or both.[104] However, a case-control study, performed to examine the hypothesis that acute HHV-6 infection occurs more commonly in children with first-time or recurrent febrile seizures than in controls, failed to demonstrate a statistically significant association between HHV-6 infection positivity and febrile seizures.[105] For further discussion of a possible relationship between febrile seizure and infection, see the section Infection and Febrile Seizures.

Enterovirus Infection

Analysis of CSF from children with neurologic symptoms associated with acute febrile illness, including febrile seizures and status epilepticus, revealed enteroviruses (echovirus and coxsackievirus) in a substantial number of patients.[106] Whether seizure expression can be directly related to CNS enteroviral infection in adults requires further investigation.

Cytomegalovirus

CMV can produce an encephalitis complicated by seizures.[13] Immunocompromised patients, such as HIV patients, are at particular risk. CMV can be transmitted via blood transfusion or donor organs. Although CMV encephalitis can be protracted, immunocompetent patients recover completely; residual epileptic sequelae are uncommon. However, immunocompromised patients surviving an acute episode can have multiple long-term neurologic deficits, including epilepsy.[107]

Arboviruses

Arboviruses constitute a large and diverse group of viruses that share a common mode of human infection via insect vector, usually mosquito or tick. The virus enters the host, replicates extraneurally, and is borne hematogenously to the brain. Seasonal variation in this group of viruses reflects the period of insect proliferation and human exposure; most infections occur in spring, summer, and fall. We briefly review the major arboviruses with potential for seizure complications.

California Encephalitis

The most common North American arbovirus infection is California encephalitis, which primarily afflicts prepubertal children in the midwestern and eastern United States.[96] It is caused by the LaCrosse strain of Bunyavirus, transmitted to humans by the *Aedes triseriatus* mosquito. The illness affects men more than women, and occurs in the summer months among children in rural areas. Seizures occur in the majority of patients, along with fever, headache, vomiting, and abdominal pain. Most cases recover uneventfully, but up to 20% experience sequelae including residual seizure disorders or cognitive deficits, or both.[13] Symptomatic infection of adults is uncommon.[13,108]

Eastern Equine Encephalitis

Eastern equine encephalitis causes fewer than 1% of U.S. encephalitis cases (there are frequently less than 10 total cases per year), but carries the highest mortality rate of any arboviral disease.[108] It is caused by an alphavirus transmitted by the *Culiseta melanura* mosquito. Wild birds are important in maintaining the virus life cycle; deaths in these animals often precede a human epidemic. All age groups can be affected. The disease is geographically confined to the eastern coastal United States.[108] Patients usually have an acute illness with seizures, high fever, and a declining mental status that progresses to coma, although a milder influenzalike form can occur. Death can occur in up to one-third of afflicted patients (a 1955 report described a death rate as high as two-thirds of cases; improved outcome is likely due to improved intensive-care management). Only one-third of patients survive without sequelae, which can include epilepsy, cognitive impairment, focal neurologic deficits, and even a persistent vegetative state. A prolonged prodrome may portend a favorable outcome.[13]

Western Equine Encephalitis

Western equine encephalitis is also caused by an alphavirus borne by the *Culex tarsalis* mosquito. Subclinical infections occur as much as 50 times more frequently than symptomatic cases, and children are affected more often than adults.[109] The illness has an incubation period of 5–20 days and usually begins with fever, malaise, pharyngitis, and vomiting.[108] As it progresses, focal convulsive seizures occur in 5–10% of cases (along with focal neurologic deficits and declining sensorium).[13,108] In large epidemics, mortality rate has ranged from 5% to 15%.[108] Adults generally recover without neurologic sequelae; however, young children can emerge with lasting neurologic sequelae, including epilepsy.[13,108]

St. Louis Encephalitis

St. Louis encephalitis is a flavivirus transmitted by several species of culicine mosquitos, with urban birds serving as principal hosts.[108] Large urban epidemics of encephalitis in the midwestern and southern United States have occurred.[110] Subclinical infections probably occur 100 times more often than symptomatic cases, which can present as three different syndromes: febrile illness with headache, aseptic meningitis, or encephalitis.[109] Older age groups have a higher attack rate and experience more severe illness and greater mortality risk than younger patients.[110] An influenzalike prodrome can precede a typical encephalitic picture of which seizures are

occasionally a complicating feature.[13] Up to 10% of cases evolve with neurologic sequelae, including epilepsy; the disease is fatal in up to 10% of patients.[110]

Japanese Encephalitis

Japanese encephalitis is a mosquito-borne flavivirus responsible for the most common form of arboviral encephalitis worldwide. The illness occurs throughout Asia and is seen more often in children than adults.[108] Convulsions can occur as part of a severe encephalitis.[13] Neurologic sequelae, including epilepsy, are present in a significant proportion of survivors; mortality rates are high (20–40%).[13,108]

West Nile Virus

On August 23, 1999, an infectious disease physician in Queens, New York, reported two cases of presumptive viral encephalitis to the New York City Department of Health. Initial epidemiologic investigation identified eight more patients. Results of serologic testing for common North American arboviruses were initially reported as consistent with St. Louis encephalitis. Concurrent with the human outbreak, there was an increase in certain bird fatalities, but these were initially thought to be unrelated to the human outbreak (although birds are the primary reservoir hosts for arboviruses such as St. Louis encephalitis, infected birds are usually asymptomatic). When it was recognized that many birds had pathologic evidence of viral encephalitis, brain specimens were sent to the CDC, where a flavivirus was isolated and identified as West Nile (WN) virus.[111] Sequence analysis of genes from mosquitoes and two fatal human cases confirmed WN virus as responsible for the human disease, and phylogenetic analysis confirmed these viruses as most closely related to a WN virus isolated from a dead goose in Israel in 1998.[112,113] Active surveillance in New York City confirmed 62 human cases of WN viral disease during the 1999 outbreak; there were seven deaths.[111]

Before the 1999 New York outbreak, WN virus had not been detected in the western hemisphere; outbreaks of WN fever and WN encephalitis had previously been identified only in Africa, Asia, the Middle East, and, rarely, Europe. Wild birds are the primary reservoir hosts, and *Culex* species are the major mosquito vectors. Humans are incidental hosts not involved in the normal transmission cycle. Incubation period is usually 6 days (range, 5–125 days). Symptomatic to asymptomatic infection ratio varies between 1 to 140 and 1 to 300.[111] In endemic areas overseas, asymptomatic infections and mild constitutional syndromes are more common than CNS disease. Symptoms in the New York outbreak included fever, headache, arthralgias, lymphadenopathy, and a maculopapular or roseolar rash.[111] Although encephalitis was the syndrome heralding the arbovirus' presence in New York, CNS involvement was relatively rare, predominantly affecting older adults.[111] Seizures were not among the multiple CNS-related signs reported.[111] However, convulsions are one of many possible representative features of CNS involvement included in the criteria for reporting a viral encephalitis case to health authorities. WN virus was isolated in mosquitoes and birds during summer 2000 again in New York City and in Boston.

Rabies Virus

Rabies, caused by a rhabdovirus, presents approximately 30 days after contact with a rabid animal. A nonspecific prodrome of fever, headache, sore throat, and abdominal pain progresses to an agitated, hallucinatory delirium followed by coma and death. Seizures occur in approximately 10% of cases.[13] Without postexposure immunoprophylaxis treatment, survival is rare.

Human Immunodeficiency Virus

Up to 70% of HIV patients develop neurologic complications.[114] Although neurologic disease typically occurs within the context of other AIDS-defining illnesses, neurologic symptoms can herald AIDS in up to 20% of HIV patients.[115] The spectrum of neurologic disorders that complicate HIV-1 infection is extremely diverse. CNS complications, including seizures, can be divided into those due to HIV infection itself and those due to HIV-related secondary etiologies (e.g., opportunistic infections consequent to HIV-induced immunosuppression). HIV-1 infection neurologic complications with seizure risk are outlined in Table 6-21.

Table 6-21. Neurologic Complications of Human Immunodeficiency Virus (HIV) 1 Infection with Seizure Risk

Disorders directly related to HIV:
Acute meningitis
Chronic meningitis
    Persistent or recurrent meningeal pleocytosis with/without meningeal symptoms
Acute encephalitis
Chronic encephalitis
    HIV-1 minor encephalopathy (cognitive/motor abnormalities)
    HIV-1 major encephalopathy (cognitive/motor abnormalities)
        Acquired immunodeficiency syndrome dementia complex
Secondary neurologic syndromes:
Opportunistic infections
    Cytomegalovirus
    Toxoplasmosis
    Cryptococcus
    Progressive multifocal leukoencephalopathy
    Herpes simplex virus encephalitis
    Candidiasis
    Herpes zoster virus encephalitis
    Histoplasmosis
    Tuberculosis
    Aspergillosis
Neoplasms
    Primary central nervous system (CNS) lymphoma
    Metastatic disease (including Kaposi's sarcoma)
Vascular disease
    CNS hemorrhage (secondary to thrombocytopenia, vasculitis, etc.)
    CNS ischemic stroke
Metabolic disorders
Drug toxicity
    Antiretroviral drugs
    Neuroleptic malignant syndrome

Source: Data from JR Berger, DM Simpson. Neurologic Complications of AIDS. In WM Scheld, RJ Whitley, DT Durack (eds), Infections of the Central Nervous System. Philadelphia: Lippincott–Raven, 1997;255–271; and CB Britton. Acquired immunodeficiency syndrome. In LP Rowland (ed), Merritt's Textbook of Neurology. Baltimore: Williams & Wilkins, 1995;179–193.

Epidemiology

Seizures can occur at any disease stage. For example, although seizures were the presenting symptom of HIV infection in 18 of 100 cases described by Holtzman et al.,[116] all seven patients with status

Table 6-22. Leading Causes of New-Onset Generalized Seizures in Acquired Immunodeficiency Syndrome

Etiology	Frequency (%)
Idiopathic	31
Human immunodeficiency virus encephalopathy	31
Central nervous system (CNS) toxoplasmosis	18
Alcohol withdrawal	8
Progressive multifocal leukoencephalopathy	8
CNS lymphoma	4

Source: Adapted from GR Pesola, RE Westfal. New-onset generalized seizures in patients with AIDS presenting to an emergency department. Acad Emerg Med 1998;5:905–911.

epilepticus described by Aronow et al. died within 1 month of the episode.[117]

Early work suggested that approximately half of seizures associated with HIV infection were due to the direct toxic effects of HIV infection of the brain, whereas secondary-process complications of AIDS contributed to the remainder. However, more recent studies have emphasized that several potential seizure-causing processes can operate simultaneously.[118]

Reviewing together 276 patients described in four large series, Labar and Harden found that generalized convulsions constituted 75% of seizures.[13] Status epilepticus, typically generalized convulsive, occurred in 13% of cases.[13]

Pesola and Westfal conducted a retrospective review of all patients with new-onset generalized seizures presenting to an academic medical center emergency department (ED) in New York City over 2 years to determine the etiologic profile of new-onset generalized seizures in AIDS patients.[119] The results are outlined in Table 6-22. (In a comparison group of HIV negative patients similarly presenting with new-onset seizures, idiopathic [36%] and alcohol withdrawal [24%] were the most common etiologies.[119])

The same study tested the applicability of American College of Emergency Physicians guidelines for ED workup of new-onset seizures to AIDS patient populations. Using those guidelines, only one-third of patients with admission-requiring

CNS lesions (e.g., toxoplasmosis and lymphoma) manifested findings meeting those guidelines' threshold criteria for admission. Thus, two-thirds of HIV-positive patients with admission-requiring CNS lesions contributing to their seizure presentation would have been inappropriately discharged under then-existing American College of Emergency Physicians guidelines. Based on such studies, guidelines have been amended with neuroimaging and LP requirements in the ED or admission for in-patient workup for all patients with AIDS or suspected AIDS presenting with new-onset seizure.[119]

In a related study performed at Johns Hopkins Medical Center, aiming to formulate a decision guideline for ED use of noncontrast head CT in HIV-infected patients, investigators sought to determine which neurologic signs or symptoms are predictive of new focal lesions on head CT in HIV-infected patients. Among the findings associated with new focal lesions revealed on head CT, new-onset seizure was the most strongly associated (relative risk of 73.5%).[120] (Of note, the most common intracranial lesion among patients with cluster of differentiation 4 [CD4] counts less than 200 was toxoplasmosis, whereas strokes [ischemic or hemorrhagic] were most common in those with CD4 counts greater than 200.[120])

Pascual-Sedano et al. also performed a prospective study of new-onset seizures in an HIV-infected patient cohort (n >500) to determine etiologic frequency of new-onset seizures.[121] Three percent of subjects had a new-onset seizure during the study period. Of these, 82% had AIDS per the 1993 CDC AIDS definition. Mean latency between HIV diagnosis and first seizure was 60.7 months. Seizure cause was drug toxicity in 47% and intracranial lesion in 35%; the remainder was secondary to metabolic derangement or unknown cause. First seizure was generalized in 71%, simple partial motor in 12%, and simple partial with secondary generalization in 18%. Partial seizures occurred in 67% of patients with an intracranial lesion.[121]

Consistent with AIDS' protean character, seizure comorbidity can also have varied phenomenology. There are multiple reports of epilepsia partialis continua (EPC) complicating HIV infection. In an HIV patient with chronic focal myoclonus described by Bartolomei et al., serial MRI demonstrated increasing left rolandic T2-weighted signal, and histopathologic study of a brain biopsy specimen demonstrated inflammation characterized by perivascular mononuclear cell infiltration; the only detectable cause was HIV infection. An EEG-electromyography back-averaging study demonstrated that focal motor activity was indeed of cortical origin. High-dose steroid and antiretroviral therapy led to marked radiologic and clinical improvement. This first reported case of HIV-related "inflammatory" EPC emphasizes the importance of including CNS-HIV involvement in the differential diagnosis of EPC.[122] More commonly, HIV-1 infection presenting with new-onset EPC can be an early manifestation of PML or secondary focal mass lesion.[123]

Seizure Diagnosis in Human Immunodeficiency Virus

Neurodiagnostic testing (neuroimaging, LP) demonstrates abnormalities compatible with HIV infection and associated secondary complications. EEGs in HIV infection and AIDS frequently show epileptiform features.[13] Harden et al. found low-amplitude, slow, monotonous EEGs associated with AIDS dementia complex.[124] Gabuzda et al. described EEGs in a series of AIDS patients; routine EEGs showed generalized slowing in 38%, focal slowing in 19%, and epileptiform activity in 6% (the remainder were unremarkable). Approximately 13% of patients had clinically diagnosed seizures; of these, half had EEGs with sharp waves, and 17% had focal slowing (the remainder had unremarkable interictal EEGs).[125]

Treatment of Seizures in Human Immunodeficiency Virus

Multidrug HIV regimens frequently include medications with a high potential for drug-drug interactions with anticonvulsants (see Tables 6-1 and 6-2). Meticulous attention to these interactions and tight anticonvulsant level monitoring is required. Of note, it has been demonstrated that valproate may increase viral burden by potentiating replication; thus, clinicians should exercise caution when using valproate in HIV-positive patients.[126]

The relatively high risk of seizure recurrence imposed by HIV or AIDS and secondary compli-

Table 6-23. Prion Diseases

Slow Virus	Host
Creutzfeldt-Jakob Disease	Humans
Gerstmann-Straussler-Scheinker disease	Humans
Fatal familial insomnia	Humans
Kuru	Humans
Scrapie	Sheep, goats
Bovine spongiform encephalopathy	Cattle, humans
Chronic wasting disease	Mule deer, elk
Transmissible mink encephalopathy	Mink
Feline spongiform encephalopathy	Cats

Source: Adapted from B Jubelt, S Ropka. Infectious Diseases of the Nervous System. In R Rosenberg (ed), Atlas of Clinical Neurology. Boston: Butterworth–Heinemann, 1998;44–46.

cations imposes increased need for anticonvulsant maintenance therapy. In one series of HIV patients with new-onset seizure, the average number of seizures per HIV patient was 2.3 during a mean follow-up interval of 4 months.[116] Other reports note seizure recurrence rates of 30–50%.[127] However, this has to be balanced with reports of the greater tendency of HIV or AIDS patients to develop adverse drug effects; 26% of patients studied by Wong et al.[127] and 14% of patients in the Holtzman et al. series[116] treated with phenytoin had to discontinue that medication secondary to toxicity (e.g., dermatologic, hematologic, hepatic). This is compared to a maximum of 12% of non-HIV or AIDS patients treated with anticonvulsants having to discontinue an anticonvulsant secondary to adverse effects. In contrast, Koppel et al. found that rashes, hepatic dysfunction, and hematologic abnormalities were equally common in AIDS patients on anticonvulsants compared to matched control subjects with AIDS without seizures and not on anticonvulsants.[128] Whether to institute maintenance anticonvulsant treatment after first seizure in an HIV patient remains a clinical decision to be made on a case-by-case basis.

Epileptic Complications of Slow Virus Infections

Slow virus infections are also known as *prion diseases*, after the presumed infectious agent, as

Table 6-24. Clinical Characteristics of Major Human Slow Virus Infections

Slow Virus	Onset	Manifestations	Laboratory Findings
Creutzfeldt-Jakob disease			
Sporadic		See Table 6-23	Typical electroencephalogram (EEG) changes (generalized periodic sharp wave complexes); 14-3-3 usually present
Hereditary	Earlier age of onset	More protracted course	Missing typical EEG changes; protein 14-3-3 absent in 50%
New-variant	Earlier age of onset	More prolonged course; early psychiatric manifestations; cerebellar ataxia, paraesthesias, dysesthesias	Variable EEG changes
Gerstmann-Straussler-Scheinker disease	Midlife onset (mean age at death = 48 yrs)	Prolonged course (5–11 yrs) Early: cerebellar ataxia Late: spastic paraparesis, limb ataxia, dysarthria, nystagmus, parkinsonism, deafness, blindness, gaze palsies, dementia, corticospinal tract signs	No typical EEG changes
Fatal familial insomnia	Mid- to late life onset	Insomnia, dysautonomia, ataxia	No typical EEG changes

Source: Adapted from B Jubelt, S Ropka. Infectious Diseases of the Nervus System. In R Rosenberg (ed), Atlas of Clinical Neurology. Boston: Butterworth–Heinemann, 1998;44–46; and DM Asher. Slow Viral Infections. In WM Scheld, RJ Whitley, DT Durack (eds), Infections of the Central Nervous System. Philadelphia: Lippincott–Raven, 1997;199–221.

well as *transmissible spongiform encephalopathies* (TSEs), after the histopathologic changes associated with these infections. The major prion diseases are listed in Table 6-23. Clinical characteristics of human TSEs are summarized in Table 6-24.

Prions are proteinaceous infectious particles (PrPs). Brain pathology of prion diseases consists of a vacuolar (spongiform) degeneration of the neuropil, cortical neurons, and subcortical gray matter with neuronal loss and gliosis. Early diagnosis is difficult, in part because prions do not have nucleic acids, making conventional nucleic acid–based viral detection systems ineffective. Additionally, PrP eludes detection by not producing a humoral immune response.[130,131]

Prion diseases are categorized into three groups: sporadic, inherited, and acquired. Most slow virus infections—approximately 85%—are sporadic. The remaining 15% consist of hereditary forms (genetic Creutzfeldt-Jakob disease [CJD], Gerstmann-Straussler-Scheinker disease, fatal familial insomnia) and acquired forms (iatrogenically transmitted [human growth hormone therapy, dura mater grafts, other neurosurgical procedures] and cannibalism [Kuru]). CJD is the most common human TSE. A new variant of sporadic CJD, likely caused by the same agent as bovine spongiform encephalopathy, was described in 1996.[131]

Variability in CJD diagnostic criteria sets relying solely on clinical manifestations led to different incidence rates in different series.[132] The introduction of 14-3-3 CSF protein Western blot immunodetection greatly improved diagnostic accuracy (sensitivity up to 99% and specificity up to 96%).[133] Further facilitating CJD diagnosis was the recognition of characteristic MRI abnormalities on diffusion-weighted imaging (cortical "ribboning").[134]

Sporadic CJD has an annual incidence of approximately 1 per 1 million in the general population and occurs randomly worldwide.[131] Inherited prion diseases have an annual incidence of approximately 1 per 10 million in the general population.[131]

Inherited prion diseases are associated with coding mutations in the prion protein gene, located on the short arm of chromosome 20. Analysis of these more than 20 mutations has broadened the recognized phenotypes of human prion disease. Pathogenic prion protein gene mutations do not occur with sporadic and acquired prion diseases. Genetic susceptibility to prion disease is conferred by homozygosity of a PrP polymorphism at residue 129, an encoding site for methionine or valine.

Although seizures are not a common complication, the slow virus most commonly associated with seizures is CJD. Sporadic CJD is most often diagnosed in patients aged 50–70 years. Initial complaints in approximately one-third of patients are systemic, consisting of fatigue, disordered sleep, or decreased appetite. Another one-third have nonfocal neuropsychiatric features at onset (e.g., confusion or atypical behaviors). The remainder can present with focal neurologic features, including ataxia, visual loss, aphasia, hemiparesis, or focal amyotrophy, sometimes leading to an erroneous initial clinical impression of stroke or motor neuron disease.[130,135] Diagnosis becomes clearer with onset of cognitive decline and startle myoclonus to abrupt sound or touch. Pyramidal, extrapyramidal, and cerebellar signs eventually occur in the majority of patients.[130,135] Seizures occur in fewer than 20% of patients and were reported to occur in as few as 9% in a series of 124 CJD patients.[13] See Table 6-25, which summarizes the principal clinical features of sporadic CJD.

Although seizures are not a common complication of slow virus infection, there can be characteristic EEG changes. Early in sporadic CJD course, the EEG may show nonspecific slowing. Later, periodic, biphasic, or triphasic synchronous sharp-wave complexes are superimposed on a slow-background rhythm in most patients. These characteristic complexes may disappear as myoclonus subsides in the terminal phase of the disease. Periodic complexes have shown a sensitivity and specificity of 67% and 86%, respectively, for CJD detection; if repeated recordings are obtained, more than 90% of patients may show periodic complexes. Generalized periodic sharp-wave complexes (Figure 6-2) appear on EEG in more than 90% of cases, usually within 12 weeks of onset.[130–132]

Table 6-25. Incidence of Neurologic Features of Sporadic Creutzfeldt-Jakob Disease

Sign/Symptom	Frequency (%)
Memory loss	100
Behavioral disturbance	57
Other neuropsychiatric dysfunction	73
Myoclonus	78
Cerebellar ataxia	71
Pyramidal signs	62
Extrapyramidal signs	56
Lower motor neuron signs	12
Visual disturbances	42
Periodic electroencephalogram complexes	60

Source: Adapted from P Brown, F Cathala, D Sadowsky, et al. Creutzfeldt-Jacob disease in France: clinical characteristics of 124 consecutive verified cases. Ann Neurol 1979;6:430–437.

With typical presentation, rapid course, an EEG showing periodic complexes, and the presence of 14-3-3 protein in CSF, CJD diagnosis is reasonably assured. CJD is uniformly fatal, with progression to death within 12 months.[137] Management is supportive; there is no cure. Any seizure complications are treated routinely.

Epileptic Complications of Fungal Infections

Most patients with a CNS fungal infection have some predisposing flaw in their immune response that allows invasion by relatively nonvirulent fungi. Conditions associated with such deficiencies are summarized in Table 6-26. CNS syndromes associated with specific fungi are summarized in Table 6-27; epidemiologic, diagnostic, and therapeutic data are outlined in Table 6-28.

Fungal Meningitis

Clinical manifestations of fungal meningitis are less stereotyped than bacterial meningitis. Patients often present with a chronic meningitis syndrome (defined as meningitis that persists for at least 1 month); in fact, fungal meningitis is always a consideration in the differential diagnosis of any patient with a chronic

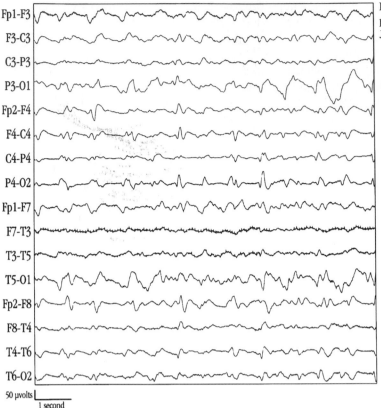

Figure 6-2. Generalized periodic complexes in a patient with Creutzfeldt-Jakob disease.

meningitis syndrome. Of fungal CNS infections, cryptococcal meningitis is the easiest to diagnose via CSF analysis. CSF cultures are frequently negative. Because fungal meningitis often involves the base of the brain more prominently than the spinal cord, cisternal CSF may yield organisms when lumbar CSF is negative. Repeated examinations of lumbar CSF or aspirates of cisternal or ventricular fluid may be needed before a diagnosis is made.[139,140]

Space-Occupying Fungal Lesions

Increased use of immunosuppressive drugs, increasingly potent broad-spectrum antibiotics, and the spread of AIDS have made fungal infections of the CNS not only no longer the rare entity they once were, but also, now, frequently, predictable events.[141] As indicated in Table 6-27, molds tend to cause most fungal CNS abscesses.

The full range of seizure semiology can occur secondary to CNS fungal infections. Multiple reports exist of patients presenting with new-onset seizures of unclear etiologies who deteriorated or died before fungal etiology was diagnosed,[142] underscoring the importance of liberal inclusion of fungal infection in the differential diagnosis of new-onset seizure, especially when any predisposing clinical context exists.[143] Anticonvulsant therapy follows routine guidelines with awareness of frequent antifungal-anticonvulsant interactions. Maintenance anticonvulsant therapy is usually required, even after definitive antifungal treatment.

Epileptic Complications of Parasitic Infections

Protozoal

Malaria

Malaria is caused by the protozoal parasite *Plasmodium* transmitted to humans via the *Anopheles*

Table 6-26. Conditions Predisposing to Fungal Infection of the Central Nervous System

Immune Risk/Deficit	Representative Fungi
Prematurity	*Candida albicans*
Inherited immune defects (e.g., chronic granulomatous disease, severe combined immunodeficiency)	*Candida, Cryptococcus, Aspergillus*
Acquired immune defects	
Steroids	*Cryptococcus, Candida*
Cytotoxic agents	*Aspergillus, Candida*
Human immunodeficiency virus infection	*Cryptococcus, Histoplasma*
Alcoholism	*Sporothrix*
Iron chelator therapy	*Zygomycetes*
Intravenous drug abuse	*Candida, Zygomycetes*
Ketoacidosis	*Zygomycetes*
Trauma, foreign body	*Candida*

Source: Adapted from JR Perfect, DT Durack. Fungal Meningitis. In WM Scheld, RJ Whitley, DT Durack (eds), Infections of the Central Nervous System. Philadelphia: Lippincott–Raven, 1997;721–739.

mosquito. The disease is endemic to large parts of Africa, South America, and Southeast Asia.[144] Cerebral malaria is an encephalopathy occurring in approximately 2% of outpatients and 10% of inpatients infected with *Plasmodium falciparum* (*P. malariae* and *P. vivax* are infrequent causes of CNS malaria).[145] The World Health Organization definition of cerebral malaria requires the following: (1) unarousable coma, (2) evidence of acute infection with *P. falciparum*, and (3) no other identifiable cause of coma.[145] Clinical manifestations of cerebral malaria are diverse. Fever is nearly universal, as is comorbidity with clinical features of *P. falciparum* systemic infection. Clinicians working in tropical and subtropical regions regard any new CNS-attributable sign developing within the context of *P. falciparum* parasitemia as evidence of possible cerebral malaria.[144] The cardinal feature is disturbed level of consciousness, usually ranging from lethargy to stupor to coma, although an agitated delirium can also occur. Generalized tonic-clonic seizures occur in more than 40% of adult patients; partial seizures are uncommon.[13] A variety of EEG abnormalities have been described. To conform to the strict diagnosis of cerebral malaria, the patient must remain comatose for more than 6 hours after seizure to distinguish from postictal-consciousness suppression. Possible seizure causes include cerebral hypoxia associated with cerebral malaria, fever, hypoglycemia, lactic acidosis, drugs (including antimalarials such as chloroquine and mefloquine), and other metabolic disturbances secondary to malarial systemic effects.[13,144] In children, cerebral malaria tends to progress more rapidly, and convulsions are a common early feature (in Malawian children, 82% of childhood cases had a history of convulsions; almost one-

Table 6-27. Central Nervous System Syndromes Associated with Specific Fungi

Species	Relative Incidence	Clinical Syndrome		
		Meningitis	Abscess	Infarct
Cryptococcus	Common	Common	Infrequent	Infrequent
Coccidioides	Common	Common	Infrequent	Infrequent
Candida	Common	Occasional	Occasional	Rare
Molds (e.g., *Aspergillus*)	Occasional	Infrequent	Occasional	Common
Zygomycetes	Occasional	Infrequent	Occasional	Common
Histoplasma	Occasional	Infrequent	Infrequent	Infrequent
Blastomyces	Occasional	Infrequent	Infrequent	Rare
Sporothrix	Occasional	Infrequent	Rare	Rare

Source: Adapted from JR Perfect, DT Durack. Fungal Meningitis. In WM Scheld, RJ Whitley, DT Durack (eds), Infections of the Central Nervous System. Philadelphia: Lippincott–Raven, 1997;721–739.

Table 6-28. Epidemiologic, Diagnostic, and Therapeutic Aspects of Central Nervous System Fungal Infections That Can Be Complicated by Seizures

Fungus	Geographic Distribution	Opportunistic Infection?	Clinical Setting	Cerebrospinal Fluid	Systemic Involvement	Treatment
Cryptococcus	Nonspecific	Sometimes	Community acquired	↑ Protein nl/↓ glucose ↑WBC (N, M) + India ink + *Cryptococcus* antigen + Latex agglutination	Lungs, skin, bones, joints	Amphotericin B + flucytosine
Coccidioides	Southwestern United States	No	Community acquired	↑ Protein nl/↓ glucose ↑WBC (N, M) + Complement fixation	Lungs, skin, bones, joints	Amphotericin B (i.v. and i.t.)
Candida	Nonspecific	Yes	Prolonged broad-spectrum antibiotics Indwelling catheters Abdominal surgery Intravenous drug abuse (IVDA)	↑ Protein nl/↓ glucose ↑WBC (N, M) + Gram's stain	Mucous membranes, skin, esophagus, genitourinary	Amphotericin B
Molds *Aspergillus* *Mucorales*	Nonspecific	Yes	Diabetes Hematologic neoplasms Transplant Near-drowning IVDA	↑ Protein nl/↓ glucose ↑WBC (N, M) + Red blood cell	Lungs, skin, orbits, paranasal sinuses	Amphotericin B
Histoplasma *Sporothrix*	Eastern/midwestern United States	Sometimes	Community acquired	↑ Protein nl/↓ glucose ↑WBC (N)	Lungs, skin, mucous membranes, heart	Amphotericin B
Blastomyces	Mississippi River Valley	No	Community acquired	↑ Protein nl/↓ glucose ↑WBC (N, M)	Lungs, skin, bones, joints, viscera	Amphotericin B
Nocardia	Nonspecific	Yes	Community acquired	↑ Protein nl/↓ glucose ↑WBC (N, M) + Gram's stain + Acid-fast bacillus	Lungs, skin	Sulfonamides

M = monocyte; N = neutrophils; nl = normal; WBC = white blood cell; ↑ = increased; ↓ = decreased; + = positive.

Adapted from JR Perfect, DT Durack. Fungal Meningitis. In WM Scheld, RJ Whitley, DT Durack (eds), Infections of the Central Nervous System. Philadelphia: Lippincott–Raven, 1997;721–739; JP Posner. Neurologic Complications of Cancer. Philadelphia: FA Davis Co, 1995;230–263.

fourth of cases had seizures within 3 hours of admission).[146] Because subclinical seizure activity is frequent, a low threshold for initiating EEG monitoring should be maintained.[13,144] Seizures are associated with prolonged coma and increased risk of neurologic sequelae and death.[13,144] Neurologic sequelae of cerebral malaria, including epilepsy, affect approximately 10% of survivors; for unclear reasons, children tend to be more frequently affected than adults.[146,147]

Diagnosis. Demonstration of parasitemia and species confirmation is by blood smear. CSF profile in cerebral malaria is notable for occasional lymphocytic pleocytosis; protein concentration may be slightly elevated, whereas glucose is usually normal.

Treatment. Cerebral malaria is a medical emergency. Treatment is tripartite: (1) specific antimalarial therapy (via quinine, quinidine, etc.), (2) management of coexistent malarial complications including seizures, and (3) treatment of associated superinfections.[144] At least initial management should be in an intensive care unit. Generalized seizures can be followed by rapid neurologic deterioration; therefore prompt treatment is required. Subclinical or nonconvulsive seizures should be suspected in patients with persistent coma. Convulsions can be prevented by controlling fever and through judicious use of prophylactic anticonvulsants.[13,144]

Toxoplasmosis

Toxoplasma gondii is an intracellular protozoan parasite. Most human infections with *T. gondii* are asymptomatic. However, CNS infection can potentially cause four syndromes: (1) meningoencephalitis during primary infection of an immunocompetent host; (2) intracerebral mass lesions or encephalitis in immunocompromised hosts; (3) retinochoroiditis associated with primary infection or reactivation of an earlier infection; and (4) congenital toxoplasmosis, encephalitis, and retinochoroiditis as a result of transplacental fetal infection.[148,149] The only definitive host for *T. gondii* is domestic cats.[148]

Transmission of *T. gondii* to humans occurs commonly, usually by eating undercooked meat or by inadvertent ingestion of oocysts from cat feces. Systemic parasitemia occurs after invasion of the gut lining by *Toxoplasma*.[148]

Toxoplasmosis in Immunocompetent Hosts. Primary infection with *T. gondii* in the immunocompetent host is usually asymptomatic. The most common sign is generalized lymphadenopathy, which occurs in up to 20% of patients.[149] Symptomatic CNS toxoplasmosis rarely develops during primary infection in normal hosts, but unusual cases of CNS involvement in immunocompetent patients can be associated with drowsiness, confusion, seizures, and even coma.[149] CSF analysis reveals mild pleocytosis, elevated protein, and normal glucose. Diagnosis is usually made on the basis of either increasing or markedly elevated serum and CSF antibody titers.[148]

Toxoplasmosis in Immunocompromised Hosts. Before AIDS, reactivation of CNS toxoplasmosis occurred most often in patients with hematologic malignancies (because many of these patients receive immunosuppressive therapy, the relative contribution of malignancy-associated vs. drug-associated immune dysfunction predisposing to toxoplasmosis is difficult to define).[148] CNS toxoplasmosis can also occur in patients receiving immunosuppressive chemotherapy after organ transplantation or for collagen vascular disorders.[148–150] Since 1981, CNS toxoplasmosis cases have increased dramatically as toxoplasmosis became one of the most common opportunistic infections in AIDS. Toxoplasmosis is responsible for over one-third of neurologic symptoms in AIDS patients[148] (in contrast, both primary CNS and metastatic lymphoma account for approximately 5% each). More than 95% of toxoplasmic encephalitis in patients with AIDS is due to reactivation of chronic latent infection.[150] For most HIV-infected patients, toxoplasmic encephalitis develops after the CD4 count falls below 100.[148] In the United States, 10–40% of AIDS patients are latently infected, and 30–50% of these will develop toxoplasmic encephalitis.[148] Clinical manifestation is variable, ranging from insidious process to acute confusional state. Partial, partial complex, and generalized seizures can occur; reported seizure rates range from 18 to 29%.[151,152] Differential diagnosis is wide, including cryptococcal meningitis, TB, nocardial or bacterial abscess, PML, and malignancies including primary CNS lymphoma. Indeed, resolving the differential diagnosis of toxoplasmosis versus primary CNS lymphoma, as the etiology of intracranial mass in the context of

AIDS, remains a difficult clinical challenge, requiring consideration of a constellation of data (see the next section).

Diagnosis

SEROLOGY. In the immunocompetent host, acute acquired toxoplasmosis is usually established by a fourfold rise in IgG antibody titer.[148] Although the presence of high IgG titer suggests acute infection, such titers can persist for years after acute infection. Therefore, immunoglobulin M is used as part of the diagnostic criteria of acute-acquired toxoplasmosis. Serologic diagnosis of toxoplasmic encephalitis in the immunocompromised host depends on the pathophysiology particular to the specific immunocompromised population. In the transplant patient, prior seronegativity or positivity can help inform the significance of serology testing after transplantation. In many immunocompromised patients, instead of rising or high titers, low or absent antitoxoplasmic antibody titers occur secondary to recrudescence of latent infection in the context of suppressed humoral immunity.[148,150] In sum, interpretation of serologic tests for toxoplasmosis is dependent on prior probability of disease and the underlying condition driving pathogenesis of the CNS toxoplasmosis complication.

NEUROIMAGING. MRI is the imaging modality of choice, revealing rounded isodense or hypodense lesions with ring enhancement. In approximately 75% of cases, lesions are multiple, with a predilection for basal ganglia and brain stem. However, in up to 80% of cases, toxoplasmosis and lymphoma are indistinguishable on standard neuroimaging studies.[148,150] Because they respond to different treatments, differentiation is essential. Toxoplasmosis and CNS lymphoma both appear as single or multiple ring or nodular-enhancing mass lesions on standard CT and MRI, and both can localize to the basal ganglia and brain stem (lymphoma can also localize to the corpus callosum, subependymal region, or periventricular regions; hence, lesions in these regions are more likely to be lymphoma[153]). Although there are subtle clues that can help distinguish toxoplasmosis from lymphoma, reliable differentiation by CT or MRI alone is impossible. To assist lesion identification, Thallium-201 single photon emission computerized tomography (SPECT) is used.[153] Thallium-201 SPECT shows uptake in CNS lymphomas but not infections, including toxoplasmosis.[153] Also, steroids that can affect appearance of lymphoma on CT and MRI do not affect SPECT results.[148,150,153]

The combination of serologic testing, contrast-enhanced CT or MRI, and SPECT should provide sufficient data for diagnostic differentiation. Definitive diagnosis of toxoplasmic encephalitis requires brain biopsy and subsequent histopathologic analysis.

Treatment. Therapy for toxoplasmic encephalitis is the combination of pyrimethamine and sulfadiazine; clindamycin can be used as an alternative to sulfadiazine.[154] Serial neuroimaging provides the best follow-up to assess treatment progress. Maintenance anticonvulsant therapy is usually required. Newborns of women contracting toxoplasmosis during pregnancy should be treated with clindamycin to reduce likelihood of developing late neurologic sequelae including seizures.[13,154]

Trypanosomiasis

Trypanosomiasis encompasses two distinct entities. African trypanosomiasis, or sleeping sickness, is caused by *Trypanosoma brucei*; the tsetse fly is the arthropod vector. CNS involvement is the principal clinical consequence of African trypanosomiasis. American trypanosomiasis, also known as Chagas' disease, is caused by *Trypanosoma cruzi*; CNS involvement is rare (cardiac and intestinal disease are primary). Reduviid bugs of genus *Triatoma* are the vector.

African Trypanosomiasis. An inflammatory nodule, a chancre, appears within several days at the site of parasite inoculation by the biting tsetse fly. Parasite replication and local tissue invasion is followed by lymphatic (causing a diffuse lymphadenopathy) and bloodstream entry causing parasitemia with high fever. Recurrent cycles of hemo-lymphatic parasitemia follow, with corresponding bouts of fever alternating with periods of well-being (African trypanosomiasis and malaria are two of the few causes of true intermittent fever).[155] Trypanosomes eventually enter the CNS to cause meningoencephalitis, causing a full range of neuropsychiatric signs and symptoms, including sleep-wake cycle abnormalities (e.g., daytime drowsiness and nocturnal insomnia) from which the disease derived its name. Frequent episodes of awakening during sleep, blurring of sleep stages, and irregular bursts of rapid EEG activity during stage 4 sleep occur.[155] Generalized convulsions become common as the disease progresses to later stages.[155] If untreated, mortality approaches 100%. Definitive diagnosis of African trypanosomiasis depends on demonstration of the parasite in chancre fluid, lymph nodes, blood, or CSF. LP should be performed in all cases of suspected trypanosomiasis (after confirming absence of increased intracranial pressure risk). Of the three drugs usually used for treatment (suramin, pentamidine, and melarsoprol), only melarsoprol penetrates the blood-brain barrier to be effective in CNS disease. Melarsoprol's use is complicated by an up to 18% incidence of severe, reactive arsenic encephalopathy that can result in permanent neurologic damage or death.[156,157] Consequently, melarsoprol should only be used in patients with CNS involvement. There are three characteristic syndromes of arsenic encephalopathy: status epilepticus with acute cerebral edema, rapidly progressive coma without seizures, and nonfatal cognitive abnormalities without other neurologic signs.[155] Steroids may help prevent or treat drug-induced encephalopathy, especially in higher risk patients (those with trypanosomes demonstrable in CSF or greater than 100 WBC, or both).[155] In a study of melarsoprol effects, patients with *T. gambiense* in the meningoencephalitic stage had waking EEGs before treatment, and then at 1 to 3 months after treatment. Before treatment, EEG tracings showed marked abnormalities in the form of periodic delta outbursts. Post-t120treatment EEGs showed improvement in 56% of patients but failed to return to normal in any patient.[155,158]

American Trypanosomiasis. American trypanosomiasis, or Chagas' disease, is an acute or chronic infection caused by *Trypanosoma cruzi*, transmitted by reduviid bugs of the genus *Triatoma*. *T. cruzi* infection occurs only in the western hemisphere. Symptomatic CNS disease is rare in immunocompetent patients; of well-described case reports, seizures can occur in both acute CNS infection as well as chronic Chagas' disease.[155] Immune response to American trypanosomiasis is mediated by T cells; thus, AIDS can alter the natural history of infection, leading to disease reactivation. A review of Chagas' disease within the context of AIDS revealed that 87% of cases had severe, multifocal, or diffuse meningoencephalitis[159]; seizures, partial and generalized, can accompany any of these forms of CNS Chagas' disease. Diagnosis is via demonstration of parasites in blood, CSF, or tissue. Treatment via trypanocides (nifurtimox) has shown to decrease parasitemia, symptoms, and mortality. Routine anticonvulsant treatment principles apply.

Amebic Infections

Amebae can invade the CNS, causing rare but fatal infections. Table 6-29 summarizes key features of the principal amebae that can cause CNS infection.

As indicated, seizures can complicate any of the ameba-caused syndromes; there is inadequate epidemiologic data to comment on seizure incidence.

Helminthic Infections

Several different helminth species can invade the CNS, as summarized in Table 6-30.

Neurocysticercosis

Pork tapeworm infection, taeniasis, results from small intestine infestation by the adult tapeworm *Taenia solium*. Cysticercosis is caused by presence of *Cysticercus*, the larval form of *T. solium*. Humans can acquire either disease, sometimes simultaneously. When the CNS or eye is involved in cysticercosis, then neurocysticercosis exists. *T. solium* is a common intestinal tapeworm, widely distributed around the world. Neurocysticercosis is the most common parasitic infection of the CNS; prevalence varies greatly according to region. Autopsy studies from Mexico suggest that up to 3.6% of the population is affected. Humans are both the definitive and intermediate hosts for *T. solium*. Ingestion of raw or undercooked pork infested with cysticerci leads to taeniasis. Ingested cysticerci are activated by gastric acid, penetrate the small intestine mucosa, and then develop to adulthood.[162]

Cysticerci have a predilection to migrate to the CNS (as well as striated muscle and eyes). Once situated, cysticerci evolve continuously through four stages: (1) edema generation, (2) development of a thin-walled cyst containing fluid and

Table 6-29. Amebic Infections of the Central Nervous System

Amebic Parasite	Geographic Distribution	Host Factors	Clinical Syndrome	Signs/Symptoms	Cerebrospinal Fluid
Entamoeba histolytica	Widespread distribution, tropics more virulent	Nonspecific	*Entamoeba* brain abscess (resembles brain abscess, tumor, or chronic meningitis, or a combination of these)	Meningitic symptoms Focal signs Seizures	↑ protein ↓ glucose
Naegleria fowleri	Southeastern United States	Freshwater swimming	Primary amebic meningoencephalitis (acute meningoencephalitis)	Acute Meningitic symptoms Seizures Stupor/coma	↑ protein ↓ glucose WBC (N) Motile trophozoites on wet mount
Acanthamoeba or *Hartmannella*	Widespread	Chronic illness, immunosuppression	Granulomatous amebic encephalitis (resembles brain abscess, tumor, or chronic meningitis, or a combination of these)	Subacute-chronic meningitic symptoms Seizures Focal deficits Stupor/coma	↑ protein ↓ glucose WBC (N, L) Wet mount: sluggish organisms

N = neutrophils; L = lymphocytes; WBC = white blood cell; ↑ = increased; ↓ = decreased.
Source: Adapted from MJ Aminoff, DA Greenberg, RP Simon. Clinical Neurology. Stamford, CT: Appleton & Lange, 1996;37; and DT Durack. Amebic infections. In WM Scheld, RJ Whitley, DT Durack (eds), Infections of the Central Nervous System. Philadelphia: Lippincott–Raven, 1997;831–844.

larvae, (3) inflammatory filling of the cyst with caseous material and consequent larvae destruction, and (4) cyst degeneration into an inactive calcified nodule with release of antigenic contents.[162]

Taeniasis (presence of the adult tapeworm in small bowel) is usually asymptomatic. But cysticercosis can be symptomatic; if acute symptoms are present, fever and headache are primary.[163] Neurocysticercosis can become symptomatic from 1 to 30 years after infection, with a median onset at 3–7 years.[164] Neurocysticercosis is associated with a wide variety of symptoms determined by pathogen burden, encystment location, whether encysted-parasite organisms are alive or dead, and host infection response. Differing encystment locations give rise to six clinical syndromes: (1) asymptomatic neurocysticercosis, (2) parenchymal neurocysticercosis, (3) subarachnoid cysticercosis, (4) intraventricular neurocysticercosis, (5) ocular neurocysticercosis, and (6) spinal neurocysticercosis. Mixed permutations of these syndromes can occur within a single patient.[162]

Parenchymal neurocysticercosis occurs when cysticerci develop within the brain, predominantly at the gray-white junction. Seizures are the most common presenting sign, affecting up to 92% of patients.[13, 164, 165] In Mexico, parenchymal neurocysticercosis is the single most common cause of adult-onset seizures (up to 50%).[165] Reports have varied regarding seizure-type frequency: partial seizures were most common in two series (up to 72%),[165] whereas another study reported a predominance of generalized seizures (60%).[164] Generalized seizures are preceded by focal symptoms in two-thirds of cases.[166] Partial complex seizures and status epilepticus are less common.[166] Seizure risk can increase during therapy as death of cysticerci causes larval antigen release, exacerbating the host's inflammatory response.[162]

In cysticercotic subarachnoiditis, patients usually present with signs of meningitis and increased intracranial pressure; seizures are not a significant complication. Intraventricular cysticercosis usually presents as subacute hydrocephalus and increased intracranial pressure; seizures are also not a frequent complication.

Diagnosis

Because symptoms can be numerous and varied, differential diagnosis is wide. Neurocysticercosis can mimic tumors, strokes, hemorrhage, abscess, meningitis, pseudotumor cerebri, pheochromocytoma, and assorted neuropsychiatric diseases. Neurologic examination can be deceptive; one study reported normal neurologic exams in 80% of cases.[13, 164] Clinical suspicion based on patient history of potential exposure is key (e.g., travel to endemic area). Tests for cysticercotic antigen and antibody exist; sensitivity and specificity depend on fluid tested (serum or CSF), cyst activity, and detection method.[162] Neuroimaging is central. Parenchymal neurocysticercosis can have four different appearances on CT: parenchymal calcifications or granulomas (representing inactive cysts), predominantly at the gray-white junctions; nonenhancing low-density rounded lesions; hypodense or isodense rounded masses with surrounding edema and ring or nodular enhancement; and diffuse brain edema with small ventricles and multiple enhancing nodular lesions.[167] MRI provides a varying amount of increased diagnostic data depending on cyst location and status; increased resolution identifies noncalcified cysts and helps define parenchymal cyst stage, whereas calcified cysts are visualized less well than on CT. EEG is abnormal in up to 50% of cases, demonstrating a variety of findings (diffuse slowing, focal paroxysmal activity, generalized spike waves) depending on lesion number, size, and location.[164] Definitive diagnosis often requires biopsy analysis.

Treatment

Principal anticysticercotic drugs include praziquantel and albendazole. Appropriate therapy for neurocysticercosis depends on the specific clinical syndrome, degree of neurologic impairment, cysticerci location, cysticerci activity, and host immune response.[162] For therapeutic decision making, it is useful to differentiate between benign and malignant neurocysticercosis.[168] Benign neurocysticer-

Table 6-30. Prominent Helminthic Infections of the Central Nervous System

Helminth	Disease
Cestodes:	
Echinococcus	Echinococcosis, hydatid disease
Taenia solium	Taeniasis
Cysticercus (larva)	Cysticercosis
Nematodes:	
Angiostrongylus	Eosinophilic meningitis
Strongyloides	Strongyloidiasis
Toxocara	Visceral larva migrans
Trichinella	Trichinosis
Trematodes:	
Schistosoma	Schistosomiasis

Source: Data from MJ Aminoff, DA Greenberg, RP Simon. Clinical Neurology. Stamford, CT: Appleton & Lange, 1996;37; and ML Cameron, DT Durack. Helminthic Infections. In WM Scheld, RJ Whitley, DT Durack (eds), Infections of the Central Nervous System. Philadelphia: Lippincott–Raven, 1997;845–878.

cosis is a chronic condition that is either asymptomatic or associated only with easily controlled seizures. Parenchymal neurocysticercosis is usually benign if the cyst number is small and predominantly calcified and with minimal edema. Anticysticercotic treatment, together with anticonvulsants, can reduce seizure activity by greater than 90%.[169] Calcified parenchymal cysticerci neither require nor respond to anticysticercotic treatment[162]; however, symptomatic-antiepileptic treatment is effective. Malignant neurocysticercosis refers to the acute or subacute disease associated with arachnoiditis, encephalitis, multiple or large cysts, or both, intraventricular cysts, hydrocephalus, increased intracranial pressure, or some combination thereof.[168] Surgical therapy is often required in addition to medical treatment. Anticysticercotic drugs are effective, reducing cyst number by up to 90% and seizure frequency by up to 95%.[170] However, exacerbation of CSF pleocytosis, acute increases in intracranial pressure, and other neurologic sequelae can follow use of praziquantel or albendazole in up to 60% of cases; thus, treatment should only be given when clinically necessary, and preferably in a hospital.[171] Solitary cysts causing treatment-refractory seizures should be surgically resected.[172] If seizures persist even after surgical and multidrug anticonvulsant therapy, the epileptogenic focus can sometimes be electrocorticographically ablated.[172]

Vazquez and Sotelo investigated seizure occurrence in 225 neurocysticercosis patients. Of 118 patients with vesicular cysts on CT-maintained anticonvulsant therapy, mean-baseline seizure rate was 11.3 seizures per year before anticysticercotic therapy; after anticysticercotic treatment, mean seizure rate decreased to 0.6 per year.[169] In contrast, in 49 patients with vesicular cysts treated only with anticonvulsants, seizure rate remained constant at 10.9 per year (over a mean follow-up of 7 years).[13,169]

Echinococcosis

Echinococcosis is caused by tapeworms of the genus *Echinococcus*, common parasites of dogs and cats, who are the definitive hosts; humans can be intermediate hosts. The disease is endemic in countries around the Mediterranean; Greece, Turkey, and Lebanon have the highest prevalences.[162] The small adult worms live in the definitive host's gut and discharge eggs into feces. If inadvertently ingested by a human, the eggs hatch in the human's gut, enabling the organism to penetrate the human's gut wall and hematogenously spread. Once located in a final tissue site, the organism forms a slowly enlarging cyst, a hydatid. When in the CNS, cysts usually locate in brain parenchyma; clinical manifestations are secondary to this mass lesion or raised intracranial pressure, or both. In addition to headache, nausea, papilledema, and focal deficits, partial and generalized seizures can result.[162] Although rare, CNS echinococcosis should be included in the differential diagnosis of any patient with a CNS mass lesion who has lived in an endemic area. Diagnosis is made by neuroimaging, which usually reveals a single, large spherical cystic lesion; there is usually no ring enhancement or associated edema.[173] Although praziquantel has activity against these organisms, primary treatment of CNS hydatids is surgical.[173] Antiepileptic management is a crucial adjunctive treatment.[162]

Angiostrongyliasis

Infection of humans by larvae of the nematode *Angiostrongylus* can cause an eosinophilic menin-

gitis, characterized by headache and paraesthesias; seizures can occur as an epiphenomenon of the meningitis. The principal hosts are rats; mollusks are the intermediate hosts, and humans can become accidental hosts if they eat infected mollusks. There is no established antiparasitic treatment. Comorbid seizures are managed routinely.[162]

Trichinosis

Trichinosis is caused by the nematode *Trichinella spiralis*. For humans, the most important source of infection is eating undercooked pork containing *Trichinella* cysts from pigs fed intreated garbage containing infected rodents. Following ingestion, larvae hematogenously disseminate and invade skeletal muscle—the only tissue of encystment. The most common symptoms and signs of infection are gastrointestinal distress, muscular pain, and periorbital edema. However, an inflammatory response can be evoked that can affect other organ systems, including the CNS, where a meningoencephalitis can result; approximately 5% of cases demonstrate neurologic signs, including seizures.[174] The clinical syndrome of fever, periorbital and peripheral edema, and firm and tender muscles in a patient who has eaten pork within the past 2–10 days are suggestive of trichinosis. Eosinophils or larvae, or both, can be found in CSF in up to 28% of cases.[162] Muscle biopsy can confirm diagnosis. Treatment is thiabendazole and steroids; seizure management is routine.

Strongyloidiasis

Strongyloides stercoralis is a small nematode that can parasitize the small bowel of humans. Larvae living freely in moist soil invade rapidly through contacted skin and migrate into lymphatics to reach the venous system, where they travel to the lungs, migrate up airways to the glottis, and then down the esophagus to the small intestine. The CNS can become involved in disseminated strongyloidiasis, which can occur within the context of compromised immune function (e.g., HIV or AIDS). CNS manifestations can be secondary to larvae infestation or, more commonly, bacterial meningitis caused by gut bacteria transmitted by the migrating parasite. Seizures can be an epiphenomenon of these complications. Thiabendazole can be helpful if started early in the disease process, but disseminated strongyloidiasis is usually fatal. Again, comorbid seizure management is routine.[162]

Toxocariasis

Toxocariasis is caused by nematodes of the genus *Toxocara*. Adult worms live in the intestines of dogs and cats, which fecally discharge millions of eggs daily. These eggs become widely distributed (up to 30% of soil samples contain them),[175] and humans become infected when they ingest ova-containing soil. Ova hatch in the small intestine, producing larvae that traverse the intestinal wall and migrate to various tissues. Immune response to migrating larvae produces the disease called visceral larva migrans, which sometimes affects the brain. Most infections are asymptomatic. If symptomatic, headache is the most common CNS complaint, although meningoencephalitis with seizures has been described.[176] Interestingly, children with idiopathic epilepsy have the antitoxocaral antibody more often than controls, prompting the hypothesis that toxocariasis may be an etiologic factor in epilepsy[177]; this remains unsettled.

Schistosomiasis

Schistosomiasis is an important parasitic disease, occurring in more than 200 million people worldwide.[162] Schistosomes are trematodes with a complicated life cycle. Humans are the definitive hosts; snails are intermediate hosts. CNS schistosomiasis usually follows egg migration into the brain or spinal cord vasculature, leading to microinfarction or granuloma formation.[178] Clinical manifestations occur in three phases: dermatitis, then fever (Katayama fever, a serum sickness reaction to schistosomal antigens), and finally chronic schistosomiasis, potentially involving multiple organ systems, including the CNS. Neurologic manifestations are rare, occurring in only 1–2% of cases, but can include a wide range of focal and nonfocal CNS symptomatology, including seizures.[179]

Diagnosis is by history and supporting lab data, including blood and CSF eosinophilia, fecal and urine analysis for schistosome eggs, and serologic enzyme-linked immunoassay directed against parasite antigens (most specific test). Neuroimaging can demonstrate cerebral edema and multiple focal lucencies.[162]

Neurologic disease during Katayama fever responds to steroids with or without antischistosomal therapy.[162] Cerebral schistosomiasis may require surgical resection of granulomalike masses. Praziquantel is the primary antischistosomal agent. Antiepileptics are used as needed.

Intracranial Epidural Abscess

Abscesses confined to epidural spaces are usually associated with infection of overlying cranial bone. Etiologies include sinusitis (most common), mastoiditis, head trauma, and neurosurgical complication. Infection spreads to produce subdural and intraparenchymal abscesses, and meningitis can occur. Clinical manifestations, in addition to headache and fever, are generally referable to the abscess' mass effect, including increased intracranial pressure and seizures. Neuroimaging usually reveals an extradural collection. LP is risky secondary to increased intracranial pressure, and CSF analysis is usually nonspecific anyway (mildly elevated protein, mild pleocytosis, with negative Gram's stain and cultures). Antibiotic therapy is targeted to the likely infectious source (e.g., sinusitis); surgical evacuation is usually necessary. Seizure management is routine; maintenance-anticonvulsant therapy after successful abscess cure is usually not required.[180]

Subdural Empyema

SDE is a focal-intracranial suppurative collection, usually in supratentorial subdural space. Etiologies include paranasal sinusitis (most common cause), otitis, postoperative neurosurgical infection, posttraumatic complication, and meningitis. An additional 10% of patients have middle ear or mastoid disease, and 5% develop SDE from hematogenous spread.[181] Infrequently, SDE is a complication of meningitis. *Streptococci* are causative half the time, and *Staphylococcus aureus* in 10% of cases; polymicrobial infection is frequent, including anaerobic organisms. Although loculation is common, infection can spread over the convexities and along the falx. A progressively severe headache often related to the sinusitis is the most consistent clinical complaint. Malaise, fever, and declining mental status can occur rapidly. Complications can include dural venous thrombosis, parenchymal abscess, epidural abscess, and meningitis; mass effect or secondary venous infarction can cause focal neurologic deficits. Seizures are one of the most common presenting signs of SDE, occurring in up to 50% of patients.[13] Seizures are usually focal, relating to empyema site.

Diagnosis relies on clinical manifestations, especially the dyad of fever and focal seizures, and brain imaging, which usually reveals a crescent-shaped hypodensity along the dura or falx.[181] LP is risky, secondary to mass effect of the SDE. Antibiotics appropriate to suspected etiology (similar to epidural abscess) and prompt neurosurgical empyema evacuation are required.[182] Seizure management is mandatory, especially given the frequent complication of increased intracranial pressure.[13] Untreated patients can die within days, and, even with treatment, the mortality rate remains as high as 40%. Maintenance-anticonvulsant therapy after successful empyema cure is often necessary, secondary to epileptogenic potential of residual scarring.

Intraparenchymal Brain Abscess

Intraparenchymal brain abscess accounts for approximately 2% of intracranial masses.[183] Brain abscesses arise, in order of frequency, by metastatic spread from infection elsewhere (e.g., pneumonia, endocarditis), direct extension from cranial and parameningeal infection (e.g., paranasal sinuses, mastoiditis, osteomyelitis), unknown source, direct seeding via trauma or neurosurgical procedure, and history of congenital heart disease.[181] The most common pathogens are bacterial, specifically *Streptococci*, *Staphylococci*, *Bacteroides*, *Proteus*, and anaerobes. *Actinomyces*, *Nocardia*, and *Candida* are also common abscess-generating pathogens. Infection is often polymicrobial.[181]

Clinical course is consistent with that of an expanding intracranial mass lesion. Seizures are the presenting manifestation in at least one-third of cases.[181,183] Although headache and fever are the most frequent initial symptoms, common signs of infection can be missing (e.g., WBC count is normal in 20% of cases).[181,183]

Neuroimaging usually confirms diagnosis by revealing a typically ring-enhancing lesion on contrast CT or MRI.[181,184] EEG can demonstrate a high-voltage slow wave over the affected brain region.[181,183] LP is usually contraindicated secondary to mass-related increased intracranial pressure.

Antibiotics can be used alone or in combination with surgical drainage.[185] The threshold for neurosurgical evacuation is lowered by the presence of significant mass effect or location near ventricular surface (with risk of rupture into ventricular system causing florid ventriculitis or meningitis).[185] Antibiotic selection is based on knowledge of likely infection source; often broad-spectrum (including anaerobes) antibiotics are used (e.g., penicillin plus chloramphenicol or metronidazole).[181,183] Serial neuroimaging is usually performed to assess treatment response.[186] Seizure management is important, especially given a context of intracranial pressure complications. Epilepsy is a frequent long-term sequela of intraparenchymal abscess secondary to residual epileptogenic encephalomalacia.[181] Anticonvulsant therapy (e.g., phenytoin) is often maintained for at least 1 year after abscess treatment.[181]

Special Clinical Syndromes

Infection and Febrile Seizures

Febrile seizures are generalized convulsions that occur during a fever. Most febrile seizures occur between the ages of 6 months and 4 years. Febrile seizure is the most common cause of seizure in children, with up to 5% of all children having at least one febrile seizure by age 5 years. There is a strong genetic predisposition (first degree relatives have up to three times greater risk of febrile seizure than the general population).[187]

The challenge of febrile seizures is a product of their frequency and benign status and the need to distinguish them from seizures of identical phenomenology, representing potentially deadly etiologies requiring acute intervention, including infection. A single, brief generalized seizure occurring concurrently with fever is likely to be a simple febrile seizure.[187] Complex febrile seizures can also occur; they frequently have focal features, last longer than 15 minutes, and recur within 24 hours.[187] Children with simple febrile seizures are usually normal postictally (in contrast, 90% of seizures secondary to meningitis are followed by postictal stupor, and most of the remaining 10% demonstrate other meningitic signs [e.g., nuchal rigidity]).[187] Approximately one-third of children who have a febrile seizure have another seizure during a subsequent febrile illness.[187] However, only 2% of children whose first seizure is associated with fever will develop true epilepsy.[187]

Because up to 30% of children with bacterial meningitis have a seizure, it is frequently taught that LP is mandatory for children who have fever and seizure, because the convulsion may represent the sole manifestation of bacterial meningitis. However, there are data suggesting that this is an excessive invasive heuristic.

Green et al. reviewed over 500 consecutive cases of meningitis in children aged 2 months to 15 years. They found that meningitis was associated with seizures in 23% of cases, but all of these patients presented with signs in addition to the fever and seizure: Approximately 91% of these cases presented with significant sensorium change, and approximately 9% presented with straightforward indications for LP (e.g., nuchal rigidity). No cases of occult bacterial meningitis were found, that is, no patients were found to have bacterial meningitis manifesting solely as a simple seizure. The authors concluded that commonly taught decision rules requiring LP in children with fever and seizure are unnecessarily restrictive.[188]

A retrospective study of pediatric patients presenting to a pediatric ER for evaluation of febrile seizures was performed to determine the incidence of bacteremia, urinary tract infections, and unsuspected bacterial meningitis. (Children with initial lab evidence of meningoencephalitis in the ED [greater than 8 WBC in CSF], known seizure disorders, chronic neurologic disease, or documented immunodeficiencies were excluded.[189]) Blood cultures were performed on approximately 85% of patients, and of these 2.9% were positive, all for *Streptococcus pneumoniae*. Urine cultures were performed in approximately 50% of cases, and only 0.7% of these yielded a bacterial pathogen. CSF cultures were performed in 27% of encounters and none yielded bacterial pathogens. The investigators concluded that patients presenting for evaluation of febrile seizures are not at increased risk for bacteremia or urinary tract infection. Furthermore, in the absence of initial lab evidence of meningoencephalitis, bacterial meningitis is very uncommon in children diagnosed with febrile seizures.[189]

Al-Eissa prospectively studied frequency and yield of LPs performed in children with fever and seizure to identify criteria used by ED physicians in selecting patients for LP. Of 200 previously healthy children aged 3 months to 5 years brought to a pediatric ED with fever and seizure, LP was performed in 51% of cases and resulted in detection of seven (3.5%) cases of meningitis, three (1.5%) of which were bacterial. Seizures with complex partial features had significant influence on the decision of performing an LP.[190]

To determine whether complicated febrile seizures occur more often in children with viral infection, especially HHV-6, Rantala et al. studied 144 children with febrile convulsions, of whom 112 had simple and 32 had complex partial seizures. A diagnosis of virus infection was verified in 46% of simple partial seizure cases and 53% of complex partial seizures. In a follow-up of 2–4 years, children with positive evidence for a viral infection (even with virus isolated from CSF) had no more recurrences than those without any proven viral infection. The investigators concluded that children with febrile convulsions who have proven viral infection have no worse prognosis than those without.[191]

Epileptic Complications of Immunosuppressed Cancer Patients

In the immunocompromised patient, even subtle neurologic signs must prompt evaluation for possible CNS infection as etiology. Although a presentation of new-onset seizure obviously prompts such a workup, seizure occurring in an iatrogenically immunosuppressed cancer patient with a known seizure disorder secondary to known brain tumor (either primary or metastatic) still mandates an expedited search for infection. In one series, 60% of immunosuppressed cancer patients died secondary to CNS infection, despite many having malignancies with less than fatal prognoses.[139,192]

Epileptic Complications of Para- or Postinfectious and Postvaccinal Encephalomyelitides

Acute disseminated encephalomyelitis (ADE), para- or postinfectious encephalomyelitis (PIE), and postvaccinal encephalomyelitis (PVE) can occur in the course of or after various infections (particularly acute childhood exanthematous diseases) and after vaccinations. Clinical symptoms and pathologic changes are similar in all of these cases, regardless of precipitating infection or vaccination.[96]

Common infectious states that can be accompanied or followed by signs and symptoms of an encephalomyelitis include measles, rubella, VZV, mumps, influenza, parainfluenza, CMV, mycoplasma, and upper respiratory infections. Vaccinations that can precipitate PVE include measles, mumps, rubella, influenza, and rabies. CNS reactions can also occur after inoculations with sera, particularly against tetanus.[96,193]

CNS damage after acute exanthematous infection occurs most commonly following measles, for which the incidence is approximately 1 per 1,000 cases.[193] However, in regions with high vaccination rates, measles is no longer a common cause of PIE. Incidence of PVE following measles vaccination is only approximately 1 per 1 million recipients.[193] VZV is now probably the most common specific etiology of PIE, although exact incidence is unknown. Nonspecific upper respiratory infections are probably the most common cause overall.[96,193]

Pathogenesis of ADE, PIE, and PVE is unknown; an allergic or autoimmune reaction is most likely. Presumably a pathogen, usually a virus, triggers an immune-mediated reaction against CNS myelin, causing a disease similar to experimental allergic encephalomyelitis.[193] The characteristic pathologic change is demyelination.[96,193] Lesions are usually numerous and diffusely distributed. Although concentrated in white matter, a few patches can be found in cortical gray matter, with consequent epileptogenic potential. Acute hemorrhagic leukoencephalo-myelitis appears to be a fulminant form of ADE, PIE, and PVE; pathology is similar to ADE, PIE, and PVE plus microscopic hemorrhages and perivascular neutrophilic infiltrates.[96,193]

Clinical manifestations of AED, PIE, and PVE correspond to the CNS component most damaged; spinal cord, meningeal, basal ganglial, cerebellar, and cortical syndromes are well described. Meningitic signs (e.g., headaches, nuchal rigidity) are common early in the course of all types of ADE, PIE, and PVE.[96] Acute toxic encephalopathy and Reye's syndrome are seen more frequently after VZV, influenza, and rubella. In encephalitic forms, focal and generalized seizures can occur and can constitute the initial presentation.[194–198]

Diagnosis

On LP, CSF pressure can be slightly elevated, protein is normal or slightly elevated, glucose is normal, there is a moderate lymphocytic pleocytosis, and CSF myelin basic protein is usually increased. EEG is abnormal in most cases, usually with slow frequency (4–6 Hz) and high voltage.[96] Abnormalities are usually generalized and symmetric, but focal and unilateral changes can be found that can persist for weeks after apparent clinical recovery.[96] Persistent EEG abnormalities correlate with persistent neurologic abnormalities, including residual epilepsy.[96] MRI can reveal assorted white matter lesions.[196–198] Because there is no specific diagnostic test, ADE, PIE, and PVE should be considered when neurologic signs develop within 1 month of onset of acute exanthemata, upper respiratory tract infection, or vaccination. Differential diagnosis includes practically all acute infectious and inflammatory diseases of the CNS, including acute diffuse multiple sclerosis.[96,197,198]

There is no definitive treatment; steroids can ameliorate symptomatology. Maintenance anticonvulsant treatment, according to routine guidelines, is often required.[194]

Two viral syndromes partially related in their pathology to ADE, PIE, and PVE are discussed in the following sections.

Subacute Sclerosing Panencephalitis

Subacute sclerosing panencephalitis (SSPE) is caused by a defective measles virus. Children younger than 12 years of age are predominantly affected, boys more than girls. After natural measles infection, SSPE incidence is 5–10 cases per 1 million. After vaccine, the rate is less than 1 case per 1 million vaccine recipients. SSPE has a gradual onset, with a full range of subtle to severe neuropsychiatric phenomenology. Initial symptoms tend to be mild cognitive deficits; these can be followed by ataxia, myoclonic jerks, and seizures. CSF profile is usually normal except for marked elevation of CSF immunoglobulin: oligoclonal IgG bands, representing measles virus-specific antibodies, can be demonstrated. EEG often shows widespread cortical dysfunction with a burst-suppression pattern of high-amplitude slow wave or spike and slow wave complexes occurring at a rate of every 4–20 seconds synchronous with or independent of myoclonic jerks. MRI can reveal multifocal white matter lesions. SSPE course is variable, but can last years. There is no definitive treatment. Long-term seizure management is often required.[96,193]

Progressive Multifocal Leukoencephalopathy

PML is a subacute demyelinating disease caused by an opportunistic papovavirus, usually the Jamestown Canyon strain. PML typically occurs in patients with defective cell-mediated immunity. Patients with lymphomas, leukemias, and drug-induced immunosuppression were primary target populations until AIDS became the most common clinical setting. PML is characterized by the presence of multiple, in part confluent, areas of CNS demyelination, primarily in subcortical white matter. As the disease progresses, demyelinated plaques coalesce to form large lesions. Onset is subacute to chronic. Clinical manifestations are diverse and related to lesion location and size; focal and generalized seizures are an infrequent complication. CSF is usually normal. EEG often demonstrates nonspecific diffuse slowing. CT and MRI reveal white matter abnormalities. There is no definitive treatment. Seizure management, if needed, is routine.[96]

Aseptic Conditions: Noninfectious Causes of Meningitis

A diverse group of noninfectious processes can involve the CNS and mimic infection; clinical

Table 6-31. Noninfectious Causes of Meningitis

Acute meningitis	Drugs
	Seizures
	St. Louis encephalitis (SLE)
Recurrent meningitis	Mollaret's syndrome
	SLE
	Tumor
	Migraine
Chronic meningitis	Behçet's disease
	Leptomeningeal metastases
	Primary central nervous system angiitis
	SLE
	Sjögren's syndrome

Source: Data from BM Gripshover, JJ Ellner. Chronic Meningitis Syndrome and Meningitis of Noninfective or Uncertain Etiology. In WM Scheld, RJ Whitley, DT Durack (eds), Infections of the Central Nervous System. Philadelphia: Lippincott–Raven, 1997;881–896.

manifestation is primarily in the form of a chronic meningitic syndrome. (This is distinguished from acute meningitis, defined as symptoms of less than 2 weeks' duration, and recurrent meningitis, defined as at least two clinically similar episodes with an interval of clinical and CSF normalization.) Chronic meningitis, which is most typical of noninfectious disease etiology, usually presents with subacute onset, headache, fever, and stiff neck; encephalitic signs can also occur, and seizures are not uncommon. CSF is marked by elevated protein, decreased glucose, and usually lymphocytic pleocytosis. Most authors define chronic meningitis as the persistence of these signs and symptoms with abnormal CSF for at least 4 weeks.[199] See Table 6-31 for a summary of the major noninfectious chronic meningitis syndromes.

Mollaret's meningitis is a rare syndrome characterized by recurrent episodes of aseptic meningitis. Symptoms resolve spontaneously within days, only to recur weeks to months later. Recurrences can go on for years, then cease as suddenly and inexplicably as they began. Each episode of Mollaret's meningitis presents fulminantly with high fever, severe headache, and meningitic signs; focal and generalized seizures can be an unpredictable component of each episode. Although most commonly seen in young adults, age range is potentially wide. LP reveals a neutrophilic and lymphocytic pleocytosis; protein is mildly elevated, and glucose is usually normal. CSF generally normalizes by 1 week. Recent studies have shown a possible link with HSV.[199]

Behçet's disease is a systemic inflammatory disease characterized by recurrent oral and genital aphthous ulcers, uveitis, and skin lesions. CNS involvement occurs in up to 29% of cases, manifested by aseptic meningitis, meningoencephalitis, cranial nerve palsies, and seizures. There is no specific diagnostic test for Behçet's disease; instead, diagnostic criteria have been established. MRI reveals small foci of high signal activity on T2 images. CSF shows a mild pleocytosis. Immunosuppressive therapy has been used in neuro–Behçet's disease: cytoxic agents, such as chlorambucil or cyclophosphamide, are added to glucocorticoid therapy to improve results. Comorbid seizure management is routine.

Seizures, although not causing an acute meningitis syndrome, can by themselves cause a mild postictal CSF pleocytosis. CSF glucose and protein are normal. Cell counts usually normalize within one week.[200]

A full discussion of inflammatory causes of encephalitis and meningitis with potential seizure comorbidity (e.g., neurosarcoidosis, systemic lupus erythematosus, etc.) appears in Chapter 7.

Anticonvulsant and Antimicrobial Drug Interactions

Coincident administration of dual therapy targeting comorbid seizure and infection requires diligent consideration of potential drug-drug interactions to optimize treatment of comorbid seizure and infection and avoid iatrogenic complications. See Table 6-31, which summarizes the effects of antimicrobials and anticonvulsants on cytochrome P-450 metabolic enzyme systems, and Table 6-2, which summarizes the major specific known interactions.

References

1. Lacy CF, Armstrong LL, Goldman MP. Drug Information Handbook. Hudson, OH: Lexi-Comp, 2000;1092–1100.
2. Hantson P, Leonard F, Maloteaux JM, Mahieu P. How epileptogenic are the recent antibiotics? Acta Clin Belg 1999;54:80–87.
3. Gilbert DN, Moellering RC, Sande MA. Guide to Antimicrobial Therapy. Hyde Park, VT: Antimicrobial Therapy, 2000;129–133.
4. Durack DT, Whitley RJ, Scheld WM. Approach to the patient with central nervous system infection. In WM Scheld, RJ Whitley, DT Durack (eds), Infections of the Central Nervous System. Philadelphia: Lippincott–Raven, 1997;3.
5. Annegers JF, Hauser WA, Beghi E, et al. The risk of unprovoked seizures after encephalitis and meningitis. Neurology 1988;38:1407–1410.
6. Iavanainen M, Hietala J, Malkamaki M, et al. An association between epileptic seizures and increased serum bacterial antibody levels. Epilepsia 1983;24:584–587.
7. Yuhas Y, Weizman A, Dinari G, et al. An animal model for the study of the neurotoxicity of bacterial products. J Infect Dis 1995;171:1244–1249.
8. Guess HA, Resseguie LJ, Melton LJ, et al. Factors predictive of seizures among intensive care unit patients with gram negative infections. Epilepsia 1990;31:567–573.
9. Jackson AC, Gilbert JJ, Young GB, et al. The encephalopathy of sepsis. Can J Neurol Sci 1985;12:303–307.
10. Roos KL, Tunkel AR, Scheld WM. Acute bacterial meningitis in children and adults. In WM Scheld, RJ Whitley, DT Durack (eds), Infections of the Central Nervous System. Philadelphia: Lippincott–Raven, 1997;336–401.
11. Durand ML, Calderwood SB, Weber DJ, et al. Acute bacterial meningitis in adults. A review of 493 episodes. N Engl J Med 1993;328:21–28.
12. Plum F, Posner JB. Infectious and Inflammatory Disorders of the Nervous System. In TE Andreoli, CC Carpenter, F Plum, et al. (eds), Cecil Essentials of Medicine. Philadelphia: Saunders, 1990;806–816.
13. Labar DR, Harden C. Infection and Inflammatory Diseases. In J Engel Jr, TA Pedley (eds), Epilepsy: a Comprehensive Textbook. Philadelphia: Lippincott–Raven, 1997;2587–2596.
14. Rosenberg NM, Meert K, Marino D, et al. Seizures associated with meningitis. Pediatr Emerg Care 1992; 8:67–69.
15. Mylomakis E, Hohmann EL, Calderwood SB. Central nervous system dysfunction with Listeria monocytogenes. Medicine 1992;77:313–336.
16. Kim JH, Durack DT. Rickettsiae. In WM Scheld, RJ Whitley, DT Durack (eds), Infections of the Central Nervous System. Philadelphia: Lippincott–Raven, 1997;403–416.
17. Ries S, Schminke, Fassbender K, et al. Cerebrovascular involvement in the acute phase of bacterial meningitis. J Neurol 1997;244:51–55.
18. Chequer RS, Tharp BR, Dreimane D, et al. Prognostic value of EEG in neonatal meningitis. Pediatr Neurol 1992;8:417–422.
19. Inoue S, Nakazawa T, Takahashi H, et al. Seizures in the acute phase of aseptic and bacterial meningitis. No To Hattatsu 1998;30:494–499.

20. Grimwood K, Nolan TM, Bond L, et al. Risk factors for adverse outcomes of bacterial meningitis. J Paediatr Child Health 1996;32:457–462.

21. Baraff LJ, Lee SI, Schriger DL. Outcomes of bacterial meningitis in children: a meta-analysis. Pediatr Infect Dis J 1993;12:389–394.

22. Cascino GD, Luckstein RR, Sharbrough FW, et al. Facial asymmetry, hippocampal pathology, and remote symptomatic seizures: a temporal lobe epileptic syndrome. Neurology 1993;43:725–727.

23. Rowland LP. Spirochete Infections: Neurosyphilis. In LP Rowland (ed), Merritt's Textbook of Neurology. Baltimore: Williams & Wilkins, 1995;200–212.

24. Hook EW. Syphilis. In WM Scheld, RJ Whitley, DT Durack (eds), Infections of the Central Nervous System. Philadelphia: Lippincott–Raven, 1997;669–684.

25. Reik L. Lyme Disease. In WM Scheld, RJ Whitley, DT Durack (eds), Infections of the Central Nervous System. Philadelphia: Lippincott–Raven, 1997;685–718.

26. Rahn DW, Felz MW. Lyme disease update. Postgraduate Medicine 1998;103:51–70.

27. Miller JR. Spirochete Infections: Lyme Disease. In LP Rowland (ed), Merritt's Textbook of Neurology. Baltimore: Williams & Wilkins, 1995;209–211.

28. Coyle PK, Deng Z, Schutzer SE, et al. Detection of Borrelia burgdorferi antigens in cerebrospinal fluid. Neurology 1993;43:1093–1097.

29. Lerner PI. Neurologic complications of infective endocarditis. Med Clin North Am 1985;69:385–398.

30. Pruitt AA, Rubin RH, Karchmer AW, et al. Neurologic complications of bacterial endocarditis. Medicine 1978;57:329–343.

31. Hantson P, Leonard F, Maloteaux JM, Mahieu P. How epileptogenic are the recent antibiotics? Acta Clin Belg 1999;54:80–87.

32. Calandra G, Lydick E, Carrigan J, et al. Factors predisposing to seizures in seriously ill, infected patients receiving antibiotics: experience with imipenem/cilastatin. Am J Med 1988;84:911–918.

33. Drug-induced convulsions. Report from Boston Collaborative Drug Surveillance Program. Lancet 1972;2:677–679.

34. Hodgman T, Dasta JF, Armstrong, et al. Ampicillin-associated seizures. South Med J 1984;77:1323–1325.

35. Grondahl TO, Langmoen IA. Epileptogenic effect of antibiotic drugs. J Neurosurg 1983;78:938–943.

36. Gerald MC, Massey J, Spadaro DC. Comparative convulsant activity of various penicillins after intracerebral injection in mice. J Pharm Pharmacol 1973;25:104–108.

37. Kamei C, Sunami A, Tasaka K. Epileptogenic activity of cephalosporins in rats and their structure-activity relationship. Epilepsia 1983;24:431–439.

38. Bechtel TP, Slaughter RL, Moore TD. Seizures associated with high cerebrospinal fluid concentrations of cefazolin. Am J Hosp Pharm 1980;37:271–273.

39. Yost RL, Lee JD, O'Leary JP. Convulsions associated with sodium cefazolin: a case report. Am Surg 1977;43:417–420.

40. Gardner ME, Fritz WL, Hyland RN. Antibiotic-induced seizure: a case attributed to cefazolin. Drug Intell Clin Pharm 1978;12:268–271.

41. Thompson JW, Jacobs RF. Adverse effects of newer cephalosporins: an update. Drug Saf 1993;9:132–142.

42. Jackson GD, Berkovic SF. Ceftazidime encephalopathy: absence status and toxic hallucinations. J Neurol Neurosurg Psychiatry 1992;55:333–334.

43. Hillsley RE, Massey EW. Truncal asterixes associated with ceftazidime, a third generation cephalosporin. Neurology 1991;41:2008.

44. Ceftazidime, penicillin, and the epilepsies [Editorial]. Lancet 1992;340:400–401.

45. Neu HC. Safety of cefepime: a new extended-spectrum parenteral cephalosporin. Am J Med 1996;100:68S–75S.

46. De Sarro A, Naccari F, Imperatore C, De Sarro GB. Comparative epileptogenic properties of two monobactam derivatives in C57, Swiss, and DBA/2 mice. J Antimicrob Chemother 1996;38:475–484.

47. Alvan G, Nord CE. Adverse effects of monobactams and carbapenems. Drug Saf 1995;12:305–313.

48. Ayroza Galvao PA, Milstein TM, Mimica IM, et al. Aztreonam in the treatment of bacterial meningitis. Chemotherapy 1989;35[Suppl 1]:39–44.

49. Brothrton TJ, Kelber RL. Seizure-like activity associated with imipenem. Clin Pharmacy 1984;3:536–540.

50. Tse ST, Vera FH, Desai DV. Seizure-like activity associated with imipenem-cilastatin. Drug Intell Clin Pharm 1987;21:629–660.

51. Eng RH, Munsif AN, Yongco BG, et al. Seizure propensity with imipenem. Arch Intern Med 1989;149:1881–1883.

52. Leo RJ, Ballow CH. Seizure activity associated with imipenem use: clinical case reports and review of the literature. Ann Pharmacother 1991;25:351–354.

53. De Sarro GB, Ammendola D, De Sarro A. Effects of some excitatory amino acid antagonists on imipenem-induced seizures in DBA/2 mice. Brain Res 1995;671:131–140.

54. Norrby SR, Gildon KM. Safety profile of meropenem: a review of nearly 5,000 patients treated with meropenem. Scand J Infect Dis 1999;31:3–10.

55. Hellinger WC, Brewer NS. Carbapenems and monobactams: imipenem, meropenem, aztreonam. Mayo Clin Proc 1999;74:420–434.

56. Day IP, Goudie J, Nishiki K, Williams PD. Correlation between in vitro and in vivo models of proconvulsive activity with the carbapenem antibiotics biapenem, imipenem/cilastatin, and meropenem. Toxicol Lett 1995;76:239–243.

57. Ball P. Adverse reactions and interactions of fluoroquinolones. Clin Invest Med 1989;12:28–34.

58. Halkin H. Adverse effects of fluoroquinolones. Rev Infect Dis 1988;10[Suppl 1]:S258–S261.

59. Anastasio GD, Menscer D, Little JM. Norfloxacin and seizures [Letter]. Ann Intern Med 1988;108:169–170.

60. Slavich IL, Gleffe RF, Haas EJ. Grand mal epileptic seizures during ciprofloxacin therapy. JAMA 1989;261:558–559.
61. Bader MB. Role of ciprofloxacin in fatal seizures. Chest 1992;101:883–884.
62. Akahan K, Sekiguchi M, Une T, Osada Y. Structure-epileptogenicity relationship of quinolones with special reference to their interaction with gamma-aminobutyric acid receptor sites. Antimicrob Agents Chemother 1989;33:1704–1708.
63. Vancutsem PM, Schwark WS. Effects of fluoroquinolone antimicrobials alone and in conjunction with theophylline on seizures in amygdaloid kindled rats: mechanistic and pharmacokinetic study. Epilepsy Res 1992;13:59–71.
64. Robson RA. The effects of quinolones on xanthine pharmacokinetics. Am J Med 1992;92:22S–25S.
65. Akahane K, Kimura Y, Tsutomi Y, et al. Possible intermolecular interaction between quinolones and biphenylacetic acid inhibits gamma-aminobutyric acid receptor sites. Antimicrob Agents Chemother 1994;38:2323–2329.
66. Akaike N, Shirasaki T, Yakushiji T. Quinolones and fenbufen interact with GABAA receptor in dissociated hippocampal cells of rat. J Neurophysiol 1991;66:497–504.
67. Segev S, Rehavi M, Rubinstein E. Quinolones, theophylline, and diclofenac interactions with the GABA receptor. Antimicrob Agents Chemother 1988;32:1624–1626. 68. Wallace KL. Antibiotic-induced convulsions. Crit Care Clin 1997;13:741–762.
69. Schliamser SE, Cars O, Norrby SR. Neurotoxicity of beta-lactam antibiotics: predisposing factors and pathogenesis. J Antimicrob Chemother 1991;27:405–425.
70. Zuger A, Lowy FD. Tuberculosis. In WM Scheld, RJ Whitley, DT Durack (eds), Infections of the Central Nervous System. Philadelphia: Lippincott–Raven, 1997; 417–443.
71. Sumaya CV, Simek M, Smith MH, et al. Tuberculous meningitis in children during the isoniazid era. J Pediatr 1975;87:43–49.
72. Haas EJ, Madhava T, Quinn EL, et al. Tuberculous meningitis in an urban general hospital. Arch Intern Med 1977;137:1518–1521.
73. Clark WC, Metcalf JC, Muhlbauer MS, et al. Mycobacterium tuberculous meningitis: report of 12 cases and literature review. Neurosurgery 1986;18:604–610.
74. Tseng MY, Kao MC, Chiu CT. Isolated leptomeningeal tuberculoma. J Formos Med Assoc 1999;98:361–364.
75. Tosomeen AH, Berbari EF, Levy NT, et al. Case report: a 26 year-old woman with seizures and multiple intracranial mass lesions. J Med Liban 1998;46:349–352.
76. Whitener DR. Tuberculous brain abscess: report of a case and review of the literature. J Neurosurg 1982;56:597–600.
77. Lesprit P, Zagdanski AM, de La Blanchardiere A, et al. Cerebral tuberculosis in patients with the acquired immunodeficiency syndrome (AIDS). Report of six cases and review. Medicine 1997;76:423–431.
78. Martinez-Vazquez C, Bordon J, Rodriguez-Gonzalez A, et al. Cerebral tuberculoma—a comparative study in patients with and without HIV infection. Infection 1995;23:149–153.
79. Brennan RW, Deheija H, Kutt H, et al. Diphenylhydantoin intoxication attendant to slow acetylation of isoniazid. Neurology 1970;21:383–385.
80. Valsdon VC, Cooper GL. Carbamazepine intoxication caused by interaction with isoniazid. BMJ 1982;285:261–262.
81. Sullivan EA, Geoffroy P, Weisman R, et al. Isoniazid poisonings in New York City. J Emerg Med 1998;16:57–59.
82. Clyde WA. Mycoplasmal Diseases. In WM Scheld, RJ Whitley, DT Durack (eds), Infections of the Central Nervous System. Philadelphia: Lippincott–Raven, 1997;603–612.
83. Caceres ME, de los Reyes EC, Khan R, et al. Acute encephalopathy and intractable seizures in a 10 year-old boy. Semin Pediatr Neurol 1999;6:229–231.
84. Aminoff MJ, Greenberg DA, Simon RP. Clinical Neurology. Stamford, CT: Appleton & Lange, 1996;29–30.
85. Cassady KA, Whitley RJ. Pathogenesis and Pathophysiology of Viral Infections of the Central Nervous System. In WM Scheld, RJ Whitley, DT Durack (eds), Infections of the Central Nervous System. Philadelphia: Lippincott–Raven, 1997;7–22.
86. Summary of notifiable diseases, United States. 1990. MMWR Morb Mortal Wkly Rep 1991;39:1–61.
87. Weber T, Frye S, Bodemer M, et al. Clinical implications of nucleic acid amplification methods for diagnosis of viral infections of the nervous system. J Neurovirol 1996;2:175–190.
88. Whitley RJ. Herpes Simplex Virus. In WM Scheld, RJ Whitley, DT Durack (eds), Infections of the Central Nervous System. Philadelphia: Lippincott–Raven, 1997;73–89.
89. Whitley R. Viral encephalitis. N Engl J Med 1990;323:242–250.
90. Whitley R, Lakeman F. Herpes simplex virus infections of the central nervous system: therapeutic and diagnostic considerations. Clin Infect Dis 1995;20:414–420.
91. Barnett E, Jacobsen G, Evans G, et al. Herpes simplex encephalitis in the temporal cortex and limbic system after trigeminal nerve inoculation. J Infect Dis 1994;169:782–786.
92. Twomey J, Barker C, Robinson G, et al. Olfactory mucosa in herpes simplex encephalitis. J Neurol Neurosurg Psychiatry 1979;42:983–987.
93. Stroop WG, Schaefer DC. Neurovirulence of two clonally related HSV-1 strains in a rabbit seizure model. J Neuropathol Exp Neurol 1989;48:171–183.
94. Jay V, Becker LE, Blaser S, et al. Pathology of chronic herpes infection associated with seizure disorder: a

report of HSV-1 detection by PCR. Pediatr Pathol Lab Med 1995;15:131–146.

95. Jay V, Hwang P, Hoffman HJ, et al. Intractable seizure disorder associated with chronic herpes infection. Childs Nerv Syst 1998;14:15–20.

96. Jubelt B, Miller JR. Viral Infections. In LP Rowland (ed), Merritt's Textbook of Neurology. Baltimore: Williams & Wilkins, 1995;142–179.

97. Schlitt M, Bucher AP, Stroop WG, et al. Neurovirulence in an experimental focal encephalitis: relationship to observed seizures. Brain Res 1988;440:293–298.

98. Cornford ME, McCormick GF. Adult-onset temporal lobe epilepsy associated with smoldering herpes simplex 2 infection. Neurology 1997;48:425–430.

99. Ross JP, Cohen JI. Epstein-Barr Virus. In WM Scheld, RJ Whitley, DT Durack (eds), Infections of the Central Nervous System. Philadelphia: Lippincott–Raven, 1997;117–127.

100. Domachowske JB, Cunningham CK, Cummings DL, et al. Acute manifestations and neurologic sequelae of Epstein-Barr virus encephalitis in children. Pediatr Infect Dis J 1997;16:336–337.

101. Kimberlin DW, Whitley RJ. Human herpesvirus 6: neurologic implications of a newly-described viral pathogen. J Neurovirol 1998;4:471–473.

102. Suga S, Yoshikawa T, Asano Y, et al. Clinical and virological analyses of 21 infants with exanthem subitum (roseola infantum) and CNS complications. Ann Neurol 1993;33:597–603.

103. Hall S, Long CE, Schnabel KC, et al. Human herpesvirus 6 infection in children: a prospective study of complications and reactivation. N Engl J Med 1994; 331:432–438.

104. Barone SR, Kaplan MH, Krilov LR. Human herpesvirus 6 infection with first febrile seizures. J Pediatr 1995;127:95–97.

105. Hukin J, Farrell K, MacWilliam LM, et al. Case-control study of primary human herpesvirus 6 infection in children with febrile seizures. Pediatrics 1998;101:E3.

106. Hosoya M, Honzumi K, Suzuki H. Detection of enterovirus by PCR and culture in CSF of children with transient neurologic complications associated with acute febrile illness. J Infect Dis 1997;175:700–703.

107. Griffiths PD, McLaughlin JE. Cytomegalovirus. In WM Scheld, RJ Whitley, DT Durack (eds), Infections of the Central Nervous System. Philadelphia: Lippincott–Raven, 1997;107–115.

108. Whitley RJ. Arthopod-Borne Encephalitides. In WM Scheld, RJ Whitley, DT Durack (eds), Infections of the Central Nervous System. Philadelphia: Lippincott–Raven, 1997;147–168.

109. Tsai T. Arboviral infections in the United States. Infect Dis Clin North Am 1991;5:73–102.

110. Bale J. Viral encephalitis. Med Clin North Am 1993;77:25–42.

111. City Health Information 2000 (pamphlet). New York: New York City Department of Health, 2000;19(1):1–5.

112. Outbreak of West Nile-like viral encephalitis—New York, 1999. MMWR Morb Mortal Wkly Rep 1999;48:845–849.

113. Lanciotti RS, Roehrig JT, Deubel V, et al. Origin of the West Nile virus responsible for an outbreak of encephalitis in the northeastern United States. Science 1999;286:2333–2337.

114. Berger JR, Simpson DM. Neurologic Complications of AIDS. In WM Scheld, RJ Whitley, DT Durack (eds), Infections of the Central Nervous System. Philadelphia: Lippincott–Raven, 1997;255–271.

115. Britton CB. Acquired immunodeficiency syndrome. In LP Rowland (ed), Merritt's Textbook of Neurology. Baltimore: Williams & Wilkins, 1995;179–193.

116. Holtzman D, Kaku D, So Y. New-onset seizures associated with HIV infection: causation and clinical features in 100 cases. Am J Med 1989;87:173–177.

117. Aronow H, Feraru E, Lipton R. New-onset seizures in AIDS patients: etiology, prognosis, and treatment. Neurology 1989;39[Suppl 1]:428.

118. van Paesschen W, Bodian C, Maker H. Metabolic abnormalities and new-onset seizures in HIV-seropositive patients. Epilepsia 1995;36:146–150.

119. Pesola GR, Westfal RE. New-onset generalized seizures in patients with AIDS presenting to an emergency department. Acad Emerg Med 1998;5:905–911.

120. Rothman RE, Keyl PM, McArthur JC, et al. A decision guideline for emergency department utilization of noncontrast head CT in HIV-infected patients. Acad Emerg Med 1999;6:1010–1019.

121. Pascual-Sedano B, Iranzo A, Marti-Fabregas J, et al. Prospective study of new-onset seizures in patients with HIV infection: etiologic and clinical aspects. Arch Neurol 1999;56:609–612.

122. Bartolomei F, Gavaret M, Dhiver C, et al. Isolated, chronic, epilepsia partialis continua in an HIV-infected patient. Arch Neurol 1999;56:111–114.

123. Ferrari S, Monaco S, Morbin M, et al. HIV-associated PML presenting as epilepsia partialis continua. J Neurol Sci 1998;161:180–184.

124. Harden C, Daras M, Tuchman A et al. Low amplitude EEGs in demented AIDS patients. Electroencephalogr Clin Neurophysiol 1993;87:544–546.

125. Gabuzda D, Levy S, Chiappa K. EEG in AIDS and AIDS-related complex. Clin Electroencephalogr 1988;19:1–6.

126. Jennings HR, Romanelli F. The use of valproic acid in HIV-positive patients. Ann Pharmacother 1999;33:1113–1116.

127. Wong M, Suite N, Labar D. Seizures in HIV infection. Arch Neurol 1990;47:640–642.

128. Koppel B, Harden C, McCoy B, et al. Antiepileptic drug treatment in patients with AIDS. Epilepsia 1992;33:69.

129. Jubelt B, Ropka S. Infectious Diseases of the Nervous System. In R Rosenberg (ed), Atlas of Clinical Neurology. Boston: Butterworth–Heinemann, 1998;44–46.

130. Asher DM. Slow Viral Infections. In WM Scheld, RJ Whitley, DT Durack (eds), Infections of the Central Nervous System. Philadelphia: Lippincott–Raven, 1997;199–221.

131. Johnson RT, Gibbs CJ. Medical progress: Creutzfeldt-Jakob disease and related transmissible spongiform encephalopathies. N Engl J Med 1998;339:1994–2004.

132. Brandel J-P, Delasnerie-Laupretre N, Laplanche J-L, et al. Diagnosis of Creutzfeldt-Jakob disease. Neurology 2000;54:1095–1099.

133. Zerr I, Bodemer M, Geller O, et al. Detection of 14-3-3 protein in the cerebrospinal fluid supports the diagnosis of Creutzfeldt-Jakob disease. Ann Neurol 1998;43:32–40.

134. Bahn MM, Parchi P. Abnormal diffusion-weighted magnetic resonance images in Creutzfeldt-Jakob disease. Arch Neurol 1999;56:577–583.

135. Brown P, Cathala F, Sadowsky D, et al. Creutzfeldt-Jacob disease in France: clinical characteristics of 124 consecutive verified cases. Ann Neurol 1979;6:430–437.

136. Brown P, Gibbs CJ Jr, Rodgers-Johnson P, et al. Human spongiform encephalopathy: the National Institutes of Health series of 300 cases of experimentally transmitted disease. Ann Neurol 1994;35:513–529.

137. Aminoff MJ, Greenberg DA, Simon RP. Clinical Neurology. Stamford, CT: Appleton & Lange, 1996;58–59.

138. Perfect JR, Durack DT. Fungal Meningitis. In WM Scheld, RJ Whitley, DT Durack (eds), Infections of the Central Nervous System. Philadelphia: Lippincott–Raven, 1997;721–739.

139. Posner JP. Neurologic Complications of Cancer. Philadelphia: FA Davis Co, 1995;230–263.

140. Prockop LD. Fungal and Yeast Infections. In LP Rowland (ed), Merritt's Textbook of Neurology. Baltimore: Williams & Wilkins, 1995;193–198.

141. Sepkowitz K, Armstrong D. Space-Occupying Fungal Lesions. In WM Scheld, RJ Whitley, DT Durack (eds), Infections of the Central Nervous System. Philadelphia: Lippincott–Raven, 1997;741–762.

142. Sutton DA, Slifkin M, Yakulis R, et al. U.S. case report of cerebral phaeohyphomycosis caused by Ramichloridium obovoideum (R. mackenziei): criteria for identification, therapy, and review of other known dematiaceous neurotropic taxa. J Clin Microbiol 1998;36:708–715.

143. Bhagatm K, Ibrahim H, Naik K. Not everything acid-fast is Mycobacterium tuberculosis—a case of Nocardia. Cent Afr J Med 1999;45:217–220.

144. Cegielski JP, Warrell DA. Cerebral Malaria. In WM Scheld, RJ Whitley, DT Durack (eds), Infections of the Central Nervous System. Philadelphia: Lippincott–Raven, 1997;765–784.

145. Warrell D, Molyneux ME, Beales PF. Severe and complicated malaria (2nd ed). (World Health Organization Malaria Action Program). Trans R Soc Trop Med Hyg 1990;84[Suppl 2]:1–65.

146. Molyneux ME, Taylor TE, Wirima JJ, et al. Clinical features and prognostic indicators in pediatric cerebral malariae: a study of 131 Malawian children. Q J Med 1989;71:441–459.

147. Marsden PD, Bruce-Chwatt LJ. Cerebral malaria. Contemp Neurol Ser 1975;12:29–44.

148. Dukes CS, Luft BJ, Durack DT. Toxoplasmosis. In WM Scheld, RJ Whitley, DT Durack (eds), Infections of the Central Nervous System. Philadelphia: Lippincott–Raven, 1997;785–806.

149. McCabe RE, Brooks RG, Dorfman RF, et al. Clinical spectrum in 107 cases of toxoplasmic lymphadenopathy. Rev Infect Dis 1987;9:754–774.

150. Jubelt B, Miller JR. Parasitic Infections. In LP Rowland (ed), Merritt's Textbook of Neurology. Baltimore: Williams & Wilkins, 1995;212–222.

151. Porter S, Sande M. Toxoplasmosis of the central nervous system in AIDS. N Engl J Med 1992;327:1643–1648.

152. Ragnaud J, Morlat P, Dupon M, et al. Cerebral toxoplasmosis in AIDS. Presse Med 1993;22:903–908.

153. Ketonen LM, Berg MJ. Clinical Neuroradiology. New York: Oxford University Press, 1997;118–120.

154. Georgiev V. Management of toxoplasmosis. Drugs 1994;48:79–88.

155. Cegielski JP, Durack DT. Trypanosomiasis. In WM Scheld, RJ Whitley, DT Durack (eds), Infections of the Central Nervous System. Philadelphia: Lippincott–Raven, 1997;807–829.

156. Wery M. Drugs used in treatment of sleeping sickness. Int J Antimicrob Agents 1994;4:227–238.

157. Pepin J, Milord F, Khonde AN, et al. Risk factors for encephalopathy and mortality during melarsoprol treatment of Trypanosoma brucei sleeping sickness. Trans R Soc Trop Med Hyg 1995;89:92–97.

158. Hamon JF, Camara P. Electroencephalographic study of meningoencephalitis from Trypanosoma gambiense before and after treatment with melarsoprol. Neurophysiol Clin 1991;21:173–181.

159. Rocha A, de Meneses AC, da Silva AM, et al. Pathology of patients with Chagas' disease and AIDS. Am J Trop Med Hyg 1994;50:261–268.

160. Aminoff MJ, Greenberg DA, Simon RP. Clinical Neurology. Stamford, CT: Appleton & Lange, 1996;37.

161. Durack DT. Amebic infections. In WM Scheld, RJ Whitley, DT Durack (eds), Infections of the Central Nervous System. Philadelphia: Lippincott–Raven, 1997;831–844.

162. Cameron ML, Durack DT. Helminthic Infections. In WM Scheld, RJ Whitley, DT Durack (eds), Infections of the Central Nervous System. Philadelphia: Lippincott–Raven, 1997;845–878.

163. Dixon HBF, Lipscomb FM. Cysticercosis: an analysis and follow-up of 450 cases. Medical Research Council Special Report Series 1961;299:1–58.

164. del Brutto O, Santibanez R, Noboa C, et al. Epilepsy due to neurocysticercosis: analysis of 203 patients. Neurology 1992;44:1706–1709.

165. Medina M, Rosas E, Rubio-Donnadieu F, et al. Neurocysticercosis as the main cause of late-onset epilepsy in Mexico. Arch Intern Med 1990;150:325–327.

166. Wei GZ, Li CJ, Meng JM, Ding MC. Cysticercosis of the central nervous system. A clinical study of 1,400 cases. Chin Med J 1988;101:493–500.

167. del Brutto OH, Sotelo J. Neurocysticercosis: an update. Rev Infect Dis 1988;10:1075–1087.

168. Estnol B, Carona T, Abad P. A prognostic classification of cerebral cysticercosis: therapeutic implications. J Neurol 1986;49:1131–1134.

169. Vazquez V, Sotelo J. The course of seizures after treatment for cerebral cysticercosis. N Engl J Med 1992;327:696–701.

170. Botero D, Uribe C, Sanchez J, et al. Short course albendazole treatment for neurocysticercosis. Trans R Soc Trop Med Hyg 1993;87:576–577.

171. Takayanagui O, Jardim E. Therapy for neurocysticercosis. Arch Neurol 1992;49:290–294.

172. Rueda-Franco F. Surgical considerations of neurocysticercosis. Childs Nerv Syst 1987;3:212.

173. Schantz PM, Okelo GB. Echinococcosis. In KS Warren, AA Mahmoud (eds), Tropical and Geographic Medicine. New York: McGraw-Hill, 1990;505–518.

174. Mawhorter S, Kazura J. Trichinosis of the central nervous system. Semin Neurol 1993;13:148–152.

175. Arpino C, Gattinara GC, Piergili D, et al. Toxocara infection and epilepsy in children: a case-control study. Epilepsia 1990;31:33–36.

176. Mikhael NZ, Montpetit VJ, Orizaga M, et al. Toxocara canis infestation with encephalitis. Can J Neurol Sci 1974;1:114–120.

177. Glickman L, Cypress R, Crumrine I, et al. Toxocara infection and epilepsy in children. J Pediatr 1979; 94:75–78.

178. Scrimgeour EM, Gajdusek DC. Involvement of the central nervous system in Schistosoma mansoni and S. hematobium infection. Brain 1985;108:1023–1038.

179. Liu L. Spinal and cerebral schistosomiasis. Semin Neurol 1993;13:189–200.

180. Miller JR, Jubelt B. Bacterial Infections. In LP Rowland (ed), Merritt's Textbook of Neurology. Baltimore: Williams & Wilkins, 1995;119.

181. Berg L, Klebanoff LM. Focal infections. In LP Rowland (ed), Merritt's Textbook of Neurology. Baltimore: Williams & Wilkins, 1995;136–142.

182. Pathak A, Sharma BS, Mathuriya SN, et al. Controversies in the management of subdural empyema. Acta Neurochir (Wien) 1990;102:25–32.

183. Aminoff MJ, Greenberg DA, Simon RP. Clinical Neurology. Stamford, CT: Appleton & Lange, 1996;297–298.

184. Britt RH, Enzmann DR, Yaeger AS. Neuropathological and CT findings in experimental brain abscess. J Neurosurg 1981;55:590–603.

185. Mampalam TJ, Rosenblum ML. Trends in the management of bacterial brain abscesses. Neurosurgery 1988;23:451–458.

186. Whelan MA, Hilal SK. CT as a guide in diagnosis and follow-up of brain abscesses. Radiology 1980;135:663–671.

187. Fenichel GM. Clinical Pediatric Neurology. Philadelphia: Saunders, 1997;18–19.

188. Green SM, Rothrock SG, Clem KJ, et al. Can seizures be the sole manifestation of meningitis in febrile children? Pediatrics 1993;92:527–543.

189. Teach SJ, Geil PA. Incidence of bacteremia, urinary tract infections, and unsuspected bacterial meningitis in children with febrile seizures. Pediatr Emerg Care 1999;15:9–12.

190. Al-Eissa YA. Lumbar puncture in the clinical evaluation of children with seizures associated with fever. Pediatr Emerg Care 1995;11:347–350.

191. Rantala H, Uhari M, Tuokko H. Viral infections and recurrences of febrile convulsions. J Pediatr 1990;117:510–511.

192. Pruitt AA. Central nervous system infections in cancer patients. Neurol Clin 1991;9:867–888.

193. Griffen DE. Measles. In WM Scheld, RJ Whitley, DT Durack (eds), Infections of the Central Nervous System. Philadelphia: Lippincott–Raven, 1997;47–56.

194. Patel SP, Friedman RS. Neuropsychiatric features of acute disseminated encephalomyelitis. J Neuropsychiatry Clin Neurosci 1997;9:534–540.

195. Hirtz DG, Nelson KB, Ellenberg JH. Seizures following childhood immunizations. J Pediatr 1983;102:14–18.

196. Kesselring J, Miller DH, Robb SA. Acute disseminated encephalomyelitis—MRI findings and the distinction from multiple sclerosis. Brain 1990;113:291–302.

197. Kepes JJ. Large tumor-like demyelinating lesions of the brain: intermediate entity between multiple sclerosis and acute disseminated encephalomyelitis? Ann Neurol 1993;33:137–141.

198. Kimberlin DW, Plotkin SA. Vaccines for Viral Diseases with Significant CNS Manifestations. In WM Scheld, RJ Whitley, DT Durack (eds), Infections of the Central Nervous System. Philadelphia: Lippincott–Raven, 1997;983–1012.

199. Gripshover BM, Ellner JJ. Chronic Meningitis Syndrome and Meningitis of Noninfective or Uncertain Etiology. In WM Scheld, RJ Whitley, DT Durack (eds), Infections of the Central Nervous System. Philadelphia: Lippincott–Raven, 1997;881–896.

200. Schmidley JW, Simon RP. Postictal pleocytosis. Ann Neurol 1981;9:81–84.

Chapter 7

Inflammatory Noninfectious Disorders

Lawrence Seiden and Allan Krumholz

Inflammatory disorders are characterized by their systemic effects, and the immune response in these illnesses may cause dysfunction in tissues other than the typically affected organs. When the central nervous system (CNS) is involved, neurologic symptoms ranging from mild to severe occur, including headaches, confusion, coma, and, as this chapter stresses, epileptic seizures. Sometimes, these seizures or other neurologic abnormalities may be the initial or even the only manifestation of a systemic inflammatory disorder.

In other instances, these systemic inflammatory disorders indirectly cause neurologic symptoms, including seizures, by their influence on other organ systems. For example, inflammatory or connective tissue disorders, such as systemic lupus erythematosus (SLE), can cause failure of multiple organ systems, including vital organs such as the kidney or lung, thereby precipitating metabolic encephalopathies and seizures.

This chapter outlines some of the more common inflammatory noninfectious disorders that affect the CNS and can cause seizures. These include collagen vascular or connective tissue disorders (e.g., SLE and Sjögren's syndrome [SS], granulomatous disorders) (e.g., Crohn's disease [CD], Wegener's granulomatosis [WG], primary angiitis of the CNS [PACNS], and sarcoidosis), and demyelinating disorders (e.g., multiple sclerosis [MS]).

Systemic Lupus Erythematosus

SLE is a multisystem autoimmune disease characterized by circulating autoantibodies and immune complexes.[1] The disorder most commonly affects young, nonwhite women. The overall prevalence is approximately 50 per 100,000, but the prevalence among young women approaches 1 in 1,000.[2] The neurologic diagnoses associated with SLE include stroke, seizure, dementia, psychosis, and peripheral neuropathy.[3] CNS involvement has been reported in up to 75% of SLE patients,[3] with seizures occurring in up to 50% of patients by the time of death.[3,4]

The systemic effects of SLE are widespread, most commonly involving the joints and the skin. A symmetric arthritis occurs in both large and small joints. A malar "butterfly" rash is considered characteristic. Renal involvement occurs in up to 50% of cases, with glomerulonephritis the most common cause of morbidity. Cardiopulmonary involvement may include pericarditis or myocarditis, pleurisy, and pneumonitis. Hematologic manifestations commonly include anemia, leukopenia, or thrombocytopenia. Constitutional symptoms consist of fever, fatigue, and myalgia.

SLE exerts its widespread effects predominantly via immune mediated mechanisms. Autoantibodies in SLE form immune complexes that activate inflammatory cascades. This may ultimately cause tissue damage by the activation of complement leukocytes and macrophages, the end products of which may damage vasculature. Deposition of immune complexes in blood vessels may also cause a vasculopathy causing a variety of end organ effects.[2] In the brain, these mechanisms may result in cerebral edema or ischemia.

Antiphospholipid antibody is one of the more common autoantibodies associated with SLE. It

Table 7-1. The 1982 American College of Rheumatology Criteria for the Diagnosis of Systemic Lupus Erythematosus

Malar rash
Discoid rash
Photosensitivity
Oral or nasopharyngeal ulcers, or both
Nonerosive arthritis
Pleuritis or pericarditis
Renal dysfunction; proteinuria above 0.5 g/dl or cellular
  casts
Seizures or psychosis
Hematologic disorder; hemolytic anemia, leukopenia, or
  thrombocytopenia
Immunologic disorder; anti–double-stranded DNA or
  anti-Sm antibodies
Antinuclear antibodies

Note: A diagnosis of systemic lupus erythematosus can be made if four or more of these criteria are present at any time during the course of illness.
Source: Adapted from EM Tan, AS Cohen, JF Fries, et al. The 1982 revised criteria for the classification of systemic lupus erythematosus. Arthritis Rheum 1982;25:1271–1277.

has been frequently reported as a potential risk factor for stroke and described as a potentially prothrombotic factor.[1]

Neurologic Manifestations

Despite the relatively common involvement of the CNS in SLE, presentation of this disorder with neurologic signs or symptoms appears to be uncommon.[5]

The exact frequency of stroke in SLE is not known, but the risk of recurrence may be 50% or higher, and the occurrence of stroke increases the risk of seizures.[3] The mechanism for stroke in SLE is also not known, but it is often believed to be related to cardiac involvement (as a source of embolic phenomena) and a prothrombotic state.[3] The presence of anticardiolipin antibody and lupus anticoagulant, both procoagulant substances in vivo, may contribute to this risk. Strokes may occur in any distribution and may be related to immune-mediated microvascular disease. Clinical features are variable and can present with focal deficits or a more global syndrome of dysfunction, such as encephalopathy.[2]

Cognitive changes with SLE are quite variable. Presentation may be acute or subacute with clinical manifestations of agitation, altered awareness, dementia, or overt psychosis. Although dementia is not considered one of the most common presentations, formal neuropsychological testing has suggested that 66% of SLE patients experience cognitive impairment.[6]

The true incidence of seizures in SLE is difficult to determine, owing to the multiple potential etiologies in SLE. In one series of 91 patients, 22 (24%) had seizures. Two of these patients probably had idiopathic epilepsy, one with probable post-traumatic seizures, nine with active systemic infections, and four with significant azotemia. All of these seizures were generalized, with focal onset in five.[3] In another series of 161 SLE patients, 16 (10%) had seizures during the entire course of illness. Seven (4.4%) of these patients had onset of their seizures before developing the required diagnostic criteria for SLE.[7]

Both partial and generalized seizures occur in SLE. They can occur as the only manifestation of CNS involvement or as a complication of the cerebrovascular manifestations. Seizures that occur secondary to strokes most commonly are focal in onset but may secondarily generalize. Seizures may also occur in association with encephalopathy that may be due to a metabolic cause, particularly uremia from liver failure.[8]

Differential Diagnosis

The diagnosis of SLE is based on a combination of clinical and laboratory data. The diagnostic criteria for the disorder are summarized in Table 7-1. When any four of these criteria are met at any point during the disease, the diagnosis of SLE is established. Early in the course of illness, the diagnosis may be difficult to make, owing to a failure of the patient to fulfill all the necessary criteria.

SLE may be confused with disorders whose manifestations are included in its diagnostic criteria. These include rheumatoid arthritis; various forms of dermatitis; hematologic disorders, such as idiopathic thrombocytopenic purpura; and neurologic disorders, such as MS.

Several drugs can cause syndromes with some clinical features similar to SLE. The most common is procainamide, but it can also occur with hydralazine, isoniazid, chlorpromazine, methyldopa, quinidine, and just about all of the antiepileptic medications.

The most common symptoms in these cases are arthralgias, dermatitis, and systemic complaints, with rare CNS involvement. Drugs, including antiepileptics, can also cause false-positive serologic tests for SLE. In drug-induced lupus, antibodies to the histone complex of DNA are found, but antibodies to native DNA (anti–double-stranded DNA) are negative, and complement levels are normal.[4–6] Discontinuation of the offending drug results in prompt resolution of symptoms, but serologic abnormalities may persist somewhat longer.

The laboratory evaluation of SLE should include a screen for antinuclear antibodies, anti–double-stranded DNA, and anti-Sm antibodies. Hematologic evaluation typically reveals anemia, leukopenia, and thrombocytopenia. Urinalysis typically reveals proteinuria, hematuria, and casts.

Magnetic resonance imaging (MRI) should be performed in patients with neurologic manifestations. Abnormalities have been reported in up to 75% of patients with active disease.[9] These most commonly include subcortical and periventricular T2 signal abnormalities. Imaging may also demonstrate areas of infarction, new or old.

Electroencephalographic (EEG) abnormalities tend to be nonspecific and may occur in up to 50% of SLE patients.[10] In one series of 42 SLE patients, 11 with seizures, no epileptiform activity was reported on EEG. However, 29% had focal slowing, and 26% had generalized slowing.[11] In another series of 120 patients, one-third had epileptiform activity on EEG, but no seizures were reported in the entire group.[12]

Elevated spinal fluid protein may be seen, as well as an increase in the number of mononuclear cells. Oligoclonal bands and increased immunoglobin synthesis may be found as well.

Treatment

There is no cure for SLE. Patients may be treated symptomatically with nonsteroidal anti-inflammatory drugs for the arthralgias, myalgias, fever, and arthritis. Rashes may respond well to antimalarials or topical preparations.

If severe or disabling manifestations are present, immunosuppression may be necessary. High-dose glucocorticoids are commonly used with close monitoring for the undesirable side effects. In severe disease states with frequent flares, the use of cytotoxic agents, such as cyclophosphamide or azathioprine, should be considered.

Anticoagulation is recommended in SLE patients that have had a stroke. This is because of the high recurrence rate, associated with anticardiolipin antibody and lupus anticoagulant, in these patients.

Seizures occurring in association with flares in disease may not require treatment with antiepileptic drugs. Treatment of the underlying inflammatory pathology may be adequate to control convulsions, or, when present, metabolic derangement can be corrected. In some instances, seizures may be controlled with pulse steroid treatments alone. When recurrent, seizures will typically respond well to most antiepileptic therapies, although long-term treatment is frequently unnecessary once the systemic inflammatory disorder or metabolic derangement is brought under control.

Prognosis

The 5-year survival rate for SLE is between 75% and 98%, but in those patients with CNS involvement, such as seizures, the 5-year survival may be as low as 55%.[13,14] This may be owing to the presence of CNS involvement, representing a marker of more severe disease.

Sjögren's Syndrome

SS is defined by a triad of signs and symptoms, including xerophthalmia, xerostomia, and nondeforming arthritis. It occurs in 0.5–2.0% of the population and is more common in women. Onset is usually in middle age. SS can occur in association with other connective tissue diseases, such as SLE, rheumatoid arthritis, or scleroderma. Approximately 50% of cases occur in isolation and represent primary SS.[15]

In primary SS, exocrine glands are the most affected, with evidence of lymphocytic proliferation and fibrosis of lacrimal and salivary glands. The result is decreased tear and saliva production, causing ocular and oral signs and symptoms.

Extraglandular manifestations occur in one-fourth to one-third of patients. Arthritis of the small joints is common, with more than 80% of patients affected. Lymphadenopathy, hepatosplenomegaly, and cutaneous vasculitis are also commonly present. Forty percent of patients may manifest renal disease with an interstitial nephritis. Clinically significant pulmonary involvement with interstitial pneumonitis is relatively uncommon.

Neurologic involvement in primary SS has been reported to affect the CNS and peripheral nervous system (PNS) with differing frequencies. CNS involvement is reported in up to 25% of cases[16] and PNS disease in up to 32%.[17]

Primary SS is an autoimmune disease characterized by lymphocytic infiltration of the exocrine glands and B-lymphocyte hyperactivity. Autoantibodies against non–organ-specific antigens are identifiable in the sera of these patients. More specifically, these are directed against rheumatoid factors and the extractable nuclear and cytoplasmic antigens (Ro/SSA and La/SSB).

The pathophysiology of the neurologic complications of SS is not known. It is presumed to be related to autoimmune-mediated vascular damage.[18] Vasculitis is thought to be present, but other mechanisms, such as immune complex deposition and vasospasm, have not been excluded.

Neurologic Manifestations

PNS manifestations usually include a sensory or mixed sensorimotor polyneuropathy characterized by numbness, paraesthesias, and, rarely, pain. Distal weakness may occur and is usually mild.[19] Carpal tunnel syndrome is well described with this disorder, and cranial neuropathies have been reported, especially of the trigeminal nerve.[19]

CNS symptoms tend to be quite variable and diffuse. SS can affect any part of the neuraxis, and the manifestations are typically multifocal, recurrent, and progressive.[20] Focal strokelike or brain stem deficits may be seen, as well as a more global encephalopathy.

The characteristics of CNS or SS have frequently led to the misdiagnosis of MS.[20] In a series of 20 patients ultimately diagnosed with SS, 13 had CNS symptoms identified before the correct diagnosis. Patients experienced such symptoms as spinal cord disease, cerebellar dysfunction, and optic neuropathy. Most experienced a relapsing-remitting course.

Atypical for MS was the presence of peripheral neuropathy in more than 50% of patients.

Seizures occur in up to 1.5% of patients with SS and are usually partial, with or without secondary generalization. They are typically attributed to the vascular complications of the disease.[21]

Differential Diagnosis

The diagnosis of SS is based on the presence of two of the three characteristic clinical manifestations: xerophthalmia, xerostomia, or nondeforming arthritis. Serologic evaluation for autoantibodies to Ro/SSA and La/SSB may help to confirm the diagnosis, but it is not necessary.

In SS patients with CNS disease, MRI will be abnormal in up to 80%. Findings include multiple subcortical white matter and periventricular T2-weighted signal abnormalities. These can be difficult to distinguish from those seen in MS. Generalized cortical atrophy or discrete cerebral infarcts may also be seen. White matter lesions may not resolve with treatment.

EEG is abnormal in more than 50% of patients.[20] This includes both epileptiform abnormalities and slowing. In two-thirds of patients, at least one or more abnormalities are seen in visual, auditory, or somatosensory-evoked potentials.[20]

During active CNS disease in SS, spinal fluid may reveal a mild pleocytosis with reactive lymphoid cells. There is also evidence for increased intrathecal immunoglobulin G (IgG) synthesis. These findings may be indistinguishable from those in MS.[20]

Pathologic studies from SS patients with active CNS disease reveal several types of inflammation, including meningitis, small to medium vessel vasculitis, and mononuclear cell infiltration.[20] Demyelination has not been described.

Treatment

Treatment is directed toward symptomatic relief by artificially replacing deficient body fluids. Artificial tears or other ocular lubrication is important to avoid corneal damage from dryness.

Glucocorticoids or other immunosuppressive agents may be used when the extraglandular involvement is severe, especially for clinically significant renal, pulmonary, or CNS involvement.

Seizures, when they occur, are treated with antiepileptic drugs and usually respond well. Treatment of the underlying inflammatory disorder is necessary for the long-term control of seizures.

Prognosis

There is no cure for SS, and it is a progressive disease in many cases. It is not known whether the use of immunosuppressive drugs alters the course of the disease.

Crohn's Disease

CD is an immune-mediated disorder that affects primarily the terminal ileum but may also affect the small and large intestines in a segmental fashion.[22] The disease is more common in whites than nonwhites and is much more common in patients of Jewish descent. The incidence of CD is 2 cases per 100,000 with a prevalence of 20–40 per 100,000.

Clinically, CD presents as abdominal pain, diarrhea, fever, and generalized fatigue. Frequent systemic complications of CD include arthritis, ankylosing spondylitis, iritis, erythema nodosum, and pyoderma gangrenosum.[22] Neurologic and psychiatric complications have been reported in up to 15% of CD patients.[22] These include seizures, stroke, peripheral neuropathy, myopathy, headache, and depression, among others. Seizures are reported to be the most common CNS complication, occurring in almost 6% of patients.[22]

The increased frequency of CD in whites who are also Jewish suggests that there may be a genetic predisposition for the disorder. No markers have been clearly established. The possibility of an infectious etiology has also been extensively evaluated without any consistently identified organism.

An immune-mediated mechanism was first postulated because of the common extraintestinal manifestations and the response of the disease to immune-modulating drugs. Both immune complexes and cell-mediated immunity have been implicated in the etiology of CD, but no definitive evidence is yet available.

Neurologic Manifestations

In a review of 263 patients with confirmed CD, the most common neurologic complications seen with a direct relationship to the illness included seizure, stroke, peripheral neuropathy, and myopathy, occurring in 15%.[22] Other neurologic complications, including headache, cerebellar dysfunction, Parkinson's disease, optic neuritis, and sixth nerve palsy, were also seen but are not clearly related to CD.

Seizures were identified in 15 patients (5.9%). The majority was generalized tonic-clonic, but partial seizures also were seen. Autoimmune phenomena, involving small vessels in the CNS, may be related to the seizures, but others have reported seizures associated with dehydration, sepsis, or metabolic disturbances.[23,24]

In a series of 253 patients, 12 (4.7%) had cerebral infarcts, four with bilateral subcortical infarcts. The presence of a hypercoagulable state in CD is well accepted, with evidence for increased platelet counts, coagulation factor VIII, and fibrinogen levels.[25] The role of dehydration, common in CD, in addition to the hypercoagulable state, is not clearly established. Prophylactic trials with anticoagulation have not been reported, possibly owing to the increased risk of bleeding complications from the intestinal tract in CD.

An inflammatory myopathy may be seen in as many as 1.5% of CD patients.[22] This is predominantly axonal and has been reported to respond well to steroids.

Differential Diagnosis

Extraintestinal manifestations of CD may present several years before its diagnosis.[22,24,26,27] The details of a differential diagnosis are guided by the organ system primarily involved and the symptoms. When neurologic complications occur, evaluation should be guided by the nature of the specific neurologic problem.

When CNS manifestations are evident, MRI may be normal or demonstrates nonspecific subcortical and periventricular T2 signal abnormalities. Strokes in large vessel distribution have been identified,[22] as well as aseptic abscesses.[24]

Spinal fluid examination may reveal mildly elevated protein in cases with neuropathy and myelopathy.[26] Moderately elevated cell counts, predominantly polymorphonuclear leukocytes, were seen in the presence of aseptic abscesses.[24]

The diagnosis of CD is most reliably made with endoscopic evaluation, biopsy, and the exclusion of other etiologies. Endoscopic examination typically reveals ulcerations in a segmental pattern, separated by normal mucosa. Pseudopolyps, strictures, and edema may be seen. Granulomas are present in 30–50% of biopsies taken from areas with active ulceration.

Treatment

The principal medical therapy of CD is anti-inflammatory agents, such as sulfasalazine or glucocorticoids. Surgical therapy is reserved for those patients with complications, which occur in up to 70% of patients. Surgery may be required for bowel obstruction due to narrowing or strictures, symptomatic fistulae, persistent anal fissures or abscesses, or for intraabdominal abscesses or perforation. Surgical therapy is not curative, with relapses occurring frequently.[28]

Treatment of neurologic complications is symptomatic and includes immune-modulating drugs, when indicated. Cases of myelopathy and aseptic brain abscesses have responded to glucocorticoids or cytotoxic agents.[22,24]

None of the reported seizure patients required long-term therapy with antiepileptic drugs.[22] In a case report of a patient with well-established CD and seizures (not clearly related to her CD), higher than expected dosages of phenytoin were required to maintain therapeutic levels.[29] This was postulated by the authors to be related to increased excretion of phenytoin in the bowel, related to CD.

Prognosis

The course of CD is chronic and intermittent. Over time, it responds less well to medications, and a majority of patients require surgery at some point during the illness. Mortality from CD increases with longer duration of illness and ranges between 5% and 10%.[28] Death is usually related to peritonitis or sepsis.

Seizures respond well to therapy of the underlying condition, as does the neuropathy and myelop-

athy. It is unclear whether immune modulation affects the hypercoagulable state in these patients, so the risk of recurrent strokes is unknown. As previously mentioned, treatment with anticoagulants may be risky in these patients, because they are predisposed to intestinal bleeding.

Primary Angiitis of the Central Nervous System

PACNS is a rare subacute vasculitis restricted to the vasculature of the CNS.[30] Vessels of any size may be affected, but small vessel vasculitis is always present.[31] Other than constitutional symptoms, such as fever, malaise, and anorexia, there is no consistent evidence for systemic disease related to this disorder.

The most common clinical features of the disease include seizure, stroke, headache, intellectual deterioration, or spinal cord syndromes.[31] Seizures occur in up to 44% of patients.[32,33]

The pathophysiology of PACNS is not known. It is presumed to have an immune-mediated basis, based on its response to immune-modulating drugs. The similarities in histopathologic findings in the brain between this disorder and others, such as sarcoidosis and disseminated herpes zoster, suggest the possibility of an underlying process that is yet to be identified.[30]

Neurologic Manifestations

The most common presenting symptoms of PACNS are cognitive changes and headache, present at disease onset in 45% and 42% of patients, respectively.[30] Headaches may be diffuse or focal, but they are typically severe and throbbing.[31] Focal neurologic signs may be present at onset in up to 16% of patients.

Seizures are the presenting sign in approximately 10% of cases,[30] but, at any time during the illness, they can occur in up to 44%.[32,33] The incidence of seizures is more frequent than can be explained on the basis of focal strokes, occurring in approximately 15%. Seizures may be focal or generalized.

The course of PACNS is consistent with a progressive encephalopathy, with both focal and generalized manifestations becoming more common as the disease progresses. Up to one-half of the cases develop coma during some part of the illness.

Differential Diagnosis

The diagnosis of PACNS is based on clinical suspicion and the absence of other diseases. Serologic studies to rule out systemic disorders, as well as antibody titers for some of the other immune mediated diseases, are necessary. Unlike other disorders associated with a peripheral vasculitis, erythrocyte sedimentation rates are usually normal.[31]

MRI of the brain might demonstrate strokes with extensive signal abnormalities in the white matter. These findings are nonspecific and do not aid in finalizing a diagnosis.

Examination of the spinal fluid usually reveals elevated protein and a normal to moderately elevated lymphocytosis.[30] Red cells may be present, with up to 200–400 cells per mm^3.[31] EEG is also nonspecific with a variety of findings, from generalized slowing to focal sharp waves.

Cerebral angiography has been reportedly normal in up to 40% of cases.[30] When angiography is positive, typical findings include segmental and nonsegmental narrowing or beading of small and medium size vessels.[30,31]

Biopsy may be diagnostic, but, given the scattered, segmental nature of the vasculitis, it may be missed. A diagnostic biopsy reveals evidence of small vessel vasculitis.

Treatment

Treatment is based on immunosuppressant therapy. High-dose corticosteroids or cytotoxic agents, such as cyclophosphamide, are commonly used. There is little evidence at this time that these drugs are effective in altering the outcome of the disease.

Control of seizures may be difficult and relies on aggressive treatment of the underlying disorder.

Prognosis

Based on a review of 78 patients, mortality was close to 80%,[30] with a mean survival of 6 months from onset of symptoms to death. The accuracy of these numbers is not clear, given the difficulty in unequivocally establishing the diagnosis.

Wegener's Granulomatosis

WG is a systemic necrotizing granulomatous vasculitis, typically involving the upper and lower respiratory tracts and kidneys.[34] The incidence of the disease is not well established but is reported at approximately 0.4 cases per 100,000 population.[35] The usual age of onset is 30–40 years, but it can start at any age. Men are affected more often than women.

The common presenting feature of WG is sinus pain with purulent or bloody nasal discharge. Nasal mucosal ulcers are common, and nasal septal perforation is a common complication. Respiratory involvement may begin as a cough, with or without hemoptysis and chest pain.[36] Renal involvement is prominent and frequently dominates the patient's clinical picture. Glomerulonephritis with proteinuria, hematuria, and red cell casts typically precedes functional renal impairment.

Neurologic involvement has been reported in 30–55% of patients.[37–39] Most common is peripheral neuropathy, followed by cranial neuropathy, ophthalmoplegia, stroke, and seizures. Neurologic complications were not considered to represent a major contribution to mortality in this group.

WG is histologically characterized by a necrotizing vasculitis of both small arteries and veins. This is seen in association with intravascular or extravascular granuloma.[40] The lungs demonstrate bilateral nodular infiltrates. Renal involvement is characterized by segmental glomerulitis with granuloma formation.

Circulating and deposited immune complexes have been demonstrated in WG, but their role in pathogenesis of the disease is unclear. The presence of cytoplasmic antineutrophil cytoplasmic antibodies serves as a marker of active disease.[40]

Neurologic Manifestations

Neurologic manifestations have been reported in up to 55% of WG patients, but in a recent series of 324 cases, 33.6% of patients experienced neurologic complications.[36–39] The most frequent complication was peripheral neuropathy, occurring in 16% of patients in that series, but with as many as 28.6% affected in another.[39] Mononeuropathy multiplex predominates.

Cranial neuropathies have been reported in up to 11.7% of patients with WG,[36] with the ophthalmic nerve being the most commonly affected. The other more commonly affected cranial nerves were the abducens and facial nerves.[37]

Strokes are considered rare events in WG and are thought to be related to a cerebral vasculitis when they occur.[34] Large and small arteries, as well as venous structures, are thought to be involved.[39] Coincident with evidence for cerebral infarcts, other features of cerebral vasculitis, such as confusion, encephalopathy, and seizure, have been documented.[37]

Seizures are also considered rare in WG, occurring in only 2–3% of cases. Seizures are believed to be associated with the cerebral vasculitis that occurs in these patients as a complication of the disease.[37] It is often considered a preterminal occurrence in these patients.

Differential Diagnosis

The diagnosis of WG is made on the basis of clinical presentation of typical signs and symptoms, described previously. Presentation with neurologic manifestations has not been described. The demonstration of necrotizing granulomatous vasculitis on biopsy of involved tissue secures the diagnosis. Lymphomatoid granulomatosis is an infiltrative disorder with clinical signs and symptoms that might be confused with WG. The biopsy findings of WG and seropositivity for cytoplasmic antineutrophil cytoplasmic antibodies help to differentiate the two.

Treatment

The treatment of choice for WG is oral cyclophosphamide, usually with the addition of oral prednisone.[36,40] Treatment continues for several months up to a year, after complete remission of symptoms. The use of azathioprine has been preliminarily evaluated and has not found to be as effective as cyclophosphamide.[36] Management of seizures is dependent on control of the underlying inflammatory disorder.

Prognosis

Before the routine use of cyclophosphamide for WG, the disease was universally fatal within several months. Using the treatment regimen previously discussed, complete remission is reported as high as 93%,[36] with a mean duration of remission reaching 4 years. The majority of neurologic complications is thought to be related to the vasculitic complications of the disease, and, by controlling the primary disorder, neurologic manifestations are controlled.

Sarcoidosis

Sarcoidosis is a multisystem granulomatous disorder of unknown etiology. Typical presentations include bilateral hilar adenopathy, pulmonary infiltration, and skin and eye lesions.[41] Neurologic manifestations of sarcoidosis occur in approximately 5% of sarcoidosis patients and are the presenting feature of sarcoidosis for approximately 50% of these patients.[42,43] Neurosarcoidosis manifests in diverse ways, including cranial neuropathy, aseptic meningitis, mass lesions, encephalopathy, vasculopathy, myelopathy, seizures, hypothalamic pituitary disorders, hydrocephalus, peripheral neuropathy, and myopathy.[30,44–47] Seizures are reported to occur in approximately 20% of patients with neurosarcoidosis and indicate the presence of more severe disease.[48]

Although the precise etiology of sarcoidosis remains unknown, there is evidence that sarcoidosis is caused by heightened immune processes at the sites of disease activity.[49] Sarcoidosis can be thought of as an inflammatory response to an as-yet unidentified foreign antigen.[49–54] The central pathologic hallmark of sarcoidosis, the granuloma (Figure 7-1), consists of macrophages, macrophage-derived epithelioid cells, and multinucleated giant cells that secrete cytokines. Around this central core exist CD4 and CD8 lymphocytes, B lymphocytes, plasma cells, and fibroblasts. The lymphocytes are thought to be stimulated by antigen presentation by activated macrophages present at sites of inflammation.[55–60]

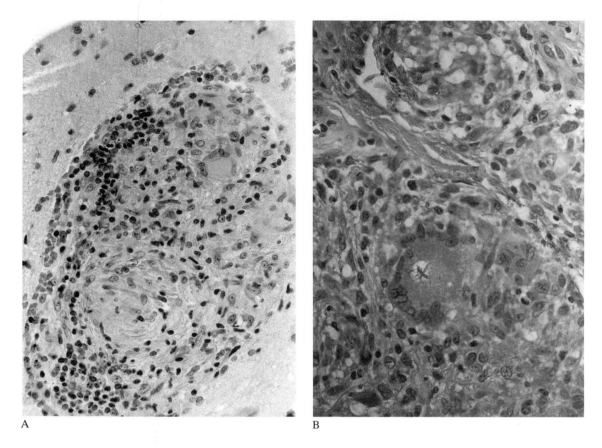

A   B

Figure 7-1. A. Photomicrograph at 200× magnification of a brain showing an intraparenchymal noncaseating or non-necrotizing sarcoid granuloma. **B.** Photomicrograph at 400× magnification of a sarcoid granuloma in the brain, demonstrating a multinucleated giant cell.

In reaction to an antigen, monocytes and macrophages form granulomas, and ultimately irreversible obliterative fibrosis can develop. Furthermore, small foci of ischemic necrosis can be found, probably as a consequence of vascular compromise due to perivascular inflammation. Importantly, these granulomas are not specific for sarcoidosis, and indistinguishable or nearly identical lesions occur in a variety of other conditions that must be excluded before a diagnosis of sarcoidosis can be made with certainty.

Sarcoidosis usually presents between the ages of 20 and 40 years. However, it also occurs in children and older populations. It appears to have similar clinical manifestations in all age groups. Intrathoracic structures are most commonly affected (87% of patients), followed by lymph node, skin, and ocular disease in 15–28% of patients (Table 7-2). Although it is generally understood that a diagnosis

of sarcoidosis is most secure when it is based on histologic confirmation, on average, 30% lack histologic confirmation, and the diagnosis is often based solely on clinical and radiologic findings.[50]

Involvement of any organ by sarcoidosis is possible and may occur with or without major symptoms. Sarcoidosis may be asymptomatic, or it can present with constitutional symptoms and pulmonary or extrapulmonary manifestations. Anatomic presence of the disease in an organ often occurs without overt clinical evidence of dysfunction. It is estimated that 20–40% of patients are asymptomatic at presentation, with their disease being discovered by routine chest radiography.[50]

Active sarcoidosis may cause an elevation in serum angiotensin–converting enzyme (SACE), which can then serve as a marker of the disease.[51] SACE, however, is neither highly sensitive, with just 50–

Table 7-2. Percentage Frequency of Organ Involvement in Sarcoidosis

Manifestation	Frequency (%)
Intrathoracic	87
Hilar nodes	72
Lung parenchyma	46
Upper respiratory tract	6
Dermatologic	—
Skin	18
Erythema nodosum	15
Ocular	15
Lacrimal	3
Parotid	6
Splenomegaly	10
Peripheral lymphadenopathy	28
Bone	3
Cardiac	3
Hepatomegaly	10
Hypercalcemia	13
Neurologic	5
Hematologic	Rare
Endocrinologic	—
Gastrointestinal and genitourinary	—

Table 7-3. Neurosarcoidosis

Clinical Manifestation	Approximate Frequency (%)
Cranial neuropathy	50–75
Facial palsy	25–50
Aseptic meningitis	10–20
Hydrocephalus	10
Parenchymal disease	—
Endocrinopathy	10–15
Mass lesion(s)	5–10
Encephalopathy/ vasculopathy	5–10
Seizures	5–10
Neuropathy	5–10
Myopathy	10

60% of active sarcoidosis patients showing abnormalities, nor very specific, because it is also often elevated in patients with other conditions, such as liver disease, diabetes mellitus, hyperthyroidism, systemic infection, malignancy, and Gaucher's disease.[51]

Neurologic Manifestations

Neurologic symptoms are the presenting feature of sarcoidosis in one-half of individuals with neurosarcoidosis.[42,43] The approximate frequency of the various neurologic complications is presented in Table 7-3. Only rarely do patients with neurosarcoidosis have no evidence of disease in other organ systems, such as the lung.[42,44–47,61,62] However, systemic disease may not always be evident early in a patient's clinical course, and, in some instances, it can be difficult to find.

Although the range of clinical manifestations of sarcoidosis is exceptionally varied, most patients present in characteristic ways that can be systematically organized (see Table 7-2). Similarly, the neurologic manifestations of sarcoidosis can be classified (see Table 7-3). However, one-third to one-half of neurosarcoidosis patients develop more than one neurologic manifestation of their disease.

Neurosarcoidosis, because of its varied manifestations, is in the differential diagnosis of many unexplained neurologic syndromes. The diagnosis of sarcoidosis is most secure when based on pathology and when more than one organ system can be documented to be involved. However, because tissue from the nervous system is difficult to secure for pathologic analysis, and other tests are not diagnostic of neurosarcoidosis, the diagnosis of neurosarcoidosis must sometimes remain tentative.

Peripheral facial seventh cranial nerve palsy is the single most frequent neurologic manifestation of sarcoidosis. It develops in 25–50% of all patients with neurosarcoidosis. Although usually unilateral, bilateral facial palsy also can occur, presenting with either simultaneous or sequential paralysis. More than half of all patients with facial palsy also have other forms of nervous system involvement. In general, the prognosis for the facial palsy is good, with more than 80% of patients having a good outcome in terms of recovery of function.[42,47]

Hydrocephalus is noted in approximately 10% of neurosarcoidosis patients and can pose great danger. Hydrocephalus is a potentially lethal complication of sarcoidosis. Patients with acute hydrocephalus may die suddenly from increased intracranial pressure, and even patients with chronic hydrocephalus have the potential to acutely decompensate. Patients with acute hydrocephalus characteristically present with headache, altered mentation or consciousness, and impaired gait. On examination, papilledema or other signs of raised intracranial pressure can be found. Acute decompensating hydrocephalus is a medical emergency that necessitates prompt diagnosis and treatment.

Parenchymal brain disease is reported in approximately 50% of patients with neurosarcoidosis and can present in several forms. Hypothalamic dysfunction is the most common manifestation of CNS parenchymatous disease. When hypothalamic dysfunction occurs, it usually involves the neuroendocrinologic system or "vegetative functions," such as temperature regulation, appetite, thirst, sleep, and libido. However, neuroendocrinologic disease in sarcoidosis can also occur secondary to pituitary disease. Any of the neuroendocrinologic systems can be affected by sarcoidosis.[42] Potential endocrinologic manifestations of neurosarcoidosis include thyroid disorders, disorders of cortisol metabolism, and sexual dysfunction. An elevated serum prolactin level, found in 3–32% of patients with sarcoidosis, may be an indication of hypothalamic dysfunction.

Hypothalamic disorders that affect vegetative functions vary considerably. A disorder of thirst is the most common hypothalamic disorder related to neurosarcoidosis and is attributed to a change in the hypothalamic "osmostat." More rarely, the syndrome of inappropriate secretion of antidiuretic hormone can occur.[43,63] These hypothalamic disorders can lead to severe hyponatremia, which can cause seizures. Neurosarcoidosis-induced disruptions of hypothalamic function also have been described to cause disorders of appetite, libido, temperature control, weight regulation, and sleep.[43,63]

Intraparenchymal mass lesions due to sarcoidosis may present as an isolated mass (Figure 7-2) or masses occurring in any cerebral area or multiple cerebral nodules. Subdural plaquelike masses may also occur and mimic meningiomas. Calcifications may also be seen. Although historically, intraparenchymal mass lesions were considered rare, computed tomography and MRI have shown parenchymatous disease to be more frequent than previously thought (see Figure 7-2).

The diffuse encephalopathy and vasculopathy associated with neurosarcoidosis are not well-under-

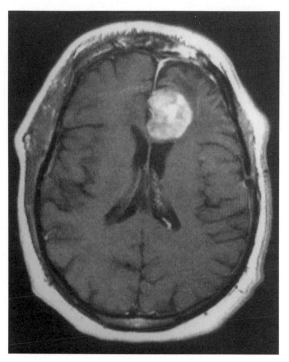

Figure 7-2. Magnetic resonance imaging, axial, T1 with gadolinium, demonstrating a frontal intracerebral mass that was proven by biopsy to be neurosarcoidosis.

stood manifestations of sarcoidosis. Moreover, it is often difficult, both clinically and pathologically, to separate clearly between these entities. In fact, these two manifestations of neurosarcoidosis frequently coexist. For these reasons, they can be considered as a single overlapping entity, but an individual patient may present with one form, or the other may dominate.[42] An example of the MRI changes in a patient with neurosarcoid encephalopathy is shown in Figure 7-3.

Seizures are an important manifestation of CNS parenchymal disease due to neurosarcoidosis, and their significance has recently been better understood.[48] They have been reported in up to 20% of patients with neurosarcoidosis and may be focal or generalized. Seizures have been correlated with a poor prognosis in neurosarcoidosis.[64] However, the cause of this poor prognosis is not directly due to seizures. Instead, the poor prognosis of neurosarcoidosis patients with seizures is due to the fact that seizures are an indicator for the presence of severe CNS parenchymal disease or hydroceph-

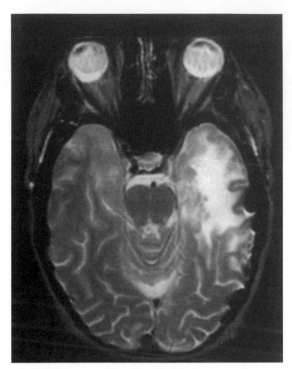

Figure 7-3. Magnetic resonance imaging, axial, T2-weighted image, which shows a large area of abnormality in the temporal lobe that proved at biopsy to be sarcoidosis manifesting with a focal encephalopathy or vasculopathy. This patient presented with seizures.

alus. This more severe pathology actually accounts for the poor outcomes because of its higher risk for progressive or recurrent disease or death.[48,64]

Importantly, seizures in patients with neurosarcoidosis are usually relatively easy to control, if the underlying CNS inflammatory process can be effectively treated.[48] Once the sarcoid inflammatory disorder is adequately controlled with anti-inflammatory or immunosuppressive therapy, consideration can be given to reducing or even discontinuing antiepileptic medications. If seizures recur, emphasis should be placed on assessing and treating the underlying inflammatory disorder rather than just focusing on antiepileptic medications.

Differential Diagnosis

When a patient without documented systemic sarcoidosis develops a clinical syndrome suggestive of neurosarcoidosis, confirming evidence for sarcoidosis should be sought in other organ systems.

Such systemic disease can best be documented when a thorough, systematic evaluation based on the known natural history of sarcoidosis is undertaken (see Table 7-1). In particular, sarcoidosis most frequently affects intrathoracic structures (87% of patients), followed by lymph node, skin, and ocular disease in 15–28% of patients. Consequently, histologic support for a diagnosis of sarcoidosis should be pursued following leads obtained from the patient's clinical evaluation and those statistics. Pulmonary involvement is so common in sarcoidosis that this should be the first organ system to consider when attempting to establish the presence of systemic sarcoidosis. Indeed, nearly 90% of patients with sarcoidosis are reported to show radiographic evidence of pulmonary involvement.[65] However, although an abnormal chest roentgenogram is often seen in sarcoidosis and can be supportive evidence for that diagnosis, these chest x-ray findings are not necessarily specific or pathognomonic for sarcoidosis. Additional evidence to support pulmonary involvement can be obtained from pulmonary function testing, including diffusion capacity. Moreover, when chest x-rays or pulmonary function studies suggest pulmonary involvement, a diagnosis of sarcoidosis is confirmed by obtaining histologic evidence of sarcoidosis with a transbronchial biopsy. To better define the extent of lung or lymph node involvement, chest computed tomography can also be useful.

The most specific laboratory test associated with sarcoidosis is the SACE. However, its sensitivity is not that high, with just 50–60% of active sarcoidosis patients showing abnormalities. In addition, SACE is not very specific, because it is abnormal in other conditions, such as liver disease, diabetes mellitus, hyperthyroidism, systemic infection, malignancy, and Gaucher's disease.[66]

Another category of neurosarcoidosis patients, those with well-documented systemic sarcoidosis who develop neurologic disease suspected to be neurosarcoidosis, still merits careful appraisal to exclude causes other than sarcoidosis for their neurologic problems. Neurosarcoidosis can be confused with many other neurologic diseases, and because it is often not possible or judicious to biopsy affected tissue from the nervous system to confirm neurosarcoidosis, good clinical judgment becomes critical. In particular, sarcoidosis and seizures are relatively common disorders, and, there-fore, sarcoidosis should not always be presumed as the cause of seizures in a patient with both disor-ders—their coexistence may merely be incidental. In general, patients with sarcoidosis who develop neurologic problems deserve consideration of dis-ease entities that may mimic neurosarcoidosis, par-ticularly infection and neoplasia.

Although not specifically diagnostic, there are tests that can support a presumptive diagnosis of neurosarcoidosis. Brain-imaging studies can be par-ticularly helpful to confirm the presence, classify the nature, and monitor the treatment of neurosarcoido-sis. The preferred imaging technique is now MRI with contrast enhancement,[67] and T2-weighted images are most useful, showing areas of increased signal intensity, especially in the periventricular dis-tribution. Contrast administration helps by demon-strating leptomeningeal enhancement (Figure 7-4) as well as parenchymal abnormalities (see Figures 7-2 and 7-3). Enhancement presumably reflects a breakdown of the blood-brain barrier and implies active inflammation.

Spinal fluid analysis is another useful method for assessment, diagnosis, and staging of neurosar-coidosis. More than 50% of patients with CNS sarcoidosis have some cerebrospinal fluid (CSF) abnormality.[42] CSF angiotensin-converting enzyme (ACE) activity tends to be raised in some 50% of untreated patients with CNS sarcoidosis,[68] although abnormalities are also seen in the presence of infection and malignancy. The CSF-ACE level may be abnormal even with steroid therapy but less consistently than in untreated patients. The degree of elevation of CSF ACE may parallel the clinical course.[68–70] A normal CSF-ACE assay does not exclude the diagnosis of neurosarcoidosis. More-over, diagnostic value of CSF ACE is further lim-ited, because assay methodology and normative values have not yet been well standardized.

Treatment

There are no rigorous studies that compare various treatments for neurosarcoidosis. However, most experts agree that corticosteroid therapy is the mainstay of treatment and is indicated for any patient without a specific contraindication to it. However, the patient's clinical course, expected

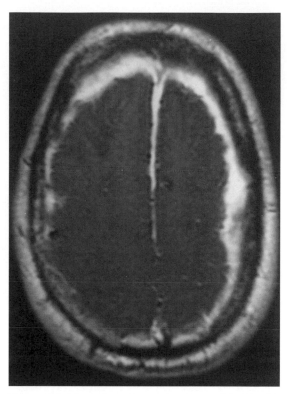

Figure 7-4. Magnetic resonance imaging, axial, T1 with gadolinium, which demonstrates marked dural enhance-ment due to sarcoidosis.

natural history or prognosis, and adverse treatment effects or side effects should guide decisions about issues, such as the optimal therapeutic dose and duration of therapy. A treatment paradigm is given in Figure 7-5.

In sarcoidosis patients with seizures, the seizures are generally not a major limiting problem and can usually be well controlled with antiepileptic medica-tion, if the underlying CNS inflammatory reaction can be effectively treated. However, seizures have been shown to be an indication of or marker for the presence of parenchymatous involvement of the brain, which is in itself a very serious manifestation of neurosarcoidosis.[47,48] Consequently, it is impor-tant to recognize the clinical relevance of seizures in patients with neurosarcoidosis. Seizures are useful, often early, warning signs that a patient may have one of the more serious forms of neurosarcoidosis, such as an intracranial mass lesion.[48]

Treatment alternatives to corticosteroids must sometimes be considered for patients with neuro-

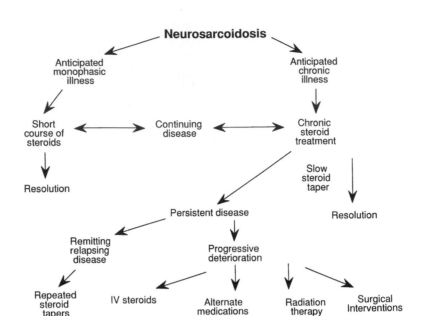

Figure 7-5. A treatment paradigm for patients with neurosarcoidosis.

sarcoidosis. Experience in this area is limited, and there is not a single established alternative treatment to corticosteroids, but there are several choices. Indications for the use of alternate treatments include contraindications to corticosteroids as initial therapy, serious adverse chronic corticosteroid effects, and progressive disease activity, in spite of aggressive corticosteroid therapy. Medication alternatives to corticosteroids that have been used to treat sarcoidosis include methotrexate, cyclophosphamide, cyclosporine, azathioprine, chlorambucil, hydroxychloroquine, pentoxifylline, and thalidomide.[43,71] One nondrug treatment that has also been reported to have some limited success is radiation therapy.[71,72]

Practically, consideration should be given to introducing alternative therapy whenever a patient shows signs of serious corticosteroid side effects or requires frequent large increases in corticosteroid dosage to control symptoms. Alternative treatment with an immunosuppressive agent or irradiation is a logical adjunctive therapy for refractory neurosarcoidosis, given what is understood of the immunopathogenic mechanisms of the disease. Alternative therapy may allow a gradual decrease in corticosteroid dosage to prevent or minimize corticosteroid complications,

often without deterioration in clinical status. Rarely, however, can corticosteroids be completely eliminated.

Recent series describe promising results with methotrexate to treat patients with refractory sarcoidosis or those who could not tolerate the side effects of corticosteroids.[73,74] This same group reports good results treating neurosarcoidosis patients with methotrexate.[75] In that series, many patients who failed treatment with methotrexate were then treated with intravenous cyclophosphamide. Although these findings reported with methotrexate are promising and deserve consideration, the observations are based on nonrandomized and uncontrolled trials.

Prognosis

The clinical course and prognosis for neurosarcoidosis varies but is somewhat predictable. For example, some two-thirds of patients have a monophasic neurologic illness; the remainder has a chronically progressive or remitting-relapsing course. Those with a monophasic illness typically have an isolated cranial neuropathy, most often involving the facial nerve, or an episode of aseptic meningitis. Those with a chronic course usually have CNS parenchymal disease, hydrocephalus, multiple cranial neuropathies (especially involving the second and eighth cranial nerves), peripheral neuropathy, and myopathy.[47]

In particular, sarcoidosis patients with seizures have a higher risk of progressive disease, a poorer prognosis, and a higher mortality. This is because seizures have been demonstrated to be associated with a higher incidence of parenchymal brain involvement in sarcoidosis,[48] and such parenchymal disease or hydrocephalus correlates with the poorest prognosis and the greatest risk of death.[48] Mortality of neurosarcoidosis is approximately 5–10% percent.[42,43,47,48]

Despite limitations in our understanding of the natural history of sarcoidosis, treatment with corticosteroids does seem to benefit many patients with neurosarcoidosis. Even more important, patients benefit most from a comprehensive approach to care based on an understanding of the full clinical spectrum of neurosarcoidosis, an appreciation of the whole range of treatment options, and the anticipation of complications, such as those relating to corticosteroid treatment.

Multiple Sclerosis

MS is a demyelinating disorder of the CNS characterized clinically by episodes of focal disturbance of the optic nerves, brain, or spinal cord. The duration of discrete episodes is quite variable, with remissions common. Classic features include motor weakness, sensory loss, paraesthesias, impairment or loss of vision, eye movement abnormalities, cerebellar dysfunction, bladder dysfunction, and cognitive or emotional changes.[76] Seizures have been reported in up to 5% of patients with MS.[77]

The prevalence of MS varies greatly by region. Worldwide prevalence rates range from approximately one case per 100,000 in the Far East to more than 150 cases per 100,000 in parts of the United Kingdom.[77] Within the United States, prevalence ranges from approximately 10 cases per 100,000 to 170 cases per 100,000. MS presents most commonly in young adults, with a mean age of 30 years.[78] Women are affected more commonly than men.

A detailed discussion on the pathophysiology of MS is beyond the scope of this chapter. The primarily affected cells in the CNS are oligodendrocytes, cells that produce a myelin sheath, surrounding axons and aiding conduction. It is not entirely clear whether the primary event in MS is an attack on the oligodendrocyte, the myelin sheath, or both.[79] The classic lesion in the CNS in MS is a focal region of demyelination, referred to as a *plaque*. Large numbers of plaques may be found throughout the white matter of the brain or spinal cord. Clinical symptoms are determined by the location of the plaques. When they become numerous, plaques may become confluent. The areas in the brain most commonly affected are the subcortical white matter and periventricular regions. In the spinal cord, subpial plaques are most common. Lesions throughout the brain stem and cerebellum are also common. Given the frequency of visual symptoms in MS, it is not surprising that the optic nerves are affected in virtually every case.[80]

Although less common, plaques located at the junction of the cortex and white matter, or even in the gray matter itself, are present in almost 25% of cases.[81] These cortical or subcortical plaques may act as seizure foci. There are several reports of seizure onset or recurrent seizures correlating with new MS lesions or with active exacerbation of older plaques.[82,83] Others have found no clear correlation.[84]

Neurologic Manifestations

As described, MS can cause virtually any neurologic deficit based on the location of new and old plaques. For the purpose of this chapter, discussion is limited to seizures.

Seizures can occur at any time during the course of illness. In some cases, it may be the only clinical manifestation.[83] Partial-onset seizures clearly predominate and occur with a higher frequency than would be expected when compared to the global epilepsy population.[77,82]

Differential Diagnosis

The diagnosis of MS requires signs or symptoms of multiple CNS lesions, separated in time and space, as well as the exclusion of other disorders that may

Table 7-4. Conditions That May Be Confused with Multiple Sclerosis

Cerebral vasculitis
Multiple cerebral emboli
Mitochondrial encephalomyopathies
Acute disseminated encephalomyelitis
Progressive multifocal leukoencephalopathy
Subacute combined degeneration of the spinal cord
Neurosarcoidosis
Lyme disease
Systemic lupus erythematosus
Cerebral lymphoma

produce a similar clinical picture (Table 7-4). Diagnosis may be difficult at the time of presentation, owing to a lack of the duration of illness required to produce multiple lesions and, therefore, multiple signs or symptoms. The use of diagnostic testing for the demonstration of additional lesions and possibly subclinical signs may be helpful in making an early diagnosis in these cases.

Diagnostic testing includes MRI of the brain or spinal cord, or both. MS plaques are typically iso- to hypodense on T1-weighted scans and hyperintense on T2-weighted scans. Periventricular lesions are seen in up to 85% of MS patients,[85] with involvement of the corpus callosum in up to 90%.[86] Acute lesions usually demonstrate enhancement, presumably owing to disruption of the blood-brain barrier.

Evoked potential studies can be useful in defining subclinical visual pathway, brain stem, or spinal cord lesions. These tests, when abnormal, typically reveal slowed central conduction, consistent with demyelination. Visual evoked potentials have been reported to be abnormal in up to 80% of MS cases.[87]

Examination of the spinal fluid usually demonstrates oligoclonal bands and increased intrathecal synthesis of IgG. During acute attacks, a mild pleocytosis may be present.

Many of the disorders that may present in a similar manner to MS do not manifest seizures frequently. Sarcoidosis and PACNS manifest seizures more frequently than MS and should be considered earlier in the evaluation.

Between 1% and 4% of patients with MS may experience paroxysmal dysarthria and ataxia.[88] These are multiple brief episodes marked by sudden onset of slurred speech and ataxia in one or more limbs. This entity may be confused with epileptic events based on its clinical characteristics. Interestingly, it responds well to anticonvulsive therapy, particularly carbamazepine.

Brief episodes of marked dystonic posturing of the arm, leg, or face on one side have also been reported.[89] Often triggered by movement or tactile sensation, episodes may start abruptly and last for 30 seconds to several minutes. The movements are frequently painful and may be successfully treated with anticonvulsant drugs as well.

Treatment

Treatment of acute exacerbations of MS is aimed at shortening the duration of individual attacks. The more commonly used immunosuppressive agents in MS are daily methylprednisolone intravenously for several days, followed by a short course of oral prednisone, oral prednisone alone, or intravenous adrenocorticotropic hormone. Relapses of prior symptoms may also be due to a metabolic or infectious cause, the treatment of which yields resolution. Treatment of acute relapses frequently results in the resolution of acute seizures.

Chronic therapy is directed more toward the prevention of relapses and progression of disease. The relatively recent introduction of interferon beta-1b, interferon beta-1a, and copolymer-1 has reduced the frequency of relapses over time. However, no currently available treatment has been shown to significantly alter the long-term outcome of the disease.

Seizures not related to an acute relapse of the underlying disorder typically respond well to traditional antiepileptic medications.

Prognosis

MS can cause significant morbidity but tends to have a much lesser effect on mortality. Given the wide variability and unpredictable nature of clinical signs and symptoms in MS, prognosis is based on a patient's own clinical history. If the disease has been mild for 5–10 years, it is likely to remain mild for the next decade. If severely affected early on in the illness, there tends to be higher disability.[90]

Some have suggested that the occurrence or frequency of seizures does not significantly correlate with MS severity or evolution.[91] Others have suggested that these patients fall into several major groups.[77,83,92] Seizures in MS patients tend to have a good prognosis, with spontaneous resolution in almost half. In many of these cases, the seizures are thought to be related to acute exacerbations. In the group of patients who have seizures that do not clearly correlate with the course of MS itself, antiepileptic drug therapy is quite effective. In those patients with a progressive cognitive decline associated with their seizures, the prognosis is somewhat worse, with a susceptibility to status epilepticus.

Immunotherapy for Seizures

As the occurrence of seizures in these various systemic immune-mediated disorders demonstrates, epilepsy can be related to immunologic disorders. This raises the issues of whether immune mechanisms may be important in other, more common forms of epilepsy and whether immunotherapy merits further consideration.

Immunoglobulin therapy was first reported to be effective in epilepsy in 1977, when epileptic children had recurrent upper respiratory tract infections treated with intramuscular IgG.[93] Improvements in seizure frequency and behavior were noted in these patients. Subsequently, 16 children with Lennox-Gastaut syndrome were treated with intravenous IgG (IVIG), and significant improvement was seen in eight.[94] Since that time, several additional clinical trials have been published with similar results, reporting significant improvement in approximately 50% of cases.[93]

In 1994, the first double-blind, placebo-controlled trial of IVIG for the treatment of epilepsy was published.[95] Three different dosages were evaluated in 61 patients with intractable epilepsy from various etiologies. Significant clinical improvement, defined as a reduction in seizures by at least 50% after 6 months, was reported in 52.5% of the IVIG group, compared to 27.8% of the placebo group, with a p value of .095. No dose relationship was identified.

Rasmussen's syndrome, or chronic encephalitis and epilepsy, is a well-recognized and relatively stereotyped disorder, first described by Rasmussen

in 1958.[96,97] It is characterized by a progressive hemiparesis, intellectual decline, and intractable seizures, in association with pathologic changes suggestive of chronic encephalitis.[97,98] At presentation, generalized seizures are most common, followed by simple partial and complex partial seizures.[99] Approximately 20% of cases may present with status epilepticus.

As the illness evolves, partial seizures clearly predominate, occurring in 77% of cases.[99] Epilepsia partialis continua has been reported to occur in more than 50% of cases at some time during the course of the disease.

The pathogenesis of Rasmussen's syndrome is unknown, but an association with autoantibodies to glutamate receptor GluR3 has been suggested.[100,101] This has been supported by the finding of a simultaneous reduction in anti-GluR3 antibody titers, with clinical improvement in patients after total plasma exchange.[102,103] This benefit is short lived, suggesting reaccumulation of a pathogenic antibody.[104,105]

The treatment of Rasmussen's syndrome with high-dose steroid preparations has been somewhat effective, but the beneficial effects are not long lived, with periodic relapses occurring frequently.[106,107] Treatment of this disorder with IVIG has been reported with initial improvement, but it is not consistently maintained.[98,108]

There is emerging clinical evidence that IVIG may be of value in several refractory seizure conditions. The details regarding which patients and at what point of the illness it should be used need to be investigated further.

References

1. Moore PM, Lisak RP. Systemic lupus erythematosus: immunopathogenesis of neurologic dysfunction. Springer Semin Immunopathol 1995;17:43–60.
2. Moore PM. Neuropsychiatric systemic lupus erythematosus. Stress, stroke, and seizures. Ann N Y Acad Sci 1997;823:1–17.
3. Futrell N, Schultz LR, Millikan C. Central nervous system disease in patients with systemic lupus erythematosus. Neurology 1992;42:1649–1657.
4. O'Connor JF, Musher DM. Central nervous system involvement in systemic lupus erythematosus: a study of 150 cases. Arch Neurol 1966;14:157–164.
5. Tola MR, Granieri E, Caniatti L, et al. Systemic lupus erythematosus presenting with neurological disorders. J Neurol 1992;239:61–64.

6. Denburg JA, Carbotte RM, Denburg SD. Neuronal antibodies and cognitive function in systemic lupus erythematosus. Neurology 1987;37:464–467.

7. Mackworth-Young CG, Hughes GRV. Epilepsy: an early symptom of systemic lupus erythematosus [Letter]. J Neurol Neurosurg Psychiatry 1985;48:185.

8. West SG. Neuropsychiatric lupus. Rheum Dis Clin North Am 1994;20:129–158.

9. Gonzalez-Crespo MR, Blanco FJ, Ramos A, et al. Magnetic resonance imaging of the brain in systemic lupus erythematosus. Br J Rheumatol 1995;34:1055–1060.

10. Rudolph NM, Bourke BE. The value of the electroencephalogram in cerebral systemic lupus erythematosus. Electroencephalogr Clin Neurophysiol 1985;61:S189(abst).

11. Hietaharju A, Jantii V, Korpela M, et al. Nervous system involvement in systemic lupus erythematosus, Sjögren syndrome, and scleroderma. Acta Neurol Scand 1993;88:299–308.

12. Matsukawa Y, Nishinarita S, Hayama T, et al. Clinical significance of electroencephalography in patients with systemic lupus erythematosus. Ryumachi 1993;33:20–28.

13. Nadeau SE, Watson RT. Neurologic Manifestations of Vasculitis and Collagen Vascular Syndromes. In AB Baker, RJ Joynt (eds), Clinical Neurology. Philadelphia: Harper & Row, 1985;59.

14. Brick JE, Brick JF. Neurologic manifestations of rheumatologic disease. Neurol Clin 1989;7:629–639.

15. Talal N. Sjögren's syndrome: historical overview and clinical spectrum of disease. Rheum Dis Clin North Am 1992;18:507–515.

16. Alexander E. Central nervous system disease in Sjögren's syndrome. Rheum Dis Clin North Am 1992;18:637–672.

17. Alexander GE, Provost TT, Stephens MB, et al. Sjögren's syndrome: central nervous system manifestations. Neurology 1981;31:1391–1396.

18. Alexander EL. Neurologic disease in Sjögren's syndrome: mononuclear inflammatory vasculopathy affecting central/peripheral nervous system and muscle. Rheum Dis Clin North Am 1993;19:869–908.

19. Kaltreider HB, Talal N. The neuropathy of Sjögren's syndrome: trigeminal nerve involvement. Ann Intern Med 1969;70:751–762.

20. Alexander EL. Central nervous system manifestations of primary Sjögren's syndrome: an overview. Scand J Rheumatol 1986;[Suppl 61]:161–165.

21. Alexander GE, Provost TT, Stephens MB, et al. Neurologic complications of primary Sjögren's syndrome. Medicine 1982;61:247–257.

22. Elsehety A, Bertorini TE. Neurologic and neuropsychiatric complications of Crohn's disease. South Med J 1997;90:606–610.

23. Gendelman S, Present D, Janowitz HD. Neurological complications of inflammatory bowel disease. Gastroenterology 1982;82:1065.

24. Andre M, Aumaitre O, Marcheix JC. Aseptic systemic abscesses preceding diagnosis of Crohn's disease by three years. Dig Dis Sci 1995;40:525–527.

25. Talbot RW, Heppell J, Dozois RR, et al. Vascular complications of inflammatory bowel disease. Mayo Clin Proc 1986;61:140–145.

26. Lossos A, River Y, Eliakim A, et al. Neurologic aspects of inflammatory bowel disease. Neurology 1995;45:416–421.

27. Andre M, Aumaitre O, Papo T, et al. Disseminated aseptic abscesses associated with Crohn's disease: a new entity? Dig Dis Sci 1998;43:420–428.

28. Farmer RG, Whelan G, Fazio VW. Long-term follow-up of patients with Crohn's disease. Relationship between clinical pattern and prognosis. Gastroenterology 1985;88:1818–1825.

29. Lesser RP, Irace P, Kutt H, et al. Enhanced gastrointestinal excretion of phenytoin in a patient with Crohn's disease. Epilepsia 1984;25:302–307.

30. Younger DS, Hays AP, Brust JC, et al. Granulomatous angiitis of the brain. An inflammatory reaction of diverse etiology. Arch Neurol 1988;45:514–518.

31. Moore PM, Cupps TR. Neurological complications of vasculitis. Ann Neurol 1983;14:155–167.

32. Abu-Shakra M, Khraishi M, Grossman H, et al. Primary angiitis of the CNS diagnosed by angiography. QJM 1994;87:351–358.

33. Calabrese LH. Vasculitis of the central nervous system. Rheum Dis Clin North Am 1995;21:1059–1076.

34. Nishino H, Rubino F, Parisi JE. The spectrum of neurologic involvement in Wegener's granulomatosis. Neurology 1993;43:1334–1337.

35. Kurland LT, Chuang TY, Hunder GH. The Epidemiology of Systemic Arteritis. In RC Lawrence, LE Shulman (eds), Epidemiology of the Rheumatic Diseases. New York: Gower, 1984;196–205.

36. Fauci AS, Haynes BF, Katz P, et al. Wegener's granulomatosis: prospective clinical and therapeutic experience with 85 patients for 21 years. Ann Intern Med 1993;98:76–85.

37. Nishino H, Rubino FA, DeRemee RA, et al. Neurological involvement in Wegener's granulomatosis: an analysis of 324 consecutive patients at the Mayo clinic. Ann Neurol 1993;33:4–9.

38. Drachman DA. Neurologic complications of Wegener's granulomatosis. Arch Neurol 1963;8:145–155.

39. Anderson JM, Jamieson DG, Jefferson JM. Non-healing granuloma and the nervous system. QJM 1975;174:309–323.

40. Leavitt RY, Fauci AS. Wegener's granulomatosis. Curr Opin Rheumatol 1991;3:8–14.

41. Johns CJ, Michele TM. The clinical management of sarcoidosis. A 50-year experience at the Johns Hopkins Hospital. Medicine 1999;78:65–111.

42. Stern BJ, Krumholz A, Johns C, et al. Sarcoidosis and its neurological manifestations. Arch Neurol 1985;42:909–917.

43. Krumholz A, Stern BJ. Neurological Manifestations of Sarcoidosis. In MJ Aminoff, CG Goetz (eds), Systemic Diseases (part 3), Handbook of Clinical Neurology (vol 71). Amsterdam, Netherlands: Elsevier, 1998; 463–499.

44. Wiederholt WC, Siekert RG. Neurological manifestations of sarcoidosis. Neurology 1965;15:1147–1154.

45. Delaney P. Neurologic manifestations in sarcoidosis: review of the literature, with a report of 23 cases. Ann Intern Med 1977;87:336–345.

46. Pentland B., Mitchell JD, Cull RE, et al. Central nervous system sarcoidosis. QJM 1985;56:457–465.

47. Luke RA, Stern BJ, Krumholz A, et al. Neurosarcoidosis: the long-term clinical course. Neurology 1987;37:461–463.

48. Krumholz A, Stern BJ, Stern EG. Clinical implications of seizures in neurosarcoidosis. Arch Neurol 1991;48:842–844.

49. Rocklin R. Cell-Mediated Immunity in Sarcoidosis. In BL Fanburg (ed), Sarcoidosis and Other Granulomatous Diseases of the Lung. New York: Marcel Dekker Inc, 1983;203–224.

50. Teirstein AS, Lesser M. Worldwide Distribution and Epidemiology of Sarcoidosis. In BL Fanburg (ed), Sarcoidosis and Other Granulomatous Diseases of the Lung. New York: Marcel Dekker Inc, 1983;101–134.

51. Leiberman J, Katarea YP, Young JR. Historical Perspectives of Sarcoidosis. In J Lieberman (ed), Sarcoidosis. Orlando, FL: Grune & Stratton, 1985;1–5.

52. Hunninghake GW, Crystal RG. Pulmonary sarcoidosis: a disorder mediated by excess helper T-lymphocyte activity at sites of disease activity. N Engl J Med 1981;305:429–434.

53. Weissler JC. Southwestern internal medicine conference: sarcoidosis: immunology and clinical management. Am J Med Sci 1994;307:233–245.

54. Moller DR. Cells and cytokines involved in the pathogenesis of sarcoidosis. Sarcoidosis Vasc Diffuse Lung Dis 1999;16:24–31.

55. Newman LS, Rose CS, Maier LA. Sarcoidosis. N Engl J Med 1997;336:1224–1234.

56. Tanoue LT, Zitnik R, Elias JA. Systemic Sarcoidosis. In GL Baum, E Wolinsky (eds), Textbook of Pulmonary Disease. Boston: Little, Brown, 1994;745–774.

57. Desai SG, Simon MR. Epidemiology of Sarcoidosis. In J Lieberman (ed), Sarcoidosis. Orlando, FL: Grune & Stratton, 1985;25–27.

58. James DG. Genetics and Familial Sarcoidosis. In BL Fanburg (ed), Sarcoidosis and Other Granulomatous Diseases of the Lung. New York: Marcel Dekker Inc, 1983;135–146.

59. Joyce-Brady M. Tastes great, less filling. The debate about mycobacteria and sarcoidosis. Am Rev Respir Dis 1992;145:986–987.

60. Ishige I, Usui Y, Takemura T, et al. Quantitative PCR of mycobacterial and propionibacterial DNA in lymph nodes of Japanese patients with sarcoidosis. Lancet 1999;354:120–123.

61. Oksanen V. Neurosarcoidosis: clinical presentations and course in 50 patients. Acta Neurol Scand 1986;73:283–290.

62. Zajicek JP, Entzian P, Dalhoff K, et al. Central nervous system sarcoidosis—diagnosis and management. QJM 1999;92:103–117.

63. Stuart CA, Neelon FA, Lebovitz HE. Hypothalamic insufficiency: the cause of hypopituitarism in sarcoidosis. Ann Intern Med 1978;88:589–594.

64. Delaney P. Seizures in sarcoidosis: a poor prognosis. Ann Neurol 1980;7:494.

65. Rodan BA, Putman CE. Radiological Alterations in Sarcoidosis. In BL Fanburg (ed), Sarcoidosis and Other Granulomatous Diseases of the Lung. New York: Marcel Dekker Inc, 1983;37–75.

66. Leiberman J. Angiotensin-Converting Enzyme (ACE) and Serum Lysozyme in Sarcoidosis. In J Lieberman (ed), Sarcoidosis. Orlando, FL: Grune & Stratton, 1985;145–159.

67. Sherman JL, Stern BJ. Sarcoidosis of the CNS: comparison of unenhanced and enhanced MR images. AJNR Am J Neuroradiol 1990;11:915–923.

68. Oksanen V, Fyhrquist F, Somer H, et al. Angiotensin converting enzyme in cerebrospinal fluid: a new assay. Neurology 1985;35:122–123.

69. Oksanen V, Fyhrquist FC, Gronhagen-Riska C, et al. CSF angiotensin-converting enzyme in neurosarcoidosis. Lancet 1985;1;1050–1051.

70. Chan Seem CP, Norfolk G, Spokes EG. CSF angiotensin-converting enzyme in neurosarcoidosis. Lancet 1985;1:456–457.

71. Agbogu BN, Stern BJ, Swell C, et al. Therapeutic considerations in patients with refractory neurosarcoidosis. Arch Neurol 1995;52:875–879.

72. Ahmad K, Kim YH, Spitzer AR, et al. Total nodal radiation in progressive sarcoidosis. Am J Clin Oncol 1992;15:311–313.

73. Lower EE, Baughmann RP. The use of low dose methotrexate in refractory sarcoidosis. Am J Med Sci 1990;299:153–157.

74. Lower EE, Baughman RP. Prolonged use of methotrexate for sarcoidosis. Arch Intern Med 1995;155:846–851.

75. Lower EE, Broderick JP, Brott TG, et al. Diagnosis and management of neurological sarcoidosis. Arch Intern Med 1997;157:1864–1868.

76. Paty DW, Noseworthy JH, Ebers GC. Diagnosis of Multiple Sclerosis. In DW Paty, GC Ebers (eds), Multiple Sclerosis. Philadelphia: FA Davis Co, 1998;48–134.

77. Kinnunen E, Wikstrom J. Prevalence and prognosis of epilepsy in patients with multiple sclerosis. Epilepsia 1986;27:729–733.

78. Ebers GC, Sadovnick AD. Epidemiology. In DW Paty, GC Ebers (eds), Multiple Sclerosis. Philadelphia: FA Davis Co, 1998;5–28.

79. Raine CS, Scheinberg L, Waltz JM. Multiple sclerosis: oligodendrocyte survival and proliferation in an active established lesion. Lab Invest 1981;45:534–546.

80. Moore GR. Neuropathology and Pathophysiology of the Multiple Sclerosis Lesion. In DW Paty, GC Ebers (eds), Multiple Sclerosis. Philadelphia: FA Davis Co, 1998;257–327.

81. Brownell B, Hughes JT. The distribution of plaques in the cerebrum in multiple sclerosis. J Neurol Neurosurg Psychiatry 1962;25:315–320.

82. Moreau TH, Sochurkova D, Lemesle M, et al. Epilepsy in patients with multiple sclerosis: radiological-clinical correlations. Epilepsia 1998;39:893–896.

83. Thompson AJ, Kermode AG, Moseley IF, et al. Seizures due to multiple sclerosis: seven patients with MRI correlations. J Neurol Neurosurg Psychiatry 1993;56:1317–1320.

84. Engelsen BA, Gronning M. Epileptic seizures in patients with multiple sclerosis. Is the prognosis of epilepsy underestimated? Seizure 1997;6:377–382.

85. Horowitz AL, Kaplan RD, Grewe G, et al. The ovoid lesions: a new MR observation in patients with multiple sclerosis. AJNR Am J Neuroradiol 1989;10:303–305.

86. Gean-Marton AD, Vezina LG, Martin KI, et al. Abnormal corpus callosum: a sensitive and specific indicator of multiple sclerosis. Radiology 1991;180:215–221.

87. Asselman P, Chadwick DW, Marsden DC. Visual evoked responses in the diagnosis and management of patients suspected of multiple sclerosis. Brain 1975;98:261–282.

88. Taylor RS. Multiple sclerosis potpourri. Paroxysmal symptoms, seizures, fatigue, pregnancy, and more. Phys Med Rehabil Clin N Am 1998;9:551–559.

89. Tranchant C, Bhetia K, Marsde UC. Movement disorders in multiple sclerosis. Mov Disord 1995;10:418–423.

90. Kurtzke JF, Beebe JW, Nagler B, et al. Studies on the natural history of multiple sclerosis. V. Long-term survival in young men. Arch Neurol 1970;22:215–222.

91. Ghezzi A, Montanini R, Basso PF, et al. Epilepsy in multiple sclerosis. Eur Neurol 1990;30:218–223.

92. Mathews WB. Symptoms and Signs. In WB Mathews, A Compston, IV Allen, CN Martyn (eds), McAlpine's Multiple Sclerosis (2nd ed). Edinburgh, UK: Churchill Livingstone, 1991;61–63.

93. Delire M. Immunoglobulin Therapy. In J Engel, TA Pedley (eds), Epilepsy: a Comprehensive Textbook. Philadelphia: Lippincott–Raven, 1997;1665–1670.

94. Ariizumi M, Shiihara H, Hibio S, et al. High-dose gammaglobulin for intractable childhood epilepsy. Lancet 1983;2:162–163.

95. van Ryckevorsel-Harmant K, Delire M, Schmitz-Moorman W, et al. IVIG treatment of refractory epilepsy. Results of the first double blind/dose finding clinical study. Int J Clin Lab Res 1994;24:162–166.

96. Rasmussen TB. Chronic Encephalitis and Seizures: Historical Introduction. In F Andermann (ed), Chronic Encephalitis and Epilepsy—Rasmussen's Syndrome. Boston: Butterworth–Heinemann, 1991;1–6.

97. Rasmussen T, Olszewski J, Lloyd-Smith D. Focal seizures due to chronic localized encephalitis. Neurology 1958;8:435–445.

98. Hart YM, Cortez F, Andermann P, et al. Medical treatment of Rasmussen's syndrome (chronic encephalitis and epilepsy): effect of high dose steroids or immunoglobulins in 19 patients. Neurology 1994;44:1030–1036.

99. Oguni H, Andermann F, Rasmussen TB. The Natural History of the Syndrome of Chronic Encephalitis and Epilepsy: a Study of the MNI Series of 48 Cases. In F Andermann (ed), Chronic Encephalitis and Epilepsy—Rasmussen's Syndrome. Boston: Butterworth–Heinemann, 1991;7–36.

100. Grenier Y, Antel JP, Osterland CK. Immunologic Studies in Chronic Encephalitis of Rasmussen. In F Andermann (ed), Chronic Encephalitis and Epilepsy—Rasmussen's Syndrome. Boston: Butterworth–Heinemann, 1991;125–134.

101. Rogers SW, Andrews PI, Gahring LC, et al. Autoantibodies to glutamate receptor GluR3 in Rasmussen's encephalitis. Science 1994;265:648–651.

102. Andrews PI, Dichter MA, Berkovic SF, et al. Plasmapheresis in Rasmussen's encephalitis. Neurology 1996; 46:242–246.

103. Adcock JE, Oxbury JM, Beeson D, et al. Comparison of treatment of Rasmussen's encephalitis with plasmapheresis versus hemispherectomy. Epilepsia 1997;38[Suppl 8]: 189.

104. Palmer CA, Geyer JD, Keating JM, et al. Rasmussen's encephalitis with concomitant cortical dysplasia: the role of GluR3. Epilepsia 1999;40:242–247.

105. Andrews PI, McNamara JO, Lewis DV. Clinical and electroencephalographic correlates in Rasmussen's encephalitis. Epilepsia 1997;38:189–194.

106. Chinchilla D, Dulac O, Robain O, et al. Reappraisal of Rasmussen's syndrome with special emphasis on treatment with high doses of steroids. J Neurol Neurosurg Psychiatry 1994;57:1325–1333.

107. So NK, Andermann F. Rasmussen's Syndrome. In J Engel, TA Pedley (eds), Epilepsy: a Comprehensive Textbook. Philadelphia: Lippincott–Raven, 1997;2379–2388.

108. Walsh PJ. Treatment of Rasmussen's syndrome with intravenous gammaglobulin. In F Andermann (ed), Chronic Encephalitis and Epilepsy—Rasmussen's Syndrome. Boston: Butterworth–Heinemann, 1991;201–204.

Chapter 8

Contribution of Drugs and Drug Interactions (Prescribed, Over the Counter, and Illicit) to Seizures and Epilepsy

Barbara S. Koppel

Physicians should evaluate seizures in the context of an affected person's overall health and lifestyle. Among the factors that may play a role in seizure occurrence are concurrent illnesses, prescribed, herbal and over-the-counter medications, recent anesthesia, and habits, such as alcohol, cigarette, and illicit substance abuse. Seizures are a symptom of cerebral dysfunction and, as such, may be symptomatic of many conditions that alter the brain's normal milieu or physiology. Such seizures may not be manifestations of epilepsy (a chronic disorder in which seizures recur unpredictably and usually without demonstrable triggers), although, in persons with epilepsy, drugs and drug interactions may exacerbate the disorder and contribute to intractability.

Patients with epilepsy who require antiepileptic drugs must be warned of possible adverse interactions from drugs prescribed for other medical illnesses, whether these are common ailments treated with over-the-counter nostrums or serious diseases, affecting one or more major organ systems. This is especially important with regard to medications used intermittently, such as analgesics, antibiotics, and decongestants. It is also advisable for physicians to have reasonable guidelines for alcohol use and to understand the short- and long-term effects of substance abuse and how the effects of prescribed medications may be altered by, or interact in unusual ways

with, other drugs. For example, phenytoin augments the effects of cocaine; hepatic enzyme–inducing drugs, such as phenytoin or carbamazepine, increase the metabolism of methadone.

In this chapter, I review the most common ways in which drugs affect seizure susceptibility, as well as the drug interactions most commonly encountered in practice. I also review briefly the effects of chronic illnesses or procedures on antiepileptic drugs (AEDs) and their effect on seizure risk.

Effects of Metabolic Encephalopathy

Renal failure and treatment with dialysis increase the risk for seizures: Nearly one-third of patients with renal failure eventually experiences seizures.[1] The dialysis encephalopathy syndrome (aphasia, seizures, and myoclonus) has been virtually eliminated since the recognition that aluminum overload, either from excessive amounts in the dialysate or in antacids used to lower phosphorus levels, is a major cause of the disorder, although myoclonus still occurs occasionally. Clonazepam or valproate is useful in controlling myoclonus, but chelation is required to treat the dementia.[2] Dialysis dysequilibrium syndrome is characterized by seizures, headache, encephalopathy, and, sometimes, coma. The condition results from rapid fluid shifts that can be avoided by slowing the rate of peritoneal or hemodialysis. It is still seen occasionally in very uremic patients, usually after their first dialysis treatments, although today manifestations are relatively mild—typically just a few seizures and mild confusion. Structural brain lesions, which increase the risk for seizures from metabolic encephalopathy and may cause similar symptoms, must be excluded by brain imaging.

Contrast injection for radiographic procedures has been associated with partial or generalized seizures, especially in patients with renal failure. Seizures are most likely to occur in three circumstances: (1) when the contrast agent inadvertently comes in contact with the cerebral cortex, as when dye passes intracranially during myelography; (2) during cerebral angiographic procedures that require large amounts of contrast (>200 ml); or (3) when the blood-brain barrier has been disrupted.[3]

Hepatic failure can occur after the use of general anesthetics, such as halothane; after overdoses of commonly used medications, such as acetaminophen; or as the result of hepatic toxins, such as insecticides or poisonous mushrooms. Small amounts of these may be all that are required if the liver is already stressed by excessive alcohol consumption or chronic use of drugs metabolized by the liver. A careful history and toxicology screens of blood and urine are necessary to establish the diagnosis of a specific toxin.[4–7] Table 8-1 summarizes many toxins that cause seizures.[4]

Seizures and myoclonus can also result from such diverse conditions as hypoxia, ischemia, hyper- or hypoglycemia, hypomagnesemia, hyponatremia, hepatic or renal failure, and rapid fluid shifts across the blood-brain barrier.[8] Identification and correction of metabolic derangements are necessary to control seizures and prevent permanent brain damage. Anticonvulsant drugs alone are generally ineffective, and dose adjustments are needed if they are used. A metabolic encephalopathy should be suspected and appropriate screening tests ordered when seizures arise after procedures associated with significant fluid shifts, such as bladder lavage, hemodialysis, radiographic procedures using intravenous iodinated contrast material, and rapid intravenous infusions.

Surgery, Anesthesia, and Seizure Risk

Seizures that occur in close relation to surgical procedures or use of anesthetic agents raise several questions. In patients on AED therapy, interruption of treatment may result from orders to be *non per os* before anesthesia. Short procedures may only require delaying a single dose, and this delay may still be within the drug's effective half-life. In such cases, a patient can be given one dose immediately before induction of anesthesia. Regular dosing can resume immediately after the patient's gag reflex has returned. With procedures that exceed the half-life of a patient's medication, the anesthesiologist may need to give a parenteral "booster" dose of an anticonvulsant drug before the patient is allowed to emerge from anesthesia.[9] Parenteral substitution for drugs usually taken orally is reasonable if the patient has been taking phenytoin, valproic acid, or phenobarbital; there is no commercially available intravenous or intramuscular formulation for carbamazepine. Lamotrigine has been successfully delivered per rectum using a suspension of tablets, but levels were half as much as the same dose delivered orally.[10]

Although sprinkle or suspension forms of several AEDs are available, their absorption, whether from oral administration or feeding tubes, may be affected by recent general anesthesia. Under the best circumstances, phenytoin suspensions are absorbed erratically. Therefore, seizures occurring in the perioperative period may be due to inadequate blood concentrations, as a result of impaired gastrointestinal absorption of antiseizure drugs. In patients undergoing craniotomy, the risk of seizures is 6% during the first postoperative week and 17% over 5 years. Although anecdotal experience suggests that AEDs may stop perioperative seizures, neither valproic acid nor phenytoin, given intraoperatively and during the postoperative period, has been shown to prevent the development of epilepsy months to years later.[9]

In operative procedures not involving the brain, transient seizures can arise from metabolic derangements or neurotoxicity from drugs. Hypoxia, hypotension, and embolic infarction are less-common causes. In such circumstances, long-term AED therapy is usually not required. For example, seizures occurring shortly after injection of moderate to large amounts of a local

Table 8-1. Toxins and Drugs That Have Been Reported to Induce Seizures

Class	Agents	Class	Agents
Alcohols and glycols	Ethanol	Antihistamines (*continued*)	Chlorpheniramine
	Ethylene glycol		Diphenhydramine
	Methanol		Doxylamine
	Propylene glycol		Hydroxyzine
Local anesthetics	Bupivacaine		Pyrilamine
	Cocaine	Antineoplastics	Bleomycin
	Lidocaine		Busulphan
	Procaine		Carmustine
	Proparacaine		Chlorambucil
	Tetracaine		Cisplatin
General anesthetics	Enflurane		Cytarabine
	Etomidate		Mechlorethamine
	Isoflurane		Methotrexate
	Ketamine		Vinblastine
	Methohexital		Vincristine
Antibiotics	Cephalosporins	Antiparasitics	Chloroquine
	Ciprofloxacin		Oxamniquine
	Gentamicin		Pyrimethamine
	Imipenem/cilastatin	Antivirals	Acyclovir
	Isoniazid		Amantadine
	Metronidazole	Asphyxiants	Acetylene
	Nalidixic acid		Butane
	Norfloxacin		Carbon dioxide
	Penicillins		Ethane
Anticonvulsants	Carbamazepine		Methane
	Ethosuximide		Nitrogen
	Phenytoin		Propane
	Valproic acid	Cardiovascular agents	Aprindine
Anticholinergics	Atropine		Digoxin
	Cogentin		Disopyramide
	Diphenhydramine		Encainide
	Optic cyclopentolate		Ergotamine
	Scopolamine		Flecainide
Cyclic antidepressants	Amitriptyline		Lidocaine
	Amoxapine		Lorcainide
	Clomipramine		Methyldopa
	Desipramine		Metoprolol
	Doxepin		Mexiletine
	Imipramine		Osmolal
	Nortriptyline		Propafenone
	Protriptyline		Propranolol
	Trimipramine		Quinidine
Other antidepressants	Bupropion		Quinine
	Fluoxetine		Tocainide
	Maprotiline		Verapamil
	Mianserin	Drugs of abuse	Amphetamines
	Trazodone		Cocaine
Antifungals	Amphotericin		Lysergic acid diethylamide (LSD)
	Miconazole		Marijuana
Antihistamines	Astemizole		Methamphetamine ("Ice")
	Brompheniramine		Phencyclidine (PCP)

Table 8-1. *Continued*

Class	Agents	Class	Agents
Drug withdrawal	Anticonvulsants	Neuroleptics	Thiothixene
	Barbiturates		Haloperidol
	Benzodiazepines		Lithium carbonate
	Ethanol	Neuromuscular blockers	Atracurium
	Other sedative-hypnotic		Tubocurarine
	agents	Nonsteroidal anti-	Ibuprofen
Hypoglycemics	Insulin	inflammatory drugs	Ketoprofen
	Sulfonylureas		Mefenamic acid
Hydrocarbons	Acetone		Naproxen
	Benzene		Piroxicam
	Camphor		Phenylbutazone
	Ethyl ether		Salicylates
	Eucalyptus oil	Opioids	Alfentanil
	Methylene chloride		Fentanyl
	Nitromethane		Meperidine
	Phenol		Morphine
	Pine oil		Pentazocine
	Toluene		Propoxyphene
	Turpentine oil		Sufentanil
	Xylene	Plants	Akee (hypoglycins)
Immunosuppressives	Azathioprine		Angel's trumpet (bella-
	Cyclosporin		donna alkaloids)
	Glucocorticosteroids		Azalea (grayanotoxin)
Inhalants	Carbon monoxide		Bleeding hearts (isoquino-
Insecticides	Benzene hexachloride		line alkaloids)
	(Lindane)		Carolina jasmine
	Carbamates		(*Gelsemium*)
	Organochlorines		Chinaberry
	Organophosphates		Christmas rose (glycosides)
	Pyrethrins		Daffodil (narcissine, lyco-
	Rotenone		rine)
Insect repellant	N,N-diethyl-m-toluamide		Deadly nightshade (sola-
	(DEET)		nine alkaloids)
Metals chelators	Deferoxamine		Golden chain (quinolizidine
	Edetic acid (EDTA)		alkaloids)
	Penicillamine		Ground hemlock (*Taxus*)
Metals	Aluminum		Juniper (essential oils)
	Arsenic		Jimson weed (solanaceous
	Bismuth salts		alkaloids)
	Copper		Jerusalem cherry (solanine
	Iron		alkaloids)
	Lead		Mountain laurel (cytisine)
	Mercury		Mistletoe
Mushrooms	Cyclopeptides		Poison hemlock (*Conium*
	Monomethylhydrazine		*maculatum*)
	Muscimol-ibotenic acid		Rhododendron (grayano-
	Orellanine		toxin)
	Psilocybe		Rhubarb (oxalic acid)
			Strychnine nux vomicus

Table 8-1. *Continued*

Class	Agents	Class	Agents
Plants *continued*	Tobacco (nicotine)	Sympathomimetics *continued*	Picrotoxin
	Umbrella Plant (essential oils)		Prethcamide
			Pseudoephedrine
	Water Hemlock (cicutoxin)		Strychnine
	Yew (*Taxus*)		Terbutaline
Radiographic contrast media	Diatrizoic acid		Theophylline
	Iopamidol	Vaccines	Measles vaccine
	Iothalamate		Pertussis vaccine
	Meglumine	Miscellaneous	Allopurinol
	Metrizamide		Borates
	Metrizoate		Bromocriptine
Rodenticides	Fluoroacetate		Cimetidine
	Phosphorus		Colchicine
	Phosphine		Corticosteroids
	Strychnine		Cyanide
	Thallium		Cycloserine
	Vacor		Dantrolene
Sedative hypnotics reversal agents	Flumazenil		Disulfiram
			Ergonovine
Skeletal muscle relaxants	Baclofen		Ergot alkaloids
	Albuterol		Erythropoietin
Sympathomimetics	Amphetamines		Famotidine
	Aminophenzole		Fluoride
	Caffeine		Hydrogen sulfide
	Doxapram		Levamisole
	Ephedrine		Levodopa
	Etamivan		Levothyroxine
	Flurothyl		Nicotine
	Imidazoline class		Pimozide
	Lobeline		Probenecid
	Methylphenidate		Prostaglandins
	Metrazole		Thyrotropin-releasing hormone
	Phenylephrine		
	Phenylpropanolamine		

anesthetic should raise suspicion that the drug has been inadvertently introduced into the vascular supply. This is especially common with pelvic or oral surgery.[11] I was asked to see a woman who had two generalized seizures after lidocaine was injected into the perineum as caudal anesthesia for uterine dilation and curettage. The serum level of lidocaine was 4.9 μg/ml. Because the blood concentration of lidocaine drops rapidly as it is cleared, we chose to give the patient a single 2-mg dose of lorazepam intravenously, after which the procedure was completed successfully. Most anesthesiologists agree that acute symptomatic seizures due to anesthetic neurotoxicity do not usually require cancelling the procedure and that chronic AED therapy is not necessary.[11]

In patients kept *non per os* before surgery, seizures may indicate withdrawal from unsuspected chronic use of excessive amounts of alcohol, sedative medications, mood-stabilizing agents, or AEDs.[12] Such seizures are usually self limited, although occasionally, it is necessary to reintroduce the missing drug or prescribe a substitute, if appropriate. Sleep deprivation associated with early arrival for same-day surgery or lack of

Table 8-2. Effect of Drug Class on Seizure Threshold

Type of Medication	Therapeutic Level	Toxic Level	Withdrawal
Antibiotics (penicillin or quinolone)	—	↑	—
Isoniazid	—	↑	—
Antiviral	—	↑	—
Antifungal	Rare ↑	↑	—
Diuretics	↑ if hyponatremia	—	—
Asthma drugs (e.g., theophylline)	—	↑	—
Cardiac, Antihypertensive, Anticoagulant/Antiplatelet drugs	—	—	—
Analgesics (tramadol, propoxyphene)	Rare ↑	↑	↑
Headache combinations with barbiturates (Fiorinal, Fioricet)	—	—	↑
Antidepressants	—	—	—
Tricyclics	—	↑	—
Selective serotonin reuptake inhibitors (SSRI) or SSRI/ norepinephrine inhibitor	↑ if hyponatremia	—	—
Selective serotonin release and dopamine inhibitors	↑	↑	—
Others (quaternary)	↑	↑	—
Antipsychotics	—	—	—
Butyrophenones	—	↑	—
Neuroleptics	—	—	—
Clozapine	↑	↑	—
Newer atypical neuroleptics	—	—	—
Stimulants	—	—	—
Methylphenidate	—	↑	—
Herbal stimulants (ephedra)	—	↑	—
Anxiolytics	—	—	↑
Anesthetics	—	↑	↑
Acetylcholinesterase inhibitors (donepezil, rivastigmine)	↑ if pre-existing epilepsy	—	—

— = there is no effect of this drug; ↑= increased seizure risk.

sleep the night before the procedure because of anxiety may trigger isolated seizures. These are rarely recurrent and do not require treatment with AEDs.

Rapid induction of anesthesia can be associated occasionally with one or more acute seizures. Propofol,[13] flurane (a substitute for halothane),[14] and benzodiazepines (especially lorazepam)[15] seem to be the agents implicated most often. Seizures can be an adverse effect of flumazenil, a benzodiazepine antagonist that is used to facilitate recovery from anesthesia and allow early discharge after outpatient surgical or endoscopic procedures. It has also been used in treatment of hepatic encephalopathy. Flumazenil is contraindicated in patients with a history of seizures, but this may need to be re-evaluated in light of a recent study. Schulze-Bonhage and Elger[16] studied 67 patients undergoing presurgical evalua-

tions for intractable localization-related epilepsy. They were given flumazenil to induce seizures, but seizures or electroencephalogram (EEG) interictal epileptiform discharges occurred in only eight patients, all of whom had been pretreated with benzodiazepines.

Table 8-2 summarizes the effect of major drug classes on seizure threshold, which is discussed in detail in the following sections. Table 8-3 lists the patient and medication characteristics that contribute to seizure occurrence.

Antimicrobial Drugs, Immunosuppression, and Seizure Risk

Penicillin, discovered in 1926, has been used experimentally to induce focal and generalized epileptiform activity and seizures in laboratory animals. It is thus not surprising that this class of drugs and its derivatives (e.g., imipenem) have been suspected of increasing the potential for seizures. However, recent reviews stress that correction of dose for body size and renal function and consideration of the separate contribution of critical illness itself to seizure risk improves the safety record of imipenem and penicillin-type antibiotics.[17,18] Increased risk of seizures has also been attributed to other antibiotics, including the first quinolone, ciprofloxacin. Newer quinolones have less effect on other drugs used concurrently, such as caffeine, theophylline, and anticonvulsants, and the risk of seizures is correspondingly lower with these agents.[19] The choice of antibiotic should always be based on the result of culture sensitivity or the presumed pathogenic organism, without concern for its potential to cause seizures. However, it is important to remember systemic factors and co-medications that may indirectly raise the risk of seizures. Evaluation of seizures occurring during antimicrobial use should be the same as if the seizure arose de novo; even apparently obvious acute symptomatic seizures may be an indication of underlying, unsuspected cerebral pathology. Antifungal and antimycobacterial drugs generally do not provoke seizures, although the severe shivering that can accompany amphotericin infusion can sometimes be confused with seizure activity. Overdosage of isoniazid (INH) precipitates seizures[5,8] as early as 3 hours after ingestion. INH-induced seizures must be treated with pyridoxine (vitamin B_6) in addition to anti-seizure drugs.[4] In this situation, anticonvulsants that are not metabolized in the liver should be used if possible, because INH also causes hepatic failure, thus leading to unpredictable AED levels and neurotoxicity.

Antiviral drugs (e.g., acyclovir, ganciclovir) are used to treat encephalitis, which in itself causes seizures. Dideoxyiodinase and zidovudine, standard treatments for patients infected with human immunodeficiency virus (HIV), are said to increase seizure risk,[20] but it is difficult to exclude other factors, including unrecognized HIV encephalitis. Because HIV-infected patients often demonstrate hypergammaglobulinemia in the early and middle stages of their illness, they have an increased risk of hypersensitivity reactions to anticonvulsant drugs.[21] In malnourished acquired

Table 8-3. Contributing Factors to Seizure Occurrence

Patient	Medication
Inherited seizure predisposition	Drug lowers seizure threshold
Brain injury (chronic or acute)	Drug causes hyponatremia
Breakdown of blood-brain barrier	Rapid increase, accidental or deliberate
Hypoalbuminemia, hypoxia	Overdose of epileptogenic (toxic) drug
Hypomagnesemia	Drug induces metabolism of anticonvulsant
Renal or hepatic failure	Drug inhibits metabolism of toxic drug
Illicit drug or alcohol abuse	Drug shares protein binding with anticonvulsant or epileptogenic drug

immunodeficiency syndrome patients, AEDs that are highly protein bound are more likely to produce toxicity because of hypoalbuminemia. Drug interactions are common, because most HIV-infected patients take multiple medications, and many of these compete with anticonvulsants for protein-binding sites. Through shared effects on the cytochrome phosphatase (CYP) liver enzymes, antiseizure drugs decrease antiviral drug levels in HIV-infected patients receiving protease inhibitors; this increases the risk of developing viral resistance.[22] Valproate stimulates viral replication directly.[22]

Immune modulators such as interferon alpha, used to treat hepatitis C and sometimes other viral infections, have been associated with seizures.[23] Cyclosporine, part of the standard immunosuppression regimen after organ transplantation, is so sufficiently epileptogenic that it has been used to induce seizures experimentally.[24] It also induces metabolism of antiepileptic medication and can cause a leukoenceph- alopathy associated with myoclonus and seizures. Metabolic disarray is common in patients with organ rejection, which lowers seizure threshold. This situation requires careful attention to doses of antibiotic, antifungal, and immunosuppressant drugs.

Considerations When Using Psychotropic Medications

The first issue is the not-uncommon problem of misdiagnosing nonepileptic behavior as a manifestation of epilepsy and prescribing anticonvulsant drugs in error.[25,26]

Abnormal involuntary movements, including myoclonus, tremor, and dystonia, may resemble seizure activity, especially when they are intermittent. In patients without a history of movement disorder or exposure to neuroleptic drugs, EEG recorded during the movements in question usually resolves any diagnostic confusion. Paroxysmal nocturnal dyskinesia, once thought to be a movement disorder, is now recognized as a manifestation of frontal lobe epilepsy. Psychogenic seizures are frequently diagnosed as epileptic events, even by experienced observers, until careful analysis of video-EEG recordings clarifies their nature.

Occasionally, patients with epilepsy misidentify toxic effects of medication, such as diplopia, blurred vision, or nausea, as auras and self medicate with additional doses of their anticonvulsant, thus aggravating the problem. High AED levels compared to baseline concentrations should lead to the correct diagnosis. This underscores the need, however, to educate patients about symptoms they may experience—which are likely to be epileptic and which are not—and alternative techniques to abort a possible seizure.

Delirium accompanied by hallucinations can be mistaken for complex partial status epilepticus. Benzodiazepine or alcohol withdrawal can cause seizures before onset of delirium and should be treated with a drug active at the benzodiazepine-γ-aminobutyric acid type A (GABA$_A$) receptor. When neuroleptics are used to treat symptoms of delirium, there are risks of autonomic dysfunction and neuroleptic malignant syndrome. Although seizures from drug or alcohol withdrawal are usually self limited, failure to correct concurrent metabolic abnormalities, such as hypoglycemia, hypomagnesemia, and hypoxia, can perpetuate seizures and lead to permanent brain damage.[27] The choice and dosage of anticonvulsant drug are limited by side effects[28] and concern about cumulative respiratory depression. These fears are heightened when the patient continues to take antiseizure drugs while resuming alcohol use (see Alcohol).[29]

Anxiety or panic disorder may be misdiagnosed as epilepsy, especially when trembling, depersonalization, dizziness, visual changes, and tachycardia are prominent.[30] Failure to elicit seizures during forced hyperventilation in the office or during an EEG almost always excludes absence attacks. At the same time, hyperventilation may reproduce the patient's symptoms, and the nonepileptic basis of his or her symptoms becomes clear. This can be reassuring when coupled with psychotherapeutic support.[25] EEG or video-EEG monitoring is frequently required for definitive diagnosis.[24,25,31]

The incidence of psychosis is 2–7% in patients with chronic epilepsy.[32] Catatonic schizophrenia may be confused with nonconvulsive status epilepticus that produces slowed, automatic behavior, decreased responsiveness, and altered consciousness.[32] Postictal psychosis is an uncommon complication of epilepsy and is seen most often in patients with temporal lobe seizures.[33] The psychotic episode typically begins after a "lucid interval" after the seizure and may persist for several days to 2 weeks. Short-term treatment with neuroleptic drugs is often required to manage the psychosis. Antipsychotic medication should not be prescribed prophylactically, as not every seizure will be followed by psychosis.[33,34] Syndromes due to serotonin excess, such as may occur in patients using reuptake inhibitors who are exposed to excess amounts of tryptophan, triptans for migraine, or illicit drugs, like cocaine or amphetamine that act on serotonin receptors, can be misinterpreted as seizures.[35] Sleep disorders such as cataplexy, hypnagogic hallucinations, automatic behavior syndrome, and rapid eye movement behavior disorder are frequently considered to be manifestations of epilepsy.[36] AEDs can exacerbate sleep disorders, and sleep disorders can aggravate seizures.[37] Thus, video-EEG monitoring or polysomnography should be considered in patients with unexplained symptoms or in those in whom the course of the disorder is unanticipated.

Complex motor tics (stereotyped repetitive movements or vocalizations) and other physical manifestations of obsessive-compulsive disorder are occasionally confused with seizures. If treatment is necessary, antidepressant or dopamine receptor–blocking drugs should be used, not antiseizure medications. Using the lowest dosage that successfully controls tics is important, because the antidepressant used most commonly in this disorder, fluvoxamine, has been associated with seizures or EEG spikes in

Table 8-4. Psychotropic Medications and Their Metabolizing Enzymes

Psychotropics	Brand Name	Generic Name	Metabolism
Antidepressants	Elavil	Amitriptyline	CYP1A2/2D6, GT1A1
Tricyclics	Tofranil	Imipramine	CYP1A2/2C19, GT1A3
	Anafranil	Clomipramine	CYP1A2/2C19/2D6
	Norpramin	Desipramine	CYP2D6
	Sinequan	Doxepin	GT1A3/1A4
	Pamelor	Nortriptyline	CYP2D6
	Surmontil	Trimipramine	
Selective serotonin reuptake inhibitors	Celexa	Citalopram	CYP2C19/2D6
	Prozac	Fluoxetine	CYP2D6/3A3/4
	Luvox	Fluvoxamine	CYP1A2/others
	Paxil	Paroxetine	CYP2D6/others
	Zoloft	Sertraline	CYP3A3/4
Monoamine oxidase inhibitors	Nardil	Phenelzine	
	Parnate	Tranylcypromine	
Others	Ludomil	Maprotiline	
	Asendin	Amoxapine	
	Wellbutrin	Bupropion	CYP2B1/2D6/3A4
	Remeron	Mirtazapine	CYP2D6
	Serzone	Nefazodone	CYP3A3/4
	Desyrel	Trazodone	
	Effexor	Venlafaxine	CYP2D6
	Vestra	Reboxatine	CYP3A4
Antipsychotics	Haldol	Haloperidol	CYP2D6/3A4
	Trilafon	Perphenazine	CYP2D6
	Thorazine	Chlorpromazine	CYP2D6, GT1A4
	Mellaril	Thioridazine	CYP2D6
	Navane	Thiothixene	CYP2D6
	Stelazine	Trifluoperazine	
Atypical	Clozaril	Clozapine	CYP1A2/3A4, GT1A3/4
	Risperdal	Risperidone	CYP2D6
	Zyprexa	Olanzapine	CYP1A2
	Seroquel	Quetiapine	CYP3A
Anxiolytics	Valium	Diazepam	CYP3A4/2C9/1A2
	Ativan	Lorazepam	CYP3A4, GT2B7
	Xanax	Alprazolam	CYP3A4/2C19
	Klonopin	Clonazepam	CYP3A3/4
	Serax	Oxazepam	
	Librium	Chlordiazepoxide	

CYP = cytochrome P-450; GT = glucuronosyltransferase.

at least one patient.[38] Table 8-4 reviews brand and generic drug names and their main metabolic pathways for reference during the following sections.

Antidepressant Drugs and Seizure Risk

Because depression is common in the general population and occurs even more often in patients with epilepsy (up to 50%, depending on the screening tool used[39]), and because treatment of depression usually requires long-term drug treatment, the choice of antidepressant medication must be made carefully, taking into account the possible effect on seizure threshold. Evidence that several anticonvulsant drugs also function as mood stabilizers means that in some patients, epilepsy and depression can be managed using one drug. However, anticonvulsants, such as carbamazepine or valproic acid, may trigger depression or mania when discontinued, and barbiturates can initiate or exacerbate depression. Enzyme-inhibiting antidepressant drugs, such as the selective serotonin reuptake inhibitors (SSRIs) and tricyclic antidepressants (TCAs), may require downward adjustment in the dosage of concurrently administered AEDs that are also metabolized by the cytochrome P-450 (CYP450) microsomal system in the liver. In other cases, phenytoin and carbamazepine inhibit the metabolism of antidepressant drugs, like fluoxetine or the tricyclics, which leads to unintended toxicity from the antidepressant.[40,41]

The risk of seizures in patients taking antidepressant drugs depends on three factors: (1) the intrinsic epileptogenic potential of the antidepressant (or, less often considered, the antiepileptic potential of the antidepressant[42]); (2) the amount of active drug that enters the brain (which depends on the dose, pharmacokinetics, and transport across the blood-brain barrier of the antidepressant); and (3) the patient's seizure threshold, including genetic factors, remote brain injury, previous febrile or acute symptomatic seizures, and alcohol or other substances.[41–44] The complex neurotransmitter effects of antidepressant drugs make it impossible to offer simplistic assumptions about their proconvulsant effects. Recent experimental studies of antiseizure drugs used to treat depression lead to the conclusion that it is unlikely that alterations in serotonin and norepinephrine levels are related to an increased risk of seizures.[42] In fact, some studies suggest that fluoxetine[40] and doxepine[41] may occasionally have anticonvulsant properties. By analyzing which transmitter systems are shared by proconvulsant drugs, like local anesthetics, cocaine, phenothiazines, and TCAs, and then eliminating those with unique properties, Dailey and Naritoku concluded that it is the antihistaminic, antimuscarinic, and local anesthetic properties of antidepressants that are most likely responsible for any increased susceptibility to seizures.[42] Even simple side effects of medication, however, such as drowsiness, can lower the seizure threshold in susceptible patients. Richelson[43] provides a useful review of the comparative effects of different antidepressant drugs on various neurotransmitter systems, although third-generation agents are not included.

Seizures occur with severe overdoses of TCAs just before cardiac arrest. Treatment should include alkalinization to avoid malignant arrhythmias,[4] but seizures in such circumstances may be prolonged or recurrent, despite appropriate use of AEDs.[8] At San Francisco's poison control center, overdoses of imipramine and amitriptyline accounted for 29% of the patients who had seizures.[5] Massive overdoses of newer antidepressant drugs, such as fluvoxamine in doses above 1,500 mg, have also been associated with seizures.[45]

The overall incidence of seizures in patients taking antidepressants at reasonable doses and presumed therapeutic ranges is 0.1–4.0%; this can be compared to an incident seizure risk of 0.073–0.086% in the general population of Rochester, Minnesota.[41] By class of drug, the highest risk of seizures has been reported with the heterocyclic antidepressant clomipramine, the dopamine or norepinephrine-specific reuptake inhibitor bupropion, and the quaternary antidepressant maprotiline. The TCAs have the next highest seizure risk (which is increased by toxic levels); the monoamine oxidase inhibitors carry the least risk. The newer SSRIs—fluoxetine, sertraline, fluvoxamine, citalopram, and paroxetine—and serotonin receptor modulators—trazodone and nefazodone—are intermediate in risk, as are venlafaxine, a combined norepinephrine and serotonin reuptake inhibitor, and mirtazapine, an adrenergic antagonist that releases norepinephrine and serotonin and blocks some serotonin receptors. The incidence is 0.04% for mirtazapine; less than 0.1% for imipramine and amitriptyline; 0.2% for fluoxetine, paroxetine, fluvoxamine, venlafaxine, and sertraline, when used at the higher doses generally required for obsessive-compulsive disorder; 0.4% for maprotiline and bupropion; and 0.5% for clomipramine.[41] The newest agents have not been used long enough to make realistic estimates of their epileptogenic potential. Some seizures in patients using SSRIs may be caused by hyponatremia due to syndrome of inappropriate secretion of antidiuretic hormone.[44,46] Syndrome of inappropriate secretion of antidiuretic hormone has also been reported with one of the newest antidepressants, reboxetine, a norepinephrine reuptake inhibitor.[47] The risk of seizures is increased further in elderly persons, probably owing to age-related reduction in metabolism and clearance that leads to drug accumulation, despite dosages well tolerated in younger patients.[7] Seizures are a neurotoxic effect of lithium and can occur even with plasma concentrations within the usual therapeutic range. EEG abnormalities are predictive of seizures.[48] Summary tables of seizure risk are available in reviews by Lambert[44] or Alldredge.[41]

Dose-effect relationships can be informative. For example, bupropion (now used more often as an aid to smoking cessation than as treatment for depression) has a risk of seizures as high as 2.2% in doses higher than 450 mg per day. The risk is as low as 0.4% with lower doses, and the slow-release formulation lowers seizure risk further still.[39] Although seizure rates with older antidepressants, such as maprotiline or amoxapine, are now much lower than earlier estimates of 15.6% and 24.0%, respectively,[39] their use has also decreased substantially because of the availability of safer alternatives. When clomipramine is used to treat obsessive-compulsive disorder, somewhat higher dosages are used than are typically used for depression. At doses above 350 mg per day, the risk of seizures is 2.1% but only 0.48% if the dose is kept below 250 mg per day.[41,44] Overall, estimates, based on large series of patients, of seizures in patients taking antidepressant drugs have declined, implying that figures from early case series are unreliable.[39]

Suicide attempts while using antidepressants must be considered separately from chronic therapeutic use. However, even in the absence of deliberate overdose, toxic amounts of antidepressant drugs can accumulate, as, for example, in the elderly. The active drug concentration actually within the brain is a product of many overlapping factors. These include variations in the amount taken by the patient, which, in turn, are a function of compliance with the prescribed regimen. Although physicians are most often concerned with lack of efficacy, owing to low drug levels from poor compliance, toxic concentrations can occur when patients take more than the prescribed dose. This may happen if patients realize they have missed one or more doses, become confused over their dosing schedule, or combine generic and branded formulations. After ingestion, levels of antidepressant drugs are affected by absorption (which may vary, depending on the presence of food or antacids in the gut) and the degree of protein binding (which is altered by the

presence of other drugs that compete for the same binding sites). Amino acids from proteins in food can affect transport across the blood-brain barrier. Finally, drug levels are affected by metabolic and excretory mechanisms, which themselves vary according to the genetically determined rate of acetylation (5–10% of the population are slow acetylators[42,44]), other genetic factors (e.g., reduced CYP450 enzymes),[41,43] age (slower in the elderly[7]), effects of other medications (including hormonal preparations) on the liver's CYP450 and glucuronyl transferase (GT) enzyme systems, and the degree of cigarette or alcohol use.[44]

A newly emphasized property of drugs is *chirality*: the beneficial or toxic effects of a drug depend on its chemical "handedness." The racemic (L or D) form of a drug affects its metabolism and reuptake, which, in turn, results in variable effects on antidepressant efficacy and on seizure propensity.[49] Although many women choose not to continue medication during pregnancy, drug metabolism for those taking medication is affected by gestational changes. Blood levels can be obtained for most antidepressant drugs, and these should be used to establish the steady-state baseline concentrations associated with optimal treatment effects and, in the event of a seizure, to document the associated blood level.[7] If a toxic or, at least, higher than baseline level is found, the antidepressant drug can generally be continued after lowering the dose.[50] Reference to drug interaction charts is necessary to anticipate the effects of one drug on another, as there are several isoenzymes of both the CYP450 and GT systems. In general, antipsychotic and antidepressant drugs are metabolized by CYP2D6 and CYP1A2, the enzyme systems that also metabolize carbamazepine. Most benzodiazepines and newer antipsychotic agents, as well as most other AEDs, excepting phenytoin, use CYP3A4. Phenytoin and a few benzodiazepines use CYP2C9. Valproic acid is also metabolized by the glucuronyl transferase system of enzymes, as are the tricyclic drugs. Chlorpromazine and clozapine use CYP1A3; lamotrigine, tricyclics, and clozapine use CYP1A4; and lorazepam and most narcotic drugs use CYP2B7. Narcotics are also metabolized by the GT1A1 system. Drugs can induce or inhibit individual enzymes; such information is generally readily available in the *Physicians' Desk Reference* or other medication guides.[51–54] Although it is tempting to use gabapentin and citalopram solely because of their "clean" metabolic profiles (they have no effect on hepatic enzyme systems),[54] like other drugs, they are neither risk nor side-effect free.[44,54,55] Because most drug interactions are predictable, they can usually be anticipated, especially with chronic use. The choice of antidepressant medication should be based on the needs of the individual patient, not the small risk of a seizure or fear of drug interactions.

When an AED is added to an antidepressant, induction of hepatic enzymes may decrease the antidepressant's effectiveness.[56] Sedating antidepressants may trigger seizures in patients whose seizure threshold is lowered by drowsiness.[42]

Although isolated case reports have described spontaneous seizures after electroconvulsive therapy (ECT),[57] an increased incidence has not been confirmed by larger series.[58] A seizure disorder is no longer a contraindication to ECT. In patients with epilepsy who require ECT, maintenance antiseizure drugs should be withheld the day of treatment to obtain the best response.[44] Newer technologies for treating depression, such as transcranial magnetic stimulation and vagal nerve stimulation, have not been associated with any increased risk of seizures.[59]

Antipsychotic Drugs and Seizure Risk

Although the absolute number of seizures reported with this class of psychotropic medication is less than that with antidepressants, this may reflect the smaller number of people using antipsychotics compared to antidepressants, rather than a difference in the epileptogenic potential of this class of drugs.[42] The incidence of psychosis in epileptic populations varies from 0.6% to 7.0% in general clinics and up to 27% in epilepsy centers.[32] Conversely, the problem of treatment of patients who have both epilepsy and schizophrenia is not rare, as schizophrenic patients are more prone to seizures, possibly due to shared kindling mechanisms, psychosocial disadvantages, temporal lobe plasticity, or other shared pathophysiologic mechanisms not yet specified.[32] Some anticonvulsants are associated with psychosis as an adverse event, especially when polypharmacy is used (which may also reflect more intractable epilepsy).[60] Variable mechanisms have been proposed, such as forced normalization using ethosuximide for absence seizures,

hyponatremia using carbamazepine (which can induce polydipsia), and toxicity with primidone or phenytoin.[32,60] Some of the newer anticonvulsants that raise GABA levels, such as tiagabine, topiramate, and especially vigabatrin (3.4–7.0% of patients),[60] have increased psychiatric problems. Successful seizure control with any anticonvulsant has long been suspected of causing presumed forced normalization, leading to psychosis.[34,60]

The real problem in this area is what to advise psychiatrists when psychotic patients have seizures. Neuroleptic drugs were used at fairly high doses initially after their introduction; phenothiazines were accompanied by a 1.2% incidence of seizures in a 4.5-year period of observation of 859 nonepileptic patients.[61] In this group, incidence was highest (9%) in those receiving more than 1,000 mg per day (chlorpromazine or equivalent), and seizures often occurred right after starting or increasing the dose. In patients with epilepsy, seizure incidence was surprisingly decreased in several studies of antipsychotic medication.[41] The epileptogenic potential of antipsychotics depends somewhat on the ratio of D1 to D2 blockade,[32,62] as well as the balance of glutamate and GABA activity.[63] D1 agonists and D2 antagonists are proconvulsant.[63] The first new, atypical neuroleptic medication, clozapine, was associated with EEG changes and dose dependent seizures in 3.5% of patients receiving more than 300 mg per day or undergoing rapid upward titration. The cumulative incidence was 5% at 1 year and 1.3% risk overall, even in patients without a history of prior seizures.[41] Newer, atypical neuroleptics, such as olanzapine and quetiapine, have an incidence of 0.24–0.88%, higher in patients with a history of seizures. Zotepine, an agent active at serotonin and dopamine receptors, has a dose-responsive incidence of seizures, up to 7.4% in doses higher than 3,900 mg per day.[32] Although seizures are rare in patients on risperidone or sertindole, they occasionally occur in association with hyponatremia.[41] Similar effects on the enzyme systems discussed in the preceding section Antidepressant Drugs and Seizure Risk are found with antipsychotics, allowing high drug levels to be obtained at therapeutic dose regimens when specific interactions occur.[41]

Because it is not rare for schizophrenia or bipolar disorder to occur in people with epilepsy, clinicians must familiarize themselves with appropriate drug choices and be watchful of drug interactions.[53] Postictal psychosis is self limited and does not usually require high doses of neuroleptics. In this circumstance, the risk of further seizures due to neuroleptic drug treatment is negligible.[33,34]

Anxiolytics and Hypnotics

Medications acting at the benzodiazepine-GABA$_A$ receptor site have overlapping effectiveness in the treatment of insomnia, delirium, and epilepsy.[64] In patients with primary generalized seizures or myoclonus, clonazepam is the most commonly used benzodiazepine, clorazepate is occasionally used as adjunctive treatment for complex partial seizures, and parenteral diazepam, lorazepam, and midazolam are used to treat status epilepticus.[64,65] All benzodiazepines treat symptoms of anxiety, and some shorter-acting ones are useful hypnotic agents.[66] Benzodiazepines, such as chlordiazepoxide, have long proved useful in treating delirium, especially that associated with alcohol withdrawal. Because some patients with epilepsy experience an aura resembling a panic attack (predominantly anxiety and fear),[60] and anxiety frequently accompanies depression in persons with epilepsy,[32] there are many patients who take benzodiazepines for both conditions. Adverse reactions to this class of drug are similar, regardless of the underlying condition being treated. Benzodiazepines, like barbiturates, can cause irritability or aggression in some children with attention deficit disorder or mental retardation.[60]

Abrupt or rapid withdrawal from benzodiazepines, especially after chronic use and high dosages, can cause seizures; these are usually brief and require no treatment.[12,15,67–70] Many dually dependent patients (those with a psychiatric illness and substance abuse) insist on renewing their benzodiazepine prescription, often clonazepam, because of previous seizures during withdrawal. They may self medicate to obtain relief from symptoms of anxiety and, possibly, delirium that accompany withdrawal,[60] just as alcoholic patients occasionally request long-term therapy with benzodiazepines after undergoing detoxification from the alcohol.[12,68] If benzodiazepines are used chronically, they are best supervised by psychiatrists or behavioral medicine specialists. In patients genuinely

fearful of withdrawal seizures, even with careful, prolonged tapering, it may be useful for them to keep the rectal gel form of diazepam on hand in case of generalized seizure.[71] Enzyme-inducing AEDs (e.g., phenytoin and carbamazepine) can lower benzodiazepine levels, rarely precipitating withdrawal seizures.[56]

Benzodiazepine levels are increased to varying degrees by the antidepressants nefazodone, fluoxetine, and fluvoxamine; the histamine-2 blocker cimetidine; and the antibiotics erythromycin and disulfan[53]; benzodiazepine overdose is not associated with seizures. Reversing benzodiazepine effects with the antagonist flumazenil is not recommended in patients at risk of seizures.[16,72] When benzodiazepine effects are reversed by flumazenil, other drug toxicities may be unmasked in patients with mixed overdoses (e.g., suicide attempts, drug abuses); flumazenil is ineffective against opiate overdose.[72]

Short-acting benzodiazepines, such as temazepam, flurazepam, and estazolam, are useful as hypnotics. Newer, even shorter–acting benzodiazepines, such as zolpidem and zaleplon, act at the central benzodiazepine omega-1 (type 1) site of the GABA$_A$ receptor complex; their effect on seizure threshold is unknown. Because sleep deprivation increases the risk for most types of seizures, restoring normal sleep patterns may be an important part of treatment. However, chronic use of hypnotics is not advisable. Searching for the cause of sleep disruption, if not obvious, may reveal unrecognized nocturnal seizures or adverse effects of medications.[36,37] Antihistamines, which are the main active ingredient in over-the-counter sleeping aids, lower seizure threshold and should therefore be avoided, although the magnitude of this risk is not known. In one series, overdosage with diphenhydramine was the third leading cause of seizures.[5]

Amphetamines

Amphetamines rarely cause seizures when used in therapeutic doses for treatment of attention deficit hyperactivity disorder, even in children with epilepsy. One patient with no previous history of seizures had a convulsion 3 hours after using 20 mg of methylphenidate to improve his concentration during college examinations (personal experience). Amphetamines have been reported to cause seizures when combined with an antidepressant, such as sertraline.[73] Seizures can occur with amphetamine overdose, although dyskinesias, tremors, and hallucinations are more common.[74] Benzodiazepines, such as lorazepam and diazepam, are the treatment of choice. Several neurotransmitters other than dopamine have been implicated in animal studies of overdoses from cocaine, methamphetamine, and amphetamine. Seizures were prevented by benzodiazepines and propranolol in animals given cocaine and amphetamine; the same drugs were ineffective in animals given metamphetamine.[75]

Antiepileptic Drugs That Can Cause Seizures

Increased seizures can occur for several reasons in patients with epilepsy taking antiseizure drugs. Sometimes the wrong drug is chosen for the patient's type of epilepsy, as in using carbamazepine to treat childhood absence or juvenile myoclonic epilepsy.[76,77] Gabapentin can exacerbate myoclonic epilepsy syndromes.[55] Phenytoin or carbamazepine can aggravate myoclonic seizures (and sometimes atypical absences) in Lennox-Gastaut syndrome.[76] Tonic seizures of Lennox-Gastaut syndrome may be exacerbated by phenobarbital or benzodiazepines. Many AEDs may modify seizure semiology.[76,78] Seizures can be a manifestation of neurotoxicity with most AEDs, but free levels may be required to document high levels. Abrupt overdoses, as in suicide attempts, are especially proconvulsant. Drug interactions from polytherapy commonly cause toxicity, which may include seizures, despite reasonable doses because of the AED's cumulative effects on CYP450 and GT enzyme systems. Serum phenytoin levels above 40 µg/ml or carbamazepine levels above 17 µg/ml have been associated with increased seizure frequency.[77,78] In cases in which the carbamazepine concentration is not found to be high, it is likely that the causative factor is carbamazepine-10,11 epoxide, carbamazepine's metabolite.[79] Valproate and gabapentin can cause a toxic encephalopathy with myoclonus and, uncommonly, generalized seizures.[55] Risk factors for worsening seizures with high AED levels include a pre-existing epileptiform EEG pattern, frequent seizures, childhood

seizure syndrome, mental retardation or major brain damage, and polytherapy.[77,78] In patients without these risks, Loiseau has postulated that the AED inadvertently activated a seizure pathway by disrupting a loop involved in seizure inhibition.[78] Oxcarbazepine,[79] levetiracetam,[80] and gabapentin only minimally affect the metabolism or protein binding of other drugs and are thus useful in avoiding drug interactions.

Seizure Risk Associated with Nonprescription (Over the Counter) and Herbal Medicines

Stimulants of all types are implicated in seizure induction, even in patients not at risk due to pre-existing seizure disorder. Ephedrine, pheniramine, and other antihistamines are associated with seizures, especially in overdose (13 of 43 people attempting suicide with pheniramine experienced seizures[81]). Stimulants used for weight loss or decongestion, such as phenylpropanolamine and ephedrine, also cause seizures. The herbal equivalent, ephedra or ma huang, has also caused seizures among other amphetaminelike side effects.[74] Caffeine, used to increase wakefulness or, in nonprescription combination form, to combat migraine headache, has only been associated with seizures in extremely rare circumstances, such as suicide attempts.[82] Gamma-hydroxybutyrate, an androgen steroid used by bodybuilders to stimulate growth hormone and by recreational users to induce tranquility, has been banned in several states owing to the potential for lethal overdose, its use with alcohol in date rape, and its rare seizure incidence.[83] As gamma-hydroxybutyrate overdose–induced coma is reversed by the acetylcholinesterase inhibitor physostigmine and not by flumazenil or naloxone, opiate and benzodiazepine neurotransmitters are not implicated in its activitity.[84] Botanical substances are difficult to evaluate owing to the variable content of active ingredients or biologically active impurities that may be present.[85,86]

Alcohol

Alcohol has been known to produce seizures since antiquity, but the relationship is complex. Seizures[27] and status epilepticus[87] have been reported in both acute intoxication and withdrawal or may be secondary to related complications of alcohol abuse, such as subdural or parenchymal hemorrhage, stroke, or head trauma.[27,88,89] Alcohol acts as a depressant at both $GABA_A$-benzodiazepine receptor complexes and at N-methyl-D-aspartate (NMDA)–glutamate receptors and down-regulates calcium channels, in addition to disrupting the neurotransmitter receptors embedded in myelin with chronic use.[89] Other theories of withdrawal seizures include zinc deficiency[90] and lowering of the aromatic to branched chain–amino acid ratio.[91] Withdrawal seizures generally occur 24–72 hours after last intake and precede delirium tremens in 5% of untreated cases.[88] Studies that used phenobarbital loading were most successful in avoiding recurrent seizures and delirium tremens in one emergency room series.[29] A kindling model in animals has documented spontaneous seizures after several alcohol withdrawals.[89] Although moderate amounts of alcohol that can bring out epileptiform discharges on patients' EEGs do not affect the seizure threshold of patients with epilepsy, recent reviews note an association of seizures with alcohol intoxication.[92] These patients may or may not have structural lesions, such as prior head trauma or stroke.[27,88,89] Although cessation of alcohol use is the best prevention of these seizures, some patients do need anticonvulsants. Many patients have the misconception that they cannot use any anticonvulsant while drinking (probably because prescription bottles are so labeled), and therefore those that require long-term medication add the risk of medication withdrawal to alcohol intake when they drink.[88] Because practitioners are often afraid to give alcoholics phenobarbital, as the combined central nervous system depressant effect may lead to respiratory problems in overdose,[89] and valproic acid because of potential liver and pancreas toxicity, alcoholics are often prescribed phenytoin, which has the highest incidence of seizures with noncompliance (whether deliberate or accidental).[88] Although pure withdrawal seizures should not be treated with anticonvulsants, most alcoholics have symptomatic and withdrawal seizures. By emphasizing improved compliance, including the importance of avoiding running out of medication and not deliberately stopping anticonvulsants while drinking, alcoholic patients with seizure disorders can be successfully treated. Medications such as sodium valproate[28] that have a pro-longed anticonvulsant effect despite short half-life, or those with long half-life such as phenobarbital,[29] are the safest in potentially poorly compliant alcoholic patients. In some cases, when the relationship between their seizures and drinking is pointed out to patients, they are sufficiently frightened that they voluntarily enter detoxification programs.[27–29] Magnesium deficiency should be treated as well.[27,88]

Cocaine

Cocaine use and seizures share a similarly complex relationship to alcohol use. The mode of intake greatly affects seizure threshold, inhaled (smoking of crack) or intravenously injected use being associated with de novo generalized seizures, and insufflated (snorted) use being associated with partial or idiopathic seizures.[93] Seizures are not usually seen in massive overdoses associated with the rupture of cocaine-containing condoms being used for smuggling (body packers).[94] In patients who are delirious from cocaine poisoning, benzodiazepines are useful and safer than neuroleptics that can cause neuroleptic malignant syndrome.[94] The mechanism of epileptogenesis is still uncertain. Variable rates relate to the frequency and mode of cocaine administration, with consequent variation in peak levels of the drug. Kindling of seizures has been described in rat models. Although effects on the major excitatory neurotransmitter systems that are mediated by action at NMDA and AMPA receptors affect seizure induction in rats,[95] other chemicals, such as polyamines, are also changed in animals who develop seizures after repeated cocaine injection.[96] Dopamine, implicated in the euphoric and addictive effects of cocaine, is probably not involved in seizures, but these effects do correlate with binding of cocaine at serotonin (more than muscarinic and cholinergic) receptors.[97] Other studies support activity at the $GABA_A$ channel receptor leading to abnormal excitation and seizures.[98]

Isolated seizures do not require treatment, but in patients with both cocaine-induced and spontaneous seizures, any anticonvulsant is effective. Rarely, cocaine abusers report enhancing their high by opening their phenytoin capsule and smoking it along with cocaine, which can lead to phenytoin toxicity.[99] Early reports that phenytoin can reduce relapse rates in cocaine detoxification programs[100] have not been confirmed.[101] Because many cocaine abusers are poorly compliant with anticonvulsant regimens, care must be used before initiating treatment, even in those with underlying seizure disorders exacerbated by cocaine.[102] Patients who drink alcohol or use benzodiazepines to regulate their cocaine high may require protection from withdrawal seizures or delirium tremens, as well as seizures from cocaine intoxication.[103]

Illicit Stimulants

As mentioned, overdosing with amphetamines and other sympathomimetic drugs can cause seizures similar to those seen with cocaine use.[104] Because the effects of stimulants on the central nervous system are more prolonged than those of cocaine, seizures can occur several hours after use. If they occur more than 24 hours after amphetamine use, cerebral vasculitis must be considered.[74,104] 3,4-Methylenedioxymethamphetamine (ecstasy), a serotonin uptake inhibitor that is both a stimulant and a hallucinogen, can cause seizures after ingestion of only one tablet.[105] Phencyclidine, an anesthetic agent that acts as an NMDA receptor antagonist, is frequently associated with seizures. Intravenous benzodiazepines are the most effective treatment for toxic symptoms, including seizures and agitation, associated with these drugs.[104] Doses of amphetamines used to treat children with attention deficit disorder rarely cause seizures in the absence of confounding factors, such as co-medication with antidepressants like sertraline.[73] In abuse situations, in which the drug is smoked instead of ingested orally, sleep deprivation probably contributes to seizure occurrence.

Seizures Caused by Opioids and Other Central Nervous System Depressants

Marijuana and heroin have a low relative risk of epileptogenesis, and some data suggest that marijuana has an anticonvulsant effect.[106] However, heroin in particular may be mixed with contaminants that, when injected, lower seizure threshold. In a case-control study by Ng et al.,[106] some heroin-abusing patients who were admitted with new-onset seizures

were found to have other serious conditions, including sepsis, brain abscess, and acquired immunodeficiency syndrome. Opiate withdrawal produces myoclonus and shivering that can be mistaken for seizure activity.[107] Tramadol, a synthetic narcotic used to treat pain, was associated with a high incidence of seizures shortly after it was introduced.[108] As more experience with the drug was gained, the usual dose was lowered and tramadol use was avoided in patients taking antidepressants, neuroleptics, or other opiates. Subsequent to these changes, the incidence of seizures has fallen to less than 1%.[109] Ng and Alvear[110] reported generalized seizures in more than half of those who used dextropropoxyphene, a morphine analog. Seizures have also occurred in people who abuse propoxyphene, meperidine, and "Ts and blues" (Talwin [pentazocine] and tripelennamine).[104] Former heroin addicts using methadone dislike AEDs, such as phenytoin and carbamazepine, that induce hepatic metabolizing enzymes, claiming that the anticonvulsants "eat" their methadone. If patients taking methadone require anticonvulsant drugs, valproic acid, levetiracetam, gabapentin, and lamotrigine are generally more acceptable to these patients.[107]

Summary

Seizures are always a symptom of brain dysfunction and usually reflect some degree of interaction between intrinsic (i.e., epileptic susceptibility or low seizure threshold) and extrinsic (i.e., physiological or environmental stressors) factors. Thus, drugs (whether medicinal, botanical, or recreational) can increase the risk of seizures by lowering a patient's seizure threshold below some critical level. Many of these extrinsic factors (e.g., alcohol, street drugs, and anesthetics) are transient or reversible. Others, especially those that cause permanent cerebral injury, are not. Sick patients, or those undergoing surgery, are especially vulnerable to seizures because of complex, potentially epileptogenic interactions among different drugs and between drugs and pre-existing cerebral pathology or systemic disease. All of these factors must be considered in patients who have new-onset seizures. Decisions about treatment depend on obtaining accurate information about the circumstances under which the seizure(s) occurred and whether these are both sufficient to explain the seizures and whether they are remediable. Acute symptomatic seizures do not usually require AED therapy if the precipitants can be eliminated or avoided. If AEDs must be prescribed, it is important to recognize the effect they may have on other aspects of the patient's treatment.

Acknowledgment

I thank Dr. Srivalli Denthireni, who assisted with library research.

References

1. Aminoff MJ, Parent JM. Comorbidity in Adults. In J Engel Jr, TA Pedley (eds), Epilepsy: a Comprehensive Textbook. Philadelphia: Lippincott–Raven, 1997;1957–1970.
2. Asconapé JJ, Penry JK. Use of antiepileptic drugs in the presence of liver and kidney diseases: a review. Epilepsia 1982;23:S65–S79.
3. Muruve DA, Steinman TI. Contrast-induced encephalopathy and seizures in a patient with chronic renal insufficiency. Clin Nephrol 1996;45:406–409.
4. Kunisaki TA, Augenstein WL. Drug- and toxin-induced seizures. Emerg Med Clin North Am 1994;12:1027–1056.
5. Olson KR, Kearney TE, Dyer JE, et al. Seizures associated with poisoning and drug overdose. Am J Emerg Med 1993;11:565–568.
6. Shannon M. Ingestion of toxic substances by children. N Engl J Med 2000;342:186–191.
7. Franson KL, Hay DP, Neppe V, et al. Drug-induced seizures in the elderly. Causative agents and optimal management. Drugs Aging 1995;7:38–48.
8. Delanty N, Vaughan CJ, French JA. Medical causes of seizures. Lancet 1998;352:383–390.
9. Hirsch LJ, Pedley TA. Perioperative Seizures: Prevention and Management. In H Batjer, C Loftus (eds), Techniques in Neurosurgery. Philadelphia: Lippincott Williams & Wilkins, in press.
10. Birnbaum AK, Kriel RL, Burkhardt RT, Remmel RP. Rectal absorption of lamotrigine compressed tablets. Epilepsia 2000;41:850–853.
11. Brown DL, Ransom DM, Hall JA, et al. Regional anesthesia and local anesthetic-induced systemic toxicity: seizure frequency and accompanying cardiovascular changes. Anesth Analg 1995;81:321–328.
12. Petursson H. The benzodiazepine withdrawal syndrome. Addiction 1994;89:1455–1459.
13. Sutherland MJ, Burt P. Propofol and seizures. Anaesth Intensive Care 1994;22:733–737.
14. Terasako K, Ishii S. Postoperative seizure-like activity following sevoflurane anesthesia. Acta Anaest Scand 1996;40:953–954.
15. Lane HY, Su KP, Chang WH. Seizures after discontinuation of low-dose lorazepam from originally seizure-free clozapine regimen: combined effects? J Clin Psychiatry 1999;60:408–409.
16. Schulze-Bonhage A, Elger CE. Induction of partial epileptic seizures by flumazenil. Epilepsia 2000;41:186–192.
17. Herishano YO, Zlotnik M, Mostoslavsky M, et al. Cefuroxime-induced encephalopathy. Neurology 1998;50:1873–1875.
18. Koppel B, van Duin D, Samkoff L, et al. Imipenem does not contribute to seizures in severely ill patients if dose is adjusted for renal function. Epilepsia 1997;38[Suppl 8]:S109–S110.
19. Walker RC. The fluoroquinolones. Mayo Clin Proc 1999;74:1030–1037.
20. Koppel BS. Neurologic Complications of AIDS and HIV Infection: an Overview. In: G Wormser (ed), A Clinician's Guide to AIDS and HIV Infection. Philadelphia: Lippincott–Raven, 1996;141–197.
21. Simpson DM, Olney R, McArthur JC, et al. A placebo-controlled trial of lamotrigine for painful HIV-associated neuropathy. Neurology 2000;54:2115–2119.
22. Romanelli F, Jennings HR, Nath A, et al. Therapeutic dilemma: the use of anticonvulsants in HIV-positive individuals. Neurology 2000;54:1404–1407.
23. Morris DJ. Adverse effects and drug interactions of clinical importance with antiviral drugs. Drug Saf 1994;10:281–291.
24. Wong M, Yamada KA. Cyclosporine induces epileptiform activity in an in vitro seizure model. Epilepsia 2000;41:271–276.
25. Devinsky O. The differential diagnosis of seizures and epilepsy. Semin Neurol 1990;10:321–327.
26. Hillbom M, Tokola R, Kuusela V, et al. Pseudoseizures and other nonepileptic paroxysmal disorders in children and adolescents. Neurology 1999;53[Suppl 2]:S89–S95.
27. Koppel BS, Daras M, Tuchman AJ, et al. Relationship between alcohol and seizures in a city hospital population. J Epilepsy 1992;5:31–37.
28. Hillbom M, Tokola R, Kuusela V, et al. Prevention of alcohol withdrawal seizures with carbamazepine and valproic acid. Alcohol 1989;6:223–226.
29. Young GP, Rores C, Murphy C, Daily RH. Intravenous phenobarbital for alcohol withdrawal and convulsions. Ann Emerg Med 1987;38:847–850.
30. Bowman ES. Nonepileptic seizures: psychiatric framework, treatment, and outcome. Neurology 1999;53[Suppl 2]:S84–S88.
31. Krumholz A. Nonepileptic seizures: diagnosis and management. Neurology 1999;53[Suppl 2]:S76–S83.
32. Torta R, Keller R. Behavioral, psychotic and anxiety disorders in epilepsy: etiology, clinical features, and therapeutic implications. Epilepsia 1999;40[Suppl 10]:S2–S20.

33. Blumer D. Evidence supporting the temporal lobe epilepsy personality syndrome. Neurology 1999;53[Suppl 2]:S9–S12.

34. Lancman M. Psychosis and peri-ictal confusional states. Neurology 1999;53[Suppl 2]:S33–S38.

35. Bodner RA, Lynch T, Lewis L, Kahn D. Serotonin syndrome. Neurology 1995;45:219–223.

36. Ehrenberg B. Importance of sleep restoration in co-morbid disease: effect of anticonvulsants. Neurology 2000;54[Suppl 1]:S33–S37.

37. Sammaritano M, Sherwin A. Effect of anticonvulsants on sleep. Neurology 2000;54[Suppl 1]:S16–S24.

38. Trabert W, Hohagen F, Winkelmann G, Berger M. Seizure and electroencephalographic signs of a lowered seizure threshold, associated with fluvoxamine treatment of obsessive-compulsive disorder. Pharmacopsychiatry 1995;28:95–97.

39. Pisani F, Spina E, Oteri G. Antidepressant drugs and seizure susceptibility: from in vitro data to clinical practice. Epilepsia 1999;40[Suppl 10]:S48–S56.

40. Kanner AM, Rivas Nieto JC. Depressive disorders in epilepsy. Neurology 1999;53[Suppl 2]:S26–S32.

41. Alldredge BK. Seizure risk associated with psychotropic drugs: clinical and pharmacokinetic considerations. Neurology 1999;53[Suppl 2]:S68–S75.

42. Dailey JW, Naritoku, DK. Antidepressants and seizures: clinical anecdotes overshadow neuroscience. Biochem Pharmacol 1996;52:1323–1329.

43. Richelson E. Pharmacology of antidepressants—characteristics of the ideal drug. Mayo Clin Proc 1994;69:1069–1081.

44. Lambert MV, Robertson MM. Depression in epilepsy: etiology, phenomenology, and treatment. Epilepsia 1999;40[Suppl 10]:S21–S47.

45. Garnier R, Azoyan P, Chataigner D, et al. Acute fluvoxamine poisoning. J Int Med Res 1993;21:197–208.

46. Goldstein L, Barker M, Segall F, et al. Seizure and transient SIADH associated with sertraline [Letter]. Am J Psychiatry 1996;153:732.

47. Ranieri P, Franczoni S, Trabucchi M. Reboxetine and hyponatremia [letter]. N Engl J Med 2000;342:215–216.

48. Bell AJ, Cole A, Eccleston D, Ferrier IN. Lithium neurotoxicity at normal therapeutic levels. Br J Psychiatry 1993;162:689–692.

49. Preskorn SH. Clinically relevant pharmacology of selective serotonin reuptake inhibitors. Clin Pharmacokinet 1997;32[Suppl 1]:S1–S21.

50. Preskorn SH, Fast GA. Tricyclic antidepressant-induced seizures and plasma drug concentration. J Clin Psychiatry 1992;53:160–162.

51. Baldessarini RJ. Drugs and the Treatment of Psychiatric Disorders. Depression and Mania. In JG Hardman, LE Limbird (eds), Goodman and Gilman's the Pharmacological Basis of Therapeutics. New York: McGraw-Hill, 1996;431–459.

52. Physicians' Desk Reference. Montvale, NJ: Medical Economics Co, 2000.

53. DeVane CL, Nemeroff CB. 1999 Guide to Psychotropic Drug Interactions. In DC Steffens, KR Krishnan, PM Doraiswamy (eds), The Psychotropic Drug Interactions Reference Guide (vol 4–6). Primary Psychiatry, 1997–1999. New York: McMahon Publishing Group.

54. Richelson E. Pharmacokinetic drug interactions of new antidepressants: a review of the effects on the metabolism of other drugs. Mayo Clin Proc 1997;72:835–847.

55. Asconapé J, Diedrich A, DellaBadia J. Myoclonus associated with the use of gabapentin. Epilepsia 2000;41:479–481.

56. Monaco F, Cicolin A. Interactions between anticonvulsant and psychoactive drugs. Epilepsia 1999;40[Suppl 10]:S71–S76.

57. Devinsky O, Duchowny MS. Seizures after convulsive therapy: a retrospective case survey. Neurology 1983;33:921–925.

58. Hsiao JK, Messenheimer JA, Evans DL. ECT and neurological disorders. Convulsive Ther 1987;3:121–136.

59. Harden CL, Pulver MC, Ravdin LD, et al. A pilot study of mood in epilepsy patients treated with vagus nerve stimulation. Epilepsy Behav 2000;1:93–99.

60. Schmitz B. Psychiatric syndromes related to antiepileptic drugs. Epilepsia 1999;40[Suppl 10]:S65–S70.

61. Logothetis J. Spontaneous epileptic seizures and electroencephalographic changes in the course of phenothiazine therapy. Neurology 1967;17:869–877.

62. Oliver AP, Luchins DJ, Wyatt RJ. Neuroleptic-induced seizures. An in vitro technique for assessing relative risk. Arch Gen Psychiatry 1982;39:206–209.

63. Starr MS. The role of dopamine in epilepsy. Synapse 1996;22:159–194.

64. Twyman RE, Rogers CJ, Macdonald RL. Differential regulation of γ-aminobutyric acid receptor channels by diazepam and phenobarbital. Ann Neurol 1989;25:213–220.

65. Henrickson O. An overview of benzodiazepines in seizure management. Epilepsia 1998;39[Suppl 1]:S2–S6.

66. Tassinari CA, Michelucci R. The use of diazepam and clonazepam in epilepsy. Epilepsia 1989;39[Suppl 1]:S7–S14.

67. Gillin JC, Byerley WF. The diagnosis and management of insomnia. N Engl J Med 1990;322:239–248.

68. Busto U, Sellers EM, Naranjo CA, et al. Withdrawal reactions after long-term therapeutic use of benzodiazepines. N Engl J Med 1986;315:854–859.

69. Preskorn SH, Denner LJ. Benzodiazepines and withdrawal psychosis. JAMA 1977;237:36–38.

70. Noyes R. Seizures following the withdrawal of alprazolam. J Nerv Ment Dis 1986;174:50–52.

71. Dooley JM. Rectal use of benzodiazepines. Epilepsia 1998;39:[Suppl 1]:S24–S27.

72. Fitzgerald J, Anderson M. Focus on flumazenil: a new benzodiazepine antagonist. Hosp Formul 1992;27:575–583.

73. Feeney DJ, Klykylo WM. Medication-induced seizures [Letter]. J Am Acad Child Adolesc Psychiatry 1997;36:1018–1019.

74. Brust JC. Amphetamine and Other Psychostimulants. In JC Brust (ed), Neurological Aspects of Substance Abuse. Boston: Butterworth–Heinemann, 1993;60–81.

75. Derlet RW, Albertson TE, Rice P. Antagonism of cocaine, amphetamine, and methamphetamine toxicity. Pharmacol Biochem Behav 1990;36:745–749.

76. Bauer J. Seizure-inducing effects of antiepileptic drugs: a review. Acta Neurol Scand 1996;94:367–377.

77. Perucca E, Gram L, Avanzine G, Dulac O. Antiepileptic drugs as a cause of worsening seizures. Epilepsia 1998;39:5–17.

78. Loiseau P. Do antiepileptic drugs exacerbate seizures? Epilepsia 1998;39:2–4.

79. Schacter SC, Vazquez B, Fisher RS, et al. Oxcarbazepine. Double-blind, randomized, placebo-control, monotherapy trial for partial seizures. Neurology 1999;52:732–737.

80. Cereghino JJ, Biton V, Abou-Khalil B, et al. Levetiracetam for partial seizures: results of a double-blind, randomized clinical trial. Neurology 2000;55:236–242.

81. Buckley NA, Whyte IM, Dawson AH, Cruickshank DA. Pheniramine—a much abused drug. Med J Aust 1994;160:188–192.

82. Zimmerman PM, Pulliam J, Schwengels J, MacDonald SE. Caffeine intoxication: a near fatality. Ann Emerg Med 1985;14:1227–1229.

83. Centers for Disease Control and Prevention. Adverse events associated with ingestion of gamma-butyrolactone—Minnesota, New Mexico, and Texas, 1998-1999. MMWR Morb Mortal Wkly Rep 1999;48:137–140.

84. Yates SW, Viera AJ. Physostigmine in the treatment of γ-hydroxybutyric acid overdose. Mayo Clin Proc 2000;75:401–402.

85. Cupp MJ. Herbal remedies: adverse effects and drug interactions. Am Fam Physician 1999;59:1239–1244.

86. Angell M, Kassirer JP. Alternative medicine: the risk of untested and unregulated remedies. N Engl J Med 1998;339:839–841.

87. Alldredge BK, Lowenstein DH. Status epilepticus related to alcohol abuse. Epilepsia 1993;34:1033–1037.

88. McMicken DB, Freedland ES. Alcohol-related seizures. Management of seizures in the ED. Emerg Med Clin North Am 1994;12:1057–1077.

89. Brust JC. Ethanol. In JC Brust (ed), Neurological Aspects of Substance Abuse. Boston: Butterworth–Heinemann, 1993;190–252.

90. Menzano E, Carlen PL. Zinc deficiency and corticosteroids in the pathogenesis of alcoholic brain dysfunction—a review. Alcohol Clin Exp Res 1994;18:895–901.

91. Saito T, Kobatake K, Ozawa H, Ogata M. Aromatic and branched-chain amino acid levels in alcoholics. Alcohol Alcohol 1994;29[Suppl 1]:133–135.

92. Ng SKC, Hauser WA, Brust JC, Susser M. Alcohol consumption and withdrawal in new-onset seizures. N Engl J Med 1988;319:666–673.

93. Pascual-Leone A, Dhuna A, Altafullah I, Anderson DC. Cocaine-induced seizures. Neurology 1990;40:404–407.

94. Brust JC. Cocaine. In JC Brust (ed), Neurological Aspects of Substance Abuse. Boston: Butterworth–Heinemann, 1993;82–114.

95. Barat SA, Abdel-Rahman MS. Decreased cocaine- and lidocaine-induced seizure response by dextromethorphan and DNQX in rat. Brain Res 1997;756:179–183.

96. Shimosato K, Watanabe S, Marley R, Saito T. Increased polyamine levels and changes in the sensitivity to convulsions during chronic treatment with cocaine in mice. Brain Res 1995;684:243–247.

97. Ritz MC, George FR. Cocaine-induced seizures and lethality appear to be associated with distinct central nervous system binding sites. J Pharm Exp Ther 1993;264:1333–1343.

98. Ye JH, Liu PL, Wu WH, McArdle JJ. Cocaine depresses $GABA_A$ current of hippocampal neurons. Brain Res 1997;770:169–175.

99. Koppel BS, Daras M, Samkoff L. Phenytoin neurotoxicity from illicit use. Neurology 1995;45:198.

100. Crosby RD, Pearson VL, Eller C, et al. Phenytoin in the treatment of cocaine abuse: a double-blind study. Clin Pharmacol Ther 1996;59:458–468.

101. Sofuoglu M, Pentel PR, Bliss RL, et al. Effects of phenytoin on cocaine self-administration in humans. Drug Alcohol Depend 1999;53:273–275.

102. Koppel BS, Samkoff L, Daras M. Relation of cocaine use to seizures and epilepsy. Epilepsia 1996;37:875–878.

103. Derlet RW, Albertson TE. Flumazenil induces seizures and death in mixed cocaine-diazepam intoxications. Ann Emerg Med 1994;23:494–498.

104. Abramowicz M, ed. Acute reactions to drugs of abuse. Med Lett 1996;38:43–46.

105. Holmes SB, Banerjce AK, Alexander WD. Hyponatraemia and seizures after ecstasy use. Postgrad Med J 1999;75:32–33.

106. Ng SK, Brust JC, Hauser WA, Susser M. Illicit drug use and the risk of new-onset seizures. Am J Epidemiol 1990;132:47–57.

107. Brust JC. Opioids. In JC Brust (ed), Neurological Aspects of Substance Abuse. Boston: Butterworth–Heinemann, 1993;16–59.

108. Tobias JD. Seizure after overdose of tramadol. South Med J 1997;90:826–827.

109. Petrone D, Kamin M, Olson W. Slowing the titration rate of tramadol HCl reduces the incidence of discontinuation due to nausea and/or vomiting: a double-blind randomized trial. J Clin Pharm Ther 1999;24:115–123.

110. Ng B, Alvear M. Dextropropoxyphene addiction—a drug of primary abuse. Am J Drug Alcohol Abuse 1993;19:153–158.

Chapter 9

Brain Tumors and Epilepsy

Francesco T. Mangano, Alexandra E. McBride, and Steven J. Schneider

Historical Perspective

Since Hippocratic times, diverse surgical therapies have been proposed as treatments for epilepsy. These have included venting obstructing humors or accumulations of "evil air" by such procedures as bleeding from an arm or leg, cauterizing the scalp and bone with a hot iron, cutting arteries around the ear, inserting cruciate incisions into the occiput, and placing dural "valves."[1–4]

Modern epilepsy surgery emerged with John Hughlings Jackson's studies of focal epilepsy (Figure 9-1), which introduced the concept of cortical control of specific movements. This early recognition that clinical seizure semiology related to specific cortical areas identified epileptogenic cortical regions that are potentially amenable to surgery.[5–7] Further expanding this concept, Sir Victor Horsley performed the first craniotomy for post-traumatic epilepsy in 1886 (Figure 9-2).[8–10] Since then, our understanding of the pathophysiology, etiology, and medical and surgical treatment of this disorder has undergone an extensive evolution.

Epilepsy and Neoplasms

Epilepsy is common in adult and pediatric populations. Intractable epilepsy is a seizure disorder that is pharmacoresistant to maximally tolerated antiepileptic drug (AED) therapy, occurring in 10–20% of those with chronic epilepsy.[11] Identifiable etiologies include infection, trauma, cerebral malformation, inborn errors of metabolism, neurocutaneous disorders, arteriovenous malformations, electrolyte imbalances, hereditary factors, substance abuse, and brain tumors (Table 9-1).[12–15] An incidence of 50–70 cases per 100,000 persons per year and a prevalence of 5–10 cases per 1,000 population emphasize its significance and medical, financial, and social burdens, such as lost work wages, driving disabilities, and pharmaceutical costs.[16]

Brain tumors are a common cause of epilepsy in adults. More than one-third of the 35,000 patients per year with newly diagnosed brain tumors develop epileptic seizures. If the tumor involves the cerebral hemispheres, seizures occur in at least 50% of cases.[17,18] Any brain tumor, benign or malignant, common or uncommon, can cause seizures.[19–23] Tumors associated with epilepsy in adults include oligodendrogliomas, astrocytomas, metastatic tumors, meningiomas, glioblastoma multiforme, dysembryoplastic neuroepithelial tumors (DNETs), and gangliogliomas (Table 9-2).[24–30]

Epilepsy is a common neurologic disorder in children, with an overall incidence of 4.3–9.3 cases per 1,000 children in the United States.[31] Eighty percent of children outgrow epilepsy or are successfully treated with AEDs. In contrast to adults, children with epilepsy have brain tumors less frequently. However, tumors must be considered even without neurologic deficits.[32–34] If a tumor is diagnosed, up to 46% of these patients may have intractable seizures.[32,35,36] Most tumors

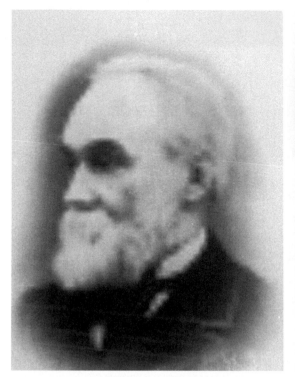

Figure 9-1. John Hughlings Jackson (1835–1911). (Reprinted with permission from H Horwitz. Library: historical perspective. Neurosurgery 1999;44:906–910.)

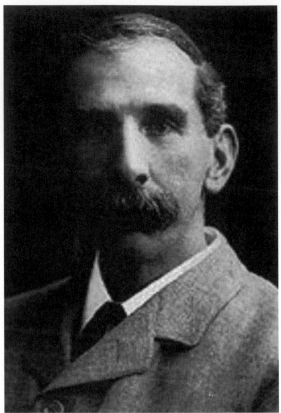

Figure 9-2. Sir Victor Horsley (1847–1916). (Reprinted with permission from H Horwitz. Library: historical perspective. Neurosurgery 1995;36:428–432.)

occur in the temporal or frontal lobes. As in adults, epileptogenic brain tumors in children may be benign or malignant. Those most common tumors are gangliogliomas, low-grade astrocytomas, DNETs, and oligodendrogliomas.[30,36–38]

Pathophysiology of Seizures in Brain Tumors

Mechanisms of tumor-related epileptogenesis remain poorly understood. In tumor-associated epilepsy, nontumoral surrounding tissue may cause seizures.[39] Abnormal growth kinetics of tumors can affect surrounding neurons morphologically and biochemically, altering neuronal structure and affecting neurotransmitter and neuromodulator release (e.g., γ-aminobutyric acid and somatostatin). These changes may cause seizures through hyperexcitability or reduced inhibition.[40,41] Hippocampal involvement, either directly, through tumor extension or, indirectly, through increased excitatory input caused by a tumor, may contribute to seizure amplification and propaga-

tion.[42] Tumors can disrupt normal electrical functional patterns, causing increased local coherence or similarity of electrical activity seen electrographically within a cortical region, which is a similar pattern observed in epileptic foci.[43] These changes, induced

Table 9-1. Common Etiology of Epilepsy

Arteriovenous malformations
Cerebral malformations
Cerebrovascular accidents
Electrolyte imbalances
Inborn errors of metabolism
Infection
Neurocutaneous disorders
Substance abuse
Trauma
Tumors

Table 9-2. Most Common Epileptogenic Tumors Presenting with Seizures

Tumor Type	Seizure Presentation (%)
Dysembryoplastic neu- roepithelial tumor	90–100
Ganglioglioma	59
Glioblastoma multiforme	34
Low-grade astrocytoma	69
Metastatic neoplasms	41
Oligodendroglioma	70–90

by a tumor in the surrounding tissue, contribute to the formation of the epileptogenic zone. Cortical connections contribute to generation and maintenance of seizures. Aggressive white matter neoplasms are less likely to cause seizures, because they do not directly irritate cortex and tumor growth and may disrupt the spread of epileptic activity.[17]

Functional Anatomy

Seizures, often complex partial, may be the first symptom of a brain tumor. Although seizure type does not reliably distinguish a tumor from a nontumor etiology,[32,36,44,45] clinical ictal characteristics, such as focal clonic activity, may suggest that a focal region of seizure onset exists and an associated lesion must be excluded. Clinical seizure semiology provides clues for the region of ictal onset and its potentially associated focal lesion. Table 9-3 summarizes the International League against Epilepsy's classification of epilepsy syndromes, which describes seizures according to anatomic location.[46] For example, very brief seizures with abundant posturing activity at onset and quick termination suggest a frontal lobe origin of seizures. Psychical symptoms with automatisms suggest temporal lobe origin. However, seizure localization is complicated by the difficulty of distinguishing seizure onset from manifestations of seizure spread. Reviews of detailed seizure classification and ictal semiology are available.[46–48]

Neuroimaging

Neuroimaging techniques for evaluating seizure localization include magnetic resonance imaging (MRI), computed tomography (CT), single photon emission computerized tomography (SPECT),

Table 9-3. General Characteristics of Seizures by Anatomic Location

Anatomic Location	General Characteristics
Frontal lobe	Usually occur several times per day, short in duration, during sleep. Tonic/postural manifestations prominent. Complex gestural automatisms common at onset.
Occipital lobe	Usually simple partial and secondarily generalized seizures. Most commonly, but not always, include visual symptoms that are contralateral to cortex. Initial signs can include tonic/clonic contraversion of eyes or head, or both; palpebral jerks; and forced closure of eyelids. Negative visual manifestations include scotoma, hemianopsia, and amaurosis. Positive manifestations include sparks, flashes, and phosphenes (more common).
Parietal lobe	Most are simple partial but can secondarily generalize. Most frequently involve hand, arm, and face with predominantly sensory features. Positive symptoms include tingling and electric feeling. Negative symptoms include numbness, absent body part, and asomatognosia. In the dominant parietal lobe, language is often involved.
Temporal lobe	Simple partial seizures: autonomic/psychic symptoms and sensory phenomena—olfactory, auditory, and, most commonly, rising epigastric sensation.
	Complex partial seizures: alteration in consciousness with behavioral arrest, often followed by oroalimentary or hand automatisms. Postictal confusion is usually followed by amnesia of the event.

Source: Adapted from Commission on Classification and Terminology of the International League against Epilepsy. Proposal for revised classification of epilepsy and epileptic syndromes. Epilepsia 1989;30:389–399.

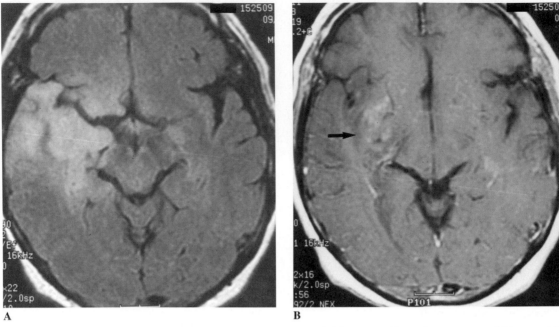

A   B

Figure 9-3. Low-grade astrocytoma. **A.** Magnetic resonance imaging, fluid-attenuated inversion recovery, axial image without gadolinium enhancement. **B.** T1-weighted axial image after gadolinium infusion. Images show an abnormal increased signal in the right anterior temporal lobe (*arrow*).

positron emission tomography (PET) scans, functional MRI (fMRI), and magnetic resonance spectroscopy (MRS). These studies help to identify structural lesions for potential resection, assess eloquent cortex, and aid in surgical planning. Brain CT scans are less sensitive than MRI in detecting structural lesions. Furthermore, middle and posterior fossa lesions can be masked by bone artifact on CT.[49] CT scan of the head is usually reserved for the acute evaluation of new-onset seizures, owing to its ready availability in settings such as the emergency room and to evaluate etiologies, such as acute hemorrhage or trauma.[50] However, MRI is the gold standard in evaluating epilepsy, because lesions, such as a neoplasm, may be missed on CT but identified on MRI. New-onset nontraumatic seizures should be evaluated with gadolinium enhanced T1-weighted, T2-weighted, and fluid-attenuated inversion recovery images, whereas evaluation of a chronic disorder may exclude the use of contrast unless there has been a recent change in seizure type, frequency, or intensity.[51] MRI is free of radiation and is therefore very safe.[52] In epilepsy surgery evaluations involving subdural and depth electrodes, MRI can verify

invasive electrode placement and location and, after surgery, document postoperative extent of cortical resection.

Some brain tumors have characteristic findings on neuroimaging that can distinguish them from non-neoplastic lesions or even suggest a specific type of tumor. However, it may be difficult to differentiate low-grade gliomas from other tumor types presenting with epilepsy. Characteristically, astrocytomas show a T2-signal increase and a nonspecific T1 signal of solid components (Figure 9-3). Cystic components are isointense to cerebrospinal fluid. Oligodendrogliomas look like astrocytomas but may have a honeycomb and stippled amorphous appearance with areas of superficially distributed calcifications.[53] Gangliogliomas have no specific MRI features distinguishing them from other gliomas (Figure 9-4). DNETs usually affect the frontal and temporal lobes in children, also appearing similar to low-grade gliomas, except that edema is rarely appreciated (Figure 9-5). Kuroiwa et al. described DNETs as hypointense on T1-weighted sequences and hyperintense and well demarcated on T2-weighted sequences with no

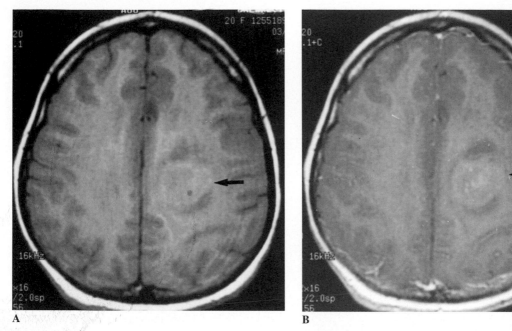

A   B

Figure 9-4. Ganglioglioma. **A.** T1-weighted axial image of a left frontoparietal space-occupying lesion (*arrow*). **B.** Note no appreciable contrast enhancement after gadolinium infusion (*arrow*).

contrast enhancement noted.[54] Glioblastoma multiforme (GBM) displays a heterogenous signal on T1- and T2-weighted imaging and inhomogeneous postgadolinium ring enhancement with nonenhancing areas representing necrosis (Figure 9-6).[55] Meningiomas are usually isodense on T1- and T2-weighted images and demonstrate intense postgadolinium enhancement in the T1 sequences (Figure 9-7).[56] Focal calcifications are seen in 25% of tumors, but hyperintensity occurs in more than 70% of CT scans.[55] To identify focal lesions, T2-weighted sequences are more sensitive to low-grade tumors, arteriovenous malformations, focal gliosis, and hamartomas.[57–59]

PET and SPECT scanning is useful in the presurgical evaluation of partial and generalized seizures, as well as the noninvasive study of brain tumors. PET scanning is a functional glucose metabolic imaging technique that assesses cerebral metabolism. Patients with low-grade epileptogenic tumors may demonstrate areas of hypometabolism interictally, and hypermetabolism may be seen during ictal events. These areas tend to be larger than the anatomic abnormality itself.[60] PET with fluoro-2-deoxy-D-glucose (FDG) uptake can have prognostic

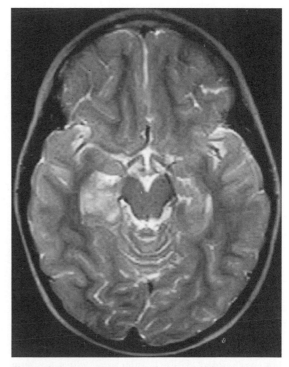

Figure 9-5. Dysembryoplastic neuroepithelial tumor. T2-weighted axial image of a right medial temporal infiltrative lesion demonstrating abnormal signal intensity.

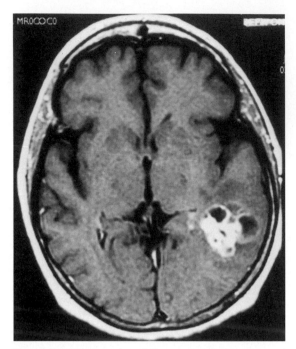

Figure 9-6. Glioblastoma multiforme. Gadolinium-enhanced axial T1-weighted image of a left-sided multicystic necrotic lesion with a solid enhancing component in the temporoparietal region.

value in low-grade gliomas.[61] Those tumors that display areas of increased FDG uptake are likely to recur or progress to higher grades. Furthermore, Derlon et al. compared metabolic patterns between astrocytomas and oligodendrogliomas using PET FDG (glucose) and ^{11}C-L-methylmethionine (amino acid) uptake.[62] Although both tumors showed glucose hypometabolism, amino acid uptake was increased only in oligodendrogliomas. This suggests that specialized PET protocols may aid in distinguishing tumor types. Continued research using this technology may help improve diagnosis, therapy, and assessment of possible tumor progression.

SPECT is a functional cerebral perfusion imaging technique used in the noninvasive physiologic evaluation of intractable seizures to help define focal areas of abnormality. Compared to PET, SPECT is less expensive and widely available in most hospitals. Electrographically, widespread blood flow changes may be seen during a seizure, but well-timed SPECT injections close to ictal onset may identify the origin of seizure onset. SPECT aids in localization by demonstrating cere-

bral areas that have decreased regional cerebral blood flow (rCBF) interictally and increased areas of rCBF ictally. Challenges in accomplishing ictal SPECT include difficulties injecting the radioisotope on time, given the unpredictability of seizures; difficulties obtaining the isotope and being limited by its half-life, particularly concerning nocturnal seizures; short duration of some seizures; and limited sensitivity and specificity of postictal data.[63] More recently, co-registered subtraction SPECT imaging from MRI can improve reliability in localizing seizure foci postictally.[64]

MRS is a noninvasive technique that measures metabolic activity, allowing for the comparison of neural and tumoral elements containing protons. Relevant metabolites are creatine, *N*-acetylaspartate, lactate, and carbohydrate (CHO)-containing phospholipids. Assessment of CHO peaks and lactate levels helps assess tumor aggressiveness and distinguish radiation damage from tumor recurrence. In a recent study of 11 pediatric patients with low-grade gliomas, Lazareff et al. showed that MRS CHO values were a viable noninvasive prognostic tool to follow tumor progression, with higher ratios correlating with more rapid tumor growth.[65] MRS has also been shown to be of prognostic value when treating recurrent malignant gliomas with radiosurgery.[66]

fMRI is another noninvasive imaging technique that maps changes in rCBF and concentrations of oxy- or deoxyhemoglobin on task performance. It is a useful tool to identify regions of eloquent cortex that need to be spared in lesion resection.[67,68]

Although SPECT, PET, MRS, and fMRI techniques are not currently the primary neurodiagnostic modalities in the evaluation of tumors and epilepsy, these studies are helpful adjuncts. They can increase the level of certainty that the region of seizure activity and eloquent cortex have been correctly identified, provide prognostic tumor data, and guide intracranial electrode placement.

Treatment of Brain Tumors

Tumors are often treated surgically with adjunctive therapies, such as chemotherapy or radiation therapy, or both, especially for aggressive histologies. When contemplating surgery, lesion location, its proximity to eloquent cortex, and involvement of vascular structures and nerves are elements that help determine surgical risks. Pathology of the lesion is the most important prognostic factor. The patient's medical condition is yet another important factor to consider. Severe cardiopulmonary or organ system disease may be a contraindication to general anesthesia. When radiologic studies fail to determine the nature of the lesion, a biopsy may be necessary.

Some tumors are best treated by observation for progression. Other tumors, such as those in deep subcortical regions, may be surgically inaccessible. Nonsurgical treatment of brain tumors can include chemotherapy, radiation, or radiosurgery.

Chemotherapeutic options include intravenous agents or local agents applied directly on the tumor bed. To control local tumor recurrence or progression in a tumor bed, surgeons may implant agents such as iodine-125 seeds or bis-chloroethyl-nitrosourea biodegradable wafers.[69–72] Theoretical advantages to such therapy include direct delivery of high concentrations of drug or radiation to the tumor bed and increasing penetration into surrounding tissue. Systemic chemotherapy may increase survival and quality of life as well. Temozolomide, for example, an oral cytotoxic alkylating agent that methylates guanine, has been beneficial in clinical trials to treat recurrent GBMs.[73] In a study of 225 patients, temozolomide delayed disease progression for a median of 12 weeks and led to 6-month survival of 60% compared to only 44% for those patients given procarbazine.[74] In treatment for recurrent anaplastic astrocytomas, it was well tolerated with a progression-free survival of 5.4 months and an overall median survival of 13.6 months in a group of 109 patients.[75]

Stereotactic radiosurgery (SRS) allows a radiation beam to be maximally and precisely focused on the tumor, with sparing of surrounding normal brain tissue. Since its inception by Lars Leskell in 1951, radiosurgery has evolved significantly. Under specific circumstances, it can be used to treat benign, malignant, and metastatic tumors of the brain, as well as vascular malformations. Several studies have recently suggested a use of this therapy for treating lesional and nonlesional epilepsy.[76–80] The role of radiosurgery and its use with other treatment modalities remains to be further clarified.

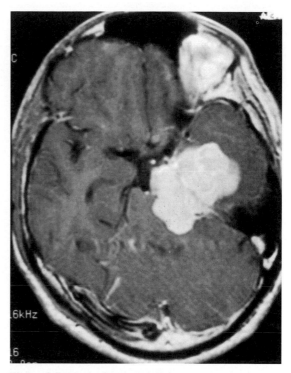

Figure 9-7. Meningioma. Gadolinium-enhanced axial T1-weighted image of a homogenously enhancing extra-axial lesion extending into the left-middle cranial fossa.

Seizure Prophylaxis

In patients with brain tumors who have not developed epilepsy, controversies exist as to the need for seizure prophylaxis. Overall, studies have found no significant difference in development of late seizures between patients receiving AED prophylaxis and those untreated.[81–84] This suggests that AEDs do not prevent epileptogenesis. Furthermore, potential AED side effects and the possibility that patients may remain seizure free without treatment may weigh against using prophylactic AED therapy. A recent practice parameter by the American Academy of Neurology recommends that AED prophylaxis is not effective in preventing seizures in patients with newly diagnosed brain tumors, and, consequently, it should not be used.[85]

Perioperative AED prophylaxis is less conclusive. Postoperative seizures for tumor and nontumor patients occur most often in the first week to first month postsurgery.[86,87] Although many patients with brain tumors are placed on AED prophylaxis in the perioperative period, no definite benefit has been demonstrated.[82,85] Patients with brain tumors who have a higher risk for development of epilepsy are often given prophylactic AEDs to avoid ictal complications in the perioperative period. However, there is no controlled evidence that perioperative AED prophylaxis is effective, and treatment is often physician dependent.[83,85,88] For patients whom physicians chose to treat perioperatively, tapering and discontinuation of AEDs after the first postoperative week is recommended.[85]

Brain Tumors and Epilepsy

Some predictive factors for seizure occurrence include tumor location in the frontal or parietal regions, evidence of cerebral hemispheric dysfunction, and incomplete tumor resection.[81,83] Tumor types that are more highly associated with the development of epilepsy include melanoma, hemorrhagic lesions, multiple metastases, slowly growing primary tumors, or tumors near the Rolandic fissure.[83,88] Epilepsy may be seen more commonly in patients with low-grade tumors, possibly owing to a longer period of time for seizures to develop, as these patients have a longer survival.[81] One retrospective study found a median interval of 8 weeks between diagnosis of a brain tumor and a first seizure.[83]

Antiepileptic Drug Considerations

Patients with cerebral neoplasms who develop epilepsy should be treated with AEDs, but there is no consensus in the literature of which AEDs are most effective. Most studies assessing the use of AEDs in this patient population involve the older AEDs, including phenytoin, phenobarbital, carbamazepine, and valproic acid.

Significant potential interactions exist between AEDs and tumor medication therapies. Enzyme-inducing AEDs, such as phenytoin, phenobarbital, and possibly carbamazepine, can induce steroid metabolism and thereby decrease the effectiveness of steroids.[89,90] One study suggests that phenytoin may have immunosuppressive potential.[91] Phenytoin and phenobarbital may decrease effective concentrations of antineoplastic drugs.[92]

Conversely, chemotherapy may alter AED blood concentrations. For example, increased phenobar-

bital and phenytoin levels and resultant clinical toxicity can occur during procarbazine therapy.[48] Subtherapeutic AED levels and an increased risk of seizures can develop in patients treated with other chemotherapeutic agents.[85,93,94] Decreased absorption of valproic acid and carbamazepine or increased metabolism of phenytoin during concurrent treatment with chemotherapeutic agents may account for these alterations.[85,93,94] Besides these alterations due to drug interactions or changes in absorption or metabolism, toxicity may occur when AEDs are adjusted in compensation, and a rebound occurs as chemotherapy cycles are concluded.

Adverse side effects are associated with AEDs and the treatment of brain tumors. Cutaneous skin reactions, including erythema multiforme and Stevens-Johnson syndrome, are more frequent in patients treated with phenytoin or carbamazepine who also receive cranial radiation therapy.[95,96] Patients with brain tumor taking phenobarbital may develop reflex sympathetic dystrophy, affecting the shoulder and hand particularly, usually contralateral to the tumor.[97] Carbamazepine rarely causes agranulocytosis and leukopenia, which could complicate use of concomitant chemotherapy agents. Valproic acid may cause hepatic toxicity, prolonged bleeding time, and thrombocytopenia.[48] Although such potential side effects have contributed to the argument against using prophylactic AEDs in seizure-free tumor patients, newer AEDs may offer similar or better efficacy with tolerance and fewer drug interactions. Studies of the newer agents, such as gabapentin, lamotrigine, tiagabine, levetiracetam, and zonisamide, in tumor patients are greatly needed.

Other AED considerations concern the route of administration, the rapidity of reaching therapeutic levels, and known idiosyncratic and dose-related AED side effects. Medications that are available in intravenous form, such as phenytoin, phenobarbital, and, recently, valproic acid, offer an alternative route of administration. These can also be loaded quickly with intravenous administration, allowing for rapid attainment of therapeutic levels, if clinically necessary.

Surgical Considerations

Surgery is indicated to decrease seizure activity, provide tissue for diagnosis and evaluate for further treatment, potentially decrease the need for AEDs, and possibly decrease the risk of sudden unexpected death.[98,99] Cranial irradiation may reduce seizures in patients with unresected, partially resected, or recurrent tumors.[47,100,101] However, acutely, cranial irradiation may worsen seizure control.

Initially, an MRI is most sensitive for identification of a structural lesion, and a routine electroencephalogram (EEG) may demonstrate correlating cerebral dysfunction and a potential epileptogenic zone. However, interictal EEG and ictal video-EEG may show mirror foci, false localization, secondary epileptogenesis, or even false lateralization with ictal onset in tumor patients.[102–104] In the majority of cases, seizures originate in the vicinity of the tumor. Focal background abnormalities with polymorphic slow wave frequencies may be seen in only 32–44% of patients.[47] Noninvasive video-EEG monitoring may identify ictal onset; however, long-term invasive video-EEG recording with extraoperative epidural, subdural, or depth electrodes may be needed to define an epileptogenic zone using ictal data at seizure onset.[47,105] The data are usually the single most reliable way of defining an epileptogenic focus via EEG.[106]

Neuropsychological testing can assess functional abilities and potential regions of dysfunction that may coincide with the location of a tumor. Language lateralization and assessment of memory can be performed with intracarotid amobarbital injection (Wada test).[107] This consists of the testing of unilateral hemispheric function after amobarbital injection into either internal carotid artery and allowing for comparison of language and memory function of each hemisphere independently. This may be crucial to know whether resection is performed near language areas. fMRI is being studied as a possible noninvasive Wada test. SPECT and PET scans can confirm a functional relationship between the radiologic lesion and epileptogenic area.

Electrocorticography (ECog) may be performed to more precisely identify dysfunctional regions as well as an epileptogenic zone. This involves recording of electrical activity through epidural, subdural, or depth electrodes on the cortex. Cortical mapping with electrical stimulation of the cortex and cortical somatosensory evoked potentials may be required to more pre-cisely determine areas of eloquent cortex, such as motor and language regions, if the ictal focus lateralizes to this region, or to guide resection of tumors involving eloquent cortex.[108,109]

The most common surgical intervention for intractable complex partial seizures associated with a temporal lobe mass is the temporal lobectomy, but techniques vary widely between institutions.[11] Some centers advocate the removal of the tumor alone, whereas others stress the importance of resecting the ictal focus, if separate from tumor pathology.[23,32,40,45,110–113] Epilepsy surgery, rather than tumor resection, may be more likely considered in patients with longer duration of epilepsy. Gross total resections are approached with standard craniotomy techniques or via computer-assisted stereotactic cranial procedures. When removal of only the tumor is advocated, gross total resection has been reported as providing greater seizure control than partial resection, with an overall range of 80–88% of patients with temporal or extratemporal lesions achieving complete relief from seizures postoperatively.[32,112–116] Conversely, from the time of Penfield and Jasper, authors have suggested that, in addition to tumor resection, epileptogenic cortical resection may be necessary to obtain seizure control, because it is the cortex adjacent to the tumor margins that is most likely responsible for epileptogenesis.[36,45,110,111,117,118] Seizure relief after resection for the tumor and the epileptogenic zone has been reported as ranging from 80% to 95% for temporal and extratemporal lesions. Surgical strategies are varied and include resection of epileptogenic cortex and mesial temporal structures, with and without the aid of extraoperative ECog.

Controversy surrounds the use of ECog data in modifying the extent of surgical resection. ECog may demonstrate slow wave activity over the tumor, whereas epileptiform activity may be seen from normal-appearing cortex. There is no clear correlation between presence of spikes on ECog over the tumor and seizure outcome postoperatively.[119] New postresection discharges are considered to be activation phenomena, unless these discharges are sustained, independent, or clearly epileptiform[120,121]; however, residual spikes do not necessarily correlate with poor seizure control

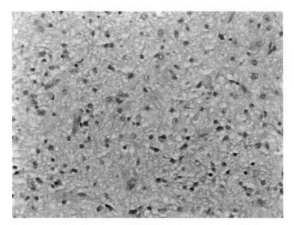

Figure 9-8. Low-grade astrocytoma. 200×. Hematoxylin-eosin stain of mildly atypical neoplastic glial cells with a fibrillar and myxoid background.

postoperatively. Only one prospective study of ECog during tumor surgery was published. Tumor resection was performed and not altered by pre- or postresection ECog findings. There was an equal frequency of spike discharges on pre- and postresection ECog between patients with postoperative seizure freedom and patients with persistent seizures.[119] ECog may not be necessary during tumor resection in patients with well-controlled preoperative seizures.[45] Further controlled prospective analyses of ECog in tumor surgery are needed.

Regardless of surgical approach, surgery provides tissue for accurate diagnosis and evaluation for possible adjuvant therapy. Additionally, early intervention may permit the developing brain of the young child to recover quickly and maximize plasticity. Postoperative follow-up, which includes a neuropsychologic assessment, EEG, and MRI, usually occurs at 1 and 6 months.

Primary Brain Tumors

Gliomas

Astrocytoma

The astrocytoma is the most common intra-axial brain tumor and is classified on a four-grade scale (Figure 9-8).[122,123] Grades I and II are considered low-grade gliomas (LGGs), grade III is anaplastic,

and grade IV is glioblastoma multiforme. Grades III and IV are considered high-grade gliomas (HGGs). Histologically, LGG diagnosis is based on minimal hypercellularity and pleomorphism, with no vascular proliferation or necrosis. These characteristics escalate to excessive pleomorphism, increased mitotic activity, necrosis, pseudopalisading, and endothelial proliferation in GBMs. Generally, most gliomas stain positively for glial fibrillary acidic protein (GFAP). In adults, LGGs have been more frequently associated with seizure disorder than GBM; however, both are epileptogenic. The majority of cases present between the ages of 21 and 40 years; however, LGGs are also a significant cause of epilepsy in children. Seizures are the most common presentation of LGG, and the LGG is the most common neoplasm responsible for tumor-related intractable epilepsy.[21] In Fried's study of 65 patients with limbic and neocortical gliomas, 63% of LGGs were temporal, 18% occipital, and 11% frontal.[124] Others have noted different distributions (Table 9-4). These tumors show indolent behavior with an average 15-year history of seizures, and, after a 17-year follow-up, only one patient died from the tumor. Gross total resection gains excellent seizure control, and subtotal resection is the most important factor in the failure to control seizures and tumor recurrence.[26,114]

Cortical astrocytomas may arise from different cell lineages rather than white matter astrocytomas. Piepmeier et al. showed that type I cortical astrocytes had different expression of GFAP and gangliosides when compared to type II fibrillary astrocytomas.[125] This may affect the differing prognosis of astrocytoma subtypes.

GBMs are less likely to cause seizures, primarily affect white matter and deeper structures, and have greater rapidity of growth associated with destruction of neural elements. In one study, only two of 24 patients became seizure free after resection.[21] Gross total resection of GBMs does not generally control seizures, and surgery alone may be inadequate treatment of the tumor without adjuvant radiation and chemotherapy. An exception may be the occurrence of HGGs in children. Although histologically identical, HGGs in the pediatric population tend to have a better prognosis, and survival seems to be based on completeness of resection. In one study of 31 children, those who received a gross total resection had a progression-free survival of 7 years, whereas

Table 9-4. Anatomic Distribution of Low-Grade Gliomas

	Anatomic Location*			
	Frontal	**Temporal**	**Parietal**	**Occipital**
Low-grade glioma	83	119	31	14

*Does not include locations that span two lobes (i.e., frontoparietal).
Source: Adapted from W Penfield, TC Erickson, I Tarlov. Relation of intracranial tumors and symptomatic epilepsy. Arch Neurol Psychiatry 1940;44:300–315; MS Berger, JR Geyer, GE Keles, GE Ojemann. Seizure outcome in children with hemispheric tumors and associated intractable epilepsy: the role of tumor removal combined with seizure foci resection. Pediatr Neurosurg 1991;17:185–191; MS Berger, S Ghatan, MM Haglund, et al. Low grade gliomas associated with intractable epilepsy: seizure outcome utilizing electrocorticography during tumor resection. J Neurosurg 1993;79:62–69; J Hirsch, C Sainte Rose, A Pierre-Kahn, et al. Benign astrocytic and oligodendrocytic tumors of the cerebral hemispheres in children. J Neurosurg 1989;70:568–572; R Soffietti, A Chio, A Giordana, et al. Prognostic factors in well-differentiated cerebral astrocytomas in the adult. Neurosurgery 1989;24:686–692; I Fried, JH Kim, DD Spencer, et al. Limbic and neocortical gliomas associated with intractable seizures: A distinct clinicopathological group. Neurosurgery 1994;34:815–824.

those who only had a biopsy or subtotal resections had a median progression-free survival of 5.0 and 11.5 months, respectively.[126] Also, patients who presented with long-standing symptoms, seizures, and tumors in the cerebral hemispheres had longer survival and better prognosis.

HGGs tend to recur. Treatment of recurrences depends on the patient's clinical status and the anatomic accessibility of the lesion. It is usually addressed with a second resection if the area is surgically accessible and adjuvant whole-brain radiation, SRS, or chemotherapy. A second resection can increase survival by an average of 36 weeks, with 28% of patients showing an improvement in the Karnofsky Performance Scale.[127] Adjuvant SRS can also improve survival.[128] When compared to brachytherapy, median survival data are similar, but SRS offers the advantage of an outpatient procedure versus the need for a 1-week hospital stay for interstitial brachytherapy.[129]

Supratentorial glial tumors in children tend to be grade I or II. Hirsch et al. reported that epilepsy was the presenting symptom in 76% of children who had astrocytomas or oligodendrocytic tumors.[113] After tumor resection alone, there was no tumor recurrence in 82% of patients, and 81% of patients were seizure free. Alternatively, Berger et al. reported 93% total seizure relief in children who underwent tumor and epileptic focus resection via ECog.[40] In a separate study comparing postoperative seizure outcome in children versus adults, all 13 pediatric patients

became seizure free, 11 of whom were able to discontinue AEDs, compared to the adult group in which 47% required AEDs to maintain seizure freedom.[45] LGG in a child has a 10-year survival of 87%.[130] In children, gross total resection of LGGs is the treatment of choice, and adjuvant radiation and chemotherapy are reserved for recurrence. For children, adjuvant whole-brain radiation therapy is not efficacious in preventing recurrence, and it is generally not prescribed because of the risk of cognitive deterioration.[130]

SRS can surgically treat incurable gliomas in children.[78] In a study by Grabb et al., 25 children who underwent surgical resection or biopsy subsequently had SRS for treatment of tumors. Eleven of 13 children with benign gliomas showed tumor control after SRS, and all 13 were alive at a median follow-up of 21 months. In the group of children with malignant tumors, seven patients died after a median survival of 6 months, and only 3 of 12 showed tumor control after SRS. This technique, although not without complications, is a promising therapy that limits radiation exposure to a developing brain.

Oligodendroglioma

Oligodendrogliomas present with seizures in 75–90% of cases.[24,25] These tumors comprise 4–5% of central nervous system neoplasms, arise in the cortical white matter, and tend to have slow growth

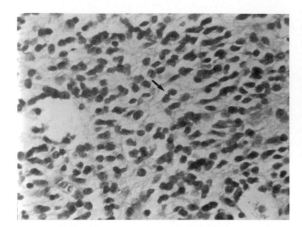

Figure 9-9. Oligodendroglioma. 200×. Microscopic section of uniform glial cells with characteristic "fried egg" appearance (*arrow*).

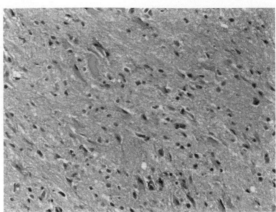

Figure 9-10. Ganglioglioma. 200×. Photomicrograph of an admixture of mildly atypical neoplastic glial cells and neurons.

kinetics.[131] Oligodendroglial tumors are closely related to the fibrillary astrocytic tumors and are generally graded as oligodendroglioma or anaplastic oligodendrogliomas if they have a high cell density, mitotic rate, and necrosis.[132] Histologically, cells have the small rounded nuclei of oligodendrocytes with variable densities in cell population and pleomorphism, display a characteristic "fried egg" appearance, and, infrequently, show necrosis (Figure 9-9). In Olson's study of 106 patients, the median age at presentation was 37 years. The overall median time to progression was 5 years, with a median survival of 17 years. Seizure patterns may be nonspecific, with one-third of patients presenting with generalized, one-third with partial, and one-third with mixed seizure types.[24] Younger patients often present with seizures and therefore are diagnosed earlier than adults who may present with neurologic symptomatology other than seizures. Presentation at a young age, seizures, and a Karnofsky Performance Status of greater than 70 are significant positive prognostic indicators for survival in low-grade tumors.[24,133,134] Those children who present with anaplastic oligodendroglioma have a significantly decreased survival time—17 months as compared to 72 months in children with low-grade neoplasms.[135] Postoperative malignant progression of a low-grade oligodendroglioma can occur but generally requires long intervals of time.[136] Surgical resection is the gold standard of treatment. A sei-

zure-free success rate between 50% and 70% was reported postoperatively by Whittle.[24] Adjuvant radiation therapy does not appear to increase survival and increases morbidity in up to 33% of patients.[25,137] Postoperative chemotherapy with procarbazine, lomustine, and vincristine for low-grade oligodendrogliomas may afford positive results in up to 62% of patients.[138] Vincristine is also effective against high-grade tumors.[139]

Ganglioglioma

In 1930, Courville defined the term *ganglioglioma* as tumors consisting of astrocytic neuronal components with rare mitotic figures (Figure 9-10).[140] Approximately 50% show focal areas of calcification. Incidence is between 0.3% and 8.0% and affects mostly children, with a mean age at presentation of 9.5 years.[30,141,142] The majority is located supratentorially, often in the temporal lobes.[143] In one study of 137 patients, 65% of gangliomas were located in the frontal, temporal, or frontotemporal regions, whereas only 8% were seen in the midline or deep structures.[141] Generally, they are benign growths that occur over a long clinical course and present with no specific radiologic characteristics, although some calcify.[144] In a study by Otsubo et al., 59% of patients presented with seizures; of those, 64% had complex partial seizures, 32% had secondarily generalized seizures, and 4% presented with generalized seizures. Optimal treatment includes gross total resection. Adjuvant chemotherapy or radiation therapy is generally not indicated.[38] Postoperative 5-year survival of hemispheric gangliogliomas has been reported as 93%, although seizure relief statistics were lower than expected.[145] Morris et al. reported freedom from seizures in 79% (30 of 38) of patients at 6 months, and 72% at 1 year postoperatively.[137] Favorable prognostic factors included younger patient age, benign histopathology, stable clinical status at admission, decreased duration of seizure disorder, and lack of generalized features of seizures.[137,141] Celli et al. reported that those patients who presented with neurologic deficits or symptoms of increased intracranial pressure fared better postoperatively if given adjuvant radiation, with a 5-year survival of 53% versus 11% for those who did not receive radiation.

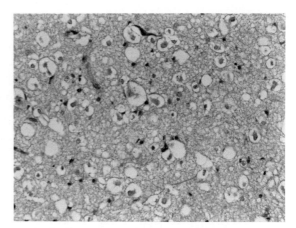

Figure 9-11. Dysembryoplastic neuroepithelial tumor. 200×. Intracortical nodule of variably sized oligodendroglial-like cells and disordered neurons demonstrating microcyst formation.

Dysembryoplastic Neuroepithelial Tumors

In 1988, Daumas-Duport described a surgically curable tumor highly associated with intractable partial epilepsy and normal neurologic examination. The majority of tumors were located in the temporal and frontal cortex, 62% and 31%, respectively. Case reports have described DNETs to occur in multifocal areas, including the caudate nuclei, midbrain, and diencephalon.[29,146,147] Histologically, DNETs are composed of neurons, astrocytes, and oligodendrocytes (Figure 9-11). Immunohistochemistry for GFAP, S-100 protein, neuronal markers, synaptophysin, neurofilament (RT97), and neuron-specific enolase establish the presence of astrocytic and neuronal components, although GFAP reactivity is negative for an oligodendrocytic component.[148,149] Although questions remain regarding the origin of this tumor, they may have a germinal origin.[29,146,147] At the time of resection, patients' ages ranged from 3 to 30 years, and patients presented with a longstanding history of symptoms, ranging from 7 to 11 years. Patients should be treated with gross total resection and considered cured after surgery.[29,149,150] In the series by Daumas-Duport, 30 of 39 patients were seizure free postoperatively, three had rare seizures, and four had significant reductions in seizures. Radiation and chemotherapy have not demonstrated a clear benefit, and withholding adjuvant therapy for this type of tumor prevents future deleterious side effects. Rarely, these tumors, as well as gangliogliomas, may be associated with a rare postoperative disorder, with schizophreniform features of paranoia, depression, and psychosis. This psychosis does not seem to accompany other tumor types resected for intractable epilepsy.[151,152]

Meningiomas

In 1614, Felix Paster described the tumor later named by Harvey Cushing as a *meningioma*.[153] Meningiomas account for 14% to 19% of all primary intracranial neoplasms, with a peak incidence around 45 years of age and a female preponderance.[28,154,155] Predisposing factors include previous radiation, type II neurofibromatosis, and monosomy or deletions of chromosome 22, or both.[156] They arise from the arachnoid cap cells and form an encapsulated mass that is usually slow growing, eventually creating mass effect on the brain. Histologically, they classically manifest a whorled cellular pattern, psammoma bodies with differing degrees of fibrous connective tissue, blood vessels, and, if malignant, mitotic activity and invasion of cortex. They most commonly arise on the brain convexity or in a parasagittal location

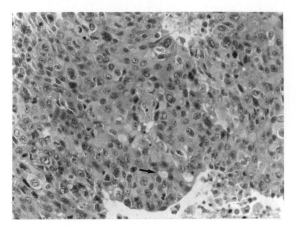

Figure 9-12. Metastatic lung adenocarcinoma. 200×. Photomicrograph of sheets of highly pleomorphic malignant cells with epithelial characteristics. Note focal glandular formation (*arrow*).

(36%), with 50% located between the coronal and lambdoid sutures and 20% anterior to the coronal suture.[157] Generally, these tumors are classified on a four-grade system. Grade I tumors are benign, grade II tumors are atypical, grade III tumors are anaplastic, and grade IV tumors are sarcomatous. The great majority of meningiomas (94%) are benign.[158] Predicting recurrence is related to tumor grade and degree of resection. Benign tumors recur in 3% at 5 years, compared to 78% recurrence at 5 years for anaplastic tumors.[159] Gross total resection has a reported recurrence rate of 7% at 5 years, compared to 37% if the resection is partial.[160]

Although headaches are a common symptom, one study found seizures to occur in 64.7% of patients.[28] Sixty-eight percent of meningiomas were associated with seizures in Penfield's series. Few studies focus on seizure outcomes after resections of meningiomas. Flyger et al. studied the neogenesis of seizure disorders postresection.[161] They observed that 41.1% of patients with no seizure disorder preoperatively developed epilepsy postoperatively. Similarly, Foy et al. reported a 22% risk of postoperative seizures after meningioma resection.[162] Parietal tumors were the most epileptogenic, followed by frontal and occipital tumors. Complete surgical resection should be the goal for accessible tumors. A 4.2-fold relative excess risk of death has been reported with partial resection compared to gross total resection.[163] Adjuvant radiation treatment, although controversial, has been used with some

success. In one study that compared nonradiated subtotal resections to radiated subtotal resections, time to recurrence was 66 versus 125 months, respectively.[164] SRS is now used to treat meningiomas that are nonoperable, small, recurrent, or a result of a subtotal resection. The goal is to prevent further tumor growth and preserve normal neurologic function. This is a safe and effective primary or adjuvant therapeutic strategy.[165–168] SRS is not indicated for large tumors (>3 cm) or those less than 5 mm from the optic nerve or chiasm.

Metastatic Brain Tumors

Metastatic disease to the brain occurs in 15–28% of all cancer patients.[169,170] Metastases occur in approximately 40% of patients, increase in frequency with prolonged survival from the primary disease, and represent a poor prognostic factor. Generally, brain metastases occur in supratentorial watershed areas, with the exception of gastrointestinal and genitourinary carcinomas that tend to metastasize to the posterior fossa.[171] Lung and breast carcinomas are the most common primary tumors that spread to the brain (Figure 9-12).[171,172] Other primary tumors that progress to involve the central nervous system include gastrointestinal cancers, pelvic cancers, melanoma, and renal cell carcinomas. Brain metastasis may be discovered serendipitously in an asymptomatic patient, or it may present as signs and symptoms of anatomic mass effect, intracranial hemorrhage, or seizures.[154] Although headaches are the most common presenting symptom, epilepsy is a common presentation of metastasis, observed in 15–25% of patients.[27] In one study, 17% of patients with brain tumors and epilepsy had metastatic disease after further evaluation, and most lesions were located in the centroparietal cortex.[173]

A patient presenting with a brain metastasis has a 1-month expected survival with no treatment, approximately 2 months with corticosteroids, and 3–6 months with whole-brain radiation.[174–177] Patchell and colleagues found that when resection and radiation therapy were compared to brain biopsy and radiation, the latter group had a better survival, 40 weeks versus 15 weeks. In addition, both local and distant recurrence rates decreased. The likelihood of death from neurologic causes also decreased with adjuvant radiation. However, this therapy does not clearly increase the duration of functional independence.[178]

Long-term survival greater than 10 years has been reported in a small subset of patients with metastatic non–small cell lung carcinoma who were treated with surgical resection and radiation. SRS is another treatment modality that has gained popularity in recent years. Patients who respond best to this treatment are those with controlled systemic disease, who experience nonmelanoma primary histology. Such patients have a median survival of 39 weeks.[79]

Multiple metastases occur in 66% of patients, with some benefiting from radiation therapy; however, most are treated medically with corticosteroids and AEDs. The overall prognosis for this subset of patients is poor, ranging from 2 to 6 months.

Patients with metastatic brain disease and epilepsy are a treatment challenge. Selection of treatment must take into account not only seizures and other neurologic dysfunction, but also the systemic disease and the potential morbidities and mortality associated with treatment.

Postoperative Complications and Future Considerations

The explanation of risks and potential complications of surgery should be part of any neurosurgical preoperative consultation. Included in this discussion should be the risk of surgical mortality, and permanent or temporary language and motor or psychologic deficits. In patients with tumor-associated epilepsy, the possibility of no improvement or worsening in seizure activity must be discussed. Other general postoperative risks of wound infection, hemorrhage, hydrocephalus, meningitis, deep venous thrombosis, pulmonary embolus, or pneumonia, or a combination of these, must also be discussed. Although specific studies on morbidity and mortality of tumor-associated epilepsy surgery have not been previously reviewed, studies have reported morbidity and mortality of epilepsy surgery based on the type of surgical procedure.[179–181] The anterior temporal lobectomy carries a 0.0–0.7% mortality, whereas extratemporal lobectomies have 0–9% mortality. Permanent hemiparesis has been reported in between 1% and 2% of cases.

In a series of 429 patients, wound infection was the most common surgical complication, occurring in 3.5% of cases. Neurologic morbidity was reported in 5.4%, with 3.03% occurring transiently and 2.33% occurring permanently.[181] These risks must be weighed against the benefits of better quality of life with relief of seizures, which is approximately 60–80% and even better, if one includes another more than 10% of patients who have a significant improvement (>90% relief) in seizure activity.

The future of epilepsy surgery for tumors depends largely on the development and practical applications of current research trends. In the operating room, the use of robotics and real-time MRI continues to decrease mortality and morbidity. Further research of invasive EEG monitoring and ECog should clarify its use for guiding surgical resection and enhancing postoperative seizure freedom. The inception of intraoperative image-guided neurosurgery has further optimized the ability to achieve the greatest area of resection and assess for potential complications.[182,183] Such technology could be applied to fMRI so that eloquent cortex can be more precisely considered intraoperatively. As surgery does not generally lead to a cure of tumor pathology, a cure for primary brain tumors and metastatic disease needs to be developed outside the operating room. Current trends include the use of boronated compounds, which would, ideally, spare normal cells, radioactive compounds attached to "cancer-seeking" molecules, gene therapy, antiangiogenesis therapy, and immunotherapy.[184] Although at this time such technology has not made a definitive impact on treatment, one must only consider what Drs. Jackson and Penfield would have thought about the medical and surgical progress that has occurred since the early twentieth century.

References

1. Aretaeus; Adams F, trans-ed. The Extant Works of Arataeus the Cappodocian. London: Printed for the Sydenham Society, 1856.
2. Galen; Daremberg C, trans. Oeuvres Anatomiques, Physiologiques, et Madicales de Galien. Paris: J. B. Bailliere, 1854.
3. Kocher T. Chirurgische beitrage zur phisiologie des gehirns und ruckenmarks. Deutsche Zeitschr F Chir 1893;35:433–494, 36:1–93.
4. Adams F. The genuine works of Hippocrates. London: Printed for the Sydenham Society, 1849.
5. Jackson JH. Selected writings of John Hughlings Jackson. London: Hodder and Stoughton Ltd, 1931.
6. Horwitz H. Library: historical perspective. Neurosurgery 1999;44:906–910.
7. Jackson JH. Localized convulsions from tumor of the brain. Brain 1882;5:364–374.

8. Horsley V. Brain surgery. BMJ 1886;2:670–675.

9. Horwitz H. Library: historical perspective. Neurosurgery 1995;36:428–432.

10. Bennett A, Godlee SR. Excision of a tumor from the brain. Lancet 1884;2:1090–1091.

11. Adelson PD. The surgical management of epilepsy in children. Contemp Neurosurg 1995;17(23):1–8.

12. Yeh HS, Kashiwagi S, Tew J, Berger T. Surgical management of epilepsy associated with cerebral arteriovenous malformations. J Neurosurg 1990;72:216–223.

13. Hauser W, Annegers J, Kurland L. Prevalence of epilepsy in Rochester, Minnesota: 1940–1980. Epilepsia 1991;32:429–445.

14. Luhdorf K, Jensen LK, Plesner AM. Etiology of seizures in the elderly. Epilepsia 1986;27:458–463.

15. Paeschel SM, Louis S, McKnight P. Seizure disorders in Down's syndrome. Arch Neurol 1991;48:318–320.

16. Brodie M, Shorvon SD, Canger R. Commission on European affairs: appropriate standards of epilepsy care across Europe. Epilepsia 1997;38:1245–1250.

17. Ketz E. Brain Tumours and Epilepsy. In P Vinken, G Bruyn (eds), Handbook of Clinical Neurology. Amsterdam: North Holland Publishing, 1974;254–269.

18. Black P. Brain tumors (First of two parts). N Engl J Med 1991;324:1471–1476.

19. Rasmussen T, Blundell J. Epilepsy and brain tumour. Clin Neurosurg 1959;7:138–158.

20. Penfield W, Erickson TC, Tarlov I. Relation of intracranial tumors and symptomatic epilepsy. Arch Neurol Psychiatry 1940;44:300–315.

21. Le Blanc FE, Rasmussen T. Cerebral Seizures and Brain Tumors. Amsterdam, Netherlands: North Holland Publishing, 1974.

22. Strobos R, Alexander E, Masland R. Brain tumor presenting as convulsive disorder. Diseases of the nervous system. 1958;19:518–522.

23. Cascino G. Epilepsy and brain tumors: implications for treatment. Epilepsia 1990;3:S37–S44.

24. Whittle I, Beaumaont A. Seizures in patients with supratentorial oligodendroglial tumors. Clinicopathological features and management considerations. Acta Neurochir 1995;135:19–24.

25. Olson J, Reidel EM, DeAngelis LM. Long-term outcome of low-grade oligodendroglioma and mixed glioma. Neurology 2000;54:1442–1448.

26. Morris H, Estes ML, Gilmore R, et al. Chronic intractable epilepsy as the only symptom of primary brain tumor. Epilepsia 1993;34:1038–1043.

27. Vecht CJ. Clinical management of brain metastasis. J Neurol 1998;245:127–131.

28. Howng SL, Kwan AL. Intracranial meningioma. Gaoxiong Yi Xue Ke Xue Za Zhi 1992;8:312–319.

29. Daumas-Duport C, Scheithauer B, Chodkiewicz J, et al. Dysembryoplastic neuroepithelial tumor: a surgically curable tumor of young patients with intractable partial seizures. Neurosurgery 1988;23:545–556.

30. Otsubo H, Hoffman H, Humphreys R, et al. Detection and management of gangliogliomas in children. Surg Neurol 1992;38:371–378.

31. Ventureyra E. Surgery for childhood epilepsy and epileptic syndromes. Contemp Neurosurg 1997;19:1–6.

32. Blume W, Girvin J, Kaufmann J. Childhood brain tumors presenting as chronic uncontrolled focal seizure disorders. Ann Neurol 1982;12:538–541.

33. Sjors K, Blennow G, Lantz G. Seizures as the presenting symptom of brain tumors in children. Acta Paediatr 1993;82:66–70.

34. Williams B, Abbott K, Manson J. Cerebral tumors in children presenting with epilepsy. J Child Neurol 1992;7:291–294.

35. Suarez J, Sfaello Z, Guerrero A, et al. Epilepsy and brain tumors in infants and adolescents. Childs Nerv Syst 1986;2:169–174.

36. Zentner J, Wolf HK, Ostertun B, et al. Surgical treatment of neoplasms associated with medically intractable epilepsy. Neurosurgery 1997;41:378–387.

37. Lee TK, Nakasu Y, Jeffree MA, et al. Indolent glioma: a cause of epilepsy. Arch Dis Child 1989;64:1666–1671.

38. Ventureyra E, Herder S, Mallya B. Temporal lobe gangliogliomas in children. Childs Nerv Syst 1986;2:63–66.

39. Haglund MM, Berger MS, Kunkel DD, et al. Changes in gamma-aminobutyric acid and somatostatin in epileptic cortex associated with low grade glioma. J Neurosurg 1992;77:209–216.

40. Berger MS, Geyer JR, Keles GE, Ojemann GA. Seizure outcome in children with hemispheric tumors and associated intractable epilepsy: the role of tumor removal combined with seizure foci resection. Pediatr Neurosurg 1991;17:185–191.

41. Petroff O, Rothman DL, Behar KL, Mattson RH. Low brain GABA levels associated with poor seizure control. Ann Neurol 1996;40:908–911.

42. Freid I, Kim JH, Spencer DD. Hippocampal pathology in patients with intractable seizures and temporal lobe masses. J Neurosurg 1992;76:735–740.

43. Towle VL, Carder RK, Khorasani L, Lindberg D. Electrocorticographic coherence patterns. J Clin Neurophysiol 1999;16:528–547.

44. Boon P, Williamson P, Fried I, et al. Intracranial, intraaxial, space-occupying lesions in patients with intractable partial seizures: an anatomoclinical, neuropsychological, and surgical correlation. Epilepsia 1991;32:467–476.

45. Berger MS, Ghatan S, Haglund MM, et al. Low grade gliomas associated with intractable epilepsy: seizure outcome utilizing electrocorticography during tumor resection. J Neurosurg 1993;79:62–69.

46. Proposal for revised classification of epilepsy and epileptic syndromes. Commission on Classification and Terminology of the International League against Epilepsy. Epilepsia 1989;30:389–399.

47. Morris H, Estes M. Brain Tumors in Chronic Epilepsy. In E Wyllie (ed), The Treatment of Epilepsy: Princi-

ples and Practice (2nd ed). Baltimore: Williams & Wilkins, 1996;637–639.

48. Weinstock A, Cohen BH. Seizures in Patients with Brain Tumors and Cancer. Philadelphia: Churchill Livingstone, 2000.

49. Jack CR. Magnetic resonance imaging in epilepsy. Mayo Clin Proc 1996;71:695–711.

50. Henry TR. Neuroimaging in epilepsy. Contemp Neurosurg 1996;18(2):1–8.

51. Bradley WG, Shey RB. MR imaging evaluation of seizures. Radiology 2000;214:651–656.

52. Sperling M. Neuroimaging in epilepsy: recent developments in MR imaging, positron emission tomography, and single-photon emission tomography. Neurol Clin 1993;11:883–903.

53. Lee C, Duncan VW, Young AB. Magnetic resonance features of the enigmatic oligodendroglioma. Invest Radiol 1998;33:222–231.

54. Kuroiwa T, Kishiawa T, Kato A, et al. Dysembryoplastic neuroepithelial tumors: MR findings. J Comput Assist Tomogr 1994;18:352–356.

55. Boyko O. Adult Brain Tumors. In DD Stark, WG Bradley Jr, (ed), Magnetic Resonance Imaging (3rd ed). St. Louis: Mosby, 1999.

56. Fujii K, Fujita N, Hirabuki N, et al. Neuromas and meningiomas: evaluation of early enhancement with dynamic MR imaging. AJNR Am J Neuroradiol 1992;13:1215–1220.

57. Kuzniecky R, de la Sayette V, Ethier R, et al. Magnetic resonance imaging in temporal lobe epilepsy: pathological correlations. Ann Neurol 1987;22:341–347.

58. Sperling MR, Wilson G, Engel J Jr, et al. Magnetic resonance imaging in intractable partial epilepsy: correlative studies. Ann Neurol 1986;20:57–62.

59. Theodore WH, Dorwart R, Holmes M, et al. Neuroimaging in refractory partial seizures: comparison of PET, CT, MRI. Neurology 1986;36:750–759.

60. Henry TR, Sutherling WW, Engel J Jr, et al. Interictal cerebral metabolism in partial epilepsies of neocortical origin. Epilepsy Res 1991;10:174–182.

61. DeWitte O, Levivier M, Violon P, et al. Prognostic value of positron emission tomography with [^{18}F] fluoro-2-deoxy-d-glucose in the low-grade glioma. Neurosurgery 1996;39:470–477.

62. Derlon JM, Petit-Taboue MC, Chapon F, et al. The in vivo metabolic pattern of low-grade brain glioma: a positron emission tomographic study using ^{18}F-fluorodeoxyglucose and ^{11}C$_1$-methylmethionine. Neurosurgery 1997;40:276–288.

63. Duncan R, Patterson J, Roberts R, et al. Ictal/post-ictal SPECT in the presurgical localization of complex partial seizures. J Neurol Neurosurg Psychiatry 1993;56:141–148.

64. O'Brien TJ, So EL, Mullan MB, et al. Subtraction SPECT co-registered to MRI improves postictal SPECT localization of seizure foci. Neurology 1999;52:137–146.

65. Lazareff JA, Bockhorst HJ, Curran J, et al. Pediatric low-grade gliomas: prognosis with proton magnetic resonance spectroscopic imaging. Neurosurgery 1998;43:809–818.

66. Graves EE, Nelson SJ, Vigneron DB, et al. A preliminary study of the prognostic value of proton magnetic resonance spectroscopic imaging in gamma knife radiosurgery of recurrent malignant gliomas. Neurosurgery 2000;46:319–328.

67. Nimsky C, Ganslandt O, Kober H, et al. Integration of functional magnetic resonance imaging supported by magnetoencephalography in functional neuronavigation. Neurosurgery 1999;44:1249–1256.

68. Atlas SW, Howard RS, Maldjian J, et al. Functional magnetic resonance imaging of regional brain activity in patients with intracerebral gliomas: findings implications and clinical management. Neurosurgery 1996;38:329–338.

69. Patel S, Breneman JC, Warnick RE, et al. Permanent iodine-125 interstitial implants for the treatment of recurrent glioblastoma multiforme. Neurosurgery 2000;46:1123–1130.

70. Valtonen S, Timonen U, Toivanen P, et al. Interstitial chemotherapy with carmustine-loaded polymers for high-grade glioma: a randomized double-blind study. Neurosurgery 1997;41:44–49.

71. Wang CC, Li J, Lee T. The delivery of BCNU to brain tumors. J Control Release 1999;61:21–41.

72. Westphal M, Daumas-Duport C, Thoron L, et al. Gliadel (polifeprosan 20 with carmustine 3.85% implant): a multinational phase III randomized double-blind trial in newly diagnosed malignant glioma. Proc Ann Meet Am Soc Clin Oncol 1999;18:A594.

73. Osoba D, Brada M, Yung WK, Prados M. Health-related quality of life in patients treated with temozolomide versus procarbazine for recurrent glioblastoma multiforme. J Clin Oncol 2000;18:1481–1491.

74. Yung WK, Albright RE, Olson J, et al. A phase II study of temozolomide vs. procarbazine in patients with glioblastoma multiforme at first relapse. Br J Cancer 2000;83:588–593.

75. Prados M, Yung A, Chang S, et al. A phase II trial of Temodal (temozolamide) in patients with anaplastic astrocytoma at first relapse. Proc Ann Meet Am Soc Clin Oncol 1999;18:A533.

76. Niranjan A, Lunsford LD. Radiosurgery: where we were, are, and may be in the third millennium. Neurosurgery 2000;46:531–543.

77. Consensus statement on stereotactic radiosurgery quality improvement. Neurosurgery 1994;34:193–199.

78. Grabb PA, Lunsford LD, Albright AL, et al. Stereotactic radiosurgery for glial neoplasms of childhood. Neurosurgery 1996;38:696–702.

79. Chen JC, Petrovich Z, O'Day S, et al. Stereotactic radiosurgery in the treatment of metastatic disease of the brain. Neurosurgery 2000;47:268–281.

80. Rutigliano MJ, Lunsford LD, Kondziolka D, et al. The cost effectiveness of stereotactic radiosurgery versus sur-

gical resection in the treatment of solitary metastatic brain tumors. Neurosurgery 1995;37:445–455.

81. Boarini D, Beck D, VanGilder J. Postoperative prophylactic anticonvulsant therapy in cerebral gliomas. Neurosurgery 1985;16:290–292.

82. Foy P, Chadwick D, Rajgopalan N, et al. Do prophylactic anticonvulsant drugs alter the pattern of seizures after craniotomy? J Neurol Neurosurg Psychiatry 1992;55:753–757.

83. Cohen N, Strauss G, Lew R, et al. Should prophylactic anticonvulsants be administered to patients with newly diagnosed cerebral metastases? A retrospective analysis. J Clin Oncol 1988;6:1621–1624.

84. Mahaley M, Dudka L. The role of anticonvulsant medications in the management of patients with anaplastic gliomas. Surg Neurol 1981;16:399–401.

85. Glantz MJ, Cole BF, Forsyth PA, et al. Practice parameter: Anticonvulsant prophylaxis in patient with newly diagnosed brain tumors. Neurology 2000;54:1886–1893.

86. North J. Anticonvulsant prophylaxis in neurosurgery. Br J Neurosurg 1989;3:425–428.

87. North J, Hanieh A, Challen R, et al. Postoperative epilepsy: a double-blind trial of phenytoin after craniotomy. Lancet 1980;1:384–386.

88. Posner J. Neurologic Complications of Cancer. Philadelphia: FA Davis Co, 1995.

89. Wong DD, Longenecker RG, Liepman MI, et al. Phenytoin-dexamethasone: a possible drug-drug interaction. JAMA 1985;254:2062–2063.

90. Chalk J, Ridgeway K, Brophy T, et al. Phenytoin impairs the bioavailability of dexamethasone in neurological and neurosurgical patients. J Neurol Neurosurg Psychiatry 1984;47:1087–1090.

91. Kikuchi K, McCormick C, Neuwelt E. Immunosuppression by phenytoin: implication for altered immune competence in brain-tumor patients. J Neurosurg 1984;61:1085–1090.

92. Muller PJ, Tator CH, Bloom M. The effect of phenobarbital on the toxicity and tumoricidal activity of CCNU in a murine brain model. J Neurosurg 1980;52:359–366.

93. Neef C, Voogd-van derStraaten I. An interaction between cytostatic and anticonvulsant drugs. Clin Pharmacol Ther 1988;43:372–375.

94. Grossman SA, Sheilder VR, Gilbert MR. Decreased phenytoin levels in patients receiving chemotherapy. Am J Med 1989;87:505–510.

95. Momon HJ, Wen PY, Burns AC, Loeffler JS. Allergic skin reactions to anticonvulsant medication in patients receiving cranial radiation therapy. Epilepsia 1999;40:341–344.

96. Hoang-Xuan K, Delattre JY, Poisson M. Stevens-Johnson syndrome in a patient receiving cranial irradiation and carbamazepine. Neurology 1990;40:1144–1145.

97. Taylor L, Posner J. Phenobarbital rheumatism in patients with brain tumor. Ann Neurol 1989;25:92–94.

98. Leestma J, Annegers JF, Brodie MJ. Sudden unexplained death in epilepsy: observations from a large clinical development programme. Epilepsia 1997;38:47–55.

99. Buttner A, Gall C, Mall C, Weis S. Unexpected death in patients with symptomatic epilepsy due to glial brain tumors—a report of two cases. Forensic Sci Int 1999;100:127–136.

100. Rogers LR, Morris HH, Lupica K. Effect of cranial irradiation on seizure frequency in adults with low-grade astrocytoma and medically intractable epilepsy. Neurology 1993;43:1599–1601.

101. Moriarty GL, Dunn ME, Frost MD, et al. Contribution of radiotherapy and chemotherapy to seizure outcome after brain tumor resection. Epilepsia 1999;40:209–210(abst).

102. Cibula JE, Gilmore RL. Secondary epileptogenesis in humans. J Clin Neurophysiol 1997;14:111–127.

103. Blume W, Pillay N. Electrographic and clinical correlates of secondary bilateral synchrony. Epilepsia 1985;26:636–641.

104. Sammaritano M, De Lotbiniere A, Andermann F, et al. False lateralization by surface EEG of seizure onset in patients with temporal lobe epilepsy and gross focal cerebral lesions. Ann Neurol 1987;21:361–369.

105. Rosenbaum TJ, Laxer KD, Vessely M, Brewster Smith W. Subdural electrodes for seizure focus localization. Neurosurgery 1986;19:73–81.

106. Jayakar P, Duchowny M, Resnick TJ, et al. Localization of seizure foci: pitfalls and caveats. J Clin Neurophysiol 1991;8:414–431.

107. Wada J. Intracarotid injection of sodium amytal for the lateralization of cerebral speech dominance: experimental and clinical observation. J Neurosurg 1960;17:266–282.

108. Khajavi K, Comair YG, Wyllie E, et al. Surgical management of pediatric tumor-associated epilepsy. J Child Neurol 1999;14:15–25.

109. Morris H, Luders H, Hahn J, et al. Neurophysiological techniques as an aid to surgical treatment of primary brain tumors. Ann Neurol 1986;19:559–567.

110. Spencer D, Spencer S, Mattson R, Williamson P. Intracerebral masses in patients with intractable partial epilepsy. Neurology 1984;34:432–436.

111. Drake J, Hoffman H, Kobayashi J. Surgical management of children with temporal lobe epilepsy and mass lesions. Neurosurgery 1987;21:792–797.

112. Awad I, Rosenfeld J, Ahl J. Intractable epilepsy and structural lesions of the brain: mapping, resection strategies and seizure outcome. Epilepsia 1991;32:179–186.

113. Hirsch J, Sainte Rose C, Pierre-Kahn A, et al. Benign astrocytic and oligodendrocytic tumors of the cerebral hemispheres in children. J Neurosurg 1989;70:568–572.

114. Soffietti R, Chio A, Giordana MT, et al. Prognostic factors in well-differentiated cerebral astrocytomas in the adult. Neurosurgery 1989;24:686–692.

115. Fried I, Kim JH, Spencer DD, et al. Limbic and neocortical gliomas associated with intractable seizures: A dis-

tinct clinicopathological group. Neurosurgery 1994;34: 815–824.

116. Cascino GD, Kelly PJ, Hirschorn KA, et al. Stereotactic resection of intraaxial cerebral lesions in partial epilepsy. Mayo Clin Proc 1990;65:1053–1060.

117. Gonzalcz D, Elvidge AR. On the occurrence of epilepsy caused by astrocytoma of the cerebral hemispheres. J Neurosurg 1962;19:470–482.

118. Otsubo H, Hoffmann HJ, Humphreys RP, et al. Evaluation, surgical approach and outcome of seizure patients w,8–212.

119. Tran TA, Spencer SS, Javidan M, et al. Significance of spikes recorded on intraoperative electrocorticography in patients with brain tumor and epilepsy. Epilepsia 1997;38:1132–1139.

120. Pilcher WH, Sybergeld DL, Berger MS, Ojemann GA. Intraoperative electrocorticography during tumor resection: impact on seizure outcome in patients with gangliogliomas. J Neurosurg 1993;78:891–902.

121. Penfield W. Epilepsy and the Functional Anatomy of the Human Brain. Boston: Little, Brown, 1954.

122. Kleihues P, Burger PC, Scheithauer BW. Histological Typing of Tumors of the Central Nervous System. Berlin: Springer, 1993.

123. Greenberg M. Handbook of Neurosurgery (4th ed). Lakeland, FL: Greenberg Graphics, 1997.

124. Freid I, Kim JH, Spencer DD, et al. Limbic and neocortical gliomas associated with intractable seizures: a distinct clinicopathological group. Neurosurgery 1994;34:815–824.

125. Peipmeier JM, Freid I, Makuch R. Low-grade astrocytomas may arise from different astrocyte lineages. Neurosurgery 1993;33:627–632.

126. Campbell JW, Polack IF, Martinez AJ, et al. High-grade astrocytoma in children: radiologically complete resection is associated with an excellent long-term prognosis. Neurosurgery 1996;38:258–264.

127. Barker FG, Chang SM, Gutin PH, et al. Survival and functional status after resection of recurrent glioblastoma multiforme. Neurosurgery 1998;42:709–723.

128. Kondziolka D, Flickinger JC, Bissonette JD, et al. Survival benefit of stereotactic radiosurgery for patients with malignant glial neoplasms. Neurosurgery 1997;41:776–785.

129. Shrieve DC, Alexander E III, Wen PY, et al. comparison of stereotactic radiosurgery and brachytherapy in the treatment of recurrent glioblastoma multiforme. Neurosurgery 1995;36:275–284.

130. Laws ER, Taylor WF, Clifton MB, et al. Neurosurgical management of low-grade astrocytomas of the cerebral hemispheres. J Neurosurg 1984;61:661–673.

131. Reis Filho JS, Netto MR, Sluminsky BG, et al. Oligodendroglioma—a pathological and clinical study of 15 cases. Arq Neuropsiquiatr 1999;57:249–254.

132. Burger PC, Rawlings C, Cox EB, et al. Clinicopathologic correlations in the oligodendroglioma. Cancer 1987;59:1345–1352.

133. Bauman G, Lote K, Larson D, et al. Pretreatment factors predict overall survival for patients with low grade glioma—a recursive partitioning analysis. Int J Radiat Oncol Biol Phys 1999;45:923–929.

134. Salu J. Oligodendrogliomas—current state V–clinical peculiarities of the oligodendrogliomas. Neurochirugie 1999;10:394–396.

135. Rizk T, Mottolose C, Bouffett E, et al. Cerebral oligodendrogliomas in children: an analysis of 15 cases. Childs Nerv Syst 1996;12:527–529.

136. Saito A, Nakazato Y. Evaluation of malignant features of oligodendroglial tumors. Clin Neuropathol 1999;18:61–73.

137. Morris H, Matkovic, Z, Estes ML, et al. Ganglioglioma and intractable epilepsy: clinical and neurophysiologic features and predictors of outcome after surgery. Epilepsia 1998;39:307–313.

138. Soffietti R, Ruda R, Bradac GB, Schiffer D. PCV chemotherapy of recurrent oligodendrogliomas and oligoastrocytomas. Neurosurgery 1998;43:1066–1073.

139. Craincross J, Ueki K, Zlatescu MC, et al. Specific genetic predictors of chemotherapeutic response and survival in patients with anaplastic oligodendrogliomas. J Natl Cancer Inst 1998;90:1473–1479.

140. Courville CB. Ganglioglioma: tumor of the central nervous system: review of the literature and report of two cases. Arch Neurol Psychiatry 1930;24:438–491.

141. Celli P, Nofrone I, Palma L, et al. Cerebral oligodendroglioma: prognostic factors and life history. Neurosurgery 1994;35:1018–1035.

142. Mork S, Lindeggard KF, Halvorsen TB, et al. Oligodendroglioma: incidence and biological behavior in a defined population. J Neurosurg 1985;63:881–889.

143. Johnson JH Jr, Hariharan S, Berman J, et al. Clinical outcome of pediatric gangliogliomas: ninety-nine cases over 20 years. Pediatr Neurosurg 1997;27:203–207.

144. Zimmerman RA, Bilaniuk LT. Computed tomography of intracerebral gangliogliomas. J Comput Tomogr 1979;2:63–66.

145. Lang FF, Epstein FJ, Ransohoff J, et al. Central nervous system gangliogliomas, part two: clinical outcome. J Neurosurg 1993;79:867–873.

146. Cervera-Pierot P, Varlet P, Chodkiewicz JP, Daumas-Duport C. Dysembryoplastic neuroepithelial tumors located in the caudate nucleus area: report of four cases. Neurosurgery 1997;40:1065–1070.

147. Whittle IR, Dow GR, Lammie GA, Wardlaw J. Dysembryoplastic neuroepithelial tumour with discrete bilateral multifocality: further evidence for a germinal origin. Br J Neurosurg 1999;13:508–511.

148. Taratuto A, Pomata H, Sevlever G, et al. Dysembryoplastic neuroepithelial tumor: morphological, immunocytochemical, and deoxyribonucleic acid analysis in a pediatric series clinical study. Neurosurgery 1995;36:474–481.

149. Honavar M, Janota I, Polkey CE. Histological heterogeneity of dysembryoplastic neuroepithelial tumors:

identification and differential diagnosis in a series of 74 patients. Histopathology 1999;34:342–356.

150. Kirkpatrick P, Honaver M, Janota I, Polkey C. Control of temporal lobe epilepsy following en bloc resection of low-grade tumors. J Neurosurg 1993;78:19–25.

151. Taylor DC, Falconer MD. Clinical, socioeconomic, and psychological changes after temporal lobectomy for epilepsy. Br J Psychiatry 1968;114:1247–1261.

152. Andermann LF, Savard G, Meencke HJ, et al. Psychosis after resection of ganglioglioma or DNET: evidence for an association. Epilepsia 1999;40:83–87.

153. Black PM. Meningiomas. Neurosurgery 1993;32:643–657.

154. Black PM. Brain tumors (second of two parts). N Engl J Med 1991;324:1555–1564.

155. Wara W, Sheline GE, Newman H, et al. Radiation therapy for meningiomas. AJR Am J Roentgenol 1975;123:435–438.

156. Collins VP, Mordenskjold M, Dumanski JP. The molecular genetics of meningiomas. Brain Pathol 1990;1:19–24.

157. Yamashita J, Handa H, Iwaki K, et al. Recurrence of intracranial meningiomas with special reference to radiotherapy. Surg Neurol 1980;14:33–40.

158. Jaaskelainen J. Seemingly complete removal of histologically benign intracranial meningioma: late recurrence rate and factors predicting recurrence in 657 patients. A multivariate analysis. Surg Neurol 1986;26:461–469.

159. Jaaskelainen J, Haltia M, Servo A. Atypical and anaplastic meningiomas: radiology, surgery and radiotherapy outcome. Surg Neurol 1986;25:233–242.

160. Mirimanoff RO, Dosoretz DE, Linggood RN, et al. Meningioma: analysis of recurrence and progression following neurosurgical resection. J Neurosurg 1985;62:18–24.

161. Flyger G. Epilepsy following radical removal of parasagittal and convexity meningiomas. Acta Psychiatr Neurol Scand 1956;31:245–251.

162. Foy PM, Copeland GP, Shaw MD. The incidence of postoperative seizures. Acta Neurochir 1981;55:253–264.

163. Kallio M, Sankilo R, Hakulinen T, et al. Factors affecting operative and excess long-term mortality in 935 patients with intracranial meningioma. Neurosurgery 1992;31:2–12.

164. Barbaro NM, Gutin PH, Wilson CB, et al. Radiation therapy in the treatment of partially resected meningiomas. Neurosurgery 1987;20:525–528.

165. Hakim R, Alexander E III, Loeffler JS, et al. Results of linear accelerator-based radiosurgery for intracranial meningiomas. Neurosurgery 1998;42:446–454.

166. Subach BR, Lunsford LD, Kondziolka D, et al. Management of petroclival meningiomas by stereotactic radiosurgery. Neurosurgery 1998;42:437–445.

167. Chang SD, Adler J Jr. Treatment of cranial base meningiomas with linear accelerator radiosurgery. Neurosurgery 1997;41:1019–1027.

168. Kondziolka D, Flickinger JC, Perez B, et al. Judicious resection and/or radiosurgery for parasagittal meningiomas: outcomes from a multicenter review. Neurosurgery 1998;43:405–414.

169. Zimm S, Wampler G, Stablein D, et al. Intracerebral metastases in solid-tumor patients: natural history and results of treatment. Cancer 1981;48:384–394.

170. Sorensen JB, Heine HH, Hansen M, Dombernowsky P. Brain metastases in adenocarcinoma of the lung: frequency, risk groups, and prognosis. J Clin Oncol 1988;6:1474–1480.

171. Delattre JY, Krol G, Thaler ST, Posner JB. Distribution of brain metastases. Acta Neurol 1988;45:741–744.

172. Tsukada Y, Fouad A, Pickren JW, Lane WW. Central nervous system metastasis from breast carcinoma. Cancer 1983;52:2349–2354.

173. Neundorfer B. Epileptic seizures in brain metastases. Adv Neurosurg 1984;12:19–24.

174. Markesbery WR, Brooks WH, Gupta GL, Young AB. Treatment for patients with cerebral metastases. Arch Neurol 1978;35:754–756.

175. Ruderman NB, Hall TC. Use of glucocorticoids in the palliative treatment of metastatic brain tumors. Cancer 1965;18:298–306.

176. Cairncross JG, Kim JH, Posner JB. Radiation therapy for brain metastasis. Ann Neurol 1980;7:529–541.

177. Borgelt B, Gelber R, Kramer S. The palliation of brain metastasis: final results of the first two studies by the Radiation Therapy Oncology Group. Int J Radiat Oncol Biol Phys 1980;6:1–9.

178. Patchell RA, Tibbs PA, Regine WF. Postoperative radiotherapy in the treatment of single metastases to the brain: a randomized trial. JAMA 1998;280:1485–1489.

179. Pilcher W, Rusyniak WG. Complications of epilepsy surgery. Neurosurg Clin North Am 1993;4:311–325.

180. Hennessy M, Langan Y, Elwes RD, et al. A study of mortality after temporal lobe epilepsy surgery. Neurology 1999;53:1276–1283.

181. Behrens E, Schramm J, Zentner J, Konig R. Surgical and neurological complications in a series of 708 epilepsy surgery procedures clinical study. Neurosurgery 1997;41:1–10.

182. Black PM, Moriarty T, Eben A, et al. Development and implementation of intraoperative magnetic resonance imaging and its neurosurgical applications. Neurosurgery 1997;41:831–845.

183. Rubino GJ, Farahani K, McGill D, et al. Magnetic resonance imaging-guided neurosurgery in the magnetic fringe fields: the next step in neuronavigation. Neurosurgery 2000;46:643–654.

184. Gutin P, Posner JB. Neurooncology: diagnosis and management of cerebral gliomas—past, present, and future. Neurosurgery 2000;47:1–8.

Chapter 10

Metabolic Disorders

Steven C. Schachter and María Raquel Lopez

Although all patients with epilepsy have seizures, the converse is not necessarily true, particularly for patients with seizures from metabolic disturbances. Metabolic disorders cause seizures because of intracellular accumulation of toxic substances, depletion of substrates essential for cellular metabolism or membrane function, or alteration of intracellular osmolality.[1–3] With the exception of certain inborn errors of metabolism, most acute metabolic derangements that present with seizures are treatable and reversible with specific interventions.

This chapter reviews the clinical presentation, evaluation, and treatment of patients with seizures caused by electrolyte abnormalities, endocrinopathies, and selected inborn errors of metabolism. Seizures due to renal and hepatic disorders are covered in Chapters 3 and 4, respectively.

Electrolyte Abnormalities

Acute electrolyte disorders that cause seizures typically present with rapidly progressive neurologic symptoms and signs, therefore requiring emergency treatment. In general, the short-term prognosis for seizure control and neurologic recovery is related to the correction of the specific metabolic derangements; the long-term prognosis depends on correction of the underlying condition.

Water homeostasis and disorders of electrolytes, particularly sodium, are interrelated. Intracellular fluid (ICF) and extracellular fluid (ECF) are the two components of total body water.[4] The ECF is further divided into the intravascular (plasma water) and extravascular (interstitial) compartments. The concentrations of particles (osmoles) in the ECF and ICF determine their osmolalities (expressed in mOsm per kilogram water). Because water moves along osmolality gradients and can pass freely across cell membranes, the osmolality of each compartment of the ECF equilibrates. Secondarily, the osmolality of the ECF equilibrates with the ICF. Because the ECF compartment has a considerably larger volume than the ICF compartment, ECF osmolality determines the volume of ICF once osmotic equilibrium is achieved.

Although water freely passes across cell membranes, some solutes may not because of active transporters or pumps that maintain different solute concentrations between the inside and outside of cells. These solutes determine CF (and, in turn, the ICF volume). Consequently, the main cause of serum hypoosmolality is hyponatremia.

The normal range of plasma osmolality is 275–290 mOsm/kg, which is maintained as long as the volume of water absorbed equals the volume of water excreted. Water excretion occurs predominantly through the kidneys but also through insensible water loss (e.g., sweat, respiration) and stool. Renal water excretion is regulated by antidiuretic hormone (ADH; also called *arginine vasopressin*), which acts on the kidney to reabsorb water. The secretion of ADH from the posterior pituitary in healthy subjects depends on serum osmolality or tonicity, which is sensed by hypothalamic osmoreceptors as a function of cell volume.[5]

Table 10-1. Major Causes of Syndrome of Inappropriate Secretion of Antidiuretic Hormone

Malignant neoplasia
 Carcinoma: bronchogenic, pancreatic, duodenal, ureteral, prostatic, bladder
 Lymphoma and leukemia
 Thymoma and mesothelioma
Central nervous system disorders
 Trauma
 Infection
 Tumors
 Porphyria
Pulmonary disorders
 Tuberculosis
 Pneumonia
 Fungal infections
 Lung abscesses
 Ventilators with positive pressure
Drug induced
 Desmopressin
 Oxytocin
 Vincristine
 Chlorpropamide
 Nicotine
 Cyclophosphamide
 Morphine
 Amitriptyline
Selective serotonin reuptake inhibitors

Source: Reproduced with permission from JP Kokko. Fluids and Electrolytes. In L Goldman, JC Bennett (eds), Cecil Textbook of Medicine (21st ed). Philadelphia: Saunders, 2000;540–567.

In healthy subjects, a water load causes plasma osmolality to fall. The release of ADH is suppressed, resulting in the rapid excretion of water from the kidneys as dilute urine. Conversely, circulatory volume loss, such as through bleeding, vomiting, diarrhea, and use of diuretics, or in association with edematous states (e.g., nephrotic syndrome, congestive heart failure) elevates ADH secretion, resulting in increased absorption of water from the kidneys (urine becomes concentrated).[4]

Sodium

Hyponatremia

Hyponatremia, a relatively common electrolyte disturbance in hospitalized patients, occurs when an imbalance between the intake and excretion of water results in excess water relative to sodium. This imbalance may be the consequence of impaired water excretion or fluid intake that exceeds the excretory capacity of the kidneys, as in primary polydipsia[6] or iatrogenic administration.[7] Water excretion may be deficient because of renal dysfunction or may be inhibited by the persistent release of ADH induced by volume depletion or by inappropriate ADH secretion (syndrome of inappropriate secretion of antidiuretic hormone [SIADH]; Table 10-1).[8,9]

Hyponatremia may also be seen in cerebral or renal salt-wasting conditions. Sodium depletion from the kidneys is associated with adrenal insufficiency (Addison's disease) and the use of thiazide diuretics. Extrarenal sodium loss occurs with vomiting, diarrhea, or third spacing. Other causes of hyponatremia are hypothyroidism; hyperlipidemia and hyperproteinemia, in which serum osmolality is normal; and hyperglycemia, in which the serum is hyperosmolar.

Because acute hyponatremia causes plasma osmolality to fall, water moves into cells to maintain osmotic equilibrium between the ECF and ICF. In the brain, water entry into neurons results in cerebral edema. Consequently, the symptoms of acute hyponatremia are predominantly neurologic and parallel the severity of cerebral edema.[10]

Early symptoms include nausea and malaise, followed by headache, confusion, lethargy, obtundation, muscle twitching, and seizures,[11,12] which may be partial or generalized tonic-clonic. In one retrospective series, hyponatremia was the cause of seizures in 70% of infants younger than 6 months who lacked other findings suggesting a cause.[13] Coma and respiratory arrest may occur if the plasma sodium concentration rapidly falls below 115–120 mEq/liter,[14] with an associated mortality rate of more than 50%[10] and risk of permanent neurologic damage in survivors.

The diagnostic evaluation of hyponatremia requires a search for causes of water retention or sodium loss, or both. Besides serum sodium concentration, other key laboratory studies are the plasma osmolality, the urine osmolality, and the urine sodium concentration. If plasma osmolality is low, the urine osmolality can be used to distinguish between impaired water excretion (inappropriately high urine osmolality) and primary polydipsia (appropriately low urine osmolality). SIADH is confirmed by inappropriately elevated urine osmolality (often above 300 mOsm/kg) and urine sodium concentration (usually above 40 mEq/liter). Other tests that may be indicated are plasma creatinine concentration and assays of adrenal and thyroid function to evaluate for renal dysfunction or an endocrinopathy, respectively.

The treatment of hyponatremia should be guided by the clinical setting. Patients with chronic hyponatremia require no specific therapy other than restricting water intake. Rapid sodium correction in patients with chronic asymptomatic hyponatremia may be hazardous.[15] When chronic hyponatremia is associated with heart failure, cirrhosis, SIADH, primary polydipsia, and advanced renal failure, water restriction to below the level of water output is the primary therapy. If fluid must be given to patients with SIADH, then the osmolality of the administered fluid must exceed the osmolality of the urine; otherwise, the hyponatremia may worsen. Consequently, isotonic saline has a limited role in the correction of the hyponatremia, because the urine osmolality is usually above 300 mOsm/kg in SIADH.

Because of the high associated mortality, acute symptomatic hyponatremia represents a medical emergency. Isotonic saline should be administered to patients with true volume depletion, diuretic therapy, or adrenal insufficiency, in which cortisol replacement is also indicated. Although sodium concentrations should generally not be increased faster than 1.5–2.0 mmol/liter per hour or 12 mmol/liter per day,[16,17] higher correction rates have been well tolerated in children.[18] The risks of fast correction are central pontine and extrapontine myelinolysis, characterized by spastic quadriparesis, pseudobulbar palsy, and an encephalopathy ranging from confusion to coma.[15–17,19]

Hypernatremia

As plasma sodium concentrations rise in healthy subjects, thirst is stimulated and eventually quenched, and ADH is released. Both actions lower the plasma sodium concentration back to normal. Hypernatremia, a relative deficit of water to sodium solute, may occur in patients who do not respond to thirst by drinking fluids. Infants, confused adults, and the elderly are at particularly high risk.[20] Other causes of hypernatremia are iatrogenic administration of hypertonic sodium solutions, such as sodium bicarbonate; solute-free water losses from the urinary (e.g., diabetes insipidus [DI], osmotic diuresis), gastrointestinal (GI; e.g., osmotic diarrhea), or respiratory tracts; or hypothalamic lesions that affect thirst or osmoreceptor function.

Generalized tonic-clonic seizures, particularly those that result in lactic acidosis, may transiently elevate serum sodium. Intracellular glycogen is metabolized to lactate in muscles during seizures. Intracellular osmolality increases, because lactate is more osmotically active than glycogen. As a result, water moves into cells, causing hypernatremia. Sodium concentrations normalize within 5–15 minutes after the cessation of exertion.

The rise in plasma sodium concentration and therefore plasma osmolality causes acute water movement out of brain cells. Consequently, the symptoms of hypernatremia are primarily neurologic and are related to the severity of the hypernatremia and the rapidity with which it develops.[21] As brain volume decreases, there may be rupture of cerebral veins, focal intracerebral and subarachnoid hemorrhages, and irreversible neuronal damage.[21,22] If hypernatremia is untreated, lethargy, weakness, and irritability progress to twitching, seizures, coma, and death, especially with severe hypernatremia.[23]

The cause of hypernatremia is usually apparent from the history of the patient and can be confirmed by measuring urine osmolality.[21] If urine osmolality exceeds 700–800 mOsm/kg, then both hypothalamic and renal function are intact, and the hypernatremia is likely due to incompletely replaced insensible or GI fluid losses, sodium overload, or insufficient oral water intake. These possible causes can be distinguished by measuring the urine sodium concentration: If less than 25 mEq/liter, water loss and volume depletion are the primary problems; if above 100m Eq/liter, the cause is ingestion or administration of hypertonic sodium solution.[24]

Alternatively, plasma osmolality that exceeds that of urine is consistent with DI, either central (i.e., ADH is deficient) or nephrogenic (i.e., the kidney resists the action of ADH). The site of the problem can be determined by administering exogenous ADH. In central DI, the urine osmolality rises by 50% or more; in nephrogenic DI, there is no response.[21] Nephrogenic DI in adults is associated with chronic lithium use and hypercalcemia.

Patients with chronic hypernatremia are generally asymptomatic. Lowering their plasma sodium concentrations too rapidly can be dangerous because of the possibility of inducing cerebral edema.[25]

Table 10-2. Causes of Fasting Hypoglycemia

Overuse of glucose
  Hyperinsulinism
    Insulinoma
    Exogenous insulin
    Sulfonylureas
    Immune disease with insulin or insulin receptor
      antibodies
    Drugs (e.g., quinine, disopyramide, pentamidine)
    Sepsis
  Appropriate insulin levels
    Extrapancreatic tumors
    Systemic carnitine deficiency
    Deficiency in enzymes of fat oxidation
    3-Hydroxy-3-methylglutaryl-CoA lyase deficiency
    Cachexia with fat depletion
Impaired production of glucose
  Hormone deficiencies:
    Hypopituitarism
    Adrenal insufficiency
    Catecholamine deficiency
    Glucagon deficiency
  Enzyme defects
    Glucose-6-phosphatase
    Liver phosphorylase
    Pyruvate carboxylase
    Phosphoenolpyruvate carboxykinase
    Fructose-1,6-bisphosphatase
    Glycogen synthetase
  Substrate deficiency
    Ketotic hypoglycemia of infancy
    Severe malnutrition, muscle wasting
    Late pregnancy
  Liver disease
    Hepatic congestion
    Severe hepatitis
    Cirrhosis
    Uremia
    Hypothermia
  Drugs
    Alcohol
    Propranolol
Salicylates

Source: Reproduced with permission from DW Foster, AH Rubenstein. Hypoglycemia. In AS Fauci, E Braunwald, KJ Isselbacher, et al. (eds), Harrison's Principles of Internal Medicine (14th ed). New York: McGraw-Hill, 1998;2081–2087.

In patients with hypernatremia caused by water loss or inadequate fluid intake, 120 ml of free water per hour should be administered orally or intravenously (IV), while carefully monitoring the plasma and urine sodium concentrations, as well as central venous pressure when necessary.[23] In patients with DI, the goals of therapy are to decrease the urine output and give specific therapy for the underlying cause.

Glucose

Hypoglycemia

The generally accepted normal range for fasting plasma glucose is 70–100 mg/dl; therefore, patients with a fasting plasma glucose concentration less than 60 mg/dl may have a hypoglycemic disorder. Symptomatic hypoglycemia is usually associated with concentrations less than 50 mg/dl and most often results from an excessive dose of insulin or other hypoglycemic agents.[26] Other, less common, causes are insulinoma, sepsis, and inborn errors of metabolism (Table 10-2).[27]

The clinical manifestations of hypoglycemia parallel the rate of decline in serum glucose concentration, more so than the absolute glucose concentration. Early symptoms may include sweating, a sensation of warmth, fatigue, headache, anxiety, nausea, visual disturbances, dizziness, hunger, and tremor. Few patients have every symptom. Later findings are confusion, drowsiness, delirium, seizures, and coma. Seizures are usually generalized, although partial seizures may occur.[27] Lateralized weakness, even in the absence of a structural brain lesion, may be seen.

Symptomatic hypoglycemia should be suspected when patients under treatment for diabetes have a change in mental status or new-onset seizures. To confirm the diagnosis, serum glucose concentrations should ideally be measured when patients are symptomatic.[28] Further evaluation usually discloses the underlying cause.[29] An electroencephalogram (EEG) while patients are symptomatic from hypoglycemia may show background slowing with or without epileptiform features.

Early or mild symptoms resolve with oral sugar. Patients presenting with altered mental status or seizures should be treated with intravenous glucose once blood samples have been drawn. Diabetic patients with recurrent symptomatic hypoglycemia require modification in their treatment regimen and instruction on the use of oral glucose to prevent the onset or worsening of hypoglycemic symptoms.

Nonketotic Hyperglycemia

Nonketotic hypoglycemia (NKH) is characterized by hyperglycemia—glucose concentrations typically exceed 1,000 mg/dl—hyperosmolality, dehydration (from hyperglycemia-induced osmotic diuresis), and neurologic manifestations.[30] Unlike diabetic ketoacidosis, there is no ketoacid accumulation. Older patients with type 2 diabetes are most likely to present with NKH. Precipitating factors include infection, surgery, dialysis, tube feedings, and stress.

Neurologic signs include focal seizures, epilepsia partialis continua (EPC), myoclonus, opsoclonia, hemiparesis, increased motor tone, and impaired consciousness.[31,32] Focal seizures may present variably from patient to patient. Stereotypic tonic changes in body posture and speech arrest, associated with supplementary motor area seizures, have been well described.[33] The syndrome of transient focal reflex epilepsy and neurologic deficits in elderly patients is highly suggestive of NKH.[34] Relatively late symptoms are reduced consciousness and cessation of seizures as hyperglycemia and hyperosmolality worsen.[35]

EPC can be an early symptom and persist in association with the presence of hyponatremia.[35] The pathogenesis of EPC is thought to require metabolic disturbances including hyperglycemia, mild hyperosmolality, hyponatremia, lack of ketoacidosis, and an area of pre-existing focal cerebral damage.[35]

Laboratory findings confirm the hyperglycemia and hyperosmolality and may also demonstrate a mild metabolic acidosis, as well as hypokalemia, hyponatremia, and elevations of blood urea nitrogen and creatinine.

The mortality rate is more than 50%, typically from circulatory collapse, and therefore NKH represents a medical emergency. Treatment consists of insulin, correction of electrolyte abnormalities, and reversal of the hyperosmolality with rehydration (the average fluid deficit is 10 liters). Focal seizures are often resistant to antiepileptic drugs (AEDs) but do respond to insulin and restoration of circulatory volume.[36,37]

Hypocalcemia

Calcium homeostasis is maintained by vitamin D and parathyroid hormone (PTH). The main dietary sources of vitamin D are fatty fish and fortified foods, such as milk. Vitamin D is also synthesized from 7-dehydrocholesterol in skin, when exposed to ultraviolet light. The liver metabolizes vitamin D to calcidiol (25-hydroxyvitamin D), which is then converted to calcitriol (1,25-dihydroxyvitamin D) in the kidney by a process stimulated by PTH and hypophosphatemia and inhibited by calcium and phosphate.

As plasma calcium concentration falls, PTH secretion increases, resulting in increased calcium release from bone (a process dependent on calcitriol) and enhanced renal production of calcitriol, which in turn increases calcium absorption in the gut and feeds back and inhibits further PTH secretion.

The ionized (free) calcium fraction, not protein-bound calcium, affects the excitability of muscle cells and neurons. The normal serum-ionized calcium concentration is 4.0–5.2 mg/dl, which represents slightly less than half of total serum calcium concentration. The total serum calcium concentration is reduced approximately 0.8 mg/dl for every 1 g/dl reduction in serum albumin concentration. Therefore, symptomatic hypocalcemia is usually defined as an abnormal reduction in serum-ionized calcium concentration or as a serum calcium level less than 7.5 mg/dl in the presence of normal levels of serum proteins. Symptomatic hypocalcemia can occasionally occur with normal total serum calcium concentration. For example, acute respiratory alkalosis causes increased protein binding of ionized calcium.

The major causes of hypocalcemia are hypoparathyroidism and vitamin D deficiency. Vitamin D deficiency can result from poor dietary intake, intestinal malabsorption, decreased hepatic production of calcidiol, increased hepatic metabolism of calcidiol to inactive metabolites (a process that is stimulated by enzyme-inducing AEDs), and decreased renal production of calcitriol in patients with kidney failure. Hypocalcemia is a common finding in intensive care units, particularly among patients with pancreatitis, hypomagnesemia, and septic shock.[38,39] It is also a frequent finding in the intensive care nursery, because neonatal hypocalcemia is usually associated with premature or difficult birth or perinatal asphyxia. It may also occur in newborns of mothers with diabetes or hyperparathyroidism or in small-for-gestational-age newborns.

The symptoms of hypocalcemia generally reflect the degree of hypocalcemia and the acuteness of the fall in serum-ionized calcium concentration, although even slowly developing hypocalcemia may produce an encephalopathy, dementia, depression, or psychosis.

Acute hypocalcemia primarily causes neurologic symptoms because of increased neuromuscular excitability, including numbness and tingling of the fingers, toes, and circumoral region; muscle cramping, stiffness, carpopedal spasm, and tetany (i.e., flexor spasms in the arms and extensor spasms in the legs); laryngeal stridor; tremor and chorea, which may be misdiagnosed as seizures; and seizures. Hypocalcemic newborns may present with hypotonia, apnea, poor feeding, jitteriness, or seizures.

Seizures may or may not occur in conjunction with tetany and are generalized tonic-clonic, focal motor, and less frequently, atypical absence and akinetic seizures.[3,40,41] They occur in 20–25% of patients presenting with hypocalcemia as a medical emergency[42] and in 30–70% of patients with symptomatic hypoparathyroidism, usually in conjunction with tetany, altered mental status, and hypocalcemia.[3]

Tetany, which may be mistaken for motor seizures, results from spontaneous action potentials originating in peripheral nerves when the serum-ionized calcium concentration falls below 4.3 mg/dl, usually corresponding to a total serum calcium concentration of 7.0–7.5 mg/dl. Tetany can also be induced by respiratory alkalosis, hypomagnesemia, and hypokalemia.[43]

The examination shows mental status changes, including irritability, depression, and psychosis. Papilledema, as well as Trousseau's and Chvostek's signs, may be present. Trousseau's sign—carpal spasm due to regional ischemia to the hand—may be observed by inflating a blood pressure cuff in the upper arm above systolic pressure for 2–3 minutes. This sign is present in 6% of healthy persons and is also associated with alkalotic states, hypomagnesemia, hypokalemia, and hyperkalemia. Chvostek's sign—contraction of the facial muscles, especially the upper lip or nasal alae, elicited by lightly tapping the facial nerve below the zygomatic arch—may also be present in healthy patients and absent in patients with chronic hypocalcemia.

The diagnosis of hypocalcemia should be confirmed by repeated measurement of serum calcium, with verification by quantification of serum-ionized calcium, if the diagnosis of hypocalcemia is uncertain (e.g., if the patient has hypoalbuminemia).

In selected patients with hypocalcemia, other laboratory tests that may establish the underlying cause are serum creatinine, amylase, magnesium, phosphate, PTH, calcidiol, and calcitriol. Hyperphosphatemia with normal alkaline phosphatase and renal function are indicative of hypoparathyroidism, which may be confirmed by a low or undetectable PTH concentration. Hyperphosphatemia with elevated creatinine is suggestive of renal failure. Normal or low serum phosphorus should prompt measurement of vitamin D metabolites and assessment of GI function to check for vitamin D deficiency and malabsorption; in these situations, PTH levels are elevated because normal parathyroid glands attempt to compensate for hypocalcemia. The electrocardiogram (ECG) may show prolongation of the Q-T interval, and the EEG may demonstrate slowing and generalized bursts of spikes.[44]

Patients with symptomatic hypocalcemia should be treated immediately because of the high associated morbidity and mortality.[39] IV calcium is the most appropriate treatment, unless severe hypomagnesemia is present. Ten to 20 ml of 10% calcium gluconate (containing 10 mg of elemental calcium per ml) should be administered over 10–20 minutes. Calcium should not be given more rapidly because of the risk of serious cardiac dysfunction, including systolic arrest; patients taking cardiac glycosides are at particularly high risk. In less urgent settings, slow IV infusion (over 4–8 hours) of 20 mg of elemental calcium per kg may be given.

Hypomagnesemia is a common cause of hypocalcemia, both by inducing resistance to PTH and by diminishing its secretion.[39,45–47] Thus, if seizures continue despite adequate therapy with calcium replacement, hypomagnesemia should be investigated as the possible cause of the hypocalcemia and treated appropriately.

An infusion raises the serum calcium concentration for up to 3 hours; therefore, additional, slow infusions of calcium are usually necessary. The dose should be 0.5–1.5 mg/kg per hour. Either 10% calcium gluconate (90 mg of elemental calcium per 10-ml ampule) or 10% calcium chloride (360 mg per 10-ml ampule) can be used. The calcium should be diluted in dextrose and water or saline, because concentrated calcium solutions are irritating to veins; furthermore, calcium gluconate is less likely to cause tissue necrosis, if extravasated, than calcium chloride. Likewise, intramuscular injection of calcium gluconate is contraindicated, because it can cause local necrosis.

IV calcium should be continued until the patient is able to take an effective regimen of oral calcium and vitamin D. Calcitriol, in a dose of 0.25–0.50 μg per day, is the preferred preparation of vitamin D for patients with severe acute hypocalcemia because of its rapid onset of action. Patients with hypoparathyroidism require chronic vitamin D and calcium therapy.[40]

Hypomagnesemia

Hypomagnesemia, defined as magnesium concentration less than 1.6 mEq/liter (<1.9 mg/dl), can result from inadequate dietary intake, diminished GI absorption, and wasting from the kidneys.[48,49] GI causes include disorders or bypass of the small bowel, diarrhea, malabsorption, steatorrhea, and acute pancreatitis. Renal etiologies include inhibition of sodium reabsorption in those segments in which magnesium transport passively follows that of sodium, a primary defect in renal tubular magnesium reabsorption, and alcohol-induced tubular dysfunction.[50] Drugs that promote magnesium wasting from the kidneys are loop and thiazide diuretics, aminoglycoside antibiotics, amphotericin B, cisplatin, pentamidine, and cyclosporine. Hypomagnesemia may occur in patients undergoing prolonged parenteral feeding, especially in combination with loss of body fluids via gastric suction or diarrhea.

In neonates, hypomagnesemia is associated with prematurity, DiGeorge syndrome, familial hypoparathyroidism, and exchange transfusions. It may also occur in infants of diabetic mothers or mothers with hyperparathyroidism or magnesium deficiency.

The overall frequency of hypomagnesemia in hospitalized patients is 11%,[51] although this may be an underestimate.[52] The frequency may be as high as 65% in patients in an intensive care setting in whom major operations, poor nutrition, diuretics, hypoalbuminemia, and aminoglycosides may be factors.[49,53,54]

Magnesium, an essential cation, is involved in many enzymatic reactions and is a cofactor to adenosine triphosphatase. Consequently, magnesium

is critical in energy-requiring metabolic processes.[49] Symptoms of hypomagnesemia include irritability, agitation, confusion, anorexia, nausea, vomiting, lethargy, weakness, tetany, tremor, and muscle fasciculations. Tetany correlates with the secondary development of hypocalcemia or hypokalemia. Seizures, usually tonic-clonic, can occur in neonates and adults in association with severe hypomagnesemia.[10] Physical examination may reveal an abnormal mental status and a positive Trousseau's sign.

Once hypomagnesemia is confirmed by measurement of the serum magnesium level, the etiology can usually be obtained from the history. If there is no apparent cause, the distinction between GI and renal losses can be made by measuring 24-hour urinary magnesium excretion or the fractional excretion of magnesium on a random urine specimen. Other electrolyte disturbances may be found. For example, hypokalemia occurs in 40–60% of patients with hypomagnesemia,[52,54] and hypocalcemia and metabolic alkalosis are frequent findings. ECG changes, including widening of the QRS wave complex and peaking of T waves, may be seen.

Treatment with magnesium salts (e.g., sulfate or chloride) should be given for symptomatic hypomagnesemia. In the setting of seizures, 2–4 g of magnesium sulfate heptahydrate may be given IV (as a 10% solution in 20 to 30 ml of 5% dextrose in water) over 5–15 minutes and repeated, if seizures persist, to a total of 10 g over the next 6 hours. In neonates, 0.25–1.00 ml of 50% magnesium sulfate heptahydrate (0.125–0.500 g) injection intramuscularly or IV is given over 10–15 minutes with careful ECG monitoring. This dose may be repeated two to three times a day. Calcium gluconate should be available, because apnea from respiratory muscle paralysis can result from transient hypermagnesemia. Besides magnesium replacement, the underlying disease should also be corrected when possible.

Endocrinopathies

Hypoparathyroidism

The differential diagnosis of hypoparathyroidism includes (1) idiopathic hypoparathyroidism, a condition in which the parathyroids are absent or atrophied, that occurs sporadically or in association with genetic autoimmune syndromes or DiGeorge syndrome; (2) pseudohypoparathyroidism, characterized by bone and kidney tissue unresponsiveness to PTH; and (3) damage or accidental removal of parathyroid glands during thyroidectomy. Transient hypoparathyroidism and hypocalcemia from subtotal thyroidectomy are common,[55,56] but permanent hypoparathyroidism rarely occurs as a complication of thyroid surgery.

Seizures occur in up to 70% of patients with symptomatic hypoparathyroidism.[3,41,57] In addition, parkinsonism, dystonia, hemiballismus, choreoathetosis, and oculogyric crises occur in 5–10% of patients with idiopathic hypoparathyroidism[58] and less often in patients with surgical hypoparathyroidism or other causes of hypocalcemia.[59] Other neurologic findings may include spastic paraplegia, ataxia, dysarthria, and dysphagia.

Chronic hypocalcemia in patients with hypoparathyroidism may be associated with dry, puffy, or coarse skin; dental changes, when hypocalcemia is present during early development[60,61]; and cataracts.

PTH levels are low or undetectable in patients with hypoparathyroidism. Besides hypocalcemia, most patients with pseudohypoparathyroidism also have high serum PTH and phosphate concentrations and low serum calcitriol concentrations. Brain computed tomography scans may show basal ganglia calcification, particularly in chronic cases.[62,63]

The acute management of symptomatic hypoparathyroidism involves correction of hypocalcemia and other associated electrolyte abnormalities.

Hyperthyroidism

Common causes of hyperthyroidism are Graves' disease, toxic multinodular goiter, toxic adenoma, and subacute thyroiditis. The clinical presentation is the same regardless of underlying cause. Symptoms include anxiety, nervousness, emotional lability, sweating, heat insensitivity, palpitations, fatigue, weight loss, irregular or fast heartbeat, muscle wasting and weakness, and increased bowel movements.[64] Signs include tachycardia, warm and moist skin, enhanced physiologic tremor, lid retraction and lag, rapid speech, hyper-

activity, and proximal muscle weakness. Chorea may be seen,[65] and a goiter may be present, depending on the cause. Exophthalmos is present only in patients with Graves' disease.

The diagnosis is confirmed by low-serum thyroid-stimulating hormone and high T4 or T3 concentrations, or both. The ECG often shows atrial fibrillation.

In patients with established epilepsy (including generalized epilepsy syndromes), seizures and paroxysmal EEG abnormalities can be exacerbated by hyperthyroidism.[66,67] In other patients, focal or generalized seizures occur only during thyrotoxic episodes.[68] Seizure exacerbations usually remit when patients become euthyroid with treatment.

Adrenal Insufficiency

The clinical presentation of adrenal insufficiency varies, depending on the degree of adrenal dysfunction, the acuteness with which function is lost, the extent of mineralocorticoid production, and the magnitude of superimposed stress or medical illness. Common symptoms of adrenal insufficiency are generalized weakness, malaise, easy fatigue, loss of appetite, and weight loss. Seizures can occur in association with hyponatremia.

An adrenal crisis may result from infection or other stress superimposed on adrenal insufficiency or from bilateral adrenal infarction or hemorrhage. The usual presenting clinical picture is shock; nausea, vomiting, abdominal pain, confusion, or coma may occur as well.

Patients with chronic primary adrenal insufficiency have hyperpigmented skin, especially in areas exposed to sun or contact pressure. Other possible findings include mood instability, psychotic ideation, and an encephalopathy varying from inattention to delirium and stupor.

Hyponatremia, found in 85–90% of patients, is caused by SIADH due to cortisol deficiency and volume loss due to mineralocorticoid deficiency. Hyperkalemia, hyperchloremic acidosis, and hypoglycemia may be present.

The acute management of seizures in patients with adrenal insufficiency requires correction of serum sodium and glucose concentrations.

Inborn Errors of Metabolism

Inborn errors of metabolism are rare, genetically transmitted enzyme deficiencies that block or interfere with cellular metabolic pathways. In British Columbia, from 1969 to 1996, the incidence of diseases of amino acids, organic acids, the urea cycle, galactosemia, primary lactic acidoses, glycogen storage, and lysosomal storage and diseases specifically involving peroxisomal and mitochondrial respiratory chain dysfunction was approximately 40 cases per 100,000 live births.[69]

Symptoms and signs result when pathway intermediates proximal to the enzymatic block accumulate to toxic levels or from deficient products of the affected metabolic pathways. Most inborn errors of metabolism present with progressive neurologic and systemic symptoms, as well as seizures, which often begin in the neonatal period or during infancy.

Several relatively more common disorders are discussed in the following sections. Table 10-3 lists the inborn errors of metabolism that cause seizures in infants.

Phenylketonuria

Phenylketonuria (PKU), an aminoaciduria, is characterized by an absence or severe deficiency of phenylalanine hydroxylase, the enzyme that hydroxylates phenylalanine to tyrosine. PKU is inherited as an autosomal recessive trait. Variant forms caused by other enzyme defects have been identified.

Normal diets typically contain more than twice the amount of phenylalanine (an essential amino acid) needed for protein synthesis. Excess phenylalanine is converted to tyrosine, but in the absence of phenylalanine hydroxylase, plasma phenylalanine concentrations are elevated, and phenylalanine is excreted in the urine. Some excess phenylalanine is metabolized to phenylacetic acid, as well as other acids, and excreted in the urine and sweat.

Serum phenylalanine concentrations in infants with PKU are normal at birth but begin to rise within the first few weeks of life. Excessive phenylalanine is generally thought responsible for the brain damage that underlies the severe mental

Table 10-3. Metabolic Disorders Associated with Infantile Seizures

Amino acidopathies
  Nonketotic hyperglycinemia
  Phenylketonuria
Organic acidopathies
  Glutaric aciduria, types I and II
  3-Methylcrotonyl aciduria
  Mevalonic acidemia
  Maple syrup urine disease
  Canavan's disease
  Succinate semialdehyde dehydrogenase deficiency
  Other organic acidurias
Glucose homeostasis
  Glycogen storage diseases, types I and III
  Fructose-1,6-bisphosphatase deficiency
  Fat oxidation defects
Biotin metabolism
  Biotinidase deficiency
  Multiple carboxylase deficiency
4-Aminobutyric acid (GABA) metabolism
  GABA-transaminase deficiency
  Pyridoxine-responsive convulsions
Peroxisome biogenesis and metabolism
  Zellweger syndrome
  Neonatal adrenoleukodystrophy
  Infantile Refsum's syndrome
  Pseudo-Zellweger syndrome
  Pseudoneonatal adrenoleukodystrophy
Metal and mineral metabolism
  Primary hypomagnesemia
  Primary hypoparathyroidism
  Menke's disease
Oxidative phosphorylation
  Pyruvate dehydrogenase deficiency
  Respiratory chain complex deficiencies
  Progressive mitochondrial encephalopathy
  Leigh's disease
  Alpers' disease
Storage disorders
  Congenital Batten's disease
  Infantile Krabbe's disease
  GM_1 and GM_2 gangliosidosis
  Niemann-Pick disease, type A
Folate metabolism
  5,10-methylenetetrahydrofolate reductase deficiency
  Congenital folate malabsorption
Others
  Sulfite oxidase deficiency
  Glutathione synthase deficiency

Source: Reproduced with permission from A Hopkins. The Causes of Epilepsy, the Risk Factors for Epilepsy and the Precipitation of Seizures. In Hopkins A, Shorvon S, Cascino G (eds), Epilepsy (2nd ed). London: Chapman & Hall Medical, 1995;59–85.

retardation and seizure disorder of PKU. In untreated infants, cognitive delay becomes evident within 6 months and is progressive. The majority of affected children are unable to talk, and a significant proportion never learns to walk. Characteristic physical findings include light hair, eye, and skin pigmentation; an eczematous rash; hyperactive behavior; and a musty or mousy odor due to phenylacetic acid in the sweat.

Approximately 25% of patients have generalized or partial seizures. Infantile spasms and myoclonic seizures may occur.[70] On the EEG, all patients have slowing, epileptiform discharges or hypsarrhythmic patterns.[71]

Because newborns with PKU are usually healthy seeming, the diagnosis requires screening tests, which are mandated by law. Confirmatory tests are high plasma phenylalanine and normal or low plasma tyrosine concentrations.

Treatment consists of dietary restriction of phenylalanine and AEDs, when necessary. The goal is to provide necessary but not excessive amounts of phenylalanine in the diet (typically 250–500 mg per day). The diet should be instituted immediately in the newborn period and maintained throughout life to preserve cognitive and neuropsychologic function. Monitoring plasma phenylalanine levels is required to gauge compliance and adequacy of the prescribed diet.

Lipidoses

Niemann-Pick Disease

Niemann-Pick disease is an autosomal-recessive lipidosis in which sphingomyelin (i.e., ceramide phosphorylcholine) accumulates in the lysosomes of reticuloendothelial cells.[72] Of the subtypes, type C is most associated with seizures. Whereas types A and B result from a deficiency of acid sphingomyelinase, types C and D are characterized by abnormal cholesterol esterification and transport out of the lysosome. Two subtypes of type-C Niemann-Pick disease have been identified based on the temporal sequence of neurologic events, neurophysiologic abnormalities, and longevity.[73]

Neonates with type-C Niemann-Pick disease may be jaundiced at birth. Slowly progressive neurologic deterioration begins within 2 years. Partial, generalized tonic-clonic and atonic seizures may occur and are usually refractory to AEDs.[73] Hepatosplenomegaly is often present.

Laboratory testing may show pancytopenia from bone marrow infiltration. Sphingomyelinase activity is not reduced, but the cholesterol transport defect can be documented in cell culture.

There is currently no specific treatment for any of the Niemann-Pick disease subtypes, and care is supportive.[72]

Gaucher's Disease

Gaucher's disease is an autosomal-recessive lipidosis caused by a deficiency of acid β-glucosidase.[72] Because acid β-glucosidase hydrolyzes glucocerebroside in lysosomes to glucose and ceramide, Gaucher's disease is characterized by the lysosomal accumulation of glucocerebrosides (primarily glucosylceramide).

There are three subtypes of Gaucher's disease. Types II and III involve the central nervous system. Whereas patients with type II die in infancy, type III, the juvenile form, may present in infancy or childhood.

Glucocerebroside accumulates in cells of the liver, spleen, lymph nodes, and bone marrow, leading to organomegaly, lymphadenopathy, and skeletal pain. Neurologic signs include ataxic gait, cognitive dysfunction, and partial and generalized tonic-clonic seizures.

The diagnosis is confirmed by the presence of characteristic cells on bone marrow aspiration and the lack of acid β-glucosidase activity in cell culture.

There is no known effective treatment for the neurologic involvement in type III Gaucher's disease.

Mucopolysaccharidoses

The mucopolysaccharidoses are lysosomal storage disorders due to a lack of enzymes that normally degrade glycosaminoglycans. They are characterized by the intracellular accumulation and urinary excretion of glycosaminoglycans (i.e., mucopolysaccharides).

The seven types of mucopolysaccharidoses are each distinguished by an excess of a particular urinary mucopolysaccharide.[74] Inheritance is autosomal dominant, except for type II, which is x-linked. Clinical features vary but generally include a characteristic coarse facies (i.e., thickened lips and open mouth), short height, bony abnormalities, mental retardation, corneal opacities, and hepatosplenomegaly.

Type III (Sanfilippo's syndrome) is the most common mucopolysaccharidosis. There are four subtypes. Onset of symptoms is usually after 2 years of age, followed by rapidly progressive neurologic and cognitive deterioration. Seizures occur in nearly half of patients. The EEG shows nonspecific abnormalities, and neuroimaging studies reveal cortical atrophy and ventricular dilatation.

Laboratory studies confirm abnormalities on urine screening tests for glycosaminoglycans. Sophisticated cell culture or serum assays are available to evaluate patients for specific enzyme deficiencies.

Treatment is symptomatic. Enzyme replacement by bone marrow transplantation has produced systemic improvement in selected patients but has not prevented neurologic deterioration.

Hepatic Porphyria

The porphyrias are caused by inherited deficiencies of enzymes involved in heme synthesis.[75] Heme is used in the bone marrow and liver to make hemoglobin and cytochrome P-450 enzymes, respectively. The hepatic synthesis of heme is largely regulated by δ-aminolevulinic acid (ALA) synthase, an inducible enzyme.

The symptoms and signs of the porphyrias result from the accumulation of toxic metabolites. They are classified either as erythropoietic and hepatic or on the basis of the specific enzyme deficiency. Seizures and other neurologic manifestations only occur in the hepatic group, in which the porphyrin precursors ALA and porphobilinogen (PBG) accumulate.[76] Both compounds have been implicated as directly neurotoxic.[77]

Three acute hepatic porphyrias, all autosomal dominant, are associated with seizures: acute intermittent porphyria (AIP), hereditary coproporphyria (HCP), and variegate porphyria (VP).[78] HCP and VP, although much less common, present similarly to AIP, except that HCP and VP are also associated with cutaneous photosensitivity.

Patients with AIP have approximately 50% reduction of PBG deaminase activity.[75] This condition is particularly prevalent in Northern Europe, especially Finland.[79] When the demand for hepatic heme synthesis is increased, the reduced PBG deaminase activity leads to the accumulation of ALA and PBG in the liver, plasma, and urine.[78] Some of the PBG and ALA is converted to porphyrin.

AIP can be precipitated by drugs that induce hepatic ALA synthase, such as enzyme-inducing AEDs, or inhibit PBG deaminase, such as sulfonamide antibiotics. Other precipitating factors include hormones (e.g., estrogen, progesterone and its metabolites, and oral contraceptives), alcohol, reduced caloric intake, intercurrent infections, and major surgery.[80]

Clinical manifestations can persist for days to weeks and may be preceded by nonspecific symptoms.[76] The most common acute symptom is abdominal pain, often severe enough to require narcotic analgesia, and sometimes accompanied by nausea, vomiting, ileus, and constipation. Sympathetically mediated signs include tachycardia, hypertension, sweating, and tremors. Sleep disturbance, anxiety, delirium, hallucinations, depressed mood, and paranoid delusions may be present.[81,82] Lethargy and coma occur rarely. Peripheral motor neuropathies may lead to foot or wrist drops.

Some studies suggest that focal and generalized seizures occur in nearly one-third of pediatric cases and up to 20% of adult cases.[83–85] By contrast, a study of patients registered at the National Porphyria Center in Sweden found that the lifetime prevalence of AIP-associated seizures was 2.2% of all those with known AIP and 5.1% of all those with manifest AIP.[86] Seizures associated with AIP occur either as a direct neurologic manifestation of the condition or from hyponatremia, which may result from SIADH, vomiting, diarrhea, or poor oral intake.

The diagnosis may be suspected based on the clinical presentation and may be confirmed by the presence of photosensitive porphyrins in the urine and reduced monopyrrole PBG deaminase in red blood cells.[81,87]

After a definitive diagnosis, treatment of acute attacks consists of narcotic analgesia for pain; symptomatic therapy of nausea, anxiety, and restlessness; and oral or IV glucose and IV hematin or heme arginate. These treatments reverse the induction of ALA synthase and thereby reduce the production and accumulation of ALA and PBG.[78,88,89]

Drugs known to precipitate AIP must be avoided,[78,90] particularly when treating seizures, pain, and anxiety-acute attacks. Hahn et al. used a cell culture model of primary chicken embryo liver cells, which maintain intact heme synthesis and regulation, to study the effects of several of the more recently approved AEDs on porphyrin accumulation as possible treatments for seizures in patients with porphyria.[91] Based on the results, they recommended vigabatrin or gabapentin, for which success was reported anecdotally,[92] but not felbamate, lamotrigine, or tiagabine. Similar animal studies suggest that patients with acute porphyrias may be at greater risk for developing porphyric attacks when treated with tramadol compared to hydrocodone, oxycodone, and morphine[93]; bupropion or nefazodone compared with fluoxetine or paroxetine; and diazepam, midazolam, and triazolam compared with low doses of lorazepam and oxazepam.[94]

Complete recovery from attacks is the rule, although neuropathic deficits may take months to resolve.

Conclusion

Seizures due to metabolic disorders present diagnostic as well as therapeutic challenges. Because AEDs alone are generally of limited benefit, and acute metabolic derangements can be fatal if untreated, neurologists must consider this group of disorders in patients presenting with new-onset seizures or in patients with epilepsy with an otherwise unexplained worsening of seizure frequency or severity.[95] Close collaboration between the neurologist and the medical specialist is essential in the care of the patient with seizures of metabolic origin.

References

1. Gilmore RL. Seizures Associated with Non-Neurologic Medical Conditions. In E Wyllie (ed), The Treatment of Epilepsy: Principles and Practice. Baltimore: Williams & Wilkins, 1996;654–665.
2. Garcia-Alvarez M, Nordli DR, De Vivo DC. Inherited Metabolic Disorders. In J Engel, TA Pedley (eds), Epilepsy: a Comprehensive Textbook. Philadelphia: Lippincott–Raven, 1998;2547–2562.
3. Messing RO, Simon RP. Seizures as a manifestation of systemic disease. Neurol Clin 1986;4:563–584.
4. Singer GG, Brenner BM. Fluid and Electrolyte Disturbances. In AS Fauci, E Braunwald, KJ Isselbacher et al. (eds), Harrison's Principles of Internal Medicine (14th ed). New York: McGraw-Hill, 1998;265–277.
5. Robertson GL, Shelton RL, Athar S. The osmoregulation of vasopressin. Kidney Int 1976;10:25–37.
6. Siegel AJ, Baldessarini RJ, Klepser MB, McDonald JC. Primary and drug-induced disorders of water homeostasis in psychiatric patients: principles of diagnosis and management. Harv Rev Psychiatry 1998;6:190–200.
7. Gowrishankar M, Lin SH, Mallie JP, et al. Acute hyponatremia in the perioperative period: insights into its pathophysiology and recommendations for management. Clin Nephrol 1998;50:352–360.
8. Kokko JP. Fluids and Electrolytes. In L Goldman, JC Bennett (eds), Cecil Textbook of Medicine (21st ed). Philadelphia: Saunders, 2000;540–567.
9. Maesaka JK. An expanded view of SIADH, hyponatremia, and hypouricemia. Clin Nephrol 1996;46:79–83.
10. Riggs JE. Neurologic manifestations of fluid and electrolyte disturbances. Neurol Clin 1989;7:509–523.
11. Daggett P, Deanfield J, Moss F. Neurological aspects of hyponatraemia. Postgrad Med J 1982;58:737–740.
12. Hojer J. Management of symptomatic hyponatraemia: dependence on the duration of development. J Intern Med 1994;235:497–501.
13. Farrar HC, Chande VT, Fitzpatrick DF, Shema SJ. Hyponatremia as the cause of seizures in infants: a retrospective analysis of incidence, severity, and clinical predictors. Ann Emerg Med 1995;26:42–48.
14. Arieff AI. Hyponatremia, convulsions, respiratory arrest, and permanent brain damage after elective surgery in healthy women. N Engl J Med 1986;314:1529–1535.
15. Laureno R, Karp BI. Myelinolysis after correction of hyponatremia. Ann Intern Med 1997;126:57–62.
16. Sterns RH. Severe symptomatic hyponatremia: treatment and outcome. A study of 64 cases. Ann Intern Med 1987;107:656–664.
17. Sterns RH, Riggs JE, Schochet SS Jr. Osmotic demyelination syndrome following correction of hyponatremia. N Engl J Med 1986;314:1535–1542.
18. Sarnaik AP, Meert K, Hackbarth R, Fleischmann L. Management of hyponatremic seizures in children with hypertonic saline: a safe and effective strategy. Crit Care Med 1991;19:758–762.
19. Ellis SJ. Severe hyponatraemia: complications and treatment. QJM 1995;88:905–909.
20. Ayus JC, Arieff AI. Abnormalities of water metabolism in the elderly. Semin Nephrol 1996;16:277–288.
21. Rose BD. Clinical Physiology of Acid-Base and Electrolyte Disorders (4th ed). New York: McGraw-Hill, 1994.
22. McManus ML, Churchwell KB, Strange K. Regulation of cell volume in health and disease. N Engl J Med 1995;333:1260–1266.
23. Daggett P, Deanfield J, Moss F, Reynolds D. Severe hypernatraemia in adults. BMJ 1979;1:1177–1180.
24. Meadow R. Non-accidental salt poisoning. Arch Dis Child 1993;68:448–452.

25. Lien YH, Shapiro JI, Chan L. Effects of hypernatremia on organic brain osmoles. J Clin Invest 1990;85:1427–1435.

26. Foster DW, Rubenstein AH. Hypoglycemia. In AS Fauci, E Braunwald, KJ Isselbacher et al. (eds), Harrison's Principles of Internal Medicine (14th ed). New York: McGraw-Hill, 1998;2081–2087.

27. Malouf R, Brust JC. Hypoglycemia: causes, neurological manifestations, and outcome. Ann Neurol 1985;17:421–430.

28. Polonsky KS. A practical approach to fasting hypoglycemia. N Engl J Med 1992;326:1020–1021.

29. Rizza RA, Service FJ. Hypoglycemia/pancreatic islet cell disorders In L Goldman, JC Bennett (eds), Cecil Textbook of Medicine (21st ed). Philadelphia: Saunders, 2000;1285–1292.

30. Arieff AI, Carroll HJ. Nonketotic hyperosmolar coma with hyperglycemia: clinical features, pathophysiology, renal function, acid-base balance, plasma-cerebrospinal fluid equilibria and the effects of therapy in 37 cases. Medicine (Baltimore) 1972;51:73–94.

31. Morres CA, Dire DJ. Movement disorders as a manifestation of nonketotic hyperglycemia. J Emerg Med 1989;7:359–364.

32. Guisado R, Arieff AI. Neurologic manifestations of diabetic comas: correlation with biochemical alterations in the brain. Metabolism 1975;24:665–679.

33. Venna N, Sabin TD. Tonic focal seizures in nonketotic hyperglycemia of diabetes mellitus. Arch Neurol 1981;38:512–514.

34. Brick JF, Gutrecht JA, Ringel RA. Reflex epilepsy and nonketotic hyperglycemia in the elderly: a specific neuroendocrine syndrome. Neurology 1989;39:394–399.

35. Singh BM, Strobos RJ. Epilepsia partialis continua associated with nonketotic hyperglycemia: clinical and biochemical profile of 21 patients. Ann Neurol 1980;8:155–160.

36. Aquino A, Gabor AJ. Movement-induced seizures in nonketotic hyperglycemia. Neurology 1980;30:600–604.

37. Hennis A, Corbin D, Fraser H. Focal seizures and non-ketotic hyperglycaemia. J Neurol Neurosurg Psychiatry 1992;55:195–197.

38. Desai TK, Carlson RW, Geheb MA. Hypocalcemia and hypophosphatemia in acutely ill patients. Crit Care Clin 1987;3:927–941.

39. Desai TK, Carlson RW, Geheb MA. Prevalence and clinical implications of hypocalcemia in acutely ill patients in a medical intensive care setting. Am J Med 1988;84:209–214.

40. Tohme JF, Bilezikian JP. Hypocalcemic emergencies. Endocrinol Metab Clin North Am 1993;22:363–375.

41. Fonseca OA, Calverley JR. Neurological manifestations of hypoparathyroidism. Arch Intern Med 1967;120:202–206.

42. Gupta MM. Medical emergencies associated with disorders of calcium homeostasis. J Assoc Physicians India 1989;37:629–631.

43. Macefield G, Burke D. Paraesthesiae and tetany induced by voluntary hyperventilation. Increased excitability of human cutaneous and motor axons. Brain 1991;114:527–540.

44. Swash M, Rowan AJ. Electroencephalographic criteria of hypocalcemia and hypercalcemia. Arch Neurol 1972;26:218–228.

45. Ryzen E, Rude RK. Low intracellular magnesium in patients with acute pancreatitis and hypocalcemia. West J Med 1990;152:145–148.

46. Connor TB, Toskes P, Mahaffey J, et al. Parathyroid function during chronic magnesium deficiency. Johns Hopkins Med J 1972;131:100–117.

47. Chase LR, Slatopolsky E. Secretion and metabolic efficacy of parathyroid hormone in patients with severe hypomagnesemia. J Clin Endocrinol Metab 1974;38:363–371.

48. Agus ZS. Hypomagnesemia. J Am Soc Nephrol 1999;10:1616–1622.

49. al-Ghamdi SM, Cameron EC, Sutton RA. Magnesium deficiency: pathophysiologic and clinical overview. Am J Kidney Dis 1994;24:737–752.

50. Booth BE, Johanson A. Hypomagnesemia due to renal tubular defect in reabsorption of magnesium. J Pediatr 1974;85:350–354.

51. Wong ET, Rude RK, Singer FR, Shaw ST Jr. A high prevalence of hypomagnesemia and hypermagnesemia in hospitalized patients. Am J Clin Pathol 1983;79:348–352.

52. Whang R, Ryder KW. Frequency of hypomagnesemia and hypermagnesemia. Requested vs. routine. JAMA 1990;263:3063–3064.

53. Ryzen E. Magnesium homeostasis in critically ill patients. Magnesium 1989;8:201–212.

54. Chernow B, Bamberger S, Stoiko M, et al. Hypomagnesemia in patients in postoperative intensive care. Chest 1989;95:391–397.

55. See AC, Soo KC. Hypocalcaemia following thyroidectomy for thyrotoxicosis. Br J Surg 1997;84:95–97.

56. Yamashita H, Noguchi S, Murakami T, et al. Seasonal changes in calcium homeostasis affect the incidence of postoperative tetany in patients with Graves' disease. Surgery 2000;127:377–382.

57. Hossain M. Neurological and psychiatric manifestations in idiopathic hypoparathyroidism: response to treatment. J Neurol Neurosurg Psychiatry 1970;33:153–156.

58. Soffer D, Licht A, Yaar I, Abramsky O. Paroxysmal choreoathetosis as a presenting symptom in idiopathic hypoparathyroidism. J Neurol Neurosurg Psychiatry 1977;40:692–694.

59. Rubenstein A, Brust JC. Parkinsonian syndrome as complication of post-thyroidectomy hypoparathyroidism. N Y State J Med 1974;74:2029–2030.

60. Frensilli JA, Stoner RE, Hinrichs EH. Dental changes of idiopathic hypoparathyroidism: report of three cases. J Oral Surg 1971;29:727–731.

61. Jensen SB, Illum F, Dupont E. Nature and frequency of dental changes in idiopathic hypoparathyroidism and pseudohypoparathyroidism. Scand J Dent Res 1981;89:26–37.

62. Illum F, Dupont E. Prevalences of CT-detected calcification in the basal ganglia in idiopathic hypoparathyroidism and pseudohypoparathyroidism. Neuroradiology 1985;27:32–37.
63. Muenter MD, Whisnant JP. Basal ganglia calcification, hypoparathyroidism, and extrapyramidal motor manifestations. Neurology 1968;18:1075–1083.
64. Schimke RN. Hyperthyroidism. The clinical spectrum. Postgrad Med J 1992;91:229–236.
65. Ahronheim JC. Hyperthyroid chorea in an elderly woman associated with sole elevation of T3. J Am Geriatr Soc 1988;36:242–244.
66. Su YH, Izumi T, Kitsu M, Fukuyama Y. Seizure threshold in juvenile myoclonic epilepsy with Graves' disease. Epilepsia 1993;34:488–492.
67. Sundaram MB, Hill A, Lowry N. Thyroxine-induced petit mal status epilepticus. Neurology 1985;35:1792–1793.
68. Jabbari B, Huott AD. Seizures in thyrotoxicosis. Epilepsia 1980;21:91–96.
69. Applegarth DA, Toone JR, Lowry RB. Incidence of inborn errors of metabolism in British Columbia, 1969–1996. Pediatrics 2000;105:e10.
70. Paine RS. The variability in manifestations of untreated patients with phenylketonuria (phenylpyruvic acidosis). Pediatrics 1969;19:1007–1011.
71. Lutcke A, Bickel H. Electroencephalographic manifestations of cerebral attacks and intellectual development in phenylketonuria. Electroencephalogr Clin Neurophysiol 1969;27:625.
72. McGovern MM, Desnick RJ. Lysosomal Storage Diseases. In L Goldman, JC Bennett (eds), Cecil Textbook of Medicine (21st ed). Philadelphia: Saunders, 2000;1104–1107.
73. Higgins JJ, Patterson MC, Dambrosia JM, et al. A clinical staging classification for type C Niemann-Pick disease. Neurology 1992;42:2286–2290.
74. Andersson HC, Shapira E. The Mucopolysaccharidoses. In L Goldman, JC Bennett (eds), Cecil Textbook of Medicine (21st ed). Philadelphia: Saunders, 2000;1116–1118.
75. Anderson KE. The Porphyrias. In L Goldman, JC Bennett (eds), Cecil Textbook of Medicine (21st ed). Philadelphia: Saunders, 2000;1123–1130.
76. Bloomer JR. The hepatic porphyrias: pathogenesis, manifestations, and management. Gastroenterology 1976;71:689–701.
77. Pierach CA, Edwards PS. Neurotoxicity of delta-aminolevulinic acid and porphobilinogen. Exp Neurol 1978;62:810–814.
78. Bloomer JR, Bonkovsky HL. The porphyrias. Dis Mon 1989;35:1–54.
79. Mustajoki P, Kauppinen R, Lannfelt L, et al. Frequency of low erythrocyte porphobilinogen deaminase activity in Finland. J Intern Med 1992;231:389–395.
80. Tschudy DP, Valsamis M, Magnussen CR. Acute intermittent porphyria: clinical and selected research aspects. Ann Intern Med 1974;83:851–864.
81. Burgovne K, Swartz R, Ananth J. Porphyria: reexamination of psychiatric implications. Psychother Psychosom 1995;64:121–130.
82. Tishler PV, Woodward B, O'Connor J, et al. High prevalence of intermittent acute porphyria in a psychiatric patient population. Am J Psychiatry 1985;142:1430–1436.
83. Kaplan PW, Lewis DV. Juvenile acute intermittent porphyria with hypercholesterolemia and epilepsy: a case report and review of the literature. J Child Neurol 1986;1:38–45.
84. Birchfield RI, Cowger ML. Acute intermittent porphyria with seizures. Anticonvulsant medication-induced metabolic changes. Am J Dis Child 1966;112:561–565.
85. Reynolds NC, Miska RM. Safety of anticonvulsants in hepatic porphyrias. Neurology 1981;31:480–484.
86. Bylesjo I, Forsgren L, Lithner F, Boman K. Epidemiology and clinical characteristics of seizures in patients with acute intermittent porphyria. Epilepsia 1996;37:230–235.
87. Bonkovsky HL, Barnard GF. Diagnosis of porphyric syndromes: a practical approach in the era of molecular biology. Semin Liver Dis 1998;18:57–65.
88. Kalman DR, Bonkovsky HL. Management of acute attacks in the porphyrias. Clin Dermatol 1998;16:299–306.
89. Tenhunen R, Mustajoki P. Acute porphyria: treatment with heme. Semin Liver Dis 1998;18:53–55.
90. Sergay SM. Management of neurologic exacerbations of hepatic porphyria. Med Clin North Am 1979;63:453–463.
91. Hahn M, Gildemeister OS, Krauss GL, et al. Effects of new anticonvulsant medications on porphyrin synthesis in cultured liver cells: potential implications for patients with acute porphyria. Neurology 1997;49:97–106.
92. Krauss GL, Simmons-O'Brien E, Campbell M. Successful treatment of seizures and porphyria with gabapentin. Neurology 1995;45:594–595.
93. Lambrecht RW, Gildemeister OS, Williams A, et al. Effects of selected antihypertensives and analgesics on hepatic porphyrin accumulation: implications for clinical porphyria. Biochem Pharmacol 1999;58:887–896.
94. Lambrecht RW, Gildemeister OS, Pepe JA, et al. Effects of antidepressants and benzodiazepine-type anxiolytic agents on hepatic porphyrin accumulation in primary cultures of chick embryo liver cells. J Pharmacol Exp Ther 1999;291:1150–1155.
95. Wijdicks EF, Sharbrough FW. New-onset seizures in critically ill patients. Neurology 1993;43:1042–1044.

Chapter 11

Hematologic and Pulmonary Disorders

Jehuda P. Sepkuty and Peter W. Kaplan

Hematologic Disorders and Seizures

Hematologic disorders can affect the central and peripheral nervous system in many ways, producing a wide range of neurologic disturbances. When seizures arise because of hematologic dysfunction, the diagnosis of seizure activity is, for the most part, no different than its diagnosis in isolation. The major challenge, however, is in how to manage epilepsy with a particular antiepileptic agent, given its complicating effect on the underlying condition; the agent may worsen the condition or potentially interact with medications used to treat it. Seizures may arise from systemic disorders in a number of ways. One of the most frequently encountered manifestations is when a particular body system has been sufficiently impaired to produce a lowering of the seizure threshold within the brain and the induction of "reactive seizures." In this situation (i.e., renal insufficiency during which a seizure may occur, but where seizure threshold is restored with reversal of renal dysfunction), the problem is largely that of identifying the toxic or metabolic problem triggering seizures and addressing this cause. Once function has been normalized, there is usually little need for future antiepileptic drug (AED) prophylaxis.

A second scenario is when the underlying condition (or some other disorder) has created an enduring state of cortical neuronal instability, such as a stroke with infarction, hemorrhage, or embolus. The focal lesion itself may then trigger seizures "spontaneously" or may do so after a relatively minor degree of systemic insult. This lowering of seizure threshold might not have triggered a seizure had a structural abnormality not been present.

Finally, a number of toxic or metabolic disturbances arising from body system failures may produce impaired cognitive states or confusion by impairing mental status and inducing an encephalopathy. Here, the question may arise as to whether the patient, instead of having partial seizures, is in nonconvulsive status or postictal state.

Confusion in encephalopathy may be further complicated by the appearance of adventitious movements mistaken by the casual observer for ictal events. The movements may arise as a function of the confused state or, more pertinently, by the result of an adventitious movement disorder, such as tremor or myoclonus. In these situations, in which there is an increased clinical suspicion of seizures, the electroencephalogram (EEG) is increasingly essential to establishing a diagnosis of seizures. In our discussion, we concentrate on unique issues that arise in the setting of the combination of hematologic disorders and seizures. We split our discussion of hematologic diseases into their two standard categories—disorders of hematopoiesis and disorders of hemostasis.

Disorders of Hematopoiesis

Anemias Associated with Seizures or Antiepileptic Drugs Affecting Hematopoiesis

Folate Deficiency. Folate deficiency is one of the causes of macrocytic anemia and most commonly affects the central nervous system (CNS) by neuropsychiatric complications,[1] but it does not cause seizures. The association between epilepsy and folate deficiency may occur in the following situations:

1. AEDs, including phenytoin, carbamazepine, and barbiturates, can impair folate absorption. Folic acid levels are reduced in patients taking phenytoin, sometimes resulting in a macrocytic anemia. The mechanism of interaction is complex, but there are data suggesting that pH changes in the gut, induced by phenytoin, affect the enterohepatic circulation of folate.[2]

2. Folic acid supplementation reduces the risk for many types of birth defects. Because some AEDs may lower folic acid levels, women taking these drugs are at an increased risk for birth defects associated with folic acid deficiency. Gestational folate deficiency has been associated with abnormal growth and development in human and experimental animal studies and has been postulated as a mechanism for the teratogenic effects of AEDs. In a prospective study of women with epilepsy, folic acid levels decreased with increasing plasma AED levels and with the number of AEDs. Low blood folate levels before or early in pregnancy were significantly associated with spontaneous abortion and the occurrence of developmental anomalies in the offspring.[3]

3. Folic acid, when given as a supplement, may enhance phenytoin metabolism and break through seizures.[4,5]

PRACTICE GUIDE RECOMMENDATIONS. Folic acid supplementation of 0.8–1.0 mg per day is readily available and relatively inexpensive through over-the-counter or prescription prenatal vitamins. Higher doses of 4 mg per day have been recommended for women with family histories of birth defects or those who have previously delivered an infant with a neural tube defect. This guideline applies to all women, not just those taking AEDs. Women receiving valproate or carbamazepine also may benefit from the 4-mg-per-day dose, because these drugs are more often associated with neural tube defects. When the continued administration of phenytoin is necessary, a daily oral dose of 0.5–1.0 mg of folic acid may be required. Lifelong therapy with folate is only rarely necessary.[6,7]

Folinic acid is the preparation of choice for the treatment of toxicity caused by folate antagonists. These agents inhibit the reduction of folic acid by dihydrofolate reductase; because folinic acid is already fully reduced, it bypasses this metabolic block. The usual dose is 3–15 mg, delivered intramuscularly. Folinic acid has also been used successfully in cases involving congenital dihydrofolate reductase deficiency.[8]

Sickle Cell Disease. Sickle cell disease is an inherited disorder caused by the abnormal properties of red blood cells containing mutant sickle cell hemoglobin. Acute and chronic organ dysfunction, chronic hemolytic anemia, and recurrent painful episodes are the main features of the disease. In the deoxygenated condition, the hemoglobin tetramer polarizes, and the cell shape becomes distorted, resulting in rigid red blood cells. Cell damage leads to hemolytic anemia and to occlusion of vessels in multiple organs, including the brain. The disorder is autosomal recessive and is seen in blacks of African descent. The different sickle cell syndromes that result from distinct inheritance patterns of the sickle cell gene (beta S gene) are divided into sickle cell disease and sickle cell trait. Sickle cell disease is associated with chronic anemia and recurrent pain; the sickle cell trait is largely asymptomatic.[9,10]

FREQUENCY. The prevalence of sickle cell trait is 8–10% among black newborns in the United States and as high as 25–30% in western Africa. In the United States, there are 4,000–5,000 pregnancies at risk for sickle cell disease each year. There are approximately 50,000–60,000 patients with sickle cell disease living in the United States. The incidence of focal or generalized seizures among these sickle cell patients varies from 6% to 12%.[9,10]

ETIOLOGIES AND RISK FACTORS. Seizures can occur with complications of sickle cell disease. Seizures may

- Accompany ischemic or hemorrhagic acute strokes
- Result from a previous stroke (e.g., focal gliotic parenchymal lesion)
- Accompany CNS infections, such as meningitis or meningoencephalitis
- Accompany a systemic infection due to high fever, sepsis, or disseminated intravascular

coagulation (DIC; see section Disseminated Intravascular Coagulation)

- Accompany any metabolic abnormality due to systemic malfunction, such as acidemia or uremia due to renal insufficiency
- Be precipitated by dehydration, as it is a risk factor for sickling
- Be precipitated by medications commonly used for sickle cell disease, such as meperidine (Demerol)

Treatment for seizures may interfere with some aspects of sickle cell disease or its treatment:

1. Folic acid deficiency may arise from repeated episodes of hemolytic anemia. Patients with this condition take 1 mg per day of folic acid, regardless of any anticonvulsants they are taking and the fact that anticonvulsants tend to exacerbate folate deficiency (see preceding section). This especially needs to be taken into consideration in women of childbearing age.

2. The major reproductive concern for patients with sickle cell disease is pregnancy. Fetal complications during pregnancy pertain to impaired placental blood flow and include spontaneous abortion, intrauterine growth retardation, low birth weight, pre-eclampsia, and death.

3. Warfarin and minidose heparin have been advocated in sickle cell disease, and methylprednisolone has been reported to provide pain relief. Hepatic enzyme–inducing AEDs increase steroid and anticoagulant metabolism (see section Anticoagulant and Antiplatelet Therapy). Of concern with bone marrow transplantation (BMT) as treatment for sickle cell anemia, carbamazepine may decrease cyclosporin levels, the main immunosuppressive agent after transplants (see section Bone Marrow Transplantation).[11]

PHENOMENOLOGY. The typical patient is anemic but asymptomatic, except during painful episodes. Most organ systems are subject to vascular occlusion, resulting in the characteristic acute and chronic multisystem failure. Therapeutic interventions are directed at specific complications.

NEUROLOGIC COMPLICATIONS. Stroke is the second leading cause of death after infection, occurring in 5.5–15.0% of homozygous children. The risk of stroke in children with sickle cell disease is 250–400 times that of the general population, with the proba-

bility of stroke by age 40 years approximately 32%. Mean age of development of cerebral infarcts is 8 years, whereas hemorrhage is usually seen in older patients at a mean age of 25 years.[10]

ASSESSMENT AND TREATMENT. Magnetic resonance imaging and transcranial Doppler (TCD) flow studies are useful in detecting subclinical cerebral infarction. The ability to predict strokes by detecting arterial stenosis with TCD and to prevent the occurrence of such strokes with chronic transfusion has led to the recommendation that TCD be used for routine screening and that transfusion be instituted on detection of arterial stenosis.[12–17] Patients with sickle cell anemia may be at particular risk of ischemic cerebral injury in situations associated with hyperventilation, which produces cerebral artery constriction and cerebral hypoxia.[18] Therefore, if the assessment includes EEG, these patients should probably not be hyperventilated.

Based on the presented data, the author's choice for chronic treatment of seizures favors gabapentin, which is less likely to interfere with other drugs or medical conditions, assuming the efficacy suffices to treat as monotherapy. Other choices include lamotrigine or topiramate, based on their side effect profiles and the likelihood of interactions with other drugs commonly administered for this condition. For acute seizure management, diazepam and lorazepam are reasonable choices, and, if needed, phenytoin can be administered for a short time and later changed to another of the chronic AEDs mentioned.

Porphyria. The porphyrias are a group of disorders divided into two categories—the erythropoietic and the hepatic, with the latter marked by neurologic abnormalities and seizures—involving genetic abnormalities, for the most part affecting heme synthesis. The three autosomal-dominant forms with neurologic manifestations are acute intermittent porphyria (AIP), hereditary coproporphyria (HC), and variegata porphyria. In AIP, the most common of the hepatic porphyrias, there is a partial deficiency of porphobilinogen (PBG) deaminase and, therefore, a buildup of delta–aminolevulinic acid (ALA) and PBG, which are excreted in the urine. HC is caused by a partial deficiency of coproporphyrinogen oxidase, and variegata porphyria by a partial deficiency of protoporphyrinogen oxidase. The neurologic manifestations of these disorders are similar and include peripheral neuropathy, autonomic dysfunction, behavioral disturbances, and seizures.[19]

FREQUENCY. AIP occurs in all races. Its prevalence in most countries has not been precisely estimated but may be most common (perhaps 5 per 100,000) in northern European populations.

Seizures may affect 10–20% of patients and are most frequently seen in AIP, sometimes as the presenting feature.[20] Seizures may be focal or generalized[21,22] and typically occur during an acute attack. Status epilepticus (SE) may occur, but it is rare.[22] Seizures in childhood may precede the first attack of an acute porphyria by many years[23,24] and may obscure the diagnosis.

ETIOLOGIES AND RISK FACTORS. The causes of the acute attacks and seizures are not clearly understood. Possible causes for seizures and cerebral dysfunction include the following:

1. It may relate to γ-aminobutyric acid receptor binding by ALA,[25] which causes seizures when infused directly into rat brain.[20]
2. Defects in hepatic heme synthesis can affect levels of neurotransmitters, such as tryptophan.[20]
3. Patients with acute porphyric attacks may also have seizures because of fluid and electrolyte disturbances, usually from excessive vomiting and inappropriate secretion of antidiuretic hormone (e.g., causing hyponatremia or hypomagnesemia, or both).[19]
4. Cerebral ischemia, as evidenced by reports of cortical blindness, could provide foci for seizure activity.[26,27,28]
5. Idiopathic or symptomatic epilepsy may coexist with porphyria,[19,28] in which case AED treatment may be required as chronic treatment.
6. Most AEDs are porphyrinogenic; although the pathogenesis of acute porphyric attacks is complex and not completely understood, an obligatory feature is the induction of hepatic ALA synthase. The depletion of a small but critical regulatory heme pool in hepatocytes accounts for this induction.[29] The rate of depletion of this heme pool, in turn, is increased by induction of cytochrome P-450. Numerous drugs induce cytochrome P-450; among such agents are most of the commonly used AEDs.[31,32] This is particularly problematic, because acute porphyrias are epileptogenic,[33,34] and the AEDs are porphyrinogenic.

PHENOMENOLOGY. Symptoms rarely occur before puberty and almost never recur in adult life. Attacks last for several days or longer, often require hospitalization, and are followed by complete recovery. Abdominal pain is the most common symptom. Autonomic manifestations of sympathetic over-activity include tachycardia, hypertension, restlessness, fine tremors, and excess sweating. Other manifestations include nausea and vomiting; constipation; pain in the limbs, head, neck, or chest; muscle weakness; and sensory loss. Ileus with distention and decreased bowel sounds is common. Recurrent attacks tend to be similar in a specific patient. Peripheral motor neuropathy leads to weakness, beginning most commonly in the proximal muscles. Tendon reflexes may be little affected or hyperactive in the early stages but are usually decreased or absent with advanced neuropathy, and cranial and sensory nerves can be affected. Sudden death, presumably from cardiac arrhythmia, may also occur. Other CNS manifestations are anxiety, insomnia, depression, disorientation, hallucinations, and paranoia. (For seizures, see preceding section.) Hyponatremia may be due to CNS involvement, vomiting, diarrhea, poor food intake, or excess renal sodium loss. Pain, depression, and other symptoms are sometimes chronic. Chronic hepatic abnormalities are common in AIP, and affected patients have an increased risk of hepatocellular carcinoma. AIP may predispose to chronic hypertension and be associated with impaired renal function.[33,34]

PRECIPITATING FACTORS. Precipitating factors include drugs (mostly P-450 inducers), progesterone, dietary restriction, intercurrent infections, major surgery, and other conditions. Recognition of precipitating factors is important in management, although published information is insufficient to allow most drugs to be classified as definitely harmful or safe. The major drugs known to be harmful in the acute porphyrias are barbiturates, sulfonamides, meprobamate, carisoprodol, glutethimide, methyprylon, ethocylorvynol, pyrazolones, griseofulvin, ergots, metoclopramide, rifampin, pyrazinamide, nonsteroidal anti-inflammatory drugs, progesterone, danazol, alcohol, and most AEDs (e.g., phenytoin, succinimides [ethosuximide, methsuximide], carbamazepine, primidone, valproic acid and, from in vitro data, felbamate, lamotrigine, and tiagabine).[28] Barbiturates and sulfonamides are the most notorious, whereas benzodiazepines are much less hazardous. The major drugs known to be safe are narcotic analgesics, aspirin, acetaminophen, phenothiazines, penicillin and its derivatives, streptomycin, insulin, glucocorticoids, atropine, cimetidine, ranitidine, erythropoietin, estrogens, and the antiepileptic bromides, as well as gabapentin and vigabatrin from in vitro culture data and isolated cases.[28,33]

DIAGNOSIS AND DIFFERENTIAL DIAGNOSIS. Any patient with acute or intermittent psychiatric or neurologic disturbances, particularly in a family history, is a candidate for diagnosis with AIP. The diagnosis is established by demonstrating a marked increase in urinary PBG by quantitative assay. ALA and PBG excretions generally decrease with clinical improvement and are particularly dramatic (temporarily) after heme therapy. In screening family members, serum PBG deaminase and urinary PBG should be measured. A normal result of a quantitative test for urinary PBG virtually excludes AIP as a cause of the acute symptoms.[33]

TREATMENT AND PROGNOSIS. Seizures occurring during acute attacks of porphyria are managed by hospitalization and treatment of the underlying porphyrinogenic metabolic defect. This includes intravenous administration of 10% dextrose solution; infusions of hematin or hemearginate[20,35]; correction of underlying metabolic abnormalities; and treatment of severe pain, nausea, and vomiting, using medications from the aforementioned safe-drug list. Heme therapy and carbohydrate loading are more case-specific therapies, because they repress hepatic ALA synthase and overproduction of ALA and PBG. The standard regimen for heme therapy is 3–4 mg heme per kg body weight infused intravenously once daily for 4 days. Carbohydrate loading may suffice for mild attacks and can be administered orally as sucrose, glucose polymers, or carbohydrate-rich foods. If oral intake is poorly tolerated or is contraindicated by distention and ileus, intravenous administration of glucose (at least 300 g daily) is usually indicated. A central venous line facilitates more complete parenteral nutrition support and avoids excess fluid volumes.[33]

Most traditional AEDs, listed previously, are porphyrinogenic. Magnesium sulfate has been successfully used for acute seizures.[22,36] The target serum-magnesium concentration is 2.5–7.5 mEq/liter. Side effects of magnesium sulfate include neuromuscular blockade with weakness, loss of tendon reflexes, and, eventually, respiratory suppression. Other authors prefer lorazepam, diazepam, and paraldehyde,[37] but their use remains controversial.[36] Choices for the chronic treatment of recurrent seizures are also limited. Previously, bromides were commonly recommended, despite their toxicity and narrow therapeutic index (serum bromide target concentration should not exceed 90 mg/dl),[36] but if seizures continue, a careful trial of standard AEDs may be indicated.[19,21,36] The first choices are gabapentin or vigabatrin.[28] Gabapentin has the advantage of being excreted unmetabolized by the kidneys, and it does not induce hepatic enzymes. It was used successfully in a case of porphyria cutanea tarda.[38] Vigabatrin, like gabapentin, does not induce hepatic enzymes, but is not approved by the U.S. Food and Drug Administration. Levels of urinary ALA and PBG should be followed closely during therapy.

If acute attacks are treated appropriately, inciting factors are removed, and precautions are taken to prevent further attacks, the outlook for patients with AIP is usually excellent. Occasional chronic pain symptoms and depression increase the risk of suicide and thus require careful management.

Other types of porphyrias are less often associated with seizures. However, except for the clinical manifestations that are unique to AIP, as covered in this section, the causes for seizures, the porphyrinogenic effect of AEDs, and the management should be the same. Clinically, patients with variegate porphyria and HC patients have cutaneous lesions, in addition to the neuropsychiatric syndrome seen in AIP. In porphyria cutanea tarda and protoporphyria, the clinical manifestations reflect hepatic disease with cutaneous lesions, and in hepatoerythropoietic porphyria, only cutaneous lesions occur.

Aplastic Anemia. Total destruction of the hematopoietic elements leads to the clinical entity known as *aplastic anemia*. Aplastic anemia can arise by several mechanisms—immunologic, infectious, constitutional, idiopathic, and physicochemical. In this chapter, we limit our discussion to chemically mediated aplastic anemia induced by AEDs.

FREQUENCY. The incidence of aplastic anemia is approximately two per million in Europe and Israel, four per 1 million in Bangkok, and higher in rural Thailand.[39] Mortality statistics indicate an equal gender ratio and a preponderance in the elderly, but at referral centers the median age is approximately 25 years. Among patients treated with AEDs, the incidence is higher. A cohort study by Blackburn et al.[40] shows the overall rate of blood dyscrasias as three to four per 100,000 prescriptions over a period of almost 4 years and includes dyscrasias other than aplastic anemia only. The authors of the study concluded that the risk of serious hematologic abnormalities with AEDs was very low (it was published in 1990, before the introduction of felbamate). Thirty-one reported cases of aplastic anemia associated with the taking of felbamate were analyzed by Kaufman et al.[41] Other attributable agents were found as possible contributors in these cases. The authors calculated a best case estimate of 27 cases per million and a worst case estimate of 209 cases per million.

ETIOLOGIES AND RISK FACTORS. Drugs can cause dose-related bone marrow suppression or idiosyncratic suppression. Idiosyncratic bone marrow suppression is a life-threatening event. These reactions are not dose related or related to the duration of administration and cannot be predicted by repeated blood draws.[42–44] Patients with a history of serious drug reactions, immune-mediated diseases, or any underlying systemic abnormalities are more susceptible to idiosyncratic reactions. All major AEDs except gabapentin are listed as possibly inducing idiosyncratic aplastic anemia: felbamate, carbamazepine, phenytoin, valproate, ethosuximide, phenobarbital, lamotrigine, and primidone.[45] The AEDs that are primarily known to be associated with very rare bone marrow suppression are felbamate, carbamazepine, phenytoin, and valproate, which is usually associated with reversible damage.[46] Methylphenylethylhydantoin (mesantoin) and trimethadione have been reported[47–52] as risk factors, but these are no longer first-line AEDs. Most of the above drugs were developed primarily for epilepsy, but, with the exception of felbamate, they are also used for other disorders (e.g., bipolar and other mood disorders, painful neuropathies, trigeminal neuralgia).

The use of felbamate was the subject of an inquiry by a practice advisory panel,[53] which reviewed the drug's use, indications, and contraindications, and issued the following set of recommendations for when to use (or not use) the drug based on a risk to benefit ratio.

A. Patients for whom the risk to benefit ratio supports use because there is class I evidence for benefit:
1. Lennox-Gastaut patients over the age of 4 years who are unresponsive to primary AEDs
2. Those patients older than 18 years of age who have intractable partial seizures and in whom the use of standard AEDs at therapeutic levels has failed (data indicate a better risk to benefit ratio for felbamate used as monotherapy)
3. Patients who have been on felbamate more than 18 months

B. Patients for whom the current risk to benefit assessment does not support the use of felbamate:
1. Adults or children with new-onset epilepsy
2. Patients who have experienced significant prior hematologically adverse events
3. Patients in whom follow-up and compliance do not allow careful monitoring
4. Patients unable to discuss risks to benefits (i.e., with mental retardation, developmental disability) and for whom no parent or legal guardian is available to provide consent

C. Patients in whom the risk to benefit ratio is unclear, and based on case reports and expert opinion (class III) only, but under certain circumstances depending on the nature and severity of the patient's seizure disorder, felbamate use may be appropriate:
1. Children with intractable partial epilepsy
2. Other generalized epilepsies unresponsive to primary agents
3. Patients who experience unacceptable sedative or cognitive side effects with traditional AEDs
4. Patients with Lennox-Gastaut syndrome younger than 4 years of age who are unresponsive to other AEDs[53]

PHENOMENOLOGY. Clinically, patients with aplastic anemia present signs of bone marrow failure. They have hemorrhages and purpura secondary to thrombocytopenia, are weak and pale because of anemia, and tend to have infections as the result of leukopenia. The course of the disease is determined by the severity of the bone marrow suppression.

DIAGNOSIS. Laboratory investigations may reveal pancytopenia with normal blood cell morphology. Bone marrow biopsy reveals a fatty hypocellular marrow.

TREATMENT. Therapy entails stopping the offending drug while supporting the patient during the period of pancytopenia. Treatment dilemmas include whether to observe the patient or initiate aggressive therapies, such as immunosuppression or BMT.[54] Data suggest that transfusions increase the likelihood of graft-versus-host reaction and rejection. A compromise approach is to wait a week and repeat bone marrow biopsy to see whether there are signs of recovery. If there is no marrow recovery, then aggressive and definitive therapy is indicated. Aplastic anemia is not itself epileptogenic, but if it occurs in an epilepsy patient and the epilepsy is concurrent with the aplastic anemia, the seizures need to be treated. For the acute management of such seizures, diazepam and lorazepam are reasonable choices. Gabapentin is a good choice for chronic treatment, if it controls the seizures. Other possibilities include lamotrigine, tiagabine, topiramate, and, lately, levetiracetam and zonisamide. Although phenobarbital has been very rarely associated with aplastic anemia, and oxcarbazepine is "hematologically safe," so far they are not necessarily good choices in this particular case owing to their possibilities of interaction with the immunosuppressant medications (steroids and cyclosporine[55–57]) that are likely to be part of the treatment for aplastic anemia (see section Bone Marrow Transplantation).

Proliferative Disorders

Blood cells are classified as being myeloid (including erythrocyte, granulocyte, and monocyte cells and platelets) or lymphoid (including all leukocyte [white blood] cells). Hematologic malignancies are classified accordingly into myeloproliferative or lymphoproliferative disorders. In this chapter, we refer to disorders of the blood as a whole group and look at the associations between it and epilepsy.[58]

Frequency. The CNS is involved in an estimated 2–4% of leukemia patients per month, a poor prognostic sign.[59] The most common leukemia in the United States is B-cell chronic lymphocytic leukemia, and the occurrence of a nonzoster neurologic complication is 1 per 1,000 patients. The lymphomas (Hodgkin's and non-Hodgkin's) only rarely affect the nervous system, and only 1% or fewer of non-Hodgkin's lymphomas present with CNS involvement. In myelomatosis, the nervous system is commonly involved, but cranial myeloma is rare, and direct infiltration of myeloma cells into the brain is extremely rare.[60]

Etiologies and Risk Factors. Seizures can be a complication associated with the proliferative disorders owing to several possible etiologies: leukemia, lymphoma, and myelomatosis.

LEUKEMIA

1. Direct infiltration of the meninges by leukemia cells.[60,61]
2. Localized leukemic deposits with focal manifestations.[62]
3. Intracranial hemorrhage associated with thrombocytopenia and, occasionally, DIC. Impaired platelet production secondary to leukemic bone marrow infiltration or myelotoxic effects, or both, of chemotherapeutic agents.[59]
4. Cellular hyperviscosity.
5. Cerebral venous thrombosis, most notably superior sagittal sinus thrombosis, occurs relatively frequently in patients treated with L-asparaginase[63,64] and may cause either infarction or hemorrhage. Headache and seizures are the most common manifestations of cerebral venous thrombosis.
6. CNS infections due to immunosuppression and the underlying disease. Occasional septic fungal emboli.
7. Cranial irradiation.
8. Chemotherapy: vincristine, prednisone, intrathecal methotrexate, mercaptopurine, cytarabine, cyclophosphamide, doxorubicin, and L-asparaginase.
9. Systemic metabolic imbalance (e.g., electrolyte disorder).
10. Complication of BMT (see section Bone Marrow Transplantation).

LYMPHOMA. Risk factors for seizures are essentially the same as for leukemia:

1. Cerebrovascular complications are much less common compared to leukemia. Intracerebral

hemorrhage caused by thrombocytopenia occasionally occurs. Cerebral infarction occurs more commonly and may be associated with DIC or nonbacterial thrombotic endocarditis.

2. Septic emboli and superior sagittal sinus thrombosis from direct infiltration or compression by lymphoma may also occur. Radiation therapy is indicated for venous sinus infiltration.

3. A few unusual cerebrovascular complications can occur. Varicella zoster, which is common in patients with Hodgkin's disease, may be associated with ipsilateral hemispheric infarction when the ophthalmic division of the trigeminal nerve is affected.[65] Patients who have Hodgkin's disease may also develop focal granulomatous angiitis of the CNS.[63]

MYELOMATOSIS.   Hypercalcemia and uremia that accompany myeloma[59] can cause confusion, headaches, uremic convulsions, somnolence, myoclonic twitches, and coma.

ASSESSMENT AND TREATMENT.   Antiepileptic medications can interfere with the underlying disease process and its treatment. Before treating a patient with any AED, a thorough assessment should take place. If the underlying cause is an electrolyte disturbance alone, there is no need for AEDs. If the patient is on chemotherapy—for instance, vincristine, intrathecal methotrexate,[66,67] cytarabine, ifosfamide, L-asparaginase, or cyclosporine[68]—then consulting the hematologist regarding possible discontinuation or decrease in dosage may be sufficient. Any reversible cause for a seizure should be excluded, including other medications that are not directly associated with the underlying hematologic disease, such as a new epileptogenic antidepressant (e.g., bupropion). If the seizure is associated with structural damage (e.g., hemorrhage, septic emboli), the seizures need to be treated acutely, and long-term treatment is also recommended. Acutely, benzodiazepines may be used; for long-term therapy, valproate and phenytoin are associated with thrombocytopenia that may, theoretically, increase the risk of intracranial hemorrhage. Carbamazepine and phenytoin are associated with possible idiosyncratic reactions that are more likely in the setting of hematologic disease and underlying immune suppression; phenobarbital is a sedative; and carbamazepine and phenobarbital may interact with cyclosporine and steroids, which are crucial after BMT. Methotrex-

ate is a folate antagonist that, when given in combination with AEDs, may cause severe folate deficiency. Folinic acid is the preparation of choice for the treatment of toxicity caused by folate antagonists (see previous section Folate Deficiency). Gabapentin, lamotrigine, tiagabine, and vigabatrin (which is not approved in the United States) are good alternatives. Newer antiepileptics, such as levetiracetam, oxcarbazepine, and zonisamide, are now available in the United States, but there is little, if any, experience using them for these conditions.

Bone Marrow Transplantation

Neurologic complications occur in 50–70% of patients undergoing allogenic BMT[63,69–71] and less often in patients undergoing autologous BMT.[69,72] The most common acute neurologic complication in BMT patients is a toxic or metabolic encephalopathy.[73] Seizures are frequent in transplant recipients who are at risk because of their underlying disease, perioperative metabolic abnormalities, and postoperative complications.

Frequency.   Seizures occur in 12–16% of BMT patients,[70] but the incidence of seizures after BMT is 3.0–11.5%.[20,74] Children are at greater risk than adults for post-transplant seizures.[20,56,75–77] Seizures are more frequent in the early phase, after receiving the organ transplant.[78]

Etiology and Risk Factors.   Many factors contribute to the etiology of seizures in transplant patients. Seizures may be associated with chemotherapy, irradiation before the transplant, systemic factors, and disease relapse, as with cases of leukemia.

Risk factors may be classified into three main groups: structural, metabolic, and iatrogenic. If the seizure is focal at onset, the cause is more likely to be structural in origin. Possible structural causes in BMT patients include ischemic stroke, intracranial localized hemorrhage, venous thrombosis, and septic embolus. Seizures frequently manifest in transplanted patients without signs of structural lesions.[69] Metabolic failure, with attendant electrolyte disturbances or uremia, should be excluded. Iatrogenic causes may occur.[78] Busulfan before the transplant and cyclosporine A (CSA) treatment may have been implicated.[79–81] Seizures induced by CSA are not associated with the level of the drug and are thought to result from CSA metabolites.[82] Various potentiating factors for CSA-induced seizures reported include high-dose steroid therapy,[79,83,84] hypertension,[85] hypomagnesemia,[86] hypocholesterolemia,[87] and microangiopathic hemolytic anemia. Other immunosuppressive agents—FK506 and OkT3[20,88,89]—are associated with post-transplant seizures. Infections may result from immunosuppression and cause seizures.

Assessment and Treatment. Because of the multiplicity of causes of seizure, a careful evaluation may be required. A head magnetic resonance image can exclude structural etiologies; laboratory tests delineate possible electrolyte or metabolic disturbances, hematologic data, and drug levels; CSF analysis evaluates infection; and EEG attempts to differentiate a focal from a generalized process. AEDs should be considered only after ruling out reversible causes (see section Myeloproliferative Diseases). Older literature suggests using phenobarbital rather than phenytoin or valproate in post-transplant patients for the first 2–6 weeks after transplantation, until the successful engraftment of the bone marrow.[20,56] Carbamazepine can be associated with myelosuppression, whereas valproate is potentially hepatotoxic and can exacerbate thrombocytopenia. All hepatic enzyme inducers (e.g., phenytoin, carbamazepine, and phenobarbital) enhance the metabolism of steroids and CSA, so a 25–30% increase in corticosteroid dosage is recommended,[20,55–57] along with an increase in the CSA serum concentration.[56] Newer agents, such as gabapentin, tiagabine, lamotrigine, and vigabatrin, may be good alternatives with a relative lack of hematologic, cognitive, and sedative properties and drug interaction.

Disorders of Hemostasis

Disorders of the Platelet and Vessel Wall

Thrombotic Thrombocytopenic Purpura. Thrombotic thrombocytopenic purpura (TTP) is an uncommon but serious disorder of young adults. The disorder is characterized by hemolytic anemia due to red cell fragmentation, thrombocytopenia, and a combination of clinical findings, including CNS dysfunction, fever, and renal failure. The clinical and laboratory manifestations are the results of microvascular thrombotic lesions that characterize this disease. Hemolytic uremic syndrome (HUS), primarily a pediatric disorder, includes thrombocytopenia, hemolytic anemia, and renal disease. Fever and neurologic dysfunction occur often.[90,91] TTP and HUS can be grouped as thrombotic microangiopathies because of their similar pathophysiologies.[90] Pathologically, there is hyperplasia of endothelial cells in arterioles and capillaries, along with hyaline and platelet-rich thrombi in these vessels and occasional microaneurysms. These endothelial cells release von Willebrand factor multimers, which may play a role in the pathogenesis of TTP.[92,93] The pathologic changes of TTP are most common in the brain, pancreas, kidney, heart, spleen, and adrenal glands,[94] but may be found throughout the body; the brain stem vessels and the cortical gray matter are often affected.

FREQUENCY. The peak incidence of TTP occurs in persons in their thirties and occurs twice as often in women as in men. There is evidence to suggest a genetic susceptibility to the development of thrombotic microangiopathies manifesting as TTP or HUS in siblings.[95–98] Approximately 50% of TTP patients present with neurologic symptoms, and 90% develop neurologic manifestations during the course of the disease.[90,100] In approximately 20% of TTP patients[99] and 40% of HUS patients[101] observed, focal or generalized seizures occurred.

ETIOLOGIES AND RISK FACTORS. Seizures can be a complication associated with these disorders for several reasons:

1. Vascular damage in cortical regions may create seizure focus or foci.

2. Metabolic imbalance (e.g., uremia, hyponatremia, fever).[90,101–103]

3. Cerebral hemorrhage due to thrombocytopenia.[102]

4. Underlying cause for TTP-like infections, drugs as CSA or FK506,[100] connective tissue diseases, and cancer, among other factors, can cause seizures as a risk factor independently of their association with TTP or HUS.

5. Garrett et al. reported that among TTP patients examined, at least 10% had nonconvulsive status epilepticus (NCSE). NCSE can mimic a common manifestation of TTP marked by fluctuat-

ing mental status and level of consciousness. TTP patients are at increased risk for NCSE owing to the tendency of NCSE to develop after generalized tonic-clonic seizures.[100,104,105] Having other underlying medical complications characterized by severe encephalopathy places patients at additional risk for NCSE. The test of choice for confirming a diagnosis of NCSE, which is a treatable condition, is EEG.

PHENOMENOLOGY. CNS involvement in TTP presents frequently as fluctuating focal neurologic deficits and changes in the level of consciousness, which result from either NCSE, transient small vessel occlusions with recanalization, or underlying metabolic disorders; these common neurologic symptoms may develop and progress rapidly. Other neurologic manifestations can include headache, cranial nerve palsies, dysphasia or aphasia, paresis, confusion, stupor, coma, and seizures (see previous discussion). TTP is characterized by the pentad of microangiopathic hemolytic anemia, thrombocytopenia, neurologic symptoms, renal dysfunction, and fever.[93] Purpura and retinal are the most common types of hemorrhages.

ASSESSMENT AND DIFFERENTIAL DIAGNOSIS. TTP must be included in the differential diagnosis of any patient with intravascular hemolysis caused by red cell fragmentation. The reticulocyte count is increased and correlates with the severity of the anemia. Hemolysis laboratory parameters are typical. Lactate dehydrogenase levels and platelet count are sensitive indicators of the response to therapy. Proteinuria, microscopic hematuria, mild azotemia, and liver function test abnormalities are common. Cerebrospinal fluid usually reveals increased protein levels and xanthochromia; less often, it is bloody. Brain computed tomography shows characteristic multiple hypodense lesions.[106,107] A biopsy of skin, gingivae, and bone marrow may be examined for hyaline thrombi within arterioles.[108,109] Biopsies are diagnostic in only approximately 50% of cases and are not specific.

DIFFERENTIAL DIAGNOSIS. Eclampsia in pregnant women may present with similar manifestations. Eclampsia, however, has a favorable prognosis and may be associated with low-grade intravascular coagulation. Other mimickers of TTP include systemic lupus erythematosus with immune thrombocytopenic purpura and vasculitis and severe idiopathic thrombocytopenic purpura with autoim-

mune hemolytic anemia. However, TTP can occur in lupus patients and often carries a poor prognosis. Some authors[100,104] emphasize the importance of EEG in these cases to rule out NCSE, particularly in patients with persistent or recurrent confusion and stupor, especially after a clinically overt seizure.

TREATMENT. More than 80% of patients who are treated aggressively with exchange plasmapheresis now survive the initial episode of TTP,[93,109,110] although presenting conditions cannot predict definitively which patients have favorable outcomes. The therapeutic effects of plasmapheresis in the critically ill patient with TTP are often dramatic: Severe neurologic manifestations may disappear, and laboratory abnormalities may diminish in a few hours. In a controlled prospective therapeutic trial of this disease, plasma exchange was significantly more effective than infusion without exchange.[111] Platelet transfusions should be avoided, because patients found marked deterioration in either renal or neurologic status during platelet transfusions.[112] The treatment of seizures in such settings is the same as for other complicated hematologic disorders:

1. No treatment is necessary if a reversible cause is identified.
2. Benzodiazepines can be given acutely.
3. The nature of chronic treatment depends on the type of injured systems. If renal function is severely impaired, medications that are metabolized in the kidney—gabapentin, levetiracetam, oxcarbazepine, topiramate, and vigabatrin—are probably not good choices. Agents that can potentially cause thrombocytopenia, hemorrhage, or bone marrow suppression are more risky, such as valproic acid and carbamazepine. Side effects of medications, such as topiramate and phenobarbital, that are associated with cognitive side effects and sedation may be difficult to differentiate from the fluctuating confusion of symptoms underlying the basic disease. The side effect profiles of lamotrigine and phenytoin seem somewhat better for the considerations listed previously. If phenytoin is prescribed, protein binding needs to be taken into consideration. In the context of proteinuria or hypoalbuminemia, the bound fraction of phenytoin may decrease (normally, 90% of protein is bound) and the unbound fraction increases, which in turn can cause toxicity. Thus, the free phenytoin

levels need to be monitored; the therapeutic range of free phenytoin is 1–2 µg/ml.

Hemolytic Uremic Syndrome.

HUS is primarily a disorder of infants and young children and rarely occurs in adults. Like TTP, microangiopathic hemolytic anemia is present in HUS, but thrombocytopenia is milder, and neurologic abnormalities are not frequent. Acute renal failure is a prominent feature of HUS, with a need for frequent hemodialysis. Severe hypertension and gastrointestinal signs and symptoms are prominent features. HUS may occur in women in the post-partum period or in women taking oral contraceptives. Cancer patients receiving mitomycin or cisplatin chemotherapy may also develop HUS. Sheth et al. have shown that the most common neurologic manifestations are seizures, mainly generalized tonic-clonic convulsions, but occasionally focal ones.[91] Seizure management and evaluation are the same as for TTP. One factor that should be taken further into account is how likely the AED is to be removed from plasma during hemodialysis. Phenytoin is not significantly removed during hemodialysis, so no adjustment is needed. Twenty percent of lamotrigine is removed after 4 hours of hemodialysis; phenobarbital, ethosuximide, and gabapentin need adjustment after dialysis (source: package inserts of the listed medications).

Disorders of Coagulation

Hemorrhagic Disease of the Newborn.

A hemorrhagic disorder can occur during the neonatal period. Intracranial hemorrhage is the most severe complication of hemorrhagic disease of the newborn and occurs mainly after breech deliveries; subarachnoid and subdural are the most common among intracranial hemorrhages. In neonates born to mothers receiving AEDs, this disorder is more frequent and severe, which is thought to be the result of AEDs crossing the placenta and lowering vitamin K levels in the newborn, and occurs with the enzyme-inducing agents phenytoin, carbamazepine, phenobarbital, primidone, and ethosuximide (Zarontin), and even in women with epilepsy taking no AEDs. Among the new AEDs, lamotrigine, oxcarbazepine, tiagabine, and topiramate are mild inducers of liver enzymes. Prophylactic treatment consists of vitamin K administered orally as 10 mg daily to the mother from the thirty-sixth week of gestation, and 1 mg administered intramuscularly or intravenously to the newborn at birth.[7,59]

Disseminated Intravascular Coagulation.

DIC can be caused by many serious disorders. DIC is a process in which the coagulation system is abnormally activated to form excess fibrin. There is a consumption of clotting factors and platelets, and afterward there is activation of fibrinolysis. The fibrin-platelet thrombi cause necrosis or ischemia of tissue due to the vascular obstruction, leading to symptoms. Bleeding can also result from consumption of clotting factors in excess of the liver's capacity to synthesize them, as well as the use of platelets in excess of capacity of the bone marrow to compensate; the anticoagulant properties of fibrin degradation products may also contribute to bleeding. DIC is most frequently associated with obstetrical catastrophes (e.g., abruptio placenta, amniotic fluid embolism), massive trauma, metastatic malignancy, and bacterial sepsis.[59,113]

ETIOLOGIES AND RISK FACTORS. Seizures can be a complication associated with DIC owing to many possible etiologies:

1. Focal or multifocal thrombi or emboli causing ischemia and structural lesions.
2. Intracranial bleeding of the subarachnoid, intracerebral, or intraventricular spaces.
3. The underlying etiology of the DIC, such as head trauma, infection with spread to CNS, high fever, and leukemia, can trigger a seizure.
4. Electrolyte or metabolic abnormality due to renal or liver dysfunction.

There are reports suggesting a causal association between severe seizures, especially SE and DIC[113–116] and suggesting that DIC is possibly a result of SE and caused by seizure-induced hyperpyrexia. The authors suggest close monitoring of hyperpyrexia during severe seizures and SE to prevent the development of DIC.[116] There are occasional reports suggesting that lamotrigine might directly cause DIC.[117,118]

PHENOMENOLOGY. The most common clinical finding in acute, uncompensated DIC is bleeding. Bleeding can be limited, but it can also be generalized in more severe cases, including diffuse oozing from mucosal surfaces and orifices. Thrombotic complications of DIC occur more often with chronic underlying diseases; the coexistence of liver disease enhances the severity of DIC. Low-grade DIC is often asymptomatic and diagnosed only by laboratory-collected values.

ASSESSMENT AND DIAGNOSIS. The laboratory diagnosis of acute DIC is based on prolongation of the prothrombin time, activated partial thromboplastin time, and thrombin time, due to consumption of clotting factors and inhibition of their function. There can also exist a condition of thrombocytopenia, which is caused by the consumption of platelets. Increased titers of fibrin degradation products can be measured due to resultant fibrinolysis. Schistocytes may be seen in the peripheral blood smear, but this is neither sensitive for nor specific to DIC. A chronic DIC condition is more difficult to diagnose, and the most difficult differential diagnosis of DIC is in patients with coexisting liver disease.

TREATMENT. Identifying and eliminating the underlying cause is the key to successful treatment of DIC. In actively bleeding patients or patients with a high risk of bleeding, the supportive treatment of choice is platelet transfusion to remedy thrombocytopenia and fresh-frozen plasma to replace consumed coagulation factors.

Treatment of seizures depends on the underlying disorder causing the DIC. The possible effects of valproic acid on thrombocytes makes it theoretically a less-favorable agent for such cases; valproate may adversely affect not only the number but also the function of platelets.[119] In the case of infection as the cause for DIC, the respondent antibiotic or antifungal treatment may interfere with some of the AEDs; for example, some antifungal agents are hepatic enzyme inhibitors and therefore may slow the metabolism of AEDs, whose buildup is then more likely to cause toxicity. The same is true for some antibiotics: Erythromycin and clarithromycin inhibit hepatic metabolism and can cause carbamazepine toxicity. When anticoagulants are being considered, interactions with AEDs need to be evaluated. In the case of liver failure, an AED that is metabolized in the kidney would be preferable, such as gabapentin, topiramate, vigabatrin, oxcarbazepine, or levetiracetam.

Anticoagulant and Antiplatelet Therapy

Anticoagulation carries risks, but even more so for patients with epilepsy or on AEDs:

1. When using heparin, the patient should be monitored for thrombocytopenia. AEDs that can cause thrombocytopenia or platelet dysfunction should not be considered as a first choice, and if the patient is already taking such an agent, the platelets should be monitored even more frequently. Prescribing anticoagulants chronically to epilepsy patients is risky, regardless of the AEDs taken, because of the increased risk of falling and bleeding; a fall in which head trauma is sustained while on anticoagulants increases the likelihood of intracranial bleeding.

2. AEDs that induce hepatic enzymes (phenytoin, carbamazepine, phenobarbital, primidone, and ethosuximide and mild inducers, including lamotrigine, oxcarbazepine, tiagabine, and topiramate) enhance the metabolism of warfarin and reduce its efficacy. If an adjustment is made by increasing warfarin and the patient does not comply or forgets to take any AEDs, then the risk of bleeding can increase.

3. AEDs that inhibit hepatic metabolism (i.e., valproate, felbamate, topiramate, and vigabatrin) can theoretically increase the risk of bleeding.

4. Many patients are on aspirin, and some cardiac patients take a combination of aspirin and warfarin. In an epilepsy patient who also has an underlying vascular disease, the risks of falls and drug interactions are increased.

5. Aspirin can increase free valproic acid and phenytoin levels owing to displacement from proteins and thus increase the likelihood of these AEDs, becoming toxic.

Pulmonary Disorders and Seizures

The association between pulmonary disorders and epilepsy is bidirectional: Seizures can cause respiratory abnormalities, and primary respiratory dysfunction can cause seizures. We concentrate on the unique issues that arise in the combination of pulmonary disorders and seizures by dividing our discussion into the following sections: Seizure Disorders Affecting

Respiration and Primary Respiratory Dysfunction Interactions with Seizure Disorders.

Seizure Disorders Affecting Respiration

Generalized Seizures or Status Epilepticus Causing Pulmonary Edema or Central Apnea, or Both

At the onset of generalized seizure activity, there is a sudden significant increase in sympathetic activity, manifested by increased systemic and pulmonary vascular pressure.[120,121] Bayne et al. suggested that transient pulmonary vascular hypertension, leading to transcapillary fluid flux, may explain the pulmonary edema after seizures.[122,123] There is also an association of neurogenic pulmonary edema with sudden unexpected death in epileptic patients (SUDEP).[124] In a recent review manuscript,[125] the author refers to different possible pulmonary mechanisms in SUDEP: The presence of pulmonary edema in SUDEP led to the suggestion that neurogenic pulmonary edema is responsible for SUDEP. The mechanism is thought to be due to increased preload and pulmonary capillary permeability. The latter may be due to hydrostatic mechanisms or directly to an abnormal cortical discharge. This hypothesis is consistent with autopsy findings and reports that death may occur an hour or later after the witnessed seizure. A sheep model of death after bicuculline-induced SE[126] found that pulmonary edema was in fact more extensive in animals that died than in animals that survived. The pulmonary edema was associated with increased left atrial and pulmonary artery pressures.

However, the degree of pulmonary edema was not sufficient to explain the degree of ventilatory failure observed in the animal model of SUDEP.[126] Further studies of eight animals[127] found that central apnea was at least partially responsible for two deaths, whereas cardiac failure related to massive subendocardial necrosis was responsible for the third death. These findings, together with the time course of the ventilatory failure, led to the conclusion that profound central apnea related to the seizure was more often responsible for death than pulmonary edema, at least in this model.[127] A skeptic would point out that this is a model of SE. There is no evidence that seizures responsible for SUDEP are more severe than the patient's characteristic seizures.

Some degree of apnea is quite common during and after epileptic seizures in humans.[128,129] Apnea appears to be central in type, but duration is not particularly long, nor is degree of oxygen desaturation profound. Two case reports of video-EEG monitoring during SUDEP[130,131] have demonstrated continuing regular heart rhythms for more than 1 minute after termination of seizure. An apparent respiratory arrest was found in one case[130] that responded to brief cardiopulmonary resuscitation. In both cases, intense postictal EEG suppression was noted, more profound than had been seen in other seizures with this patient. A SUDEP case series suggested that SUDEP was far more common in an outpatient setting than in a group home setting where staff had received vigorous training in first aid treatment of tonic-clonic seizures.[132] This group has suggested that attention to positioning, aggressive treatment of seizures, stimulation after seizures, and respiratory support when necessary may help prevent SUDEP. Treatment should take into consideration the risk of suppressing the respiratory drive, as with benzodiazepines and barbiturates (see section Antiepileptic Drugs Can Cause Respiratory Depression or Arrest).

Limbic-Onset Seizures or Cortical Stimulation Can Cause Ictal Apnea

Experimental evidence in animals shows that respiratory arrest can occur on electrical or mechanical stimulation of the posterior lateral frontal cortex, the anterior part of the hippocampal gyrus, the anterior insula, the ventral and mesial planes of the temporal lobe, the anterior cingulate gyrus, the uncus, or the fornix.[133,134] Spontaneous ictal events originating from limbic regions may also cause apneic episodes.[135] The cortical motor control of the diaphragmatic contraction can also be a part of an epileptic focus (as can any other cortical region), and therefore seizures may potentially interfere with normal diaphragmatic function and respiration.[136]

Antiepileptic Drugs Can Cause Respiratory Depression or Arrest

Medications with respiratory suppressant effects, such as benzodiazepines and barbiturates, can cause acute respiratory failure. The most important risk associated with benzodiazepines and barbiturates (especially given intravenously and at a rate that is too high) is respiratory depression, apnea, or laryngospasm. Airway patency must be assured and respiration monitored closely. The combination effect of these two classes of medications during treatment of SE increases the risks of respiratory arrest. Ventilation support should be given as required.[137] Patients with chronic respiratory insufficiency who are given these drugs are at an even higher risk for acute respiratory decompensation. Another drug within the family of benzodiazepines, Klonopin (clonazepam), may produce an increase in salivation, which should be considered before initiating treatment in patients with chronic respiratory diseases because of the added risk factor to respiratory depression posed by increased oral and pulmonary secretions.

Primary Respiratory Dysfunction Affecting Seizure Disorders

Respiratory Insufficiency

Hypoxia and hypercapnia accompany respiratory insufficiency and are the primary causes for neurologic manifestations seen in this disorder. Respiratory acidosis is associated with hypercapnia if respiratory failure is acute, and acute respiratory insufficiency can occur in people with previously normal lungs. Recent abdominal surgery may cause atelectasis or spontaneous pneumothorax and pulmonary infections. Chronic respiratory insufficiency can develop as a result of many etiologies, such as mechanical and extrapulmonary musculoskeletal abnormalities, extreme obesity, or neuromuscular diseases, and intrinsic pulmonary disorders, like chronic obstructive pulmonary disease or interstitial lung disease.[138]

Etiologies and Risk Factors. Seizures are a possible complication of respiratory insufficiency owing to two factors:

1. Severe prolonged hypoxia is occasionally accompanied by generalized seizures and myoclonus,[138,139] although hypoperfusion of the brain is the usual reason for the neuropathologic changes.[140]
2. Acute hypercapnia can cause seizures in patients with CO_2 intoxication.[134] Initially, sei-

zure threshold may increase,[141] owing to inhibitory effect, then seizure threshold decreases.[142]

Phenomenology. Clinical manifestations of respiratory insufficiency include confusion, irritability, and mental status changes, including coma. Tremor, twitches and asterixis, and ocular abnormalities, including papilledema and morning headaches, can also occur as the results of increased intracranial pressure.[143,144] EEG may show diffuse slowing and no variation from other metabolic encephalopathies.

Treatment. Treatment of the respiratory insufficiency requires the improvement of gas exchange as well as treatment of the underlying cause for the insufficiency itself (e.g., by treatment of an infection or insertion of a chest tube in the case of trauma). Treatment of the underlying causes also eliminates seizures in such cases, and there is usually no need for chronic administration of AEDs. Acute seizure treatment may include carefully monitored and administered benzodiazepines or phenytoin.

Sleep Apnea Syndrome

Sleep apnea syndrome is a disorder of abnormal respiration during sleep that results in a combination of hypoxemia and hypercapnia. The syndrome can be caused by obstruction of the upper airway during sleep, by abnormality in regulation of breathing by the CNS, or by a combination of obstructive and central problems.

Etiologies and Risk Factors. Epilepsy and sleep apnea syndrome have a reciprocal influence on one another that may exacerbate the processes of both conditions. The apneic episodes lead to hypoxemia and to chronic sleep deprivation, because sleep fragmentation is the result of multiple arousals during the apneic episodes. These arousals and their association with the apneic episodes are demonstrated in polysomnographic recording, which is the "gold standard" diagnosis of sleep disorders. Sleep deprivation and hypoxia can decrease the seizure threshold in epilepsy patients. In many epilepsy patients without sleep apnea, seizures may occur on arousal. In addition to the effect of sleep apnea on seizures, AEDs also have the effect of exacerbating sleep apnea through an inhibitory effect on respiratory drive centers and a relaxing effect on upper respiratory muscle tone.[138,145]

Wyler and Weymuller showed that seizures were reduced in an epilepsy patient who continued to have sleep apnea after tracheostomy.[146] Devinsky et al.[147] also showed that in patients with epilepsy and sleep disorders (including obstructive sleep apnea), seizures were controlled after tracheostomy or initiation of nasal continuous positive airway pressure treatment.

Phenomenology Assessment and Treatment.
Sleep apnea is typically seen more commonly in men and with snoring, obesity, and a bed partner who notices periods of apnea. Often, jerking movements of the limbs, waking at night, and, occasionally, somnambulism are experienced. Patients may typically awaken the next morning with a headache. Morbidity arises from sleep deprivation, daytime hypersomnolence, and cardiac arrhythmias, some of which may be life-threatening and occasionally may lower the seizure threshold.[148,149] Treatment of sleep apnea is aimed predominantly at weight loss, the lowering of nasal oxygen flow by using continuous positive airway pressure, and occasionally the use of acetazolamide, protriptyline, or aminophylline. With an obstructive sleep apnea condition, tracheostomy or excision of the obstructing uvula may be helpful. It is very important to effectively treat the underlying sleep apnea in an intractable epilepsy patient to avoid loading with AEDs.[138] This is particularly true in children with neurodevelopmental disorders who are on multiple AEDs and may become excessively sedated.[150]

Theophylline

Theophylline is a widely used bronchodilator and a very potent CNS stimulant. Theophylline toxicity, mainly iatrogenic, can cause seizures in patients without known underlying epilepsy. The most common types of seizures are generalized and partial seizures with secondary generalization,[151,152] but SE can occur in approximately 30% of patients.[153] Peak theophylline serum concentrations are greater than 21 mg/liter in most of cases.

Seizures occur as a complication of theophylline toxicity resulting from acute over-dosage, as well as chronic use. The mechanism is not entirely clear, but it is probably associated with inhibition of phosphodiesterase, causing a reduction of CNS inhibition through adenosine receptors.[153–155] Patients with underlying CNS structural or functional abnormalities, as well as the elderly, are at an increased risk for seizures, even at usual therapeutic levels.[156] Seizures are generally benign. In one series of clinical studies, the outcome was poor, and 8 out of 12 patients died. Age, underlying brain disease or injury, advanced pulmonary disease, and possibly low serum albumin level are thought to be possible risk factors for poor outcomes in these cases. For patients with any of these conditions, theophylline levels should be kept below 10 mg/liter, or, if possible, in consultation with the internist, some alternatives to theophylline should be found.[156,157] Theophylline is also an added risk factor for seizure exacerbation in epilepsy patients and preferably should be avoided. It interacts with AEDs metabolized by the liver[19]: Theophylline reduces phenytoin levels, and, in turn, its own level is reduced by the hepatic enzyme inducers phenytoin, carbamazepine, and phenobarbital.

Conclusion

When the patient has been diagnosed with epilepsy and has been struck by another unrelated disease or is known to have another underlying disease and concurrent seizures, the situation can pose significant challenges to the primary or specialist physician. The physician is faced with the challenges associated not only with epilepsy and the second disease, but also with potential influences that one disease may exert on the other, such as the induction of seizures and interactions among medications. This chapter focuses on the clinical indications and symptomatologies of the various hematologic and pulmonary disorders considered; discusses their indications for treatment, specifically as concerns the treatment of a patient with epileptic manifestations; and flags out warnings and risks that may be involved in treating, or failing to treat properly, each condition. We have examined various AEDs and profess above all this rule: In general, after ruling out particular etiologies and finally isolating the culprit for the seizures, the medical treatment of choice should be the one that can, if at all possible, be administered as a single agent with minimal side effects or interactions and with maximal efficacy.

Acknowledgment

The authors would like to thank Jonathon Scott Feit for proofreading and editorial assistance.

References

1. Shorvon SD, Carney MW, Chanarin I, Reynolds EH. The neuropsychiatry of megaloblastic anaemia. BMJ 1980;281:1036–1038.
2. Carl GF, Smith ML. Phenytoin-folate interactions: differing effects of the sodium salt and the free acid of phenytoin. Epilepsia 1992;33:372–377.
3. Dansky LV, Rosenblatt DS, Anderman E. Mechanisms of teratogenesis: folic acid and antiepileptic therapy. Neurology 1992;42[Suppl 5]:32–42.
4. Seligman H, Potasman I, Weller B, et al. Phenytoin-folic acid interaction: a lesson to be learned. Clin Neuropharmacol 1999;22:268–272.
5. Chanarin I, Laidlow J, Longbridge LW, et al. Megaloblastic anaemia due to phenobarbitone. The convulsant action of therapeutic doses of folic acid. BMJ 1960;1:1099.
6. Lee GR. Folate Deficiency: Causes and Management. In GR Lee (ed), Wintrobe's Clinical Hematology (10th ed). Baltimore: Williams & Wilkins, 1999;965–971.
7. Zahn CA, Morrell MJ, Collins SD, et al. Management issues for women with epilepsy: a review of the literature. Neurology 1998;51:949–956.
8. Walters TR. Congenital megaloblastic anemia responsive to N-5-formyltetrahydrofolic acid administration. J Pediatr 1967;70:686.
9. Stephen HE. Sickle Cell Anemia and Associated Hemoglobinopathies. In L Goldman, JC Bennett (eds), Cecil Textbook of Medicine (21st ed). Philadelphia: Saunders, 2000;893–905.
10. Balmaceda CM, Fetell MR. Hematologic and Related Diseases. In LP Rowland (ed), Merritt's Textbook of Neurology (9th ed). Baltimore: Williams & Wilkins, 1995;903–915.
11. Abboud MR, Jackson SM, Barredo J, et al. Neurologic complications following bone marrow transplantation for sickle cell disease. Bone Marrow Transplant 1996; 17:405–407.
12. Adams RJ, McKie VC, Hsu L, et al. Prevention of a first stroke by transfusions in children with sickle cell anemia and abnormal results on transcranial Doppler ultrasonography. N Engl J Med 1998;339:5–11.
13. Steinberg MH. Management of sickle cell disease. N Engl J Med 1999;340:1021–1030.
14. Fabian R, Peters B. Neurological complications of

15. hemoglobin SC disease. Arch Neurol 1984;41:289–292.
15. Greenberg J, Massey E. Cerebral infarction in sickle cell trait. Ann Neurol 1985;18:354–355.
16. Hart RG, Kanter MC. Hematologic disorders and ischemic stroke. A selective review. Stroke 1990;21: 1111–1121.
17. Reyes M. Subcortical cerebral infarctions in sickle cell trait. J Neurol Neurosurg Psychiatry 1989;52:516–518.
18. Massey EW, Riggs JE. Neurologic manifestations of hematologic disease. Neurol Clin 1989;7:549–561.
19. Aminoff MJ, Parent JM. Comorbidity in Adults. In J Angel, TA Padley (eds), Epilepsy: a Comprehensive Textbook (1st ed). Philadelphia: Lippincott–Raven, 1997;1957–1970.
20. Kappas A, Sassa S, Galbraith RA, Nordmann Y. The Porphyrias. In CR Scriver, AL Beaudet, WS Sly, D Valle (eds), The Metabolic Base of Inherited Disease. New York: McGraw-Hill, 1989;1305–1355.
21. Bonkowsky HL, Sinclair PR, Emery S, Sinclair JF. Seizure management in acute hepatic porphyria: risks of valproate and clonazepam. Neurology 1980; 30:588–592.
22. Sadeh M, Martonovits G, Karni A, Goldhammer Y. Treatment of porphyric convulsions with magnesium sulfate. Epilepsia 1991;32:712–715.
23. Kaplan PW, Lewis DV. Juvenile acute intermittent porphyria with hypercholesterolemia and epilepsy: a case report and review of the literature. J Child Neurol 1986;1:38–45.
24. Birchfield RI, Cowger ML. Acute intermittent porphyria with seizures. Am J Dis Child 1996;112:561–565.
25. Muller WE, Snyder SH. Delta aminolevulinic acid: influences on synaptic GABA receptor binding may explain CNS symptoms of porphyria. Ann Neurol 1977;2:340–342.
26. Lai CW, Hung TP, Lin WSJ. Blindness of cerebral origin in acute intermittent porphyria. Arch Neurol 1977;34:310–312.
27. Kupferschmidt H, Bont A, Schnorf H, et al. Transient cortical blindness and biooccipital brain lesions in two patients with acute intermittent porphyria. Ann Intern Med 1995;123:598–600.
28. Hahn M, Gildemeister OS, Krauss GL, et al. Effects of new anticonvulsants medications on porphyrin synthesis in cultured liver cells: Potential implications for patients with acute porphyria. Neurology 1997;49:97–106.
29. Bonkovsky HL. Porphyrin and Heme Metabolism and the Porphyrias. In D Zakim, TD Boyer (eds), Hepatology: a Textbook of Liver Disease (2nd ed). Philadelphia: Saunders, 1990;378–424.
30. Moore MR. International review of drugs in acute porphyria—1980. Int J Biochem 1980;12:1088–1097.
31. Bonkowsky HL, Schady W. Neurologic manifestations of acute porphyria. Semin Liver Dis 1982;2:108–124.
32. Bylesjo I, Forsgren L, Lithner F, Boman K. Epidemiology and clinical characteristics of seizures in patients

with acute intermittent porphyria. Epilepsia 1996;37: 230–235.

33. Anderson KE. The Porphyries. In L Goldman, JC Bennett (eds), Cecil Textbook of Medicine (21st ed). Philadelphia: Saunders, 2000:Chapter 219, 1123–1130.

34. Anderson KE. The Porphyrias. In D Zakim, T Boyer (eds), Hepatology. Philadelphia: Saunders, 1996;417–463.

35. Shedlofsky SI, Bonkowsky HL. Seizure management in the hepatic porphyries: results from a cell-culture model of porphyria. Neurology 1984;34:399.

36. Reynolds NC, Miska RM. Safety of anticonvulsants in hepatic porphyries. Neurology 1981;31:480–484.

37. Mustajoki P, Nordmann Y. Early administration of heme arginate for acute porphyric attacks. Arch Intern Med 1993;153:2004.

38. Krauss GL, Simmons-O'Brian E, Campbell M. Successful treatment of seizures and porphyria with gabapentin. Neurology 1995;45:594.

39. Young NS. Aplastic Anemia and Related Bone Marrow Failure Syndromes. In L Goldman, JC Bennett (eds), Cecil Textbook of Medicine (21st ed). Philadelphia: Saunders, 2000:Chapter 160, 848–853.

40. Blackburn SC, Oliart AD, Garcia Rodriguez LA, Perez Gutthann S. Antiepileptics and blood dyscrasias: a cohort study. Pharmacotherapy 1998;18:1277–1283.

41. Kaufman DW, Kelly JP, Anderson T, Harmon DC, et al. Evaluation of case reports of aplastic anemia among patients treated with felbamate. Epilepsia 1997;38:1265–1269.

42. Kaufman DW, Kelly JP, Jurgelon JM, et al. Drugs in the etiology of agranulocytosis and aplastic anaemia. Eur J Haematol Suppl 1996;60:23–30.

43. Vincent PC. Drug-induced aplastic anaemia and agranulocytosis: incidence and mechanisms. Drugs 1986;31:52.

44. Young NS. Agranulocytosis [Conference]. JAMA 1994;271:935.

45. Scheuer ML. Antiepileptic Drugs. In LP Rowland, DF Klein (eds), Current Neurologic Drugs. New York: Brunner/Mazel, 1996;119–151.

46. Suchitra A, Bussel JB. Hematologic toxicity of sodium valproate. J Pediatr Hematol Oncol 2000;22:62–65.

47. Robins MM. Aplastic anemia secondary to anticonvulsants. Am J Dis Child 1962;104:614.

48. Isaacson S, et al. Fatal aplastic anemia after therapy with Nuvarone (3-methyl-5-phenylhydantoin). JAMA 1956;160:1311.

49. Tyler MW, King EQ. Phenacemide in treatment of epilepsy. JAMA 1951;147:17.

50. Brittingham TE, et al. Reversible erythroid aplasia induced by diphenyl-hydantoin. Arch Intern Med 1964;113:764.

51. Mann LB, Habenicht HA. Fatal bone marrow aplasia associated with the administration of ethosuximide (Zarontin) for petit mal epilepsy. Bull Los Angeles Neurol Soc 1962;27:173.

52. Felbamate linked to aplastic anemia; warning issued on drug's use. Am J Hosp Pharm 1994;51:2324.

53. French J, Smith M, Faught E, et al. Practice advisory: the use of felbamate in the treatment of patients with intractable epilepsy. Report of the Quality Standards Subcommittee of the American Academy of Neurology and the American Epilepsy Society. Neurology 1999;52:1540–1545.

54. Young NS, Barrett AJ. The treatment of severe acquired aplastic anemia. Blood 1995;85:3367.

55. Alvarez JS, Delm Castillo JA, Ortiz MJ. Effect of carbamazepine on cyclosporin blood level. Nephron 1991;58:235–236.

56. Gilmore RL. Seizures and antiepileptic drug use in transplant patients. Neurol Clin 1988;6:279–296.

57. Walker RW, Brochstein JA. Neurologic complications of immunosuppressive agents. Neurol Clin 1988;6:261–278.

58. Tefferi A, Silverstein MN. Myeloproliferative Diseases. In L Goldman, JC Bennett (eds), Cecil Textbook of Medicine (21st ed). Philadelphia: Saunders, 2000:Chapter 174, 935–941.

59. Davies-Jones GA. Neurological Manifestations of Hematological Disorders. In MJ Aminoff (ed), Neurology and General Medicine: the Neurological Aspects of Medical Disorders (2nd ed). New York: Churchill Livingstone, 1995;219–245.

60. Price RA, Johnson W. The central nervous system in childhood leukemia: I. The arachnoid. Cancer 1973;31:520.

61. Smith HP, Biller J, Kelly DL. Oculomotor palsy with pupillary sparing, coincidental aneurysm, and chronic lymphocytic leukemic meningeal infiltration. Surg Neurol 1981;16:26.

62. Ha K, Kanaya S, Ikeda T, et al. Cortical blindness in a child with acute leukemia. Acta Paediatr Scand 1980;69:781.

63. Schiff D, Batchelor T, Wen PY. Neurologic emergencies in cancer patients. In: Neurol Clin 1998;16:449–483.

64. Feinberg WM, Swenson MR. Cerebrovascular complications of L-asparaginase therapy. Neurology 1988;38:127.

65. Eidelberg D, Sotrel A, Horoupian DS, et al. Thrombotic cerebral vasculopathy associated with herpes zoster. Ann Neurol 1986;19:7.

66. Boogerd W, van der Sande JJ, Kroger R, et al. Effective systemic therapy for spinal epidural metastases from breast carcinoma. Eur J Cancer 1988;25:149.

67. Phillips, PC. Methotrexate toxicity. In DA Rottenberg (ed), Neurological Complications of Cancer Treatment. Boston: Butterworth–Heinemann, 1991;115.

68. O'Sullivan DP. Convulsions associated with cyclosporin A. BMJ 1985;290:858.

69. Davis DG, Patchell RA. Neurologic complications of bone marrow transplantation. Neurol Clin 1988;6:377–387.

70. Graus F, Saiz A, Sierra I, et al. Neurologic complications of autologous and allogeneic bone marrow transplantation in patients with leukemia: a comparative study. Neurology 1996;46:1004–1009.

71. Patchell RA. Neurological complications of organ transplantations. Ann Neurol 1994;36:688.
72. Gallardo D, Ferra C, Berlanga JJ, et al. Neurologic complications after allogeneic bone marrow transplantation. Bone Marrow Transplant 1996;18:1135–1139.
73. Snider S, Bashir R, Bierman P. Neurologic complications after high-dose chemotherapy and autologous bone marrow transplantation for Hodgkin's disease. Neurology 1994;44:681.
74. Patchell RA, White CL, Clark AW, et al. Neurologic complications of bone marrow transplantation. Neurology 1985;35:300–306.
75. Kahan BD, Flecher SM, Lorber MI, et al. Complications of cyclosporine-prednisone immunosuppression in 402 renal allograft recipients exclusively followed at a single center for from one to five years. Transplantation 1987;43:197–204.
76. Martin AB, Bricker JT, Fishman M, et al. Neurologic complications of heart transplantation in children. J Heart Lung Transplant 1992;11:933–942.
77. McEnery PT, Nathan J, Bates SR, Daniels SR. Convulsions in children undergoing renal transplantation. J Pediatr 1989;115:532.
78. Antonini G, Ceschin V, Morino S, et al. Early neurologic complications following allogeneic bone marrow transplant for leukemia: a prospective study. Neurology 1998;50:1441–1445.
79. Marcus RE, Goldman JM. Convulsions due to high-dose busulfan. Lancet 1984;2:1463–1464.
80. Ghany AM, Tutschka PJ, McGhee RB, et al. Cyclosporine-associated seizures in bone marrow transplant recipients given busulfan and cyclophosphamide preparative therapy. Transplantation 1991;52:310–315.
81. Sureda A, Perez de Oteyza J, Garcia-Larana J, Odriozola J. High-dose busulfan and seizures. Ann Intern Med 1989;111:543–544.
82. Cilio MR, Danhaive O, Gadisseux JF, et al. Unusual cyclosporin related neurological complications in recipients of liver transplants. Arch Dis Child 1993;68:405–407.
83. Boogaerts MA, Zachee P, Verwilghen RL. Cyclosporin, methylprednisolone, and convulsions. Lancet 1982;2:1216–1217.
84. Durrant S, Chipping PM, Palmer S, Gordon-Smith EC. Cyclosporin A, methylprednisolone, and convulsions. Lancet 1982;2:829–830.
85. Joss DV, Barrett AJ, Kendra JR, et al. Hypertension and convulsions in children receiving cyclosporin A. Lancet 1982;1:906.
86. Thompson CB, June CH, Sullivan KM, Thomas ED. Association between cyclosporin neurotoxicity and hypomagnesemia. Lancet 1984;2:1116–1120.
87. De Groen PC, Aksamit AJ, Rakela J, et al. Central nervous system toxicity after liver transplantation: the role of cyclosporine and cholesterol. N Engl J Med 1987;317:861–866.
88. Eidelman BH, Abu-Elmagd K, Wilson J, et al. Neurologic complications of FK 506. Transplant Proc 1991;23:3175–3178.
89. Shihab F, Barry JM, Bennett WM, et al. Cytokine-related encephalopathy induced by OKT3: incidence and predisposing factors. Transplant Proc 1993;25:564–565.
90. Ruggenenti P, Remuzzi G. Thrombotic thrombocytopenic purpura and related disorders. Hematol Oncol Clin North Am 1990;4:219–241.
91. Sheth KJ, Swick HM, Haworth N. Neurological involvement in hemolytic-uremic syndrome. Ann Neurol 1986;19:90–93.
92. Moake J. Thrombotic thrombocytopenic purpura. Thromb Haemost 1995;74:240–245.
93. Parker Levine S. Thrombotic Thrombocytopenic Purpura and Other Forms of Nonimmunologic Platelet Destruction. In GR Lee (ed) Wintrobe's Clinical Hematology (10th ed). Baltimore: Williams & Wilkins, 1999.
94. Asada Y, Sumiyoshi A, Hayashi T, et al. Immunohistochemistry of vascular lesion in thrombotic thrombocytopenic purpura, with special reference to factor VIII related antigen. Thromb Res 1985;38:469–479.
95. Norkin SA, Freedman HH, Evans GW. Thrombotic thrombocytopenic purpura in siblings. Am J Med 1967;43:294–303.
96. Wallace DC, Lovric A, Clubb JS, Carseldine DB. Thrombotic thrombocytopenic purpura in four siblings. Am J Med 1975;58:724–734.
97. Fuchs WE, George JN, Dotin LN, Sears DA. Thrombotic thrombocytopenic purpura: occurrence two years apart during late pregnancy in two sisters. JAMA 1976;235:2126–2127.
98. Hellman RM, Jackson DV, Buss DH. Thrombotic thrombocytopenic purpura and hemolytic-uremic syndrome in HLA-identical siblings. Ann Intern Med 1980;93:283–284.
99. Ridolfi RL, Bell WR. Thrombotic thrombocytopenic purpura: report of 25 cases and review of the literature. Medicine (Baltimore) 1981;60:413–428.
100. Blum AS, Drislane FW. Nonconvulsive status epilepticus in thrombotic thrombocytopenic purpura. Neurology 1996;47:1079–1081.
101. Bale JF, Brasher C, Siegler RL. CNS manifestations of the hemolytic-uremic syndrome: relationship to metabolic alterations and prognosis. Am J Dis Child 1980;134:869–872.
102. Kwaan HC. Clinicopathologic features of thrombotic thrombocytopenic purpura. Semin Hematol 1987;24:71–81.
103. Bukowski RM. Thrombotic thrombocytopenic purpura: a review. Prog Hemost Thromb 1982;6:287–337.
104. Garrett WT, Chang CW, Bleck TP. Altered mental status in thrombotic thrombocytopenic purpura is secondary to nonconvulsive status epilepticus. Ann Neurol 1996;40:245–246.
105. Fagan KJ, Lee SI. Prolonged confusion following con-

vulsions due to generalized nonconvulsive status epilepticus. Neurology 1990;40:1689–1694.

106. Mizock BA, Ramsey RG, Barreta T. Computed tomographic brain scan of thrombotic thrombocytopenic purpura. Scand J Haematol 1984;32:271–274.

107. Kay AC, Solberg LA, Nichols DA, Petitt RM. Prognostic significance of computed tomography of the brain in thrombotic thrombocytopenic purpura. Mayo Clin Proc 1991;66:602–607.

108. Goodman A, Ramos R, Petrelli M, et al. Gingival biopsy in thrombotic thrombocytopenic purpura. Ann Intern Med 1978;89:501–504.

109. Nishioka GJ, Chilcoat CC, Aufdemorte TB, Clare N. The gingival biopsy in the diagnosis of thrombotic thrombocytopenic purpura. Oral Surg Oral Med Oral Pathol Oral Radiol Endod 1988;65:580–585.

110. Lichtin AE, Schreiber AD, Hurwitz S, et al. Efficacy of intensive plasmapheresis in thrombotic thrombocytopenic purpura. Arch Intern Med 1987;147:2122–2126.

111. Rock GA, Shumak KH, Buskard NA, et al. Comparison of plasma exchange with plasma infusion in the treatment of thrombotic thrombocytopenic purpura. N Engl J Med 1991;325:393–397.

112. Harkness DR, Byrnes JJ, Lian EC, et al. Hazard of platelet transfusion in thrombotic thrombocytopenic purpura. JAMA 1981;246:1931–1933.

113. Schafer AI. Hemorrhagic disorders: mixed abnormalities. In L Goldman, JC Bennett (eds), Cecil Textbook of Medicine (21st ed). Philadelphia: Saunders, 2000;1013–1016.

114. Fisher SP, Lee J, Zatuchni J, et al. Disseminated intravascular coagulation in status epilepticus. Thromb Haemost 1977;38:909–913.

115. Yuen AW, Bihari DJ. Multiorgan failure and disseminated and intravascular coagulation in severe convulsive seizures [Letter]. Lancet 1992;340:618.

116. Felcher A, Commichau C, Cao Q, et al. Disseminated intravascular coagulation and status epilepticus. Neurology 1998;51:629–631.

117. Schaub JE, Williamson PJ, Barnes EW, Trewby PN. Multisystem adverse reaction to lamotrigine. Lancet 1994;344:481.

118. Chattergoon DS, McGuigan MA, Koren G, et al. Multiorgan dysfunction and disseminated intravascular coagulation in children receiving lamotrigine and valproic acid. Neurology 1997;49:1442–1443.

119. Kis B, Szupera Z, Mezei Z, et al. Valproate treatment and platelet function: the role of arachidonate metabolites. Epilepsia 1999;40:307–310.

120. Benowitz NL, Simon RP, Copeland JR. Status epilepticus: divergence of sympathetic activity and cardiovascular response. Ann Neurol 1986;19:197.

121. Bayne LL, Simon RP. Systemic and pulmonary vascular pressures during generalized seizures in sheep. Ann Neurol 1981;10:566.

122. Simon RP, Bayne LL, Tranbaugh RF, Lewis FR. Elevated pulmonary lymph flow and protein content during status epilepticus in sheep. J Appl Physiol 1982;52:91.

123. Darnell JC, Jay SJ. Recurrent postictal pulmonary edema: a case report and review of the literature. Epilepsia 1982;23:71.

124. Terrence CF, Rao GR, Perper JA. Neurogenic pulmonary edema in unexpected, unexplained death of epileptic patients. Ann Neurol 1981;9:458.

125. Walczak, T. Epilepsia (not yet published).

126. Johnston SC, Horn JK, Valnete J, Simon RP. The role of hypoventilation in a sheep model of epileptic sudden death. Ann Neurol 1995;37:531–537.

127. Johnston SC, Siedenberg R, Min J, et al. Central apnea and acute cardiac ischemia in a sheep model of epileptic sudden death. Ann Neurol 1997;42:588–594.

128. Nashef L, Walker F, Allen P, et al. Apnea and bradycardia during epileptic seizures: relation to sudden death in epilepsy. J Neurol Neurosurg Psychiatry 1996;60:297–300.

129. Walker F, Fish DR. Recording respiratory parameters in patients with epilepsy. Epilepsia 1997;38[Suppl 11]:41–42.

130. So EL, Sam MC, Lagerlund TL. Postictal central apnea as a cause of SUDEP: evidence from a case of near-SUDEP. Epilepsia 1999;40[Suppl 7]:90–91.

131. Bird JM, Dembny KA, Sandeman D, Butler S. Sudden unexplained death in epilepsy: an intracranially monitored case. Epilepsia 1997;38[Suppl 11]:52–56.

132. Nashef L, Garner S, Fish D. Circumstances of death in sudden death in epilepsy: interviews of bereaved relatives. J Neurol Neurosurg Psychiatry 1998;64:349–352.

133. Kaada BR. Somatomotor, autonomic, and electrocorticographic responses to electrical stimulation of "rhinencephalic" and other structures in primates, cat, and dog. Acta Physiol Scand 1951;24:1.

134. Kaada BR, Jasper H. Respiratory responses to stimulation of temporal pole, insula and hippocampal and limbic gyri in man. Arch Neurol Psychiatry 1952;68:609.

135. Nelson DA, Ray CD. Respiratory arrest from seizure discharges in limbic system. Arch Neurol 1968;19:199.

136. Maskill D, Murphy K, Mier A, et al. Motor cortical representation of the diaphragm in man. J Physiol (Lond) 1991;443:105.

137. Anticonvulsant Prescribing Guide. PDR Pocket Guide to Prescription Drugs. Montvale, NJ: Medical Economics Company, 2000;6,14–15.

138. Jozefowicz RF. Neurologic manifestations of pulmonary disease. Neurol Clin 1989;7:605–616.

139. Killburn KH. Neurologic manifestations of respiratory failure. Arch Intern Med 1965;116:409.

140. Brierley JB, Graham DI. Hypoxia and vascular disorders of the central nervous system. In JH Adams, JA Corsellis, LW Duchen (eds), Greenfield's Neuropathology (4th ed). New York: Wiley, 1984.

141. Sieker HO, Hickam JB. Carbon dioxide intoxication. Medicine (Baltimore) 1956;35:389.

142. Woodbury DM, Karler R. The role of carbon dioxide in the nervous system. Anesthesiology 1960;21:687.

143. Simpson T. Papilledema in emphysema. BMJ 1948; 2:639.

144. Miller A, Bader RA, Bader ME. The neurologic syndrome due to marked hypercapnia, with papilledema. Am J Med 1962;33:309.

145. Ehrenberg B. Importance of sleep restoration in comorbid disease: effect of anticonvulsants. Neurology 2000;54[Suppl 1]:S33–S37.

146. Wyler AR, Weymuller EA. Epilepsy complicated by sleep apnea. Ann Neurol 1981;9:403–404.

147. Devinsky O, Ehrenberg B, Barthlen GM, et al. Epilepsy and sleep apnea syndrome. Neurology 1994;44:2060–2064.

148. Guilleminault C, Tilkian A, Dement WC. The sleep apnea syndromes. Annu Rev Med 1976;27:465.

149. Tobin MJ, Cohn MA, Sacner MA. Breathing abnormalities during sleep. Arch Intern Med 1983;143:1221.

150. Koh S, Ward SL, Lin M, Chen LS. Sleep apnea treatment improves seizure control in children with neurodevelopmental disorders. Pediatr Neurol 2000;22:36–39.

151. Schachter SC. Iatrogenic seizures. Neurol Clinics 1998;16:157–170.

152. Paloucek FP, Rodvold KA. Evaluation of theophylline overdoses and toxicities. Ann Emerg Med 1988;17:135.

153. Gaudreault P, Guay J. Theophylline poisoning: pharmacological considerations and clinical management. Med Toxicol 1986;1:169.

154. Edvinsson L, Fredholm BB. Characterization of adenosine receptors in isolated cerebral arteries of cat. Br J Pharmacol 1983;80:631.

155. Garcia PA, Alldredge BK. Drug-induced seizures. Neurol Clin 1994;12:85–99.

156. Bahls FH, Ma KK, Bird TD. Theophylline associated seizures with "therapeutic" or low toxic serum concentrations: risk factors for serious outcome in adults. Neurology 1991;41:1309–1312.

157. Zwillich CW, Sutton FD, Neff TA, et al. Theophylline-induced seizures in adults: correlation with serum concentrations. Ann Intern Med 1975;82:784.

Chapter 12

Head Trauma and the Development of Post-Traumatic Epilepsy

L. James Willmore

Head trauma from blunt force or from penetration of the skull causes a sequence of pathophysiologic changes in brain that correlates with the severity of injury. Acute traumatic brain injury causes a cascade of changes in brain metabolism, blood flow, and homeostasis that is a threat to survival. Seizures may occur because of the acute injury and are liable to complicate management. Such immediate seizures[1] that occur either acutely or within the first 24 hours of injury may require initiation of treatment at the injury scene or may occur later in the course of treating the injured patient. Phenytoin is an anticonvulsant that is effective in preventing seizures that occur in the acute injury period.[2] Of course, occurrence of a seizure in a patient with a head injury requires immediate brain imaging to define a possible cause, such as the accumulation of blood within the cranium.

Risks for Development of Epilepsy

The risk for development of post-traumatic epilepsy (PTE) is related to the severity of injury.[3–5] Within the first year after head trauma, the incidence of seizures exceeds the population risk for the development of epilepsy by 12 times.[3] Patients experiencing severe head trauma and cortical injury with neurologic deficits on physical examination, but with the dura mater remaining intact, have an incidence of epilepsy from 7% to 39%. However, increased severity of trauma, as indi-

cated by dural penetration and neurologic abnormalities, yields an incidence range of epilepsy incidence of 20–57%.[3,6] Guidelines for identifying patients at risk for late epilepsy (Table 12-1) include those factors associated with the severity of neocortical contusion, including presence of an intracerebral hematoma and the need for surgical repair of a depressed skull fracture.[1]

An attempt was made to improve the prediction of who might be liable to develop PTE.[7] Refinement of risk factors was attempted by application of a formula using weighted trauma categories. The formula included the brain location, the agent of injury, severity, complications, and the presence of focal neurologic deficits.[7] Observed variables from the highest numeric values of risk were associated with missile wound with dural penetration, central-parietal location, occurrence of an early seizure, and presence of an intracerebral hematoma. Predictive factors associated with epilepsy risk found in the Vietnam Head Injury Survey included cortical involvement, a moderate volume of brain tissue loss, intracerebral hematoma, and retained metal fragments.[8] Other studies of patients with PTE showed prolonged post-traumatic amnesia, the presence of a cortical laceration occurring with a depressed skull fracture with dural laceration, and intracerebral hematoma to be predictive.[9,10] The risk of development of seizures is increased after hemorrhagic cerebral infarction[11,12] and spontaneous intracerebral hematoma.[13] These data resulted in the development of a hypothesis by Willmore et al. that

Table 12-1. Factors Associated with Increased Incidence of Late Epilepsy

Factor	n	%
No early epilepsy	29/868	3
Early epilepsy	59/238	25*
No hematoma	27/854	3
Hematoma	45/128	35*
No depressed fracture	27/832	3
Depressed fracture	76/447	17*

*$p < .001$.

Source: Adapted from B Jennett, G Teasdale. Management of Head Injuries. Philadelphia: FA Davis Co, 1981:271.

suggested that trauma-induced hemorrhage with blood in contact with the neuropil is an important etiologic factor in the development of PTE.[14–16]

Latency from head injury to the development of epilepsy varies, although 57% of patients have onset of seizure within 1 year of injury.[8] Whether a seizure occurs immediately after injury, within the first week, or beyond the first week may have prognostic significance for the development of epilepsy.[1] Immediate seizures, occurring within hours after trauma, or a sequence of seizures, with development of post-traumatic status epilepticus, complicate management of an injured patient by causing hypoxia, hypertension, and metabolic changes. Although an immediate seizure may be a nonspecific reaction to head trauma, an intracranial hematoma may present this way and must be excluded. An early seizure, occurring during the first week after injury, increases the incidence of late epilepsy.[1]

Closed head injury of such severity to cause hospitalization results in an overincidence of PTE of 4–7%.[1,17] The incidence of PTE is considerably higher among patients undergoing rehabilitation for head injury.[18–20] Patients with penetrating head injury have an epilepsy incidence of 35–50%.[3,8,21–23] However, not all factors are understood, because trivial head injury has been associated with development of PTE.[24]

Occurrence of a seizure after head injury is not always predictive for development of epilepsy, nor does such a complication predict an eventual enduring problem with chronic epilepsy. Between 50% and 65% of patients who have seizures do so within 12 months of injury.[8,23,25] Approximately 80% have

seizures by 2 years after injury.[26,27] Of interest, approximately 50% of all patients have single seizures, without recurrence, whereas another 25% have just two or even three seizures followed by abatement of that clinical problem. Timing of a seizure in relationship to head injury provides some predictive information. Twenty percent to 30% of patients with a seizure within 1 week of injury have late seizures, beyond 1 week of injury.[8,26,28,29] Such later seizure recurrence seems better correlated with seizure frequency during the first year. Although these observations suggest that the overall prognosis is good,[30] intractability becomes a major clinical problem for some patients. Nonepileptic seizures have complicated head trauma, with up to 32% of one series of pseudoseizure patients having a history of head injury.[31]

History of febrile seizures is found as part of the pattern of risk for development of typical mesial temporal sclerosis and the clinical problem of complex partial seizures. However, head injury, particularly during childhood, is a factor in some cases.[32] Indeed, the University of California at Los Angeles series[33,34] found head trauma as an associate event in 16% of their cases with mesial temporal sclerosis. Such an occurrence is not typically dual in pathology[35,36] but may represent the consequences of transmitted forces with selective vulnerability of the hippocampus, as has been observed in animals.[37]

Patients with PTE may develop intractable epilepsy. Because such patients are unresponsive to antiepileptic drug therapy, the usual strategy is to evaluate the patient for consideration for resective surgery. The challenge of the monitoring process and accompanying planning for potential resective surgery is the unpredictable nature of the process of lesion formation after head injury. Head trauma of sufficient intensity to result in the development of PTE causes spatial dispersion of injured cortex in temporal and extratemporal regions.[38] Location of the clinically important regions of injury causing epilepsy requires careful planning of intracranial electrode arrays. Knowledgeable observers, such as family members, should review videotaped seizures captured during epilepsy monitoring to ensure that the clinical events reflect the patient's typical seizures. The patient must understand the success rate of resective surgery and the potential for the need to pursue further assessment should the initial surgical effort fail.

Prevention and Prophylaxis

Prophylaxis is the process of guarding against the development of a specific disease by an action or treatment that affects pathogenesis. Prevention renders a process impossible by an advanced provision.[39] One example of prevention is administration of anticonvulsants to patients with severe head trauma to prevent seizures that could cause the complications of hypertension and hypoxia. Such use of antiepileptic medications for patients who are thought to be at risk to have tonic-clonic seizures is intended to prevent the complications that are associated with the occurrence of convulsive seizures. Prophylactic use of antiepileptic drugs in patients with head trauma or for patients undergoing neurosurgical procedures requiring incision of the neocortex has the intention to interfere with epileptogenesis.[40] Although prevention of acute seizures that occur after head injury is a practical goal,[2] such treatment is not likely to have a prophylactic effect against later development of epilepsy.

Clinical observations suggesting the efficacy of antiepileptic drugs as prophylactic against the development of PTE appeared within a few years of the availability of phenytoin.[40] Young et al.[41] compared the observed 6% epilepsy occurrence in their treated head-injured patients to historic controls developing post-traumatic seizures. They concluded that early administration of antiepileptic drugs prevented the development of PTE and recommended prophylactic administration of phenytoin to patients with a 15% or greater risk of developing PTE.

Rish and Caveness[42] did not detect a difference in early seizure occurrence between phenytoin-treated and -untreated patients. However, Wohns and Wyler[43] reviewed patients selected with critical trauma indicators, including depressed skull fracture, dural or cortical laceration, or a prolonged period of post-traumatic amnesia. Although the authors acknowledged the selection bias introduced in their study, they concluded that antiepileptic drug administration prevented the development of PTE.

Because the uncontrolled studies suggested that antiepileptic drugs might have a prophylactic effect, prospective placebo-controlled assessments were undertaken (Table 12-2). Penry et al.[4] administered phenytoin and phenobarbital to head-

Table 12-2. Summary of Double-Blind Placebo-Controlled Prospective Studies of the Efficacy of Antiepileptic Drugs as Prophylaxis of Post-Traumatic Epilepsy

Authors	Drug	Patients Developing Epilepsy (%)	
		Control	Treated
Penry et al. (1979)[44]	Phenytoin Phenobarbital	13 —	23 —
Young et al. (1983)[45]	Phenytoin	10.8	12.9
Temkin et al. (1990)[2]	Phenytoin	21.1	27.5
Temkin et al. (1999)[48]	Valproic acid	15	24

injured patients in a double-blind fashion with placebo control. Seizure occurrence in the treated group was 21% and 13% in controls. The lack of significant difference between the treatment and control groups suggested that anticonvulsant administration had no effect on the development of PTE in the treated patients.

Young et al.[45] used a double-blind prospective study of 179 head-injured patients treated with phenytoin or with placebo for 18 months. Eighty-five patients were included in the treated group, whereas 74 patients were enrolled as placebo control. Seizures occurred in 12.9% of the treated patients and in 10.8% of the control patients. Temkin et al.[2] reported their experience with 404 patients treated in a prospective fashion. Patients with severe head trauma were assigned to receive an intravenous loading dose of phenytoin or placebo. Serum levels were measured at regular intervals, blood levels of drug were maintained in the therapeutic range, and efforts were made to assure that evaluations were blinded. At 1 year, no difference in incidence of PTE was found between the treatment and control groups. However, they did observe that phenytoin was effective in preventing seizures during the acute period immediately after injury. By 2 years PTE had occurred in 27.5% of phenytoin treated patients and in 21.1% of controls. Thus, early post-traumatic seizures can be prevented with administration of phenytoin for 1 or 2 weeks, but reduction in seizure occurrence was not associated with a reduction of mortality.[46]

Valproic acid had an effect on kindling in animals[47] and was evaluated in humans as well.[48] Valproic acid was given for 1 month or 6 months, or patients were treated for 1 week with phenytoin as control; 379 patients were enrolled in this study. Patients were followed for 2 years after entry into the study. Phenytoin and valproic acid were effective in preventing early seizures, with 1.5% in the phenytoin arm and 4.5% in the valproic acid arm developing seizures within the first week of injury. Valproic acid failed to prevent the development of post-traumatic seizures, with late seizures developing in 15% in the phenytoin group, 16% in the 1-month valproate group, and 24% in the 6-month valproate group. A trend to higher mortality in the long-term valproate treatment group was noted; no specific cause was reported.[48]

Mechanisms of Brain Injury

Blunt impact to the head that deforms the skull causes transmission of a pressure wave through the brain that results in abrupt and transient cavitation in brain tissue. Mechanical forces propagate a pressure wave through the brain.[38,49] Mechanical forces of head injury cause the brain to accelerate with induction of rotation and shearing injury to fiber tracts and blood vessels and contusion.[50] Contusion results in hemorrhage and is an admixture of red blood cells, necrotic brain caused by coagulation necrosis, and edema caused by mechanical disruption of blood vessels or by cellular diapedesis. Histopathologic studies of material obtained from traumatized brain show formation of axonal retraction balls, reactive gliosis, wallerian degeneration, and microglial star formation within cystic white matter lesions.[51–53] Mechanical effects cause bulk displacement of tissue with secondary responses that include alterations in cerebral vasomotor regulation, vasospasm, altered cerebral blood flow, changes in intracranial pressure, and altered vascular permeability.[54] Delayed effects of acute head trauma include focal or diffuse brain edema, ischemia, necrosis, gliosis, and neuronal loss.

Biochemical Effects of Brain Injury

Contusion or cortical laceration causes bleeding within the neuropil followed by red blood cell hemolysis and deposition of hemoglobin within the neuropil. Iron, liberated from hemoglobin and transferrin and deposited as hemosiderin, is found within the brain of patients with PTE.[55] Iron is critical to biological functions, but the two stable oxidation states and the redox properties of iron pose a biological hazard. Although oxidation of ferrous iron to ferric is a simple reaction yielding insoluble hydroxide complexes, autoxidation reactions in aqueous solution, or biological fluids, with or without chelators, it causes a complicated series of one-electron transfer reactions yielding free-radical intermediates.[14] Addition of iron salts or heme compounds to solutions containing polyunsaturated fatty acids or to suspensions of subcellular organelles results in the formation of highly reactive free-radical oxidants, including perferryl ions, superoxide radicals, singlet oxygen, and hydroxyl radicals.[14,56–59] Although free-radical species may form by iron-catalyzed Haber-Weiss reactions,[60,61] these oxidants are also actively generated by iron in biologically chelated forms in heme or with adenosine 5'-diphosphate.[57,62]

Free radicals react with methylene groups adjacent to double bonds of polyunsaturated fatty acids and lipids within cellular membranes, causing hydrogen abstraction and subsequent propagation of peroxidation reactions.[57] This nonenzymatic initiation and propagation of lipid peroxidation causes a disruption of membranes of subcellular organelles, degrades deoxyribose and amino acids, and yields diene conjugates and fluorescent chromophores.[63–65] Inorganic iron salts, hematin, and hemoproteins stimulate peroxidation of lipids of microsomes and mitochondria and change cellular thiodisulfide function.[66] Alkyl hydroxyl and peroxyl species of fatty acids propagate until a termination reaction occurs with a membrane constituent capable of electron donation without formation of a free radical. Such constituents include tocopherol, cholesterol, proteins, or the sulfhydryl group of glutathione.[62,67–69] Histopathologic alterations after injection of aqueous iron into neural tissue can be prevented by pretreatment of animals with α-tocopherol and selenium, further supporting the contention that peroxidative reactions are of importance in trauma-induced brain injury responses.[67–70]

Cellular Mechanisms of Epileptogenesis

Interictal epileptiform discharges reflect a stereotyped cellular pattern of depolarization shift.[71] Transition from interictal to ictal discharge is characterized by loss of hyperpolarization and by synchronization of neurons in the focus. Amplification of excitatory postsynaptic potentials that underlie the patterns of depolarization shift may be produced by mechanisms that include withdrawal of inhibition, frequency potentiation of excitatory postsynaptic potentials, change in the space constant of the dendrites of the postsynaptic neuron, activation of the N-methyl-D-aspartate receptor, and potentiation by neuromodulators.[72]

Biochemical injury to neurons may cause a sequence of changes, ranging from cellular loss with replacement gliosis to subtle alterations in neuronal plasma membrane. Membrane changes initiated by biochemical effects of injury may alter densities and distribution of ion channels on neuronal membrane. Alteration of membrane ionotophores could affect Na^+ and Ca^{2+} currents, alter thresholds, and lead to progressive depolarization. Intrinsic cellular bursting may also develop with an increase in extracellular K^+ or reduction of extracellular Ca^{2+}. Development or recruitment of a critical mass of neurons sufficient to cause clinical manifestations requires synchronization of a critical mass of cells.[71,72]

The mechanism or critical physiologic changes causing post-traumatic epileptogenesis remains unknown. However, several processes may provide useful areas for investigation. Trauma may cause mechanical shearing of fiber tracts with loss of inhibitory interneurons after anterograde transsynaptic neuronal degeneration.[73] Trauma-induced release of aspartate or glutamate, with attendant activation of N-methyl-D-aspartate receptors,[74] elaboration of nerve growth factor,[75] or enhancement of reactive gliosis may be operant as well.[76] Assessment of hippocampal tissue obtained during surgical resection for temporal lobe seizures and stained for identification of acetylcholine esterase shows enhancement of staining in the outer portion

of the molecular layer of the dentate gyrus.[77] Histochemical staining of rodent kindled hippocampus shows abundant mossy fiber synaptic terminals in the supragranular region and the inner molecular layer of the dentate gyrus.[78] Although speculative, synaptic reorganization may increase recurrent excitation in granule cells, favoring epileptogenesis. Experimental foci have losses in the number of axosomatic γ-aminobutyric acid (GABA)–ergic terminals, as represented by asymmetric synapses. The GABA-ergic pericellular basket plexus that provides tonic inhibition was thought to be sensitive to hypoxia, given the implied dependence on aerobic metabolism evidenced by the presence of increased numbers of mitochondria within the altered synapses.[79]

Genetic and Molecular Factors

Cellular responses to the generation of free-radical oxidants after decompartmentalization of hemoglobin or iron-containing heme compounds may depend on the induction of protective mechanisms. For example, strains of *Escherichia coli* may be differentiated on observation of responses to peroxide. Induction of enzymes to repair DNA damage induced by Fenton-derived free radicals appears to be critical for cellular survival.[80,81] Although speculative, sustained membrane changes that are associated with continuing alterations causing focal epileptiform discharges may result from free-radical injury to neuronal nuclear or mitochondrial DNA. Differentiation of susceptibility to develop epilepsy after a given trauma dose may be related to the ability of repair-response induction after initiation of lipid peroxidation.

Specific brain genetic factors that cause a liability to develop PTE remain unknown. However, a possible genetic predisposition has been observed with the detection of decreased levels of serum haptoglobin in familial epilepsy.[82] Haptoglobins are acute phase glycoproteins in the alpha L–globulin fraction of serum that form stable complexes with hemoglobin.[83] Because antioxidants such as superoxide dismutase and peroxidases are not found in high concentrations in extracellular fluid, containment of initiators of oxidation must depend on binding of reactive metals to carrier proteins, including transferrin, lactoferrin, ceruloplasmin, and haptoglobins.[83] Because one mechanism of protection against the induction of oxidant stress is sequestration of free hemoglobin with haptoglobins, identification of impairment in the synthesis of these glycoproteins may identify an inherent susceptibility to the development of epilepsy after head trauma.

Regulation of glutamate may be critical in the process of epileptogenesis. Microdialysis measurements from humans with spontaneous seizures from the hippocampus show transient release of glutamate.[84] Most glutamate is cleared from the extrasynaptic space by the action of high-affinity transporters called GLAST and GLT-1. These proteins are found predominantly in glia.[85,86] Decreasing GLAST and GLT-1 expression would be the result of down-regulation, because the messenger RNAs of these proteins were decreased even though progressive gliosis is a characteristic found in the hippocampus of rats that are spontaneously seizing.[87,88] Down-regulation of glial glutamate transporter with expected increase in tissue glutamate concentration contributes to excitatory synaptic transmission, associated occurrence of seizures, and neurodegeneration in the hippocampus. Animals with spontaneous iron-induced amygdalar seizures[89] have down-regulation of glutamate transporter production as a component of their chronic epileptogenesis.[90,91]

Molecular changes appear to correlate with depolarization-induced elevation of extracellular glutamate levels in the hippocampus, as determined by in vivo microdialysis. A protein called GAT-1 transports GABA. This transporter protein is reported to be responsible for approximately 85% of GABA reuptake.[92] GAT-1 is widely distributed in neurons and astrocytes in hippocampal and limbic regions.[93–95] Alterations in GABA uptake may be of importance to the process of chronic epileptogenesis after head trauma.[96]

Alteration of Brain Injury Responses

Because antiepileptic drugs administered in a prophylactic fashion apparently fail to inhibit the process of epileptogenesis, are there biochemical strategies that could disrupt the brain injury responses associated with the development of epilepsy?

Antiperoxidants may be of value in modulating brain injury responses. Hydroxyl radicals, superoxide radicals, and peroxides generated in biological systems by oxidative chemistry or by actions of heme-containing compounds liberated within lipid systems are quenched by action of enzymes, such as catalase, peroxidase, and superoxide dismutase.[97] Glutathione peroxidase, using glutathione as a co-substrate and selenium as a metallic co-factor, reduces intracellular formation of hydrogen peroxide and free radicals. Oxidative stress increases activity of glutathione reductase, glucose-6-phosphate dehydrogenase, and glutathione peroxidase.[98,99] Selenium, a metallic co-factor of glutathione peroxidase, also seems to act synergistically with α-tocopherol in preventing peroxidation of structural membrane components.

Alpha-tocopherol prevents peroxidative injury of sulfhydryl groups of glycolipids and glycoproteins, apparently augmenting the antioxidant effects of enzyme systems, such as glutathione peroxidase. Tocopherol also prevents peroxidation of unsaturated fatty acids and lipids by reaction of phenolic hydroxyl groups with propagating lipid radicals that were initiated by oxidative carbonyl hydrogen abstraction.[100–103] Furthermore, the phytyl side chain of tocopherol may intercalate within the acyl chains of polyunsaturated phospholipids, causing lipid membrane stabilization and a reduction in membrane permeability.[104,105] Tocopherol may also act as a free-radical scavenger and singlet oxygen-quenching agent.[103] A novel nonglucocorticoid 21–aminosteroid, with properties of inhibiting iron-dependent lipid peroxidation, had a salutary effect on concussive injury to mice.[106,107]

Superoxide radicals induce cellular and vasogenic edema.[108–110] Initiation of focal edema by cold-induced injury to the cerebral cortex of rodents causes increased levels of superoxide radicals.[108] Administration of liposome-entrapped copper-zinc superoxide dismutase interferes with the development of cold-induced edema, suggesting that superoxide dismutase interruption of oxygen free-radical induced fatty acid injury may have the potential for interruption of trauma-induced brain injury.[108]

Conclusion

Decisions about how to manage head-injured patients with regard to the development of epilepsy are confounded by the lack of specific information on which to base recommendations. Using an antiepileptic drug as a prophylactic treatment must be accompanied by informed consent of patients and the members of their families. Misunderstanding about the intent of treatment with antiepileptic drugs may cause problems with compliance or leave the impression that discontinuation of such medication has caused the patient to be vulnerable to the development of epilepsy. Because long-term prophylaxis with currently available antiepileptic drugs has not been shown to be effective in preventing PTE, the following algorithm provides a rational guide for the management of these patients:

1. High-risk patients: Those patients with head injury of such severity that risk of occurrence of seizures is high and in whom the physiologic consequences would complicate management should receive preventive phenytoin treatment. The patient should receive a loading dose of phenytoin in the form of fosphenytoin of 18 mg/kg by peripheral vein at a rate not to exceed 100 phenytoin mEq per minute. A maintenance dose of 5 mg/kg per day should be given intravenously until such time that oral administration is possible. Should a nasogastric tube feeding be required, care should be taken to avoid simultaneous feeding and phenytoin administration. Blood levels should be maintained within the recognized therapeutic range of 10–20 µg/ml. Because an allergic rash may develop in as many as 10% of patients treated in this fashion, regular skin inspection must be performed. If such an allergic reaction occurs, then use another parenteral form of anticonvulsant drug, such as phenobarbital.

2. Maintenance of preventive treatment: Available data suggest that treatment with phenytoin is effective in prevention of seizures for at least 1 month after injury. One method would be to maintain therapeutic plasma levels of phenytoin for at least 1 month after injury. At that time, the drug should be tapered over the following 4 weeks. Obtain an electroencephalogram (EEG) before drug taper. Although the EEG is not predictive of the potential for development of epilepsy immediately after injury, the observation of epileptiform patterns on the EEG after injury

may be of value in making a decision about whether to continue administration of an anticonvulsant drug.

3. Discontinuation of treatment: Patients occasionally are maintained on antiepileptic drugs for 6 months or more after injury. Because long-term treatment is not as effective as prophylaxis, early taper is preferred. If a patient ends up having been maintained on long-term prophylaxis even without having a seizure, then the patient and the physician face a clinically challenging problem. A patient may be anxious about such long-term treatment and may not be willing to risk discontinuing the drug. If the patient agrees to discontinue antiepileptic drug treatment, then special cautions regarding the prohibition of driving during the time of tapering of the drug must be individualized. A realistic discussion of risk along with EEG assessment, followed by discontinuation over 6 weeks, may be best.

4. Natural history of PTE: As with other forms of epilepsy, those patients with few seizures that are easily controlled tend to have the best prognosis. Walker and Erculei[30] observed that 50% of patients identified as having PTE would be in complete remission by 15 years after injury. Assessment and decisions about discontinuation of medication after a long seizure-free interval should be governed by guidelines that apply to any patient who is a candidate for a trial off of medication.[111,112]

References

1. Jennett B, Teasdale G. Management of Head Injuries. Philadelphia: FA Davis Co, 1981:271.
2. Temkin NR, Dikmen SS, Wilensky AJ, et al. A randomized double-blind study of phenytoin for the prevention of post-traumatic seizures. N Engl J Med 1990;323:497–502.
3. Caveness WF. Epilepsy, a product of trauma in our time. Epilepsia 1976;17:207–215.
4. Weiss GH, Feeney DM, Caveness WF, et al. Prognostic factors for the occurrence of posttraumatic epilepsy. Arch Neurol 1983;40:7–10.
5. Weiss GH, Salazar AM, Vance SC, et al. Predicting posttraumatic epilepsy in penetrating head injury. Arch Neurol 1986;43:771–773.
6. Annegers JF, Hauser WA, Coan SP, Rocca WA. A population-based study of seizures after traumatic brain injuries. N Engl J Med 1998;338:20–24.

7. Feeney DM, Walker AE. The prediction of posttraumatic epilepsy. A mathematical approach. Arch Neurol 1979;36:8–12.

8. Salazar AM, Jabbari B, Vance SC, et al. Epilepsy after penetrating head injury. I. Clinical correlates: a report of the Vietnam Head Injury study. Neurology 1985;35:1406–1414.

9. Jennett B. Epilepsy and acute traumatic intracranial haematoma. J Neurol Neurosurg Psychiatry 1975;38:378–381.

10. Kaplan HA. Management of craniocerebral trauma and its relation to subsequent seizures. Epilepsia 1961;2:111–116.

11. DeCarolis P, D'Alessandro R, Ferrara R, et al. Late seizures in patients with internal carotid and middle cerebral artery occlusive disease following ischaemic events. J Neurol Neurosurg Psychiatry 1984;47:1345–1347.

12. Richardson EP, Dodge PR. Epilepsy in cerebrovascular disease. Epilepsia 1954;3:49–74.

13. Faught E, Peters D, Bartolucci A, et al. Seizures after primary intracerebral hemorrhage. Neurology 1989;39:1089–1093.

14. Aisen P. Some Physicochemical Aspects of Iron Metabolism. In Ciba Foundation Symposium (51st ed). New York: Elsevier, 1977:1–14.

15. Levitt P, Wilson WP, Wilkins RH. The effects of subarachnoid blood on the electrocorticogram of the cat. J Neurosurg 1971;35:185–191.

16. Willmore LJ, Sypert GW, Munson JB. Recurrent seizures induced by cortical iron injection: a model of post-traumatic epilepsy. Ann Neurol 1978;4:329–336.

17. Annegers JF, Grabow JD, Grover RV, et al. Seizures after head trauma: a population study. Neurology 1980;30:683–689.

18. Bontke CF, Lehmkuhl LD, Englander J, et al. Medical complications and associated injuries of patients treated in TBI Model System programs. J Head Trauma Rehabil 1993;8(2):34–46.

19. Kalisky Z, Morrison P, Meyers CA, Von Laufen AV. Medical problems encountered during rehabilitation of patients with head injury. Arch Phys Med Rehabil 1985;66:25–29.

20. Sazbon L, Groswasser Z. Outcome in 134 patients with prolonged posttraumatic unawareness. Part 1: parameters determining late recovery of consciousness. J Neurosurg 1990;72:75–80.

21. Ascroft PB. Traumatic epilepsy after gunshot wounds of the head. BMJ 1941;1:739–744.

22. Caveness WF, Liss HR. Incidence of post-traumatic epilepsy. Epilepsia 1961;2:123–129.

23. Caveness WF, Meirowsky AM, Rish BL, et al. The nature of posttraumatic epilepsy. J Neurosurg 1979;50:545–553.

24. Devinsky O. Epilepsy after minor head trauma. J Epilepsy 1996;9:94–97.

25. da Silva AM, Vaz AR, Riberiro I, et al. Controversies in posttraumatic epilepsy. Acta Neurochir (Wien) 1990;50:48–51.

26. Walker AE. Posttraumatic epilepsy in World War II veterans. Surg Neurol 1989;32:235–236.

27. Walker AE, Blumer D. The fate of World War II veterans with posttraumatic seizures. Arch Neurol 1989;46:23–26.

28. Walker AE, Jablon S. A follow-up of head injured men of World War II. J Neurosurg 1959;16:600–610.

29. Jennett WB, Lewin W. Traumatic epilepsy after closed head injuries. J Neurol Neurosurg Psychiatry 1960;23:295–301.

30. Walker AE, Erculei F. Posttraumatic epilepsy 15 years later. Epilepsia 1970;11:17–26.

31. Westbrook LE, Devinsky O, Geocadin B. Nonepileptic seizures after head injury. Epilepsia 1998;39:978–982.

32. Falconer MA, Serafetinides EA, Corsellis JA. Etiology and pathogenesis of temporal lobe epilepsy. Arch Neurol 1964;10:233–248.

33. Betz P, Eisenmenger W. Traumatic origin of a meningioma? Int J Legal Med 1995;107:326–328.

34. Mathern GW, Babb TL, Armstrong DL. Hippocampal Sclerosis. In J Engel Jr, TA Pedley (eds), Epilepsy: a Comprehensive Textbook. Philadelphia: Lippincott–Raven, 1997:133–155.

35. Cascino GD, Jack CR, Parisi JE, et al. Operative strategy in patients with MRI-identified dual pathology and temporal lobe epilepsy. Epilepsy Res 1993;33:639–644.

36. Li LM, Cendes F, Watson C, et al. Surgical treatment of patients with single and dual pathology: relevance of lesion and of hippocampal atrophy to seizure outcome. Neurology 1997;48:437–444.

37. Lowenstein DH, Thomas MJ, Smith DH, McIntosh TK. Selective vulnerability of dentate hilar neurons following traumatic brain injury: a potential mechanistic link between head trauma and disorders of the hippocampus. J Neurosci 1992;12:4846–4853.

38. Lingren SO. Experimental studies of mechanical effects in head injury. Acta Chir Scand 1966;132[Suppl 360]:1–32.

39. Willmore LJ. Prophylactic Use of Anticonvulsant Drugs. In SR Resor Jr, H Kutt (eds), Medical Treatment of Epilepsy. New York: Dekker, 1992:73–77.

40. Rapport RL, Penry JK. Pharmacologic prophylaxis of post-traumatic epilepsy: a review. Epilepsia 1972;13:295–304.

41. Young B, Rapp R, Brooks WH, et al. Post-traumatic epilepsy prophylaxis. Epilepsia 1979;20:671–681.

42. Rish BL, Caveness WF. Relation of prophylactic medication to the occurrence of early seizures following craniocerebral trauma. J Neurosurg 1973;38:155–158.

43. Wohns RN, Wyler AR. Prophylactic phenytoin in severe head injuries. J Neurosurg 1979;51:507–509.

44. Penry JK, White BG, Brackett CE. A controlled prospective study of the pharmacologic prophylaxis of posttraumatic epilepsy. Neurology 1979;29:600–601.

45. Young B, Rapp RP, Norton JA, et al. Failure of prophylactically administered phenytoin to prevent late posttraumatic seizures. J Neurosurg 1983;58:236–241.

46. Haltiner AM, Newell DW, Temkin NR, et al. Side effects and mortality associated with use of phenytoin for early posttraumatic seizure prophylaxis. J Neurosurg 1999;91:588–592.

47. Silver JM, Shin C, McNamara JO. Antiepileptogenic effects of conventional anticonvulsants in the kindling model of epilepsy. Ann Neurol 1991;29:356–363.

48. Temkin NR, Dikmen SS, Anderson GD, et al. Valproate therapy for prevention of posttraumatic seizures: a randomized trial. J Neurosurg 1999;91:593–600.

49. Pudenz RH, Shelden CH. The lucite calvarium—a method for direct observation of the brain. J Neurosurg 1946;3:487–505.

50. Gennarelli TA, Thibaulat LE, Adams JH, et al. Diffuse axonal injury and traumatic coma in the primate. Ann Neurol 1982;12:564–574.

51. Langfitt TW, Weinstein JD, Kassell NF. Vascular Factors in Head Injury. Contribution to Brain-Swelling and Intracranial Hypertension. In WE Caveness, AE Walker (eds), Head Injury. Philadelphia: Lippincott, 1966:172–194.

52. Tornheim PA, Liwnicz BH, Hirsch CS, et al. Acute responses to blunt head trauma. J Neurosurg 1983;59:431–438.

53. Unterharnscheidt F, Sellier K. Mechanisms and pathomorphology of closed head injuries. In WF Caveness, AE Walker (eds), Head Injury. Philadelphia: Lippincott, 1966:321–341.

54. Willmore LJ. Posttraumatic epilepsy: cellular mechanisms and implications for treatment. Epilepsia 1990;31[Suppl 3]:S67–S73.

55. Payan H, Toga M, Berard-Badier M. The pathology of post-traumatic epilepsies. Epilepsia 1970;11:81–94.

56. Fong KL, McCay BP, Poyer JL, et al. Evidence that peroxidation of lysosomal membranes is initiated by hydroxyl free radicals produced during flavin enzyme activity. J Biol Chem 1973;248:7792–7797.

57. Fong KL, McCay PB, Poyer JL, et al. Evidence of superoxide-dependent reduction of Fe^{3+} and its role in enzyme-generated hydroxyl radical formation. Chem Biol Interact 1976;15:77–89.

58. Svingen BA, O'Neal FO, Aust SD. The role of superoxide and singlet oxygen in lipid peroxidation. Photochem Photobiol 1978;28:803–809.

59. Willmore LJ, Hiramatsu M, Kochi H, Mori A. Formation of superoxide radicals, lipid peroxides, and edema after $FeCl_3$ injection into rat isocortex. Brain Res 1983;277:393–396.

60. Czapski G, Ilan YA. On the generation of the hydroxylation agent from superoxide radical. Can the Haber-Weiss reaction be the source of OH radicals? Photochem Photobiol 1978;28:651–653.

61. Koppenol WH, Butler J, van Leeuwen JW. The Haber-Weiss cycle. Photochem Photobiol 1978;28:655–660.

62. Aust SD, Svingen BA. The role of iron in enzymatic lipid peroxidation. In WA Pryor (ed), Free Radicals in Biology. New York: Academic, 1982:1–28.

63. Baker N, Wilson L. Water-soluble products of UV-irradiated, autoxidized linoleic and linolenic acids. J Lipid Res 1966;7:341–348.

64. Niehaus WG, Samuelsson B. Formation of malonaldehyde from phospholipid arachidonate during microsomal lipid peroxidation. Eur J Biochem 1968;6:126–130.

65. Triggs WJ, Willmore LJ. In vivo lipid peroxidation in rat brain following intracortical Fe^{2+} injection. J Neurochem 1984;42:976–980.

66. Smith GJ, Dunkley WL. Initiation of lipid peroxidation by a reduced metal ion. Arch Biochem Biophys 1962;98:46–48.

67. Anderson DK, Means ED. Lipid peroxidation in spinal cord. $FeCl_2$ induction and protection with antioxidants. Neurochem Pathol 1983;1:249–264.

68. Willmore LJ, Rubin JJ. Effects of antiperoxidants on $FeCl_2$-induced lipid peroxidation and focal edema in rat brain. Exp Neurol 1984;83:62–70.

69. Triggs WJ, Willmore LJ. Effect of [dl]-alpha-tocopherol on $FeCl_2$-induced lipid peroxidation in rat amygdala. Neurosci Lett 1994;180:33–36.

70. Willmore LJ, Rubin JJ. Antiperoxidant pretreatment and iron-induced epileptiform discharge in the rat: EEG and histopathologic study. Neurology 1981;31:63–69.

71. Prince DA, Connors BW. Mechanisms of epileptogenesis in cortical structures. Ann Neurol 1984;16[Suppl]:S59–S64.

72. Dichter MA, Ayala GF. Cellular mechanisms of epilepsy: a status report. Science 1987;237:157–164.

73. Saji M, Reis DJ. Delayed transneuronal death of substantia nigra neurons prevented by gamma-aminobutyric acid agonist. Science 1987;235:66–69.

74. Faden AI, Demediuk P, Panter SS, Vink R. The role of excitatory amino acids and NMDA receptors in traumatic brain injury. Science 1989;244:798–800.

75. Gall CM, Isackson PJ. Limbic seizures increase neuronal production of messenger RNA for nerve growth factor. Science 1989;245:758–761.

76. Nieto-Sampedro M. Astrocyte mitogen inhibitor related to epidermal growth factor receptor. Science 1988;240:1784–1786.

77. Green RC, Blume HW, Kupferschmid SB, Mesulam MM. Alterations of hippocampal acetylcholinesterase in human temporal lobe epilepsy. Ann Neurol 1989;26:347–351.

78. Sutula T, Cascino G, Cavazos J, et al. Mossy fiber synaptic reorganization in the epileptic human temporal lobe. Ann Neurol 1989;26:321–330.

79. Ribak CE, Harris AB, Vaughn JE, Roberts E. Inhibitory GABAergic nerve terminals decrease at sites of focal epilepsy. Science 1979;205:211–214.

80. Carlsson J, Carpenter VS. The recA$^+$ gene product is more important than catalase and superoxide dismutase in protecting *Escherichia coli* against hydrogen peroxide toxicity. J Bacteriol 1980;142:319–321.

81. Imlay JA, Linn S. DNA damage and oxygen radical toxicity. Science 1988;240:1302–1309.

82. Panter SS, Sadrzadeh SM, Hallaway PE, et al. Hypohaptoglobinemia associated with familial epilepsy. J Exp Med 1985;161:748–754.

83. Gutteridge JM. The antioxidant activity of haptoglobin towards haemoglobin-stimulated lipid peroxidation. Biochim Biophys Acta 1987;917:219–223.

84. During MJ, Spencer DD. Extracellular hippocampal glutamate and spontaneous seizure in the conscious human brain. Lancet 1993;341:1607–1610.

85. Rothstein JD, Dykes-Hoberg M, Pardo CA, et al. Knockout of glutamate transporters reveals a major role for astroglial transport in excitotoxicity and clearance of glutamate. Neuron 1996;16:675–686.

86. Lehre KP, Levy LM, Ottersen OP, et al. Differential expression of two glial glutamate transporters in the rat brain: quantitative and immunocytochemical observations. J Neurosci 1995;15:1835–1853.

87. Tanaka S, Kondo S, Tanaka T, Yonemasu Y. Long-term observation of rats after unilateral intra-amygdaloid injection of kainic acid. Brain Res 1988;463:163–167.

88. Tanaka T, Tanaka S, Fujita T, et al. Experimental complex partial seizures induced by a microinjection of kainic acid into limbic structures. Prog Neurobiol 1992;38:317–334.

89. Ueda Y, Willmore LJ, Triggs WJ. Amygdalar injection of FeCl$_3$ causes spontaneous recurrent seizures. Exp Neurol 1998;153:123–127.

90. Doi T, Ueda Y, Tokumaru J, et al. Sequential changes in glutamate transporter mRNA during Fe^{+++} induced epileptogenesis. Mol Brain Res 2000;75:105–112.

91. Ueda Y, Willmore LJ. Sequential changes in glutamate transporter protein levels during Fe^{+++} induced epileptogenesis. Epilepsy Res 2000;39:201–219.

92. Borden LA, Smith KE, Hartig PR, et al. Molecular heterogeneity of gamma-aminobutyric acid (GABA) transport system. J Biol Chem 1992;267:21098–21104.

93. Durkin MM, Smith KE, Borden LA, et al. Localization of messenger RNAs encoding three GABA transporters in rat brain: an in situ hybridization study. Mol Brain Res 1995;33:7–21.

94. Minelli A, Brecha NC, Karschin C, et al. GAT-1, a high affinity GABA plasma membrane transporter is localized to neurons and astroglia in the cerebral cortex. J Neurosci 1995;15:7734–7746.

95. Ribak CE, Tong WM, Brecha NC. GABA plasma membrane transporters. GAT-1 and GAT-2 display different distributions in the rat hippocampus. J Comp Neurol 1996;367:595–606.

96. Ueda Y, Willmore LJ. Hippocampal gamma-aminobutyric acid transporter alterations following focal epileptogenesis induced in rat amygdala. Brain Res Bull 2000;52:357–361.

97. Fridovich I. Superoxide dismutase. Adv Enzymol 1974;41:35–97.

98. Orlowski M, Karkowsky A. Glutathione metabolism and some possible functions of glutathione in the nervous system. Int Rev Neurobiol 1976;19:75–121.

99. Tappel AL. Lipid peroxidation damage to cell components. Fed Proc 1973;32:1870–1874.

100. McCay PB, King MM. Vitamin E: Its Role As a Biological Free Radical Scavenger and Its Relationship to the Microsomal Mixed-Function Oxidase System. In LJ Machlin (ed), Vitamin E. New York: Marcel Dekker Inc, 1980;289–317.

101. Rehncrona S, Smith DS, Akesson B, et al. Peroxidative changes in brain cortical fatty acids and phospholipids, as characterized during Fe2+- and ascorbic acid-stimulated lipid peroxidation in vitro. J Neurochem 1980;34:1630–1638.

102. Tappel AL. Vitamin E and free radical peroxidation of lipids. Ann N Y Acad Sci 1972;203:12–28.

103. Witting LA. Vitamin E and Lipid Antioxidants in Free-Radical-Initiated Reactions. In WA Pryor (ed), Free Radicals in Biology (vol 4). New York: Academic, 1980;295–319.

104. Diplock AT, Lucy JA. The biochemical modes of action of vitamin E and selenium: a hypothesis. FEBS Lett 1973;29:205–210.

105. Lucy JA. Functional and structural aspects of biological membranes: a suggested structural role for vitamin E in the control of membrane permeability and stability. Ann N Y Acad Sci 1972;203:4–11.

106. Hall ED, Yonkers PA, McCall JM, Braughler JM. Effects of the 21-aminosteroid U74006F on experimental head injury in mice. J Neurosurg 1988;68:456–461.

107. Willmore LJ. Post-traumatic epilepsy: mechanisms and prevention [Review]. Psychiatry Clin Neurosci 1995;49:S171–S173.

108. Chan PH, Fishman RA. Transient formation of superoxide radicals in polyunsaturated fatty acid-induced brain swelling. J Neurochem 1980;35:1004–1007.

109. Fishman RA, Chan PH, Lee J, Quan S. Effects of superoxide free radicals on the induction of brain edema. Neurology 1979;29:546.

110. Wagner FC, Stewart WB. Effect of trauma dose on spinal cord edema. J Neurosurg 1981;54:8802–8806.

111. Callaghan N, Garrett A, Goggin T. Withdrawal of anticonvulsant drugs in patients free of seizures for two years. N Engl J Med 1988;318:942–946.

112. Chadwick D, Reynolds EH. When do epileptic patients need treatment? Starting and stopping medication. BMJ 1985;290:1885–1888.

Chapter 13

Headache and Epilepsy

Stephen D. Silberstein and Richard B. Lipton

Migraine and epilepsy are a heterogenous family of chronic disorders with highly variable clinical features, natural histories, and patterns of treatment response.[1,2] Both are characterized by episodes of neurologic dysfunction, sometimes accompanied by headache, as well as gastrointestinal, autonomic, and psychological features. Each has an internationally recognized classification system.[3]

The International Headache Society (IHS) criteria divide headache disorders into two broad groups: primary headache disorders and secondary headache disorders.[3] In the secondary headache disorders, the headache is symptomatic of an underlying condition, such as a stroke or a mass lesion. This group is analogous to the symptomatic epilepsies. In the primary headache disorders, the headache does not have an identifiable underlying cause. This group includes migraine, tension-type headache, and cluster headache, along with a number of other rare disorders; it is analogous to the idiopathic epilepsies.

This chapter focuses on the relationship between headache and epilepsy for several reasons. First, abundant clinical and epidemiologic data demonstrate that migraine and epilepsy are highly comorbid, and individuals with one disorder are at least twice as likely to have the other.[1,4–7] Comorbid disease presents challenges in both differential diagnosis and concomitant diagnosis.[8] Second, the clinical presentation of migraine and epilepsy may overlap, creating diagnostic difficulty. Finally, the disorders have overlapping risk factors, brain mechanisms, and treatments.[8]

We begin by describing the migraine attack, dividing it into traditional stages. We then review the diagnosis of migraine using the IHS criteria, emphasizing the variants of migraine most frequently mistaken for epilepsy. Finally, we summarize the epidemiologic evidence that migraine and epilepsy are associated.

Migraine

Migraine is a relatively common disorder. Population-based studies have yielded remarkably consistent 1-year period prevalence estimates of approximately 6% in men and 15–18% in women.[9,10] Most studies find that migraine is approximately three times more common in women than in men.[9,10]

Headache diagnosis is usually based on the retrospective reporting of attack characteristics. The results of general medical and neurologic examinations, as well as laboratory studies, are usually normal and serve to exclude other, more ominous, causes of headache in migraineurs. The 1988 IHS classification of migraine subtypes is presented in Table 13-1. The most important IHS subtypes of migraine are migraine without aura (formerly common migraine; Table 13-2) and migraine with aura (formerly classic migraine; Table 13-3), the aura being the complex of focal neurologic symptoms that precedes or accompanies an attack.[11] Approximately 20–30% of migraineurs have migraine with aura.[12] The same patient may have headache with-

Table 13-1. International Headache Society Migraine Classification

1. Migraine
   1.1. Migraine without aura
   1.2. Migraine with aura
      1.2.1. Migraine with typical aura
      1.2.2. Migraine with prolonged aura
      1.2.3. Familial hemiplegic migraine
      1.2.4. Basilar migraine
      1.2.5. Migraine aura without headache
      1.2.6. Migraine with acute onset aura
   1.3. Ophthalmoplegic migraine
   1.4. Retinal migraine
   1.5. Childhood periodic syndromes that may be precursors to or associated with migraine
      1.5.1. Benign paroxysmal vertigo of childhood
      1.5.2. Alternating hemiplegia of childhood
   1.6. Complications of migraine
      1.6.1. Status migrainosus
      1.6.2. Migrainous infarction
   1.7. Migrainous disorder not fulfilling above criteria

Classification and diagnostic criteria for headache disorders, cranial neuralgias and facial pain. Headache Classification Committee of the International Headache Society. Cephalalgia 1988;8(Suppl 7):1–96.

Table 13-2. Migraine without Aura (1.1)

Diagnostic criteria
A. At least five attacks fulfilling B–D.
B. Headache lasting 4–72 hours (untreated or unsuccessfully treated).
C. Headache has at least two of the following characteristics:
   1. Unilateral location.
   2. Pulsating quality.
   3. Moderate or severe intensity (inhibits or prohibits daily activities).
   4. Aggravation by walking up stairs or similar routine physical activity.
D. During headache, at least one of the following occurs:
   1. Nausea or vomiting, or both.
   2. Photophobia and phonophobia.
E. At least one of the following occurs:
   1. History and physical and neurologic examinations do not suggest an organic disorder.
   2. History, physical examination, or neurologic examination, or a combination of these, suggests such disorder, but it is ruled out by appropriate investigations.
   3. Such disorder is present, but migraine attacks do not occur for the first time in close temporal relation to the disorder.

Classification and diagnostic criteria for headache disorders, cranial neuralgias and facial pain. Headache Classification Committee of the International Headache Society. Cephalalgia 1988;8(Suppl 7):1–96.

out aura, headache with aura, and aura without headache.

The migraine attack can be divided into four phases: the premonitory phase, which occurs hours or days before the headache; the aura, which comes immediately before the headache; the headache itself; and the postdrome. Although most people experience more than one phase, no one phase is absolutely required for a diagnosis of migraine, and most people do not experience all four phases.[13] The epilepsy attack also has premonitory, aura, attack, and postictal phases. The similarity in terminology does not imply similarity in mechanisms.

Premonitory Phase

Premonitory or prodromal phenomena occur in approximately 60% of migraineurs, often hours to days before the onset of headache.[13–15] The phenomena include constitutional, autonomic, psychological (e.g., depression, euphoria, irritability, restlessness, mental slowness, hyperactivity, fatigue, and drowsiness), and neurologic (e.g., photophobia, phonopho-

bia, and hyperosmia) features. Some patients report a poorly characterized feeling that a migraine attack is coming. Although prodromal features vary widely among individuals, they are often consistent within an individual. Premonitory symptoms have also been reported in patients before the onset of the seizure.[16]

Aura

The migraine aura consists of focal neurologic symptoms that precede or accompany an attack. Approximately 20–30% of migraineurs experience auras. Most aura symptoms develop slowly over 5–20 minutes and usually last for less than 60 minutes. The aura almost always includes visual phenomena, but may involve somatosensory or motor phenomena, as well as language or brain stem disturbances.

The most common aura is the visual aura. A visual aura often has a hemianoptic distribution and includes both positive (e.g., scintillations, fortification spectra, photopsia) and negative (e.g., scotoma) features. Elementary visual disturbances include colorless scotoma, photopsia, or phosphenes. Simple flashes, specks, or hallucinations of geometric forms (e.g., points, stars, lines, curves, circles, sparks, flashes, or flames) may occur and may be single or number in the hundreds. More complicated hallucinations include teichopsia (e.g., Greektown wall and vision) or fortification spectrum, which is the most characteristic visual aura and is almost always diagnostic of migraine. An arc of scintillating lights classically begins near the point of fixation and may form a herringbone-like pattern that expands to encompass an increasing portion of a visual hemifield. It migrates across the visual field with a scintillating edge of zigzag or flashing lights that are often black and white; on occasion, colored dots appear at the end of the white stripe. A scotoma is a negative phenomenon consisting of a blanking or graying out of vision. Scotomas are usually accompanied by a positive visual display but may occur independently. Complex disorders of visual perception include metamorphopsia, micropsia, macropsia, zoom vision, and mosaic vision.[2,17]

Numbness or tingling (paresthesia) over one side of the face and in the ipsilateral hand or arm is the most common somatosensory phenomenon. Hemiparesis and dysphasia or aphasia may develop. Olfactory hallucinations are rare, unpleasant, and short lived (5 minutes to 24 hours). Anxiety, deja vu, and jamais vu have been reported as migraine auras and are presumably of temporal lobe origin.[18] One type of aura may follow another: Sensory phenomena may occur as visual phenomena fade, or motor phenomena may develop as sensory phenomena dissipate. Although auras are relatively specific for migraine, related phenomena may occur in cerebrovascular disease, including carotid dissection, and in epilepsy, especially of the occipital lobes.

Nonvisual association cortex symptoms also occur: These include complex difficulties in the perception and use of the body (e.g., apraxia and agnosia); speech and language disturbances; states of double or multiple consciousness, associated with déjà vu or jamais vu; and elaborate, dreamy, nightmarish, trancelike, or delirious states.[18–22]

Table 13-3. Migraine with Aura (1.2)

Diagnostic criteria
A. At least two attacks fulfilling B.
B. At least three of the following four characteristics:
   1. One or more fully reversible aura symptoms indicating focal cerebral cortical or brain stem dysfunction, or both.
   2. At least one aura symptom develops gradually over more than 4 minutes or two or more symptoms occur in succession.
   3. No aura symptom lasts more than 60 minutes. If more than one aura symptom is present, accepted duration is proportionally increased.
   4. Headache follows aura with a free interval of less than 60 minutes (it may also begin before or simultaneously with the aura).
C. Not attributable to another disorder.

Classification and diagnostic criteria for headache disorders, cranial neuralgias and facial pain. Headache Classification Committee of the International Headache Society. Cephalalgia 1988;8(Suppl 7):1–96.

In epilepsy, the aura is brief and rapid in development and, at times, is associated with unusual symptoms, such as a rising abdominal sensation followed by a déjà vu illusion or a visual hallucination associated with nausea and fear.[23]

Physiology of the Aura

Cortical spreading depression (CSD) is believed to underlie the migraine aura. CSD consists of a wave of cortical excitation followed by a wave of inhibition, induced by stimulating the cortex of an experimental animal with a needle or with potassium chloride. This wave marches over the cortical mantle at a rate of 3 mm per minute, crossing vascular territories. In humans with migraine, cerebral blood flow (CBF) studies demonstrate a wave of oligemia that spreads forward from the occipital area; it precedes the aura and may persist into the headache phase.[24] The rate of progression of the oligemia is comparable to the rate of CSD.[25]

Magnetoencephalographic studies have suggested the existence of spreading depression in humans with migraine,[26] implying that spreading depression may be the mechanism that produces the aura.[27–31] Subjects who had spontaneous migraine visual auras have been studied with functional magnetic resonance imaging.[32] Interictally, using perfusion-weighted imaging, CBF, cerebral blood volume, and mean transit time were normal and symmetric. During visual auras, CBF decreased 15–53%, cerebral blood volume decreased 6–33%, and mean transit time increased 10–54% in the occipital cortex gray matter contralateral to the affected visual hemifield. When multiple perfusion images were obtained during the same aura, the margin of the perfusion defect moved anteriorly. The absence of diffusion abnormalities in these patients suggests that ischemia does not occur during the migraine aura.[33]

The epileptic aura is that portion of the seizure experienced before loss of consciousness and for which memory is retained. The aura is the entire seizure for simple partial seizures. When consciousness is lost, the aura is the simple symptom of a complex partial seizure. The aura is associated with the electroencephalographic (EEG) correlate of the seizure type in which it occurs.[34]

Headache Phase

The typical migraine headache is unilateral and described as throbbing in 85% of patients. Headache severity ranges from moderate to marked and is aggravated by head movement or physical activity. The onset is usually gradual, and the attack usually lasts 4–72 hours in adults and 2–48 hours in children.[2] To make a diagnosis of migraine, the pain must be accompanied by other features. Anorexia is common, although food cravings can occur. Nausea occurs in up to 90% of patients, and vomiting occurs in approximately one-third of migraineurs.[12] Many patients experience sensory hyperexcitability, manifested by photophobia, phonophobia, and osmophobia, and seek a dark, quiet room.[22,35] The IHS selects particular associated features as cardinal manifestations for diagnosis (see Table 13-2).[36]

Postdrome or Postictal Phase

In migraine, the patient may feel tired, washed out, irritable, and listless and may have impaired concentration. Many patients report scalp tenderness. Some

people feel unusually refreshed or euphoric after an attack, whereas others note depression and malaise. In epilepsy, during the postictal phase, there may be a depressed level of awareness or focal neurologic deficits that sometimes provide clues to the site of onset of the seizure.

Formal International Headache Society Classification

Migraine without Aura (Common Migraine)

To establish a diagnosis of IHS migraine without aura (see Tables 13-1 [1.1] and 13-2), five attacks lasting from 4 to 72 hours are required. The attacks must have two of the following four pain characteristics: unilateral location, pulsating quality, moderate to severe intensity, and aggravation by routine physical activity. In addition, the attacks must be associated with at least one of the following symptoms: nausea or vomiting or photophobia and phonophobia. No single characteristic is mandatory for a diagnosis of migraine. A patient who has photophobia, phonophobia, and severe pain aggravated by routine activity meets these criteria, as does the more typical patient with unilateral throbbing pain and nausea.[36] Attacks that persist for more than 3 days are known as *status migrainosus*. Although the frequency of attacks varies widely, the average migraineur experiences one to three headaches a month. Like epilepsy, migraine is, by definition, a recurrent phenomenon. The requirement for at least five attacks is imposed, because headaches simulating migraine may be caused by such organic diseases as brain tumors, sinusitis, or glaucoma.[36]

Migraine with Aura (Classic Migraine)

The diagnosis of migraine with aura (see Tables 13-1 [1.2] and 13-3) requires at least two attacks with any three of the following four features: one or more fully reversible aura symptoms, aura developing over a course of more than 4 minutes, aura lasting less than 60 minutes, and headache within 60 minutes after the aura. Fewer attacks are required to make a diagnosis of migraine with aura because a typical aura is highly specific for migraine. However,

Table 13-4. Symptoms Common to Both Migraine and Epilepsy

Symptom	Migraine	Epilepsy
Systemic		
Vomiting	+	±
Nausea	+	±
Diarrhea	±	−
Headache	+	±
Visual disturbances[a]		
Colored circles	−	+
Black and white lines	+	−
Blindness	±	±
Blurred vision	+	+
Visual triggering factors	+	+
Other neurologic		
Olfactory	±	+
Vertigo	+	±
Confusion	±	+
Loss of consciousness	±[b]	+
Impaired consciousness	±	+
Loss of memory	±	+
Postevent lethargy	+	+
Depersonalization	±	+
Paresthesias	+	+
Hemiparesis	±[b]	+
Hemisensory loss	±[b]	+
Aphasia	±[b]	+

+ = present; − = absent; ± = can occur.
[a] More complex.
[b] Hemiplegic migraine.

Table 13-5. Prodrome and Aura in Migraine and Epilepsy

Symptom	Migraine	Epilepsy
Premonitory	Common	Often
Duration of aura	15–60 mins	Brief, often <1 min
Automatisms	Unusual	Frequent for complex partial seizures
Gastrointestinal aura	Abdominal pain (rare); nausea (common)	"Butterflies"— rising epigastric sensation
Visual disturbances	Positive/negative	Complicated visual phenomenon
Paresthesias	Common (5–60 mins)	Common (seconds to minutes)
Altered consciousness	Usually responsive	Often unresponsive
Olfactory	Very uncommon	More common
Aphasia	Common	Common
Déjà vu	Rare	Common

usually lasts 20–30 minutes and typically precedes the headache, but occasionally it occurs only during the headache.

Migraine Variants

The variants of migraine, as classified by the IHS system, are discussed in detail in the previous section. In this section, we describe the migraine variants that are most commonly confused with epilepsy, using IHS terminology when possible.

Basilar Migraine

Basilar migraine was originally called basilar artery migraine[3]; sometimes the term Bickerstaff's syndrome is used.[37] Originally believed to be mainly a disorder of adolescent girls, it affects all age groups and both genders, with the usual female predominance. The aura often lasts less than 1 hour and is usually followed by a headache. A hemianoptic field disturbance can rapidly expand to involve both visual fields, leading, at times, to temporary blindness. The visual aura is usually followed by at least

organic causes of headache must still be excluded, at least by history and physical examination.[3,36]

Migraine with aura is subclassified into migraine with typical aura (see Table 13-1[1.2.1]) (e.g., homonymous visual disturbance, unilateral numbness or weakness, or aphasia), migraine with prolonged aura (see Table 13-1, 1.2.2) (aura lasting longer than 60 minutes), familial hemiplegic migraine (see Table 13-1, 1.2.3), basilar migraine (see Table 13-1 [1.2.4]; Table 13-4), migraine aura without headache (see Table 13-1[1.2.5]; Table 13-5), and other varieties (see Table 13-1). Some of these variants are discussed in detail, because they may be confused with epilepsy.

The headache and associated symptoms of migraine with aura are similar to those of migraine without aura but may be less severe or of shorter duration, or both. Most people who have migraine with aura also have migraine without aura. The aura one of the following symptoms: ataxia, vertigo, tinnitus, diplopia, nausea and vomiting, nystagmus, dysarthria, bilateral paresthesia, or a change in the levels of consciousness and cognition. If marked, these alterations in consciousness define confusional migraine.

The diagnosis of basilar migraine should be considered in patients with paroxysmal brain stem disturbances. Basilar migraine may be difficult to differentiate from simple or complex partial seizures and the postictal state. The aura symptoms described previously are often, but not always, followed by a severe, throbbing occipital headache and vomiting. Although attacks are usually infrequent, they can last for 1 to 3 days. These headaches can be very frightening and difficult to diagnose. On occasion, the attacks can lead to cardiac arrhythmias and brain stem stroke. The differential diagnosis, besides occipital lobe epilepsy, includes posterior fossa tumor or malformation, urea cycle defects, and mitochondrial disorders.[38]

Confusional Migraine

Confusional migraine[3,39] is characterized by a typical migraine aura, a headache (which may be insignificant), and confusion, which may precede or follow the headache. During the confused period, the patient is inattentive and distracted and has difficulty maintaining speech and other motor activities. The EEG may be abnormal during the attack. Agitation, memory disturbances, obscene utterances, and violent behavior have been reported. Single attacks are most common; multiple attacks are rare. Both may be triggered by mild head trauma. A more profoundly disturbed level of consciousness may lead to migraine stupor, which can last from hours up to 5 days. The confusional state is usually followed by sleep, resembling postictal depression of mental status. Confusional migraine may be difficult to diagnose. The differential diagnosis includes drug ingestion, metabolic encephalopathies (e.g., Reye's syndrome, hypoglycemia), viral encephalitis, and acute psychosis. Acute confusional states also occur during complex partial seizures and the postictal state. The patient may be delirious, hyperactive, restless, and, on occasion, combative. Acute migraine confusional states may recur over a period of days or months and then evolve into typical migraine episodes. A history of typical migraine aura supports a diagnosis of migraine.

Benign Paroxysmal Vertigo of Childhood

Benign paroxysmal vertigo of childhood may be a migraine equivalent (see Table 13-1 [1.5.1]). It is a disorder characterized by the sudden onset of brief attacks of severe vertigo in an otherwise healthy child. Children with this disorder cannot stand and lie silently on the floor or wish to be held. The spells are brief, lasting only a few minutes and tending to recur at irregular intervals over a period of 6–12 months. Although headache may not be present at the onset, as the disorder evolves, the vertigo may be replaced by attacks of headache and vomiting, facilitating diagnosis. When simple partial seizures give rise to vertigo, vertigo is usually less prominent than in migraine.

Aura without Headache

Migraine aura can occur without headache,[40] although, in this setting, diagnosis is more difficult. These periodic neurologic phenomena (i.e., scintillating scotomata or recurrent sensory, motor, or mental phenomena) should be accepted as migraine only after a full investigation. Headache occurring in association with some attacks helps confirm the diagnosis.[30] Ziegler and Hassanein[11] reported that 44% of their patients who had headache with aura had aura without headache at some time.

Late-life migrainous accompaniments are characterized by attacks of aura without headache, beginning in late life.[41,42] Many patients have a history of migraine in early or midlife, often with an attack-free hiatus. Because focal neurologic defects occur without headache, they can be confused with transient ischemic attacks or seizures. Late-life migrainous accompaniment remains a diagnosis of exclusion.

Epidemiologic Connections between Migraine and Epilepsy

Andermann and Andermann[4] summarized a number of studies that examined the association between migraine and epilepsy. The prevalence of epilepsy in persons with migraine ranged from 1% to 17%, with a median of 5.9%, substantially higher than epilepsy's population prevalence of 0.5%. Migraine prevalence in patients with epilepsy ranged from 8% to 15%. Many of these studies were limited by the method of patient identification, the lack of appropriate control groups, and poorly specified definitions of migraine and epilepsy. Nonetheless, these studies powerfully argue that migraine and epilepsy are associated.

Ottman and Lipton[43] examined the association between migraine and epilepsy using data from the Epilepsy Family Study of Columbia University. Subjects with epilepsy (probands) who were older than 18 years of age were identified and recruited from voluntary organizations for persons with epilepsy. Among the probands with epilepsy, migraine prevalence was 24%. Migraine prevalence was 26% in the relatives with epilepsy. In the control group of relatives without epilepsy, only 15% had migraines. The gender-adjusted rate ratio (RR) for migraine in probands with epilepsy compared to relatives without epilepsy was 2.4 (95% confidence interval [CI]; 2.0–2.9). For relatives with epilepsy compared with relatives without epilepsy the RR was also 2.4 (95% CI; 1.6–3.8). These statistics indicate that the incidence of migraine is 2.4 times higher in persons with epilepsy than in persons without epilepsy.

Risk of migraine was not associated with the age of onset of epilepsy. The risk of migraine was elevated in both partial and generalized seizures, although the risk was higher for probands with partial-onset versus those with generalized-onset seizures (RR = 1.3; 95% CI; 1.00–1.86). The risk of migraine was elevated in idiopathic and symptomatic epilepsy. Probands with epilepsy caused by head trauma had a higher risk of migraine than probands with idiopathic or cryptogenic epilepsy (RR = 1.8, 95% CI; 1.32–2.43). Nonetheless, migraine risk was elevated in every subgroup of epilepsy defined by seizure type, age of onset, and etiology of epilepsy.[44]

Although migraine and epilepsy are associated, the mechanisms of the association are complex and may be multifactorial. One possibility is a simple unidirectional causal explanation. For example, migraine may cause epilepsy by inducing brain ischemia and injury. Under this hypothesis, we would expect the incidence of migraine to be elevated before, but not after, the onset of epilepsy. Alternatively, epilepsy may cause migraine by activating the trigeminovascular system. This hypothesis leads us to expect an excess risk of migraine after, but not before, the onset of epilepsy. The data show that there is an excess risk of migraine both before and after seizure onset, leading to the rejection of both unidirectional causal models.

Marks and Ehrenberg[6] explored the timing and features of headache in patients with epilepsy. They found that of 79 of 395 patients with epilepsy, 20% also had IHS migraine. In 84% of patients with both migraine and epilepsy (66/79), the attacks were completely independent. In 16% of patients (13/79), a seizure immediately followed the migraine aura (i.e., migralepsy); 11 of 13 were women, seven of whom had a catamenial pattern. Migralepsy was also seen in refractory patients with migraine and epilepsy in Andermann's series,[1] although this phenomenon does not account for the majority of the comorbidity.

Velioglu and Özmenoglu[45] studied the relationship between migraine and epilepsy in 412 adults with epilepsy. Fourteen percent of adults with seizures had IHS migraine. Migraine-induced epilepsy (i.e., migralepsy) was found in seven patients (1.7%); all had migraine with aura. The authors, at times, found it difficult clinically to distinguish the aura of migraine from the aura of epilepsy. Patients were at increased risk for both conditions if they had migraine with aura and catamenial epilepsy. Three of the patients with refractory seizures had improved control with the combination of antimigraine and antiepilepsy drugs.

Lenaerts[46] evaluated the degree of comorbidity and tried to establish the pattern of temporal relationship between migraine and epilepsy in 201 patients from tertiary care clinics. He systematically reviewed charts, obtained additional information by telephone interviews where necessary, and applied IHS and International League Against Epilepsy diagnostic criteria. Two-tier grouping according to reason for referral (migraine or epilepsy) was done. Adequate information was obtained from 185 patients (113 women, 72 men). In the epilepsy-referred patient group (n = 103), 23% had migraine and a risk ratio of 1.9 (p = .01). In the migraine-referred group (n = 82), 11% had epilepsy and a risk ratio of 21 (p = .05). Of the 33

Table 13-6. Migraine and Epilepsy Relationships

Coexisting epilepsy and migraine
    Both disorders occur together at an increased
      prevalence, but attacks occur independently
Migraine-induced epilepsy (migralepsy)
    Seizures are triggered by migraine aura
Epilepsy-induced headache (ictal or postictal)
    Headache occurs as part of seizure or postictal state
Primary epilepsy-migraine syndromes
    Syndromes with features of both migraine and epilepsy
      without a specific underlying cause
      Occipital epilepsies (e.g., benign occipital epilepsy)
      Benign rolandic epilepsy
Secondary epilepsy-migraine syndromes
    Both migraine and epilepsy occur in the same individual
      with a common underlying cause—mitochondrial
      disorders (MELAS)
      Symptomatic (e.g., arteriovenous malformation of
      occipital lobe)
      Neurofibromatosis
Sturge-Weber

MELAS = mitochondrial encephalomyopathy, lactic acidosis, and stroke-like episodes.
Source: Adapted from F Andermann. Migraine and Epilepsy: An Overview. In F Andermann, E Lugaresi (eds), Migraine and Epilepsy. Boston: Butterworths, 1987;405–421; and KM Welch, D Lewis. Migraine and epilepsy. Neurol Clin 1997;15:107–114.

comorbid cases, 21 had their attacks in close temporal relation. The migraine attack preceded the seizure in 12 patients (57%; nine migraine with aura) and followed it in nine (43%; six migraine with aura). Migraine attacks equally precede or follow seizures, but migraine aura more often precedes the seizure (i.e., migralepsy).

Shared environmental risk factors may contribute to comorbidity. The risk of migraine is higher in subjects with epilepsy caused by head injury. Because head injury is also a risk factor for migraine,[47] comorbidity may result, in part, from an effect of head injury on the risk of both disorders. Because risk is also significantly increased in persons with idiopathic or cryptogenic epilepsy, known environmental risk factors cannot account for all of the comorbidity.

Ottman and Lipton[7] tested the alternative hypothesis that shared genetic risk factors might account for comorbidity. They argued that the risk of migraine should be higher in families with genetic versus nongenetic forms of epilepsy, if

genetic factors account for comorbidity. They further argued that the risk of epilepsy should be greater in the relatives of probands with migraine and epilepsy versus the relatives of probands with epilepsy alone. In a series of analyses, they adjusted for a number of potentially confounding factors, including age, gender, the familial aggregation of migraine, and the comorbidity of migraine and epilepsy. The analyses failed to confirm either of the authors' hypotheses, leading them to reject the idea that genetic susceptibility accounts for comorbidity.[43]

Having rejected the unidirectional model, the environmental model, and the genetic hypothesis, they proposed that an altered brain state (increased excitability) might increase the risk of both migraine and epilepsy and account for comorbidity. Enhanced neuronal hyperexcitability and a reduced threshold to attacks figure prominently in the pathophysiologic models of migraine and epilepsy. Reduction in brain magnesium or perturbations in neurotransmitter systems may provide a basis for these alterations in brain excitability. In theory, genetic or environmental factors could produce these alterations. Regardless of mechanisms, these findings are important for clinical practice.

Interrelationships between Headache and Epilepsy

Apart from the causal epidemiologic issues discussed above, there are many possible clinical interrelationships between headache and epilepsy (Table 13-6). The disorders may exist independently. Migraine may trigger epilepsy (i.e., migralepsy) or epilepsy may initiate headache. Seizure and headache seem to be associated in certain syndromes, such as benign occipital epilepsy of childhood with occipital paroxysms (BOEP). In addition, both disorders may have a common underlying cause, such as head trauma, an arteriovenous malformation,[48] or neurofribromatosis.[49,50] We now consider some of these interrelationships.

Headache as a Consequence of Seizures

Although headache is commonly associated with seizures as a preictal, ictal, or postictal phenomenon, it is often neglected because of the dramatic neurologic manifestations of the seizure. Patients with migraine-triggered epilepsy seek medical attention because of seizures, which may overshadow the migraine and be overlooked by the patient and physician. Headache can also be the sole or most predominant clinical manifestation of epileptic seizures, although this is a relatively rare situation.[51]

Preictal and Ictal Headache

Palmini and Gloor[52] presented a descriptive study of auras in partial seizures. Auras were termed cephalic if the symptoms included nonvertiginous dizziness, lightheadedness, or pressure on the head; cephalic auras occurred in 22 of 196 patients. In Blume and Young's epilepsy unit, 2.8% of 858 patients had brief ictal pain and 1.3% (11 patients) had headache. Only two patients described the pain as throbbing; the others described it as sharp or steady. Headache preceded the seizure in eight patients and accompanied the other ictal symptoms in three; all three of these patients had partial seizures, although the nature and location of EEG abnormalities varied considerably from patient to patient.

Isler et al.[53] found that hemicranial attacks of pain coincided with seizure activity and lasted for seconds to minutes (i.e., hemicrania epileptica). Two exceptions were noted: one, a case of complex partial status in which the headache lasted for hours and another in which the headache lasted most of the 20 minutes of a recorded seizure. Overall, 20% of this group of drug-resistant epileptics had cephalic symptoms.

Postictal Headache

In a telephone interview of 372 patients attending an epilepsy clinic, 45% had experienced postictal headache (PIH), and 21% always had PIH. Of those who always had PIH, it was severe 39% of the time; in contrast, it was severe in only 10% of patients with occasional PIH. Twenty-seven percent of patients had independent headaches that were usually similar to their seizure-related headaches. Headaches lasted less than 6 hours in 81%, 12–24 hours in 11%, and more than 24 hours in 8% of patients.[54] The headache was throbbing in more than two-thirds of patients.

Schön and Blau[55] reported on 100 epileptic patients, 51 of whom had PIH either always (n = 35), usually (n = 5), or 25–50% of the time (n = 11). PIH was more commonly associated with generalized tonic-clonic seizures than with focal seizures; 9% of the patients had independent migraine attacks. The headaches were either bilateral or unilateral. They were associated with photophobia and phonophobia, throbbing pain, vomiting, nausea, and visual aura, and lasted 6–72 hours. Epileptic migraineurs recognized these headaches as being similar to their migraines. Epileptic migraine responds to sumatriptan.[56]

The mechanism of ictal headache and PIH is uncertain. In recent years, the theory of migraine pathogenesis has focused on the trigeminovascular system; activation of this system gives rise to neurogenic inflammation of cranial blood vessels and pain.[44] In animal models, Moskowitz and coworkers have shown that seizures activate the trigeminovascular system, providing a potential mechanism for the associated headaches. In summary, preictal and ictal headaches are relatively rare and short lived. The seizure itself may limit the patient's ability to observe or recall the manifestations of these headaches. In contrast, PIH is common and can impact on the epileptic's quality of life. It is most common with generalized tonic-clonic seizures but is also common in complex partial seizures; it is less common with simple partial seizures.[54]

Migraine-Epilepsy Syndromes

Benign Occipital Epilepsy of Childhood with Occipital Paroxysms

BOEP is a clinical syndrome characterized by visual symptoms, followed by a partial seizure, and postictal migraine. The EEG reveals occipital spikes. A rare syndrome of childhood (mean age of onset is 7.5 years), it accounts for less than 5% of epilepsy in children.[57–59] BOEP has features of both epilepsy and migraine.[58,60,61] The seizures usually begin with visual symptoms, including amaurosis, elementary visual hallucinations (i.e., phosphenes), complex visual hallucinations, or visual illusions, including micropsia, metamorphopsia, or palinopsia.[58,62,63] The visual symptoms are often followed by hemiclonic, complex partial, or generalized tonic-clonic seizures. After the seizure, approximately 25–40% of the patients develop migrainelike headaches.[61]

The interictal EEG is characterized by normal background activity and distinct occipital discharges. The occipital spikes typically have a high voltage (200–300 μV), diphasic morphology, and a unilateral or bilateral occipital and posterotemporal distribution. The spikes disappear with eye opening and reappear 1–20 seconds after eye closure.

Gastaut reviewed the clinical and EEG features of 53 patients with BOEP. Only 55% had the complete syndrome of occipital spikes, ictal visual symptoms followed by a partial seizure, and postictal migraine. In patients with nocturnal seizures, motor symptoms predominated; in those with diurnal seizures, visual symptoms were more common. Nocturnal seizures are more common in younger children and bear a good prognosis.[58,59] Seizures starting after 8 years of age are more likely to be frequent, diurnal, and persistent,[58,59] although overall, complete seizure control is achievable in approximately 60% of patients.

Occipital spikes are not specific for BOEP. They have been reported in people with migraine and in children younger than 4 years of age, and they may not be associated with epilepsy or any other defined disorders.[64–66] Occipital spikes can also be seen in other disorders, including myoclonic, absence, and photosensitive epilepsies, as well as celiac disease.[58,67]

Benign Rolandic Epilepsy

Benign rolandic epilepsy is characterized by unilateral somatosensory or motor seizures and centrotemporal spikes; clinical and electrographic features can shift from side to side. Speech arrest, pooling of saliva, and usually, preservation of consciousness are also typical, although spread and generalization do occur. Most patients respond well to anticonvulsant medication. In one series, 75% of patients were seizure free after 5 years.[68] The seizures almost invariably disappear by age 15 years. An association with migraine has been reported in some, but not all, studies.[69,70] Rossi et al.[71] found that migraine prevalence in male controls (11.1%) was much higher than one would

expect in boys between the ages of 6 and 15 years. Giroud and colleagues,[72] in a control study, found that epilepsy with rolandic paroxysms and migraine were associated. Migraine incidence was studied in four groups of patients: patients with centrotemporal epilepsy, patients with absence epilepsy, patients with partial epilepsy, and nonepileptic patients with a history of cranial trauma. Migraine was present in 62% of the patients with centrotemporal epilepsy, 34% of the patients with absence epilepsy, 8% of the patients with partial epilepsy, and 6% of the patients with cranial trauma. These results suggest that centrotemporal epilepsy and, to a lesser degree, absence epilepsy and migraine are associated with migraine.[72] The association between benign rolandic epilepsy and migraine may be a manifestation of the comorbidity of migraine and epilepsy in general.[50]

Differential Diagnosis of Migraine and Epilepsy: Clinical and Electroencephalogram Features

The history is the most important tool in differentiating between migraine without aura and epilepsy.[59] See Table 13-4, which illustrates high levels of symptomatic overlap between migraine and epilepsy. Tables 13-5 and 13-7 present the features most useful in distinguishing them. In general, in comparison with epilepsy, attacks of migraine are of more gradual onset and of longer duration. Nausea and vomiting are more commonly associated with migraine. Prolonged confusion or lethargy after the attack favors epilepsy.

When tonic or clonic movements are absent, differentiating migraine with aura from epilepsy can be difficult. The characteristics of the aura may help[73]: the aura usually lasts longer than 5 minutes in migraine and less than 5 minutes in epilepsy (usually less than 1 minute).[4] In addition, the aura symptom profiles differ. Automatism, positive motor features, and alteration of consciousness favor an epileptic aura. A mix of positive and negative features, such as a scintillating scotoma, favors migraine.[74]

The characteristics of the elementary visual hallucinations often differ as well. Colorless glittering scotomata are typical of migraine, as are black-and-white zigzag patterns that appear concentrically around the point of fixation, usually unilaterally. (These are also termed fortification lines.) The phenomenon of a geometric pattern with expansion from the center to the periphery of the visual field (rarely in the reverse direction) and a simultaneous increase in size over a period of several minutes reflects migrainous cortical impulse propagation. The regular angular patterns in the photopsias that accompany migraine correspond to the cortical structures that generate them.[75–77] Photopsias in migraine may evolve into a scotoma or a temporary homonymous hemianopia. Resolution of the visual field defect typically occurs without any positive visual phenomena. Colors may be seen as well or spots, circles, and beads, with or without colors. When these occur, they are usually part of the scintillating scotoma or teichopsia and not a predominant independent feature of the migrainous visual hallucination.

In contrast, visual epileptic auras are predominantly multicolored with a circular or spherical pattern, as opposed to the predominantly black-and-white zigzag pattern of migraine.[78] During a seizure, hallucinations that begin unilaterally may later encompass the whole visual field, and simple hallucinations may develop into complex forms. In contrast to migraine, epileptic visual auras last for only seconds (with the rare exception of persistent visual auras),[79] thus limiting the patient's opportunity to observe and describe the hallucinations. The auras are often associated with head or eye movement and alteration of consciousness.

The sensory auras of migraine and epilepsy also differ. In migraine, the auras are paresthesias (i.e., pins and needles) that typically begin in the hand, move up the arm, skip the shoulder, and move into the face and tongue over a period of 10–15 minutes. They are often associated with a visual aura.[54] Sensory aura is typically briefer and is often described as burning, cramping, stinging, aching, electric, or throbbing.

Correctly diagnosing and separating epilepsy and migraine can be more difficult in children than in adults. Young children often give only a partial description of their symptoms, and features useful in diagnosing epilepsy or migraine in adults may not be present or may be difficult to elicit in children. Hemicranial pain and visual auras occur less often in children with migraine than in adults. In

Table 13-7. Features of Epilepsy and Migraine

Clinical Features	Migraine	Epilepsy
Consciousness	Usually clear	Usually clouded
Duration	Hours	Minutes
Aura	Usually visual, present in 20%	Variable
Family history	Often positive for migraine	Sometimes positive for epilepsy
Onset	Gradual	Sudden
Electroencephalogram	Nonspecific abnormalities	Spikes and sharp waves

children, the first symptoms of migraine may not even be associated with headaches.[80] Children are also less likely to experience or report feelings of déjà vu or have olfactory hallucinations as part of a simple partial seizure or temporal lobe epilepsy.

Although the EEG is extraordinarily useful in diagnosing epilepsy and differentiating subtypes, it is less valuable in the diagnosis of migraine. EEG findings, such as posterior slowing and response to hyperventilation, as well as other features, such as 14- and 6-Hz positive spikes, are not specific for migraine. Epileptiform discharges and focal slowing occur in the EEGs of patients with and without migraine. EEGs recorded during a migraine with aura, unlike those recorded during a clinical seizure, are usually normal. Focal slowing sometimes occurs during migraine auras, although this is not a consistent finding. Although photic driving beyond a stimulation rate of 20 Hz (the so-called harmonic response) was thought to be characteristic of migraine, it can be seen in children without a history of migraine and is not very specific.[81]

The Quality Standards Subcommittee of the American Academy of Neurology has reviewed the usefulness of the EEG in headache. They found that no study has consistently demonstrated that the EEG improves diagnostic accuracy for the patient who experiences headache. The EEG has not been convincingly shown to identify headache subtypes, nor has it been shown to be an effective screening tool for structural causes of headache. They concluded that the EEG is not useful in the routine evaluation of patients with headache (guideline). This does not exclude the use of EEG to evaluate headache patients with associated symptoms suggesting a seizure disorder, such as atypical migrainous aura or episodic loss of consciousness. Assuming head imaging capabilities are readily available, EEG is not recommended to exclude a structural cause for headache (option).[82] The incidences of spikes and paroxysmal rhythmic events (PREs) in 10-hour overnight EEGs of normal adult volunteers (n = 135) were studied at 11 sites with a computer-assisted ambulatory EEG monitoring system with automatic spike and PRE detection. Spikes were evident in the overnight EEG of one subject (0.7%), and PREs were apparent in the overnight EEG of the same subject (0.7%). The incidences of spikes in 24 other subjects with a history of migraine or a family history of epilepsy, or both, were 12.5% and 13.3%, respectively. The overnight EEGs of these subjects were significantly more likely to show spikes than the overnight EEGs of subjects without migraine or a family history of epilepsy.[83]

The EEG and 24-hour closed-circuit television EEG recording can help differentiate migraine aura and epileptic aura; these procedures can also facilitate the diagnosis of comorbid epilepsy and migraine, as well as the migralepsy syndrome. Marks and Ehrenberg[73] studied patients with migralepsy, using multiple 24-hour video-EEG telemetry recordings. In two patients, the entire migraine-epilepsy sequence was captured, showing changes during the clinical migraine aura that were atypical for electrographic epilepsy. During migraine aura, bursts of spike activity may resemble the ictal EEG during an epileptic seizure. In most reported cases, however, the EEG does not show the usual temporal evolution with progressive increases and declines in the frequency and amplitude of rhythmic, repetitive epileptiform activity typical of ictal EEGs in epilepsy. In addition, the EEG during migraine aura may show "waxing and waning" patterns, separated by completely normal EEG activity, despite the persistence of clinical symptoms.

Manzoni et al.[84] and Terzano et al.[85,86] coined the term *intercalated seizures* to denote epileptic seizures occurring between the migrainous aura and the headache phase of migraine. They found that of 450 patients with migraine, 16 (3.6%) also had seizures. The two conditions appeared to be coincidental in 4 of the 16 patients. In another five

patients, the two types of attacks were quite distinct, but often an epileptic seizure was followed by a migraine attack and vice versa. The remaining seven patients had intercalated seizures. All had a family history of migraine, and two also had relatives with epilepsy. They all had visual seizures consisting of highly stylized contours of plain figures or single or multicolored spots that often rotated. The seizures lasted for 1–2 minutes and came out of a scintillating scotoma, slowly developing in the visual field and evolving into unilateral or bilateral hemianopia. DeRomanis et al.[87,88] studied patients who had brief ictal visual hallucinations of colored dots or discs and interictal occipital paroxysms on EEG. EEG during a seizure showed that they had occipital epilepsy and not migraine with aura.[50]

Striking EEG patterns have been described in specific subtypes of migraine.[89] The brain regions most often involved in the published EEG samples in basilar migraine include the posterior temporal, parietal, and occipital regions. The posterior electrographic localization may not pertain to other forms of migraine.[90] Paroxysmal lateralizing epileptiform discharges (PLEDs) or PLED-like activity has been associated with hemiplegic migraine, prolonged migraine aura, or incipient migrainous infarction. Those patients with PLED-like activity did not have any of the usual entities associated with PLEDs, such as stroke, brain abscess, glioblastoma, or viral encephalitis; their PLEDs usually resolved within 24 hours. Certain migralepsy patients had clinical seizures when PLEDs were present on their EEGs.[6]

Conclusions and Treatment Considerations

In typical patients, the clinical history usually allows the separation of migraine and epilepsy. In more complex cases, EEG and closed-circuit television EEG monitoring are useful. Because migraine and epilepsy are associated, clinicians should be sensitive to the issue of concomitant diagnoses. When diseases are comorbid, the principle of diagnostic parsimony does not apply. Individuals with one disorder are more likely, not less likely, to have the other. In the Epilepsy Family Study, among probands with epilepsy who were classified as having migraine on the basis of their self-reported symptoms, only 44% reported physician-diagnosed migraine.[91] In the general population, 29% of men and 40% of women with migraine reported a medical diagnosis.[12] The proportion of probands reporting a physician's diagnosis of migraine was surprisingly low, given that all were already being treated for epilepsy.

Why is the comorbidity of migraine and epilepsy not recognized? Epilepsy may be viewed as a more serious disorder than migraine. As a result, the migrainous symptoms of patients with a diagnosis of epilepsy may have been overlooked or attributed to the seizure disorder. In addition, the diagnosis of atypical migraine symptoms can be quite difficult, and a number of epileptic and nonepileptic syndromes may mimic migraine. Some patients with epilepsy and migraine may not report their headaches because the headaches are being effectively treated with an antiepileptic drug without a diagnosis of migraine. Finally, the interview used in the Epilepsy Family Study may lead to the over-diagnosing of migraine in some patients.

When planning treatment strategies for epilepsy and migraine, the possibility of comorbid disease should be considered. Although tricyclic antidepressants and neuroleptic drugs are often used to treat migraine in patients with comorbid epilepsy, caution is advisable as these medications may lower seizure thresholds. When selecting drugs for migraine prophylaxis, it is sometimes advantageous to treat comorbid conditions with a single agent; for example, when migraine and hypertension occur concomitantly, a beta-blocker or calcium channel blocker is often appropriate.[36] In the same way, anticonvulsants with efficacy for both migraine and epilepsy (e.g., divalproex sodium, gabapentin, and topiramate) should be considered in patients with both disorders.

Divalproex sodium is a U.S. Food and Drug Administration–approved anticonvulsant for migraine prophylaxis. The efficacy of divalproex has been supported by open and double-blind placebo-controlled studies.[92–95] The doses that are effective in migraine are generally lower than those used for epilepsy; 500 mg a day is often sufficient. Gabapentin at a dose of 1,800–2,400 mg a day has been shown to be superior to placebo for migraine.[96] Topiramate, in both open and small placebo-controlled double-blind trials, at doses of 50–100 mg per day, has been shown to be effective for

migraine.[97] Anticonvulsants can be administered to patients with depression, Raynaud's disease, asthma, and diabetes, circumventing the contraindications to beta-blockers.[36]

Migraine and epilepsy are comorbid conditions, and the presence of one disorder increases the likelihood of the other. Because of its greater prevalence, migraine is common in epileptics, whereas epilepsy is rare in migraineurs. The diagnosis and treatment of each disorder must take into account the potential presence of the other.

References

1. Andermann F. Clinical Features of Migraine-Epilepsy Syndrome. In F Andermann, E Lugaresi (eds), Migraine and Epilepsy. Boston: Butterworths, 1987;3–30.
2. Silberstein SD, Saper JR. Migraine: Diagnosis and Treatment. In DJ Dalessio, SD Silberstein (eds), Wolff's Headache and Other Head Pain (6th ed). New York: Oxford University Press, 1993;96–170.
3. Classification and diagnostic criteria for headache disorders, cranial neuralgia, and facial pain. Headache Classification Committee of the International Headache Society. Cephalalgia 1988;8:1–96.
4. Andermann E, Andermann FA. Migraine-Epilepsy Relationships: Epidemiological and Genetic Aspects. In FA Andermann, E Lugaresi (eds), Migraine and Epilepsy. Boston: Butterworths, 1987;281–291.
5. Andermann F. Migraine and Epilepsy: an Overview. In F Andermann, E Lugaresi (eds), Migraine and Epilepsy. Boston: Butterworths, 1987;405–421.
6. Marks DA, Ehrenberg BL. Migraine related seizures in adults with epilepsy, with EEG correlation. Neurology 1993;43:2476–2483.
7. Lipton RB, Ottman R, Ehrenberg BL, Hauser WA. Comorbidity of migraine: the connection between migraine and epilepsy. Neurology 1994;44:28–32.
8. Lipton RB, Silberstein SD. Why study the comorbidity of migraine? Neurology 1994;44:4–5.
9. Lipton RB, Silberstein SD, Stewart WF. An update on the epidemiology of migraine. Headache 1994;34:319–328.
10. Silberstein SD, Lipton RB. Epidemiology of migraine. Neuroepidemiology 1993;12:179–194.
11. Ziegler DK, Hassanein RS. Specific headache phenomena: their frequency and coincidence. Headache 1990;30:152–156.
12. Lipton RB, Stewart WF, Celentano DD, Reed ML. Undiagnosed migraine: a comparison of symptom-based and self-reported physician diagnosis. Arch Intern Med 1992;156:1–6.
13. Blau JN. Migraine prodromes separated from the aura: complete migraine. BMJ 1980;281:658–660.

14. Amery WK, Waelkens J, Caers I. Dopaminergic Mechanisms in Premonitory Phenomena. In WK Amery, A Wauquier (eds), The Prelude to the Migraine Attack. London: Bailliere Tindall, 1986;64–77.
15. Amery WK, Waelkens J, Van den Bergh V. Migraine warnings. Headache 1986;26:60–66.
16. Fenwick P. Episodic dyscontrol. In J Engel Jr, TA Pedley (eds), Epilepsy: a Comprehensive Textbook. Philadelphia: Lippincott–Raven, 1997;2767–2774.
17. Silberstein SD, Young WB. Migraine aura and prodrome. Seminars Neurol 1995;45:175–182.
18. Sacks O. Migraine: Understanding a Common Disorder. Berkeley, CA: University of California Press, 1985.
19. Haas DC. Prolonged migraine aura status. Ann Neurol 1982;11:197–199.
20. Klee A, Willanger R. Disturbances of visual perception in migraine. Acta Neurol Scand 1966;42:400–414.
21. Lippman CV. Certain hallucinations peculiar to migraine. J Nerv Ment Dis 1952;116:346.
22. Selby G, Lance JW. Observation on 500 cases of migraine and allied vascular headaches. J Neurol Neurosurg Psychiatry 1960;23:23–32.
23. So NK, Andermann F. Differential Diagnosis. In J Engel Jr, TA Pedley (eds), Epilepsy: a Comprehensive Textbook. Philadelphia: Lippincott–Raven, 1997;791.
24. Olesen J, Edvinsson L. Basic Mechanisms of Headache. New York: Elsevier, 1988.
25. Leao AA. Spreading depression of activity in cerebral cortex. J Neurophysiol 1944;7:359–390.
26. Simkins RT, Tepley N, Barkley GL, Welch KM. Spontaneous neuromagnetic fields in migraine: possible link to spreading cortical depression. Neurology 1989;39:325.
27. Blau JN. Migraine pathogenesis: the neural hypothesis reexamined. J Neurol Neurosurg Psychiatry 1984;47:437–442.
28. Lance JW. The Pathophysiology of Migraine. In D Dalessio, SD Silberstein (eds), Wolff's Headache and Other Head Pain (6th ed). New York: Oxford University Press, 1993;59–95.
29. Pearce JM. Migraine: a cerebral disorder. Lancet 1984;11:86–89.
30. Raskin NH. Conclusions. Headache 1990;30:24.
31. Welch KM, D'Andrea G, Tepley N, et al. The concept of migraine as a state of central neuronal hyperexcitability. Neurol Clin 1990;8:817–828.
32. Cutrer FM, Sorenson AG, Weisskoff RM, et al. Perfusion-weighted imaging defects during spontaneous migrainous aura. Ann Neurol 1998;43:25–31.
33. Cutrer FM, O'Donnell A. Recent advances in functional neuroimaging. Curr Opin Neurol 1999;12:255–259.
34. Dreifuss R. Classification of Epileptic Seizures. In J Engel Jr, TA Pedley (eds), Epilepsy: a Comprehensive Textbook. Philadelphia: Lippincott–Raven, 1997;517–524.
35. Drummond PD. A quantitative assessment of photophobia in migraine and tension headache. Headache 1986;26:465–469.
36. Silberstein SD, Lipton RB. Overview of diagnosis and treatment of migraine. Neurology 1994;44:6–16.
37. Bickerstaff ER. Migraine Variants and Complications. In JN Blau (ed), Migraine: Clinical and Research Aspects. Baltimore: Johns Hopkins University Press, 1987;55–75.
38. Panayiotopoulos CP. Basilar Migraine: a Review. In CP Panayiotopoulos (ed), Benign Childhood Partial Seizures and Related Epileptic Syndromes. London: John Libbey & Company Ltd, 1999;303–308.
39. Hosking G. Special Forms: Variants of Migraine in Childhood. In JM Hockaday (ed), Migraine in Childhood and Other Non-Epileptic Paroxysmal Disorders. Boston: Butterworths, 1988;35–53.
40. Whitty CW. Migraine without headache. Lancet 1967;2:283–285.
41. Fisher CM. Late life migraine accompaniments as a cause of unexplained transient ischemic attacks. Can J Neurol Sci 1980;7:9–17.
42. Fisher CM. Late-life migraine accompaniments—further experience. Stroke 1986;17:1033–1042.
43. Ottman R, Lipton RB. Is the comorbidity of epilepsy and migraine due to a shared genetic susceptibility? Neurology 1996;47:918–924.
44. Moskowitz MA. The Trigeminovascular System. In J Olesen, P Tfelt-Hansen, KM Welch (eds), The Headaches. New York: Raven Press, 1993;97–104.
45. Velioglu SK, Ozmenoglu M. Migraine-related seizures in an epileptic population. Cephalalgia 1999;19:801.
46. Lenaerts ME. Migraine and epilepsy: comorbidity and temporal relationship. Cephalalgia 1999;19:418–419 (abst).
47. Appenzeller O. Posttraumatic Headaches. In DJ Dalessio, SD Silberstein (eds), Wolff's Headache and Other Head Pain (6th ed). New York: Oxford University Press, 1993; 365–383.
48. Maria BL, Neufeld JA, Rosainz LC, et al. Central nervous system structure and function in Sturge-Weber syndrome: evidence of neurologic and radiologic progression. J Child Neurol 1998;13:606–618.
49. Creange A, Zeller J, Rostaing-Rigattieri S, et al. Neurological complications of neurofibromatosis type 1 in adulthood. Brain 1999;122:373–381.
50. Panayiotopoulos CP. Differentiating Occipital Epilepsies from Migraine with Aura, Acephalgic Migraine, and Basilar Migraine. In CP Panayiotopoulos (ed), Benign Childhood Partial Seizures and Related Epileptic Syndromes. London: John Libbey & Company Ltd, 1999;281–302.
51. Laplante P, Saint JH, Bouvier G. Headache as an epileptic manifestation. Neurology 1983;33:1493–1495.
52. Palmini A, Gloor P. The localizing value of auras in partial seizures: a prospective and retrospective study. Neurology 1992;42:801–808.
53. Isler H, Wirsen ML, Elli N. Hemicrania Epileptica: Synchronous Ipsilateral Ictal Headache with Migraine

Features. In F Andermann, E Lugaresi (eds), Migraine and Epilepsy. Boston: Butterworths, 1987;246–263.

54. Schacter SC, Richman K, Loder E, Beluk S. Self-reported characteristics of postictal headaches. J Epilepsy 1995;8:41–43.

55. Schon F, Blau JN. Postepileptic headache and migraine. J Neurol Neurosurg Psychiatry 1987;50:1148–1152.

56. Jacob J, Goadsby PJ, Duncan JS. Use of sumatriptan in postictal migraine headache. Neurology 1996;47:1104.

57. Deonna T, Ziegler AL, Despland PA, VanMelle G. Partial epilepsy in neurologically normal children: clinical syndromes and prognosis. Epilepsia 1986;27:241–247.

58. Gastaut H. A new type of epilepsy: benign partial epilepsy childhood with occipital spike-waves. Clin Electroencephalogr 1982;13:13–22.

59. Panayiotopoulos CP. Benign childhood epilepsy with occipital paroxysms: a 15-year prospective study. Ann Neurol 1989;26:51–56.

60. Gastaut H. Benign Epilepsy of Childhood with Occipital Paroxysms. In J Roger, C Dravet, M Bureau et al. (eds), Epileptic Syndromes in Infancy, Childhood, and Adolescence. London: John Libbey Eurotext Ltd, 1985;150–158.

61. Talwar D, Rask CA, Torres F. Clinical manifestations in children with occipital spike-wave paroxysms. Epilepsia 1992;33:667–674.

62. Beaumanoir A. Infantile epilepsy with occipital focus and good prognosis. Eur Neurol 1983;22:43–52.

63. Newton R, Aicardi J. Clinical findings in children with occipital spike-wave complexes suppressed by eye-opening. Neurology 1983;33:1526–1529.

64. Herranz FT, Saenz LP, Cristobal SS. Occipital spike wave with and without benign epilepsy in the child. Rev Electroencephalogr Neurophysiol Clin 1984;14:1–17.

65. Lerman P, Kivity SE. Focal epileptic EEG discharges in children not suffering from clinical epilepsy: etiology, clinical significance, and management. Epilepsia 1981;22:551–558.

66. Smith JM, Kellaway P. The natural history and clinical correlates of occipital foci in children. In P Kellaway, I Petersen (eds), Neurologic and electroencephalographic correlative studies in infancy. New York: Grune & Stratton, 1965;230–249.

67. Bye ME, Andermann F, Robitaille Y, et al. Cortical vascular abnormalities in the syndrome of celiac disease, epilepsy, bilateral occipital calcifications, and folate deficiency. Ann Neurol 1993;34:399–404.

68. Bazil CW. Migraine and epilepsy. Neurol Clin 1994;12:115–128.

69. Bladin PF. The Association of Benign Rolandic Epilepsy with Migraine. In F Andermann, E Lugaresi (eds), Migraine and Epilepsy. Boston: Butterworths, 1987;145–152.

70. Bladin PF, Papworth G. Chuckling and glugging seizures at night—sylvian spike epilepsy. Proc Aust Assoc Neurol 1974;11:171–175.

71. Rossi PG, Santucci M, Giuseppe G, et al. Epidemiologic Study of Migraine in Epileptic Patients. In F Andermann, E Lugaresi (eds), Migraine and Epilepsy. Boston: Butterworths, 1987;313–321.

72. Giroud M, Couillaut G, Arnould S, et al. Epilepsy with rolandic paroxysms and migraine; a nonfortuitous association. Results of a controlled study. Pediatrie 1989;44:659–664.

73. Ehrenberg BL. Unusual clinical manifestations of migraine, and "the borderland of epilepsy" re-explored. Semin Neurol 1991;11:118–127.

74. Panayiotopoulos CP. Difficulties in Differentiating Migraine and Epilepsy Based on Clinical and EEG Findings. In F Andermann, E Lugaresi (eds), Migraine and Epilepsy. Boston: Butterworths, 1987;31–46.

75. Hubel DH, Wiesel TN. Laminar and columnar distribution of geniculocortical fibers in the macaque monkey. J Comp Neurol 1972;146:421–450.

76. Hubel DH, Wiesel TN. Receptive fields and functional architecture in two nonstriate visual areas (18 and 19) of the cat. J Neurophysiol 1965;195:229–289.

77. Hubel DH, Wiesel TN. Receptive fields and functional architecture of monkey striate cortex. J Physiol 1968;195:214–243.

78. Panayiotopoulos CP. Elementary visual hallucinations in migraine and epilepsy. J Neurol Neurosurg Psychiatry 1991;57:1371–1374.

79. Wolf P. Systematik von Satus Kleiner Anfalle in Psychopathologischer Hinsicht. In P Wolf, GK Kohler (eds), Psychopathologische und Pathogenetische Probleme Psychotischer Syndrome bei Epilepsie. Vienna, Austria: Huber, 1980;32–52.

80. Hockaday JM. Equivalents of Childhood Migraine. In JM Hockaday (ed), Migraine in Childhood and Other Non-Epileptic Paroxysmal Disorders. Boston: Butterworths, 1988;54–62.

81. Gronseth GS, Greenberg MK. The utility of the electroencephalogram in the evaluation of patients presenting with headache: a review of the literature. Neurology 1995;45:1263–1267.

82. Practice parameter: the electroencephalogram in the evaluation of headache (summary statement). Report of the Quality Standards Subcommittee. Neurology 1995;45:1411–1413.

83. Schachter SC, Ito M, Wannamaker BB, et al. Incidence of spikes and paroxysmal rhythmic events in overnight ambulatory computer-assisted EEGs of normal subjects: a multicenter study. J Clin Neurophysiol 1998;15:251–255.

84. Manzoni GC, Terzano MG, Mancia D. Possible interference between migrainous and epileptic mechanisms in intercalated attacks. Case report. Eur Neurol 1979;18:124–129.

85. Terzano MG, Manzoni GC, Parrino L. Benign Epilepsy with Occipital Paroxysms and Migraine: the Question of Intercalated Attacks. In F Andermann, E Lugaresi (eds), Migraine and Epilepsy. Boston: Butterworths, 1987;83–96.

86. Terzano MG, Parrino L, Pietrini V, Gailli L. Migraine-Epilepsy Syndrome: Intercalated Seizures in Benign Occipital Epilepsy. In F Andermann, A Beaumanoir, L Mira et al. (eds), Occipital Seizures and Epilepsies in Children. London: John Libbey & Company Ltd, 1993;93–99.

87. DeRomanis F, Buzzi MG, Cerbo R, et al. Migraine and epilepsy with infantile onset and electroencephalographic findings of occipital spike-wave complexes. Headache 1991;31:378–383.

88. DeRomanis F, Feliciani M, Cerbo R. Migraine and other clinical syndromes in children affected by EEG occipital spike-wave complexes. Funct Neurol 1988;3:187–203.

89. Beaumanoir A, Jekiel M. Electrographic Observations during Attacks of Classical Migraine. In F Andermann, E Lugaresi (eds), Migraine and Epilepsy. Boston: Butterworths, 1987;163–180.

90. Muelbacher W, Mamoli B. Prolonged impaired consciousness in basilar artery migraine. Headache 1994; 34:282–285.

91. Ottman R, Lipton RB. Comorbidity of migraine and epilepsy. Neurology 1994;44:2105–2110.

92. Jensen R, Brinck T, Olesen J. Sodium valproate has a prophylactic effect in migraine without aura. Neurology 1994;44:647–651.

93. Mathew NT. Valproate in the treatment of persistent chronic daily headache. Headache 1990;30:301.

94. Sianard-Gainko J, Lenaerts M, Bastings E, Schoenen J. Sodium valproate in severe migraine and tension-type headache: clinical efficacy and correlations with blood levels. Cephalalgia 1993;13:252.

95. Sorensen KV. Valproate: a new drug in migraine prophylaxis. Acta Neurol Scand 1988;78:346–348.

96. Mathew N, Saper J, Magnus-Miller L. Efficacy and safety of gabapentin (Neurontin®) in migraine prophylaxis. San Diego, CA: 17th Annual Meeting of the American Pain Society; 1998;(abst).

97. Silberstein SD, Saper J, Frietag F. Migraine: Diagnosis and Treatment. In SD Silberstein, RB Lipton, DJ Dalessio (eds), Wolff's Headache and Other Head Pain (7th ed). New York: Oxford University Press, 2001:121–237.

Chapter 14

Sleep Disorders and Epilepsy

Beth A. Malow and Bradley V. Vaughn

Sleep disorders are common, treatable conditions that frequently coexist with epilepsy. Understanding the relationship between epilepsy and sleep disorders is important for optimizing management of the epilepsy patient in several ways. First, epilepsy and its treatment may affect sleep organization and daytime alertness. Second, treatment of a coexisting sleep disorder may improve seizure control or daytime alertness, or both. Finally, sleep disorders may mimic epileptic seizures. Examples include sleepwalking, nocturnal panic disorder, and sleep attacks due to excessive daytime sleepiness. In this chapter, issues related to the diagnosis and management of coexisting sleep disorders in the epilepsy patient are discussed.

Sleep is an active process, resulting from the interactions of neuronal networks within the brain. These systems have some redundancy such that lesions of the central nervous system temporarily interrupt the ability to access sleep. This reduplication of systems involved in sleep activation and maintenance demonstrates the necessity of sleep, even though we do not understand the full purpose of sleep.

Sleep is divided into stages based on three physiologic parameters (electroencephalography, eye movements, and muscle tone). Sleep is divided into rapid eye movement (REM) and non–rapid eye movement (NREM) sleep. Sleep stages 1, 2, 3, and 4 are called collectively *NREM sleep*. Stage 1 is characterized by a loss of the posterior dominant rhythm, mildly slowing background activity, and the appearance of vertex sharp waves. Stage 2 is characterized by the appearance of sleep spindles or K complexes. Stage 3 is characterized by the presence of 0- to 2-Hz, greater than 70-μV, slow waves that occupy 20–50% of the 30-second epoch. Stage 4 sleep is characterized by the slow waves occupying more than 50% of the 30-second epoch. REM sleep is characterized by a low-amplitude mixed frequency pattern on electroencephalogram (EEG), absence of muscle tone in voluntary muscles, and intermittent rapid eye movements.

Sleep is a maturational process. Sleep time is greatest in infancy, divided equally between REM and NREM sleep. By the end of the first decade of life, sleep has developed its basic adult pattern. Healthy adults display a reproducible pattern of sleep organization. Normal sleep architecture is composed of progressive cycles in which the majority of delta or slow wave (stages 3 and 4) sleep occurs in the first one-third of the sleep period and the majority of REM sleep in the later one-third. At the onset of sleep, the individual displays stage 1 sleep, progresses to stage 2, and subsequently enters stage 3 and stage 4. After approximately 80–90 minutes, the first REM episode occurs, lasting approximately 5–10 minutes. The individual generally returns to stage 1 or 2 sleep before entering delta sleep. The next episodes of REM occur in approximately 60- to 90-minute cycles and gradually lengthen through the night. For most adults, approximately 50% of the sleep period is spent in stage 2 sleep, approximately 20% in stages 3 and 4, and approximately 25% in REM sleep. Adults may normally awaken 4–6 times and have several shifts to lighter stages of sleep during the night. With advancing age, there is a decrease in the amount of stage 4 (and some stage 3) sleep and an increase in sleep fragmentation owing to spontaneous arousals.

Etiologies and Risk Factors

Patients with epilepsy are at risk for sleep disorders for several reasons. Seizures, interictal epileptiform discharges (IEDs), or the epileptic state itself may alter sleep organization. Treatment with antiepileptic drugs (AEDs) may also directly contribute to daytime sleepiness and insomnia or exacerbate underlying sleep disorders, such as obstructive sleep apnea (OSA). Conversely, these drugs may also improve sleep organization. These issues are reviewed in the following discussion.

Effects of Seizures and the Epileptic State on Sleep

Seizures have immediate effects on sleep, resulting in a stage shift to a lighter stage of NREM sleep or to the awake state. Seizures also have more delayed effects on REM sleep and other sleep parameters. Seventy-seven subjects with primarily or secondarily generalized tonic-clonic seizures had reduced total sleep time, a reduced proportion of REM sleep, increased wake time after sleep onset, and an increased proportion of stage 2 NREM sleep time on nights when generalized seizures occurred, as compared to seizure-free nights.[1] In a separate study of 80 subjects with partial seizures, total sleep time and the relative proportion of NREM sleep were not different on nights when partial seizures occurred as compared to seizure-free nights. If recurrent partial seizures occurred during sleep, the relative proportion of REM sleep time but not total sleep time was reduced, suggesting that the REM-suppressing effects of seizures are independent of reductions in total amounts of sleep.

A separate group of investigators independently reported this REM-suppressing effect of seizures, as well as other effects on sleep organization, in 11 subjects with temporal lobe epilepsy. On nights when seizures occurred versus seizure-free nights, there was a disturbance in sleep architecture, con-sisting of increased wake time after sleep onset, decreased sleep efficiency, decreased proportion of stage 3 NREM sleep, decreased proportion of REM sleep, and prolonged REM sleep latency.[2] These subjects were sleepier on the day after nocturnal seizures, as assessed by the Maintenance of Wakefulness Test[3] and the Stanford Sleepiness Scale.[4] In a separate study of these 11 subjects, daytime seizures also affected sleep organization. These subjects showed a significant decrease in the amount of REM sleep and a prolongation of the REM sleep latency on nights after daytime seizures.[5]

Even on seizure-free nights, sleep was disrupted in epilepsy patients as compared to nonepileptic controls. A decrease in sleep efficiency, an increase in the number of sleep stage shifts and entries to wakefulness, and an increase in the number and duration of awakenings was noted in 80 patients with primary generalized epilepsy or complex partial seizures, as compared to 17 healthy controls.[6] Those with temporal lobe epilepsy were the most affected. The duration and percentages of the different stages of NREM and REM sleep, the number of sleep cycles, and the REM sleep latency were not statistically different from those of controls. Sleep fragmentation by awakenings was greater in untreated, newly diagnosed patients. After treatment with carbamazepine (CBZ) for 1 month, the newly diagnosed epilepsy patients showed improvement in these parameters.

Survey studies have reported similar results to polysomnographic studies. Miller, interviewing 60 patients with epilepsy, found that 68% complained of feeling sleepy during the day, 39% had difficulty falling asleep or staying asleep, and 42% complained that their sleep difficulties interfered with their work performance.[7] In a survey of 30 independently living adults with partial or generalized seizures and 23 healthy controls, night awakenings were reported more frequently in those with epilepsy.[8] Those who had at least one seizure a month were the most affected. The majority of epileptic subjects described feeling mildly tired or very tired on awakening.

Effects of Interictal Epileptiform Discharges on Sleep

Apart from seizures, IEDs that result in arousals may disrupt sleep. In one study of 14 patients, overnight-sleep EEG recordings showed bursts of generalized spike-wave complexes appearing in stages 2 and 3 of NREM sleep, at times occurring with K complexes.[9] The discharges were associated with arousals. In some patients, discharges were associated with nonconvulsive body movements and resulted in significant sleep fragmentation with increased amounts of wakefulness and decreased amounts of REM sleep. Three patients treated with antiepileptic medications showed reduced paroxysmal events during sleep, increased REM sleep, increased sleep efficiency, and a significant improvement in daytime sleepiness. However, not all IEDs result in arousals. Malow and colleagues found that IEDs in temporal lobe epilepsy were rarely associated with arousals from sleep and were most prevalent in deeper sleep stages (NREM stages 3 and 4).[10]

Effects of Antiepileptic Drugs on Sleep

AEDs affect sleep organization in highly variable ways.[11,12] Phenobarbital shortens sleep latency, and decreases the number of arousals in patients with epilepsy. Benzodiazepines decrease time to sleep onset, increase the amount of NREM stage-2 sleep, decrease the quantity and the amplitude of delta (stages 3 and 4) NREM sleep, decrease the amount of REM sleep, prolong REM sleep latency, and decrease the number and duration of awakenings and arousals. In patients with epilepsy taking phenytoin, increases in the amount of delta NREM sleep occurred subacutely (after 4–6 weeks of treatment), but the only chronic effect of phenytoin treatment was shortened sleep latency.[13] Ethosuximide decreases delta sleep and increases stage-1 NREM sleep in epilepsy patients.[14] Period analysis showed a decrease in REM activity and an increase in delta activity in healthy subjects treated with high doses of valproic acid (1,000 mg), but visual-analyzed data did not show a statistically significant difference.[15] Subjects with bipolar disease treated with CBZ had decreased sleep fragmentation, increased delta NREM sleep, and increased total sleep time.[16] As discussed previously, newly diagnosed patients with epilepsy had an improvement in the fragmentation of their sleep, owing to awakenings after treatment with CBZ for 1 month.[6] Paradoxically, in one report, initiation of controlled-release CBZ in epilepsy patients provoked a reduction and fragmentation of REM sleep and an increase in the number of sleep stage shifts.[17] These effects, however, were almost completely reversed after 1 month of treatment, and no significant difference was noted between the baseline condition and long-term follow-up.

Felbamate (FBM) can have stimulantlike effects in patients with epilepsy given the medication as part of a 2-week randomized double-blind placebo-controlled trial, followed by open FBM monotherapy.[18] Another study of the side effects of FBM reported insomnia in 25% of 60 epilepsy patients.[19] Psychiatric rating scales demonstrated stimulantlike effects of FBM (e.g., insomnia, anorexia, and anxiety) in the acute and chronic phases of treatment. Lamotrigine (LTG) can also cause insomnia.[20] Among 109 patients taking LTG, seven (6.4%) had insomnia requiring a change in therapy. The insomnia appeared to be dose dependent. In contrast, a polysomnographic study of LTG in seven subjects with epilepsy showed no effect on total sleep time, sleep efficiency, sleep latency or REM latency, or the percentage of time spent in NREM sleep stages. Stage shifts and arousal indices were reduced, whereas percent REM increased after addition of LTG.[21] The effects of the more recently introduced AEDs on sleep in epilepsy patients await further investigations. With the large number of AED choices currently available and with additional AEDs in clinical testing, clinicians may base their AED choice not only on the epilepsy syndrome, but also on its effects on sleep. For example, sedating AEDs may benefit epilepsy patients with insomnia, and stimulating AEDs may benefit epilepsy patients with daytime sleepiness (see section Treatment).

In addition to their direct pharmacologic effects on sleep, AEDs may indirectly improve sleep in the epilepsy patient through the reduction of seizures and, in some cases, IEDs. Conversely, AEDs may contribute to sleep disorders and adversely affect sleep. For example, in a patient predisposed to OSA, barbiturates and benzodiazepines may worsen the frequency of apneas and hypopneas by decreasing upper airway resistance or arousal mechanisms. AEDs that are associated with weight gain, such as valproate, may also worsen OSA. Avoiding these agents in patients with untreated OSA may be advisable, especially if alternative AEDs are available.

Table 14-1. International Classification of Sleep Disorders

Dyssomnias	Parasomnias
Intrinsic sleep disorders:	Arousal disorders:
Psychophysiologic insomnia	Confusional arousals
Sleep state misperception	Sleepwalking
Idiopathic insomnia	Sleep terrors
Narcolepsy	Sleep-wake transition disorders:
Recurrent hypersomnia	Rhythmic movement disorder
Idiopathic hypersomnia	Sleep starts
Post-traumatic hypersomnia	Sleeptalking
Obstructive sleep apnea syndrome	Nocturnal leg cramps
Central sleep apnea syndrome	Other parasomnias:
Central alveolar hypoventilation syndrome	Sleep bruxism
Periodic limb movements in sleep disorder	Sleep enuresis
Restless legs syndrome	Sleep-related abnormal swallowing syndrome
Intrinsic sleep disorder not otherwise specified	Nocturnal paroxysmal dystonia
Extrinsic sleep disorders:	Sudden unexplained nocturnal death syndrome
Inadequate sleep hygiene	Primary snoring
Environmental sleep disorder	Infant sleep apnea
Altitude insomnia	Congenital central hypoventilation syndrome
Adjustment sleep disorder	Sudden infant death syndrome
Insufficient sleep syndrome	Benign neonatal sleep myoclonus
Limit-setting sleep disorder	Other parasomnias not otherwise specified
Sleep-onset association disorder	Parasomnias usually associated with rapid eye movement
Food allergy insomnia	(REM) sleep:
Nocturnal eating (drinking) syndrome	Nightmares
Hypnotic-dependent sleep disorder	Sleep paralysis
Stimulant-dependent sleep disorder	Impaired sleep-related penile erections
Alcohol-dependent sleep disorder	Sleep-related painful erections
Toxin-induced sleep disorder	REM sleep–related sinus arrest
Extrinsic sleep disorder not otherwise specified	REM sleep behavior disorder
Circadian rhythm sleep disorders:	
Time zone change (jet lag) syndrome	
Shift-work sleep disorder	
Irregular sleep-wake pattern	
Delayed sleep phase syndrome	
Advanced sleep phase syndrome	
Non–24-hour sleep-wake disorder	
Circadian rhythm sleep disorder not otherwise specified	

Source: Reproduced with permission from American Sleep Disorders Association. The International Classification of Sleep Disorders Diagnostic and Coding Manual. Rochester, MN: American Sleep Disorders Association, 1990:15–17.

Frequency, Phenomenology, and Assessment

The International Classification of Sleep Disorders divides sleep disorders into four major categories: dyssomnias, parasomnias, sleep disorders associated with medical and psychiatric disorders, and proposed sleep disorders.[22] Table 14-1 lists the dyssomnias and parasomnias. Dyssomnias are dis-orders that result in excessive daytime sleepiness or insomnia. Categories of dyssomnias include intrinsic sleep disorders (e.g., OSA, restless legs syndrome [RLS], periodic limb movements in sleep disorder, and narcolepsy), extrinsic sleep disorders (e.g., insufficient sleep, inadequate sleep hygiene, or alcohol-dependent sleep disorder), and circadian rhythm sleep disorders (e.g., shift-work sleep disorder or jet lag syndrome). The parasomnias may mimic epileptic seizures; their distinguishing features are discussed in the section Parasomnias and Other Sleep Disorders and Their Differential Diagnosis from Seizures. Sleep disorders that are especially relevant to the epilepsy patient are discussed in the following sections, followed by a discussion of the approach to the patient with symptoms of daytime sleepiness and insomnia. For more detailed information regarding sleep disorders and the neurobiology of sleep, the reader is referred to several comprehensive sleep medicine texts.[23–25]

Sleep Apnea

One of the most well-publicized sleep disorders is sleep apnea. Sleep apnea is defined by repetitive cessation of breathing for more than 10 seconds associated with oxygen desaturation and arousals or microarousals. These patients may awaken more than 100 times per hour and are unable to obtain quality sleep owing to the frequent arousals. These patients are generally unaware of the frequent arousals.

Sleep apnea is divided into two forms: obstructive and central. Obstructive apnea is the most common form of sleep apnea. These apneas occur owing to obstruction of the upper airway. The apneas are commonly noted during stage 1 or 2, or REM sleep. Patients are generally obese and have large necks or crowded upper airways. Some patients, however, have a normal body habitus. Bed partners generally note loud snoring and periods of apnea. Overnight sleep studies reveal that these periods of apnea are associated with ventilatory effort but no air movement. Collapse of the upper airway occurs when the intraluminal pressures are lower than the extraluminal pressures. Commonly, structural abnormalities, such as a long soft palate or retroflexed mandible leading to a small airway, are believed to cause airway obstruction. However, for most patients with sleep apnea, the breathing disturbance is state dependent. Regulation of the airway dilator muscles comes from the nucleus solitarius and nucleus ambiguous, both of which are involved in the regulation of sleep state and respiration. Output from these nuclei can also be influenced by alcohol and muscle relaxants. When defined as having a frequency of apneas (i.e., complete absence of air movement) or hypopneas (i.e., decreased air movement) exceeding five per hour, the prevalence of OSA is 9% in adult women and 24% in adult men. If the frequency of apneas and hypopneas per hour exceeds five and is associated with symptoms of excessive sleepiness, the prevalence is 2% in women and 4% in men.[26] Long-term risks of sleep apnea include increased risk of myocardial infarction, stroke, motor vehicle accidents, hypertension, pulmonary hypertension, and right-sided heart failure.[27]

Central apnea is much less common than obstructive apnea. This may be caused by a neurologic abnormality in the posterior fossa or other respiratory regulatory centers. Patients may have a normal body habitus. Bed partners may note occasional snorts, but these should not be a common occurrence. If snorts or grunts at the end of the apnea periods do occur, the investigator should look for a possible obstructive component. These apneas also are associated with arousals and microarousals. Overnight sleep studies reveal periods of apnea without a ventilatory effort.

Periodic Movements of Sleep and Restless Legs Syndrome

Periodic movements of sleep are repetitive stereotyped movements of the lower extremities that occur during sleep, consisting of the extension of the great toe with dorsiflexion of the ankle and flexion of the knee and hip. These movements last 0.5–4.0 seconds and occur at 20- to 120-second intervals. These movements may be associated with arousals. Only a minority of patients with periodic movements of sleep have excessive daytime sleepiness or insomnia. Patients may be unaware of the movements, but bed partners usually note the movements. Periodic movements of sleep have been associated with uremia, peripheral vascular disease, anemia, arthritis, peripheral neuropathy, spinal cord lesions, tricyclic antidepressants, and caffeine use.[28]

RLS is characterized by the patient's complaining of an unpleasant crawling, deep, aching sensation in the legs that is improved by motion of the legs. Most individuals experience these symptoms while sitting or lying down and may complain of the need to walk or continuously move their legs. RLS usually occurs along with periodic movements of sleep. The same factors that provoke periodic limb movements increase the likelihood of RLS.

Narcolepsy

Narcolepsy is a disorder of the control of sleep, particularly REM sleep.[29] Patients with narcolepsy develop symptoms related to the inability to control the onset and offset of sleep or its fragments. The traditional tetrad of narcolepsy is excessive daytime sleepiness, cataplexy, sleep paralysis, and hypnagogic hallucinations, although patients may present with excessive daytime sleepiness alone. Excessive daytime sleepiness occurs despite relatively normal nocturnal sleep. These patients have irresistible bouts of sleep and fall asleep in inappropriate situations (e.g., in the middle of a conversation or while driving or eating). Cataplexy, a second major symptom, consists of an abrupt decrease in muscle tone without loss of consciousness. Individuals who have severe attacks may fall or experience varied degrees of weakness. Strong emotional stimuli may provoke a cataplectic attack. Cataplectic attacks are generally brief—less than 30 seconds in duration. Sleep paralysis is an inability to move during the transition into or out of sleep. These episodes may last several minutes and can be accompanied with the feeling of impending doom. Occasionally, patients may have concurrent hallucinations. Hypnagogic hallucinations are vivid dreams that are difficult to distinguish from reality. Cataplexy, sleep paralysis, and hypnagogic hallucinations are features or fragments of REM sleep.

Narcolepsy is a genetic nonprogressive disorder that appears in early adolescence and persists throughout life. Narcolepsy has a strong link to the DR2 (DR15) major histocompatability complex and a weaker link to DQW1. HLA DQB1*0602 has demonstrated an even stronger linkage for narcolepsy.[30] This gene so far appears in 36% of those who were HLA-DR2 negative. Narcolepsy is diagnosed by an appropriate history and physical examination and supported by short sleep latency and the presence of REM sleep in two or more naps on a multiple sleep latency test.

Idiopathic Central Nervous System Hypersomnia

Idiopathic central nervous system hypersomnia is characterized by prolonged periods of recurrent sleepiness that cannot be attributed to other sleep disorders.[31] These individuals have prolonged sleep periods, prolonged daytime naps, excessive daytime sleepiness, and difficulty waking. Patients may be very challenging to awaken and have aggressive and automatic behavior on awakening. These patients need to be evaluated for other possible sleep disorders, such as narcolepsy, periodic limb movements, or sleep-related respiratory disturbances. Some patients may need to have repeated evaluations to delineate the underlying disorder.

Insomnia

Insomnia is the complaint of difficulty initiating or maintaining sleep, combined with daytime sleepiness or impairment of daytime performance. For most patients, an occasional night fraught with difficulty falling asleep or having trouble maintaining sleep is not unusual. These occasional nights might be closely linked to the surrounding events of the day or sudden changes in medical condition. For a smaller group of patients, insomnia persisting for less than 3 months (subacute) or longer than 3 months (chronic) is a greater disruption of life and may lead to more significant medical symptoms. Approach to the patient with insomnia should consider that there are multiple problems causing the lack of ability to access sleep. To sleep well, one needs to be in the correct environment, be psychologically prepared for sleep, and have the ability to access the neurophysiologic mechanisms for sleep. Most patients with chronic insomnia have factors that predispose them for insomnia, initiate the insomnia, and perpetuate the insomnia. Gender, age, and coping mechanisms may predispose one to insomnia, whereas poor sleep hygiene, substance abuse, and performance anxiety may perpetuate the insomnia.

Psychiatric disorders may frequently be preceded by insomnia, and the complaint of insomnia may be the last symptom to resolve with affective disorders. Patients with medical disorders, such as congestive heart failure, renal failure, arthritis, and pain syndromes, may complain of insomnia that is related to the medical condition. Sleep disorders, such as sleep apnea, periodic leg movements of sleep, and circadian rhythm disorders, may provoke patients to complain of insomnia. Three primary insomnia disorders have been recognized. Psychophysiologic insomnia is characterized by poor sleep in the usual sleep environment but better sleep in a new environment. Idiopathic insomnia is chronic difficulty with sleep that does not improve with change in environment and has no definable etiology. In sleep state misperception syndrome, some patients perceive themselves to be awake, although the physiologic parameters show that they are asleep.

Physicians should take a thorough history, including a review of the patient's 24-hour schedule; meals; caffeine, tobacco, and medicine intake; feelings about going to bed and going to sleep; and the bed partner's report of the patient's sleep. The patient should be asked to keep a diary of his or her daily events. Clues to the cause of nighttime sleep difficulties frequently can be found in the review of daytime events.

Approach to the Epilepsy Patient with Daytime Sleepiness or Insomnia

The physician who is faced with a patient with epilepsy who has sleep difficulty should approach the complaint with several key points. The complaint should be defined into categories of excessive daytime sleepiness, insomnia, or unusual events at night. A detailed history should be obtained, including information regarding the clinical course, the degree of impact on the patient, the sleep-wake pattern, the report from the bed partner, dietary and activity changes, and drug (including over-the-counter agents) and medical conditions. The physician should look for potential causes of sleep disturbance from three groups: effects of epilepsy on sleep, effects of medication on sleep, and the presence of another sleep disorder.

Daytime sleepiness in the epilepsy patient is common and has a variety of causes (Table 14-2). Using the Epworth Sleepiness Scale, a widely used, validated subjective measure of daytime sleepiness, Malow et al. reported that 28% of 158 adult epilepsy patients surveyed had an elevated

Table 14-2. Some Causes of Sleepiness in Epilepsy Patients

Antiepileptic medications
Seizures
Depression
Insufficient sleep
Inadequate sleep hygiene
Obstructive sleep apnea
Upper airway resistance syndrome
Restless legs syndrome
Periodic limb movements in sleep disorder
Narcolepsy
Idiopathic hypersomnia

score (higher than 10 points). Specifically, 44% of subjects reported a moderate or high tendency to fall asleep while watching television and 41% while sitting or reading.[32] AEDs are often believed by patients and physicians to be the cause of their sleepiness. An Italian multicenter survey of 509 patients taking AEDs reported that somnolence was the most common complaint, experienced by 51 patients (10%).[33] However, 48 of these 51 patients were taking phenobarbital or primidone as one of their AEDs, usually in combination with at least one other AED.

Although sleepiness may result from AEDs, we believe that it is important to consider other causes before attributing sleepiness to these drugs. Unrecognized nocturnal seizures, frequent sleep disruption caused by IEDs, and arousals from sleep are other important causes of sleepiness in the epilepsy patient, and treatment with increased doses of AEDs may improve sleepiness. Video-EEG polysomnography may be useful in evaluation of such patients.[34] Symptoms of drowsiness in a patient on AEDs may also result from a coexisting sleep disorder. In a study of predictors of sleepiness in epilepsy patients, symptoms of OSA or RLS were more significant predictors of elevated scores on the Epworth Sleepiness Scale than the number or type of antiepileptic medication, seizure frequency, epilepsy syndrome, or the presence of sleep-related seizures.[32] As discussed in the section Treatment, identifying and treating coexisting sleep disorders may also improve seizure control or allow the physician to increase a patient's medication regimen to improve seizure control.

Table 14-3. Epilepsy Syndromes That Occur Exclusively or Predominantly during Sleep

---

Autosomal-dominant nocturnal frontal lobe epilepsy
Supplementary sensorimotor seizures
Nocturnal paroxysmal dystonia
Benign epilepsy of childhood with centrotemporal spikes
Lennox-Gastaut syndrome (tonic seizures)
Nocturnal temporal lobe epilepsy
Juvenile myoclonic epilepsy
Generalized tonic-clonic seizures on awakening
Continuous spike waves during slow-wave sleep

Insomnia is a less common complaint in the patient with epilepsy. Insomnia may occur on the basis of frequent arousals caused by epileptic activity. Patients have reported insomnia with FBM and LTG (see previous discussion). Patients undergoing medication tapers during video-EEG monitoring, after being seizure free, or as part of an optimization in their medication regimen may experience insomnia due to removal of sedating AEDs. In addition, depression or anxiety is common in epilepsy patients and may contribute to insomnia. Finally, other causes of insomnia, such as psychophysiologic insomnia, inadequate sleep hygiene, RLS, or periodic limb movements of sleep should be evaluated in epilepsy patients with this complaint.

Parasomnias and Other Sleep Disorders and Their Differential Diagnosis from Seizures

Epilepsy syndromes that occur exclusively or predominantly during sleep (Table 14-3) can be confused with other nocturnal events, such as parasomnias. Table 14-4 and the text in the following section describe some of the distinguishing features of common parasomnias, nocturnal seizures, and psychogenic events.

Non–Rapid Eye Movement Arousal Disorders

Disorders of arousal from NREM sleep are defined by the incomplete arousal from NREM sleep. Patients demonstrate behaviors usually associated with wakefulness while still asleep. Events such as sleepwalking, sleep terrors, and confusional arousals are common in children and to a lesser extent in adults. Approximately 30% of children have sleepwalking or sleep terror events, and the reported prevalence in adults ranges from 2% to 5%.[35–37] The decrease in NREM events with increasing age raises the question that these disorders represent an aberrance of maturation of sleep-wake regulation. Frequently, patients with a NREM parasomnia disorder have a family history.[38] First-degree relatives of a patient with sleepwalking have a tenfold greater incidence of sleepwalking. Typically, NREM events are more common in the first one-third of the night, and patients are amnestic for the event, although a brief visual or auditory perception may occur.

Sleepwalking events can be very elaborate, including behaviors such as dressing, unlocking locks, cleaning, cooking, and driving. Some patients even describe events involving firearms and other potentially dangerous items.[39] Patients can recall various feelings or impressions from the events and, rarely, some imagery. A potential variant of this behavior is nocturnal eating disorder, in which patients arise during the night and eat high-caloric food. The patients generally have different eating habits than their usual daytime habits and have no memory for the events. Patients may eat raw meats, candies with the wrappers, or boxes of cookies. Patients may describe awakening in the morning to find a messy kitchen and food particles still on their bedclothes and in their hair. Occasionally, these events coincide with time periods of restricted caloric intake.[38]

Sleep terrors are a more intense form of sleepwalking, because most patients with sleep terrors also have sleepwalking events. The predominance of autonomic expression during sleep terrors helps to distinguish these events from other partial arousals from NREM sleep. The sudden arousal from slow-wave sleep with a piercing scream or cry, accompanied by autonomic and behavioral manifestation of intense fear, is rarely forgotten by any witness. The onset of the events is abrupt, and patients have tachycardia, tachypnea, flushing, diaphoresis, and mydriasis. The patients are confused and disoriented and attempts to intercede may result in harm to the person trying to wake the patient. Patients can become violent, resulting in injury to the patient and bed partners. Approximately 3% of children and fewer than 1% of adults may have these events.[36,37] Confusional arousals can occur at any arousal from NREM sleep and are characterized by disorientation, slow speech, and mentation or inappropriate behavior.[40] The patients have memory impairment for the event, and the events can be induced with forced arousal. The course of these events usually improves with age and remains stable in adults.

The diagnosis of NREM arousal disorder is usually made by history, although video-EEG polysomnography should be performed to exclude seizure activity, if any atypical characteristics are present. Such characteristics include adult onset, lack of a family history, spells not limited to the first one-third of the night, spells that occur multiple times a night, spells that occur during naps, or stereotyped features. Treatment includes avoidance of sleep deprivation, which can precipitate events; creation of a safe environment for the patient (e.g., window locks, ground floor rooms); and, occasionally, treatment with clonazepam or tricyclic antidepressants.

Rapid Eye Movement Sleep Behavior Disorder

REM sleep behavior disorder (RBD) was predicted by Jouvet in 1965, when he showed in cats that the loss of REM sleep–induced atonia could be produced experimentally by specific pontine tegmental lesions.[41] In 1986, Schenck and Mahowald described RBD in humans.[42] The disorder is characterized by intermittent loss of REM sleep, electromyography atonia, and the appearance of elaborate motor activity associated with dream mentation. These behaviors can include punching, kicking, leaping, running, talking, yelling, and any behavior that could occur during a dream. Bed partners are frequently injured, and patients may go to great lengths to prevent injury to themselves or to bed partners. Patients usually have a vivid recall of the actual dreams that correlate to the witnessed behavior. Dream recall is not uniformly noted in our experience, and patients may not be willing to talk about the dream that led them to seek medical attention. These events occur more commonly in the latter half of the night but can occur any time the patient enters REM sleep. Most cases

begin in late adulthood, but we have seen children as young as age 2 years present with symptoms of RBD. There is a preponderance of men who have RBD.[43] RBD can be induced by medication, and cases of tricyclic antidepressants, monoamine oxidase inhibitors, and serotonin reuptake inhibitors causing RBD-like behavior have been reported. Acute forms of RBD can also occur during alcohol withdrawal and, potentially, benzodiazepine withdrawal. Approximately 60% of these patients have no clear identifiable cause for the disorder. In 40%, an identifiable neurologic disorder, such as strokes, posterior fossa tumors, demyelination, and degenerative disorders, may prevent the induction of REM sleep–related atonia.[44,45]

The diagnosis of RBD is made by a combination of historic and polysomnographic features.[43] Patients or witnesses should give the history of sleep behaviors that are disruptive, potentially harmful, or annoying, or there should be videotape documentation of excessive limb or body jerks, complex movements, or vigorous movements during REM sleep. The polysomnogram should demonstrate excessive electromyography tone in the chin or excessive twitching of the chin or limb leads during REM sleep. The addition of an extended EEG montage is important for excluding epileptic seizures. REM behavior disorder can be distinguished from seizures, because the events are longer and less stereotyped. Patients with this disorder generally respond well to clonazepam. Dopaminergic compounds, AEDs, clonidine, and even tricyclic antidepressants may be helpful in intractable cases.

Other Rapid Eye Movement Sleep–Related Events

Occasionally, patients present with the description of other REM sleep fragmentary events as nocturnal behaviors. Patients with terrifying hypnagogic hallucinations may note recurrent scary imagery just as they are falling asleep. These events may be associated with screaming, yelling, or other frightened behavior. Patients have a clear memory for the events and can recall the visual imagery.[46]

Patients with recurrent sleep paralysis may also present with complaints of unusual spells. These individuals describe complete paralysis on awakening. They cannot move their extremities, and calling out may only produce a weak whisper. They can have concurrent visual imagery and a sense of impending doom or of being chased. These episodes may last seconds to minutes and can be aborted by another individual touching the patient. Patients may note that these spells are recurrent.[47]

A rare disorder, REM sleep sinus arrest can present as events of sudden arousal with a sense of impending doom. In these patients, a sense of panic and fear can be a symptom. These patients may have histories compatible with isolated nocturnal panic attacks. Polysomnography shows sinus pauses of 2.5 seconds or greater during REM sleep. These patients need to be identified and referred for cardiac evaluation and pacemaker placement.[48]

Movement Disorders during Sleep

Patients with rhythmic movement disorder can present with complaints of repetitive movements that occur before sleep onset.[49] The movements are stereotyped, involving large muscles, usually of the head and neck, and are sustained into light sleep. Movements may include head banging, body rocking, leg rolling, humming, and chanting. Some patients are relatively unaware of the movement, and others describe the movement as a calming effect or a compulsion before sleep. This behavior is frequently seen in infants and young children, and the prevalence diminishes with age. It is more commonly seen in individuals with mental handicaps or autism and is more prevalent in men. Emotional stress may provoke the movements. Typical episodes are seen on polysomnography as episodes of rhythmic movement preceding sleep onset and during stage 1 sleep, although rhythmic movement disorder can occur out of any stage of sleep.

Sleep bruxism can also occur as a rhythmic or repetitive movement during sleep.[22,50] Grinding or clenching of the teeth during sleep may produce bizarre sounds, and patients rarely can even vocalize with the episodes. Patients may have abnormal wear of the teeth, jaw pain, headache, facial pain, or tooth pain. They may have hundreds of events per night, and the events increase with emotional stress. Some studies suggest as many as 85% of the population

grinds its teeth to some degree.[22] These events usually begin in the teen years, and occasionally a familial pattern can be ascertained. The polysomnogram demonstrates repetitive bouts of increased temporalis muscle activity, particularly occurring before sleep onset and continuing through stage 2 sleep. Patients should have a dental evaluation and be considered for bite plates.

Panic Disorder

Panic disorders range in prevalence between 1% and 3% of the general population. Approximately 6–14% of young adults report at least one episode of spontaneous panic attack.[51,52] The majority of these events occur during the day, although as many as 2.5% of the attacks may occur exclusively as nighttime events. Two-thirds of patients with panic attacks have had one or more events at night. Polysomnographic data demonstrate that panic attacks can occur at sleep onset, stage 2 sleep, or slow-wave sleep, but the hallmark is that the event occurs after awakening. On polysomnography, patients have an abrupt arousal from sleep, with subsequent associated tachycardia, tachypnea, diaphoresis, tremulousness, feelings of impending doom, and clear memory of the events.[52–55] Distinction of nocturnal panic attacks from other parasomnias, nightmares, gastroesophageal reflux, REM sleep sinus arrest, sleep-related laryngospasm, paroxysmal nocturnal dyspnea, nocturnal asthma, or seizures may require further systematic monitoring to exclude these other etiologies.

Dissociative and Conversion Disorder

Dissociative disorders can also present as nocturnal events (Table 14-4). These disorders are relatively rare and may present initially as only nocturnal events.[56] These fugue states may last hours, with loss of identity and memory. Patients usually have some diurnal symptoms and may have a history of physical or sexual abuse. They can occur in association with post-traumatic stress disorder.[57] During monitoring, patients frequently demonstrate polysomnographic findings of wakefulness before the onset of the spells.[58] Simultaneous time-synchronized video monitoring is required to correlate the

Table 14-4. Nocturnal Events

	Non-REM Parasomnia	REM Behavior Disorder	Nocturnal Seizures	Psychogenic Events
Time of occurrence	First one-third of night	During REM	Any time	Any time
Memory of event	Usually none	Dream recall	Usually none	None
Stereotypical movements	None	None	Yes	None
Polysomnogram findings	Arousals from delta sleep	Excessive electromyography tone during REM	Potentially epileptiform activity	Occur from awake state

REM = rapid eye movement.

behavior with the electrographic data. Conversion disorders also present as nocturnal events. Patients have significant underlying stressors or conflicts that initiate or exacerbate the episodes.[56] They may also have models to mimic epileptic spells. Although unintentional, events have a clear impact on the patients' abilities to function.[56] Most patients with nocturnal event and conversion disorders have arousals before their events and may or may not have memory for the events.

Sleep Attacks

Sleep attacks owing to excessive daytime sleepiness may result from a variety of causes. Intrinsic causes of daytime sleepiness resulting in sleep attacks include narcolepsy and idiopathic hypersomnia. OSA, RLS, or other causes of sleep disruption and chronic sleep deprivation may result in sleep attacks. These sleep attacks may mimic epileptic seizures or the pseudoseizures characteristic of conversion disorders.[59] A cardinal diagnostic feature of these sleep attacks is their propensity to occur in sedentary situations. Performing long-term video-EEG monitoring to exclude seizures is sometimes necessary, and it typically documents drowsiness at the onset of the attack.

Treatment

A wide variety of sleep disorders occurs in association with epilepsy, including OSA, RLS, periodic limb movements of sleep, narcolepsy, and idiopathic hypersomnia. Although subjective sleepiness is a

common side effect of AEDs, it is important to consider other causes of sleepiness before attributing sleepiness to AEDs. Diagnosis and treatment of these coexisting sleep disorders may improve not only daytime sleepiness and quality of life, but also seizure control. A dose-limiting effect of AEDs is sedation; with the improvement of a coexisting sleep disorder, the physician may be able to control the seizure disorder. In addition, seizure control may improve even without increasing AED doses. Several case series of coexisting sleep apnea and epilepsy have described improvement in seizure frequency with treatment of sleep apnea.[60–63] The mechanisms whereby treatment of a sleep disorder improves a seizure disorder are unknown. Resolution of chronic sleep deprivation, improvement in cerebral hypoxemia, and reduction in arousals from sleep have been postulated.

In patients with coexisting RLS or periodic limb movements of sleep, choosing an AED that treats the coexisting sleep disorder may be useful. Such choices include gabapentin and clonazepam. Clonazepam is also useful in treating RBD in association with seizures.

When epilepsy coexists with a sleep disorder known to cause excessive daytime sleepiness (e.g., narcolepsy) or when AEDs are the suspected cause of daytime sleepiness, removing sedating AEDs from a patient's regimen may be helpful. Such agents include barbiturates and benzodiazepines. Some newer AEDs may be less likely to cause sedation than older AEDs. In one double-blind comparison study, CBZ and LTG were equally effective in controlling seizures, but sleepiness was significantly less common in patients taking LTG.[64] Although FBM usage has been limited owing to its adverse hematologic and hepatic effects, side effects such as insomnia are potentially useful in patients with extreme daytime sleepiness. In one study, 9 of 10 epilepsy patients with hypersomnolence treated with FBM had a marked and sustained improvement in daytime wakefulness and alertness.[65] Other measures for reducing daytime sleepiness in the epilepsy patient include simplifying the AED regimen to avoid polytherapy, prescribing AEDs so that the largest dose is given at night, and using extended release preparations.

Insomnia, a rarer complaint in the epilepsy patient, can be treated behaviorally, pharmacologically, or with a combination of modalities. Caffeine use in the late afternoon and evening hours should be avoided, as should heavy exercise or meals just before bedtime. Relaxation techniques and sleep restriction may also be helpful. When AEDs are the suspected cause of insomnia, giving the AED earlier in the evening and substituting a more sedating AED are useful strategies. Addition of a sedative agent may be necessary if the insomnia-producing AED is required for optimal seizure control.

References

1. Touchon J, Baldy-Moulinier M, Billiard M, et al. Sleep Organization and Epilepsy. In R Degen, E Rodin (eds), Epilepsy, Sleep, and Sleep Deprivation (2nd ed). New York: Elsevier, 1991;73–81.
2. Castro L, Bazil C, Walczak T. Nocturnal seizures disrupt sleep architecture and decrease sleep efficiency. Epilepsia 1997;38:49.
3. Mitler M, Gujavarty K, Browman C. Maintenance of wakefulness test: a polysomnographic technique for evaluation treatment efficacy in patients with excessive somnolence. Electroencephalogr Clin Neurophysiol 1982;53:658–661.
4. Hoddes E, Dement W, Zarcone V. The development and use of the Stanford Sleepiness Scale (SSS). Psychophysiology 1972;9:150.
5. Bazil C, Castro L, Walczak T. Daytime seizures increase REM latency and decrease total REM. Epilepsia 1997;38:176.
6. Touchon J, Baldy-Moulinier M, Billiard M, et al. Sleep Instability in Temporal Lobe Epilepsy. In P Wolf, M Dam, D Janz, F Dreifuss (eds), Advances in Epileptology. New York: Raven Press, 1987;709–711.
7. Miller M, Vaughn B, Messenheimer J, et al. Subjective sleep quality in patients with epilepsy. Epilepsia 1996;36:43.
8. Hoeppner JB, Garron DC, Cartwright RD. Self-reported sleep disorder symptoms in epilepsy. Epilepsia 1984;25:434–437.
9. Peled R, Lavie P. Paroxysmal awakenings from sleep associated with excessive daytime somnolence: a form of nocturnal epilepsy. Neurology 1986;36:95–98.
10. Malow B, Lin X, Kushwaha R, Aldrich M. Interictal spiking increases with sleep depth in temporal lobe epilepsy. Epilepsia 1998;39:1309–1316.
11. Declerck A, Wauquier A. Influence of Antiepileptic Drugs on Sleep Patterns. In R Degen, E Rodin (eds), Epilepsy, Sleep, and Sleep Deprivation (2nd ed). New York: Elsevier, 1991;153–164.
12. Wolf P. Influence of Antiepileptic Drugs on Sleep. In P Wolf, M Dam, D Janz, F Dreifuss (ed), Advances in Epileptology. New York: Raven Press, 1987;733–737.
13. Roder-Wanner U, Noachtar S, Wolf P. Response of polygraphic sleep to phenytoin treatment for epilepsy. A longitudinal study of immediate, short- and long-term effects. Acta Neurol Scand 1987;76:157–167.
14. Roder-Wanner U, Wolf P. Effects of Treatment with Dipropylacetate and Ethosuximide on Sleep Organization in Epileptic Patients. In M Dam, L Gram, J Penry (eds). Advances in Epileptology: XIIth Epilepsy International Symposium. New York: Raven Press, 1981;145–157.
15. Harding G, Alford C, Powell T. The effect of sodium valproate on sleep, reaction times, and visual evoked potential in normal subjects. Epilepsia 1985;26:597–601.
16. Ballenger J, Post R. Carbamazepine in manic-depressive illness: a new treatment. Am J Psychiatry 1980;137:782–790.
17. Gigli G, Placidi F, Diomedi M, et al. Nocturnal sleep and daytime somnolence in untreated patients with temporal lobe epilepsy: changes after treatment with controlled-release carbamazepine. Epilepsia 1997;38:696–701.
18. Ketter T, Malow B, Flamini R. Felbamate has stimulant-like effects in patients with epilepsy. Epilepsy Res 1996;23:129–137.
19. Ettinger AB, Jandorf L, Berdia A, et al. Felbamate-induced headache. Epilepsia 1996;37:503–505.
20. Sadler M. Lamotrigine associated with insomnia. Epilepsia 1999;40:322–325.
21. Foldvary N, Perry M, Lisac S, et al. The effects of lamotrigine on sleep and daytime alertness. Epilepsia 1999;40:142.
22. American Sleep Disorders Association. The International Classification of Sleep Disorders Diagnostic and Coding Manual. Rochester: American Sleep Disorders Association, 1990.
23. Aldrich M. Sleep Medicine. New York: Oxford University Press, 1999.
24. Chokroverty S. Sleep Disorders Medicine. Boston: Butterworth–Heinemann, 1999.
25. Kryger MH, Roth T, Dement WC. Principles and Practice of Sleep Medicine (3rd ed). Philadelphia: Saunders, 2000.
26. Young T, Palta M, Dempsey J, et al. The occurrence of sleep-disordered breathing among middle-aged adults. N Engl J Med 1993;328:1230–1235.

27. Redline S, Strohl KP. Recognition and consequences of obstructive sleep apnea hypopnea syndrome. Clin Chest Med 1998;19:1–19.

28. Trenkwalder C, Walters A, Hening W. Periodic limb movements and restless legs syndrome. Neurol Clin 1996;14:629–650.

29. Aldrich MS. Narcolepsy. Neurology 1992;42:34–43.

30. Faraco J, Lin X, Hinton L, et al. Genetic studies in narcolepsy, a disorder affecting REM sleep. J Hered 1999;90:129–132.

31. Bassetti C, Aldrich M. Idiopathic hypersomnia. A series of 42 patients. Brain 1997;120:1423–1435.

32. Malow B, Bowes R, Lin X. Predictors of sleepiness in epilepsy patients. Sleep 1997;20:1105–1110.

33. Beghi E. Adverse reactions to antiepileptic drugs: a multi-center survey of clinical practice. Epilepsia 1986;27:323–330.

34. Aldrich MS, Jahnke B. Diagnostic value of video-EEG polysomnography. Neurology 1991;41:1060–1066.

35. Bixler E, Kalres A, Soldatos C, et al. Prevalence of sleep disorders in the Los Angeles metropolitan area. Am J Psychiatry 1979;136:1257–1262.

36. Klackenberg G. Somnambulism in childhood—prevalence, course, and behavioral correlations. A prospective longitudinal study (6–16 years). Acta Paediatr Scand 1982;71:495–499.

37. Klackenberg G. Incidence of Parasomnias in Children in a General Population. In C Guilleminault (ed), Sleep and its Disorders in Children. New York: Raven Press, 1987:99–113.

38. Kales A, Soldatos C, Bixler E. Hereditary factors in sleepwalking and night terrors. Br J Psychiatry 1980;137:111–118.

39. Mahowald M, Bundlie S, Hurwitz T, Schenck C. Sleep violence—forensic science implications: polygraphic and video documentation. J Forensic Sci 1990;35:413–432.

40. Mahowald M, Ettinger M. Things that go bump in the night: the parasomnias revised. J Clin Neurophysiol 1990;7:119–143.

41. Jouvet M, Delorme F. Locus coeruleus et sommeil paradoxal. C R Seances Soc Biol Fil 1965;159:895–899.

42. Schenck C, Bundlie S, Patterson A, Mahowald M. Rapid eye movement sleep behavior disorder: a treatable parasomnia affecting older patients. JAMA 1987;257:1786–1789.

43. Mahowald M, Schenck C. REM Sleep Behavior Disorder. In M Kryger, T Roth, W Dement (eds), Principles and Practice of Sleep Medicine (2nd ed). Philadelphia: Saunders, 1994;598–601.

44. Schenck C, Mahowald M. Polysomnographic, neurologic, psychiatric, and clinical outcome report on 70 consecutive cases with the REM sleep behavior disorder (RBD): sustained clonazepam efficacy in 89.5% of 57 treated patients. Clev Clin J Med 1990;57:S10–S24.

45. Culebras A, Moore J. Magnetic resonance findings in REM sleep behavior disorder. Neurology 1989;39:1519–1523.

46. Ohayon M, Priest R, Caulet M, Guilleminault C. Hypnagogic and hypnopompic hallucinations: pathological phenomena? Br J Psychiatry 1996;169:459–467.

47. Ohayon M, Zulley J, Guilleminault C, Smirne S. Prevalence and pathological associations of sleep paralysis in the general population. Neurology 1999;52:1194–1200.

48. Guilleminault C, Pool P, Motta J, Gillis A. Sinus arrest during REM sleep in young adults. N Engl J Med 1984;311:1006–1010.

49. Thorpy M, Glovinsky P. Headbanging (Jactatio Capitus Nocturna). In M Kryger, T Roth, W Dement (eds), Principles and Practice of Sleep Medicine (1st ed). Philadelphia: Saunders, 1989:648–654.

50. Hartmann E. Bruxism. In M Kryger, T Roth, W Dement (eds), Principles and Practice of Sleep Medicine (2nd ed). Philadelphia: Saunders, 1994:598–601.

51. Sheeham D. Current concepts in psychiatry. Panic attacks and phobias. N Engl J Med 1982;307:156–158.

52. Craske M, Barlow D. Nocturnal panic. J Nerv Ment Dis 1989;177:160–167.

53. Lesser I, Poland R, Holcomb C, Rose D. Electroencephalographic study of nighttime panic attacks. J Nerv Ment Dis 1990;173:744–746.

54. Hauri PJ, Freidman M, Ravaris CL. Sleep in patients with spontaneous panic attacks. Sleep 1989;12:323–337.

55. Mellman TA, Uhde TW. Sleep panic attacks: new clinical findings and theoretical implications. Am J Psychiatry 1989;146:1204–1207.

56. Diagnostic Criteria from DSM-IV/American Psychiatric Association. Washington: The Association, 1994.

57. Mellman T, Kulick-Bell R, Ashlock L, Nolan B. Sleep events among veterans with combat-related posttraumatic stress disorder. Am J Psychiatry 1995;152:110–115.

58. Thacker K, Devinsky O, Perrine K, et al. Nonepileptic seizures during apparent sleep. Ann Neurol 1993;33:414–418.

59. Malow BA, Fromes G, Selwa LM. Sleep attacks mimicking epileptic seizures and pseudoseizures. J Epilepsy 1997;10:232–235.

60. Wyler AR, Weymuller EA. Epilepsy complicated by sleep apnea. Ann Neurol 1981;9:403–404.

61. Devinsky O, Ehrenberg B, Barthlen GM, et al. Epilepsy and sleep apnea syndrome. Neurology 1994;44:2060–2064.

62. Vaughn BV, D'Cruz OF, Beach R, Messenheimer JA. Improvement of epileptic seizure control with treatment of obstructive sleep apnea. Seizure 1996;5:73–78.

63. Malow BA, Fromes G, Aldrich MS. Usefulness of polysomnography in epilepsy patients. Neurology 1997;48:1389–1394.

64. Brodie M, Richens A, Yuen A. Double-blind comparison of lamotrigine and carbamazepine in newly diagnosed epilepsy. Lancet 1995;345:476–479.

65. Sharp S, D'Cruz OF, Vaughn BV. Felbamate efficacy in the treatment of hypersomnia. Sleep 1999;22:S278.

Chapter 15

Seizures and Cerebrovascular Disease

Edward B. Bromfield and Galen V. Henderson

The term *stroke* refers to a neurologic deficit with sudden or rapid onset due to hemorrhagic or ischemic cerebrovascular disease, which lasts 24 hours or more. A deficit due to ischemia that lasts less than 24 hours is a transient ischemic attack (TIA). Historical references for stroke as a cause of seizures or epilepsy date back to Hippocrates, but it was not until Hughlings Jackson in 1864 that the association was clearly defined: brain damage from stroke as the cause of epilepsy.[1] In 1885, Gowers coined the term *posthemiplegic epilepsy*.[2] Subsequent studies have confirmed that cerebrovascular disease is the most common documented cause of seizures in the elderly, accounting for 22–69% of seizures in this age group.[3–5] As the population ages, cerebrovascular disease will account for an increasingly high percentage of total seizure and epilepsy cases.

An additional relationship between seizures and vascular disease concerns differential diagnosis: In some cases, it is difficult to determine whether the cause of transient neurologic dysfunction is ischemia (TIA) or seizure and, if from a seizure, whether the seizure itself results from a new vascular insult. These distinctions have major implications for treatment.

With stroke, as with other structural lesions of the brain, neuronal damage can alter the balance between excitation and inhibition and lead to acute symptomatic seizures, generally defined as occurring within 1–2 weeks of the stroke, and epilepsy, a chronic tendency toward recurrent unprovoked seizures. The occurrence of acute symptomatic sei-

zures is neither necessary nor sufficient to predict the later development of epilepsy, but in most settings, acute seizures increase the risk of subsequent epilepsy.[6] If the ischemia is of insufficient duration to produce neuronal damage, an acute symptomatic seizure is still possible, but permanent alterations leading to epilepsy should not occur. However, modern neuroimaging has established that the 24-hour definition of a TIA is insufficiently restrictive, as many TIAs lasting longer than a few minutes produce evidence of permanent neuronal damage that could potentially be epileptogenic.[7]

In addition to neuronal damage altering neuronal networks in the direction of hyperexcitability, cortical iron resulting from hemorrhagic strokes can make neuronal membranes more excitable, producing a chronic epileptic focus.[8,9] Finally, stroke treatment can result in seizures, most commonly by causing hemorrhage into an infarcted brain region (i.e., hemorrhagic conversion). Measures for treating or preventing stroke can also occasionally lead to seizures by causing new infarcts or acute elevation of blood pressure that disrupts autoregulation of cerebral blood flow and leads to localized cerebral edema.[10,11]

Etiologies

Cerebrovascular insults are generally divided into those that result from the interruption of blood flow or ischemia and those that result primarily from blood vessel rupture, causing hemorrhage.

Table 15-1. Types of Stroke

Ischemic
Thrombotic
Embolic
    Cardiac
    Artery-to-artery
Small vessel ("lacunar")
Hypoperfusion ("watershed")
Coagulation-related
Vasospastic
    Migrainous
    Vasculitic
Hemorrhagic
Related to vascular malformations
    Arteriovenous malformation
    Cavernous angioma
    Venous angioma
Subarachnoid (aneurysmal)
Spontaneous intracerebral
    Hypertensive (deep, lobar)
    Amyloid angiopathy
Coagulopathy-related
Other
Venous occlusion
Hypertensive encephalopathy
    Hypertensive crisis
    Immunosuppressant-associated
    Postendarterectomy hyperfusion syndrome
    Eclampsia

Prolonged ischemia causes neuronal death; these infarcts may secondarily undergo hemorrhagic conversion, and primary hemorrhages can cause infarcts via pressure effects (e.g., vascular compression and in situ thrombosis) or vasospasm. Stroke classification generally follows a mechanistic scheme, although lesion location is also important, especially for hemorrhagic stroke (Table 15-1).

Ischemic infarcts result in neuronal death as a result of localized loss of blood flow. Energy-dependent processes, such as maintaining ionic gradients across cellular and intracellular membranes, fail, and cell death occurs; excitotoxicity mediated by glutamate receptors also occurs.[12] In addition, as the damage heals, inflammatory processes are activated and can cause further neuronal damage. A frequent cause of ischemic infarcts is progressive atherosclerosis leading to critical stenosis or occlusion of major arteries, such as the internal carotid, vertebral, or basilar arteries; however, an unclear percentage of

such vascular lesions may actually produce infarcts by the phenomenon of artery-to-artery embolisms arising from unstable plaques or thromboses.[7,13] Cardiogenic emboli most often arise from a friable clots occurring on a diseased valvular or myocardial surface. They frequently lodge in large arteries at branching points, such as the origin of the middle cerebral artery (MCA) and its major subdivisions or the basilar bifurcation at the origin of the posterior cerebral arteries (PCAs). Less common are clots that result from nonbacterial thrombotic endocarditis or septic emboli from infectious endocarditis. Embolic strokes usually affect the cortex of gray-white junction, where blood flow is highest and end arteries predominate; cortical involvement would more likely be expected to precipitate seizures and epilepsy than subcortical lesions. Arterial dissection, occurring because of trauma (sometimes trivial or forgotten) to the vessel or connective tissue disorders, or both, can cause embolic or thrombotic stroke in the involved vascular territory.

A common cause of ischemic stroke is progressive stenosis of small vessels, classically from damage to the vascular media caused by chronic hypertension, a process termed *lipohyalinosis* (probably a form of atherosclerosis). This usually affects the penetrating arteries that branch off the MCA or basilar artery, causing "lacunar" infarcts of the basal ganglia, deep white matter, or brain stem. Damage to these areas is less likely to cause acute symptomatic seizures or epilepsy than are strokes that affect cortex directly.

Global cerebral hypoperfusion that occurs in the setting of stenotic vessels can result in focal infarcts, usually occurring at cortical and subcortical border zone or "watershed" areas between territories of the major blood vessels, especially the anterior cerebral artery and MCA or MCA and PCA. Severe hypoperfusion or cardiac arrest can also cause selective damage to these areas, particularly if large vessels are narrowed from atherosclerosis, but more commonly results in widespread damage, sometimes diffusely affecting the middle layers of cortex, termed *laminar necrosis*. Less complete insults may cause selective damage of the hippocampus and cerebellum. Acute symptomatic seizures or status epilepticus (SE), especially myoclonic status, is common after hypoxic-ischemic insults.[14]

Hypercoagulable states, such as may be associated with malignancy, collagen vascular diseases, or genetic abnormalities of the thrombolytic system, cause in situ thrombosis of small or large vessels, often multiple. They are also associated with cardiogenic emboli from nonbacterial thrombotic endocarditis.[13] Certain types of coagulation defects may promote venous rather than arterial thrombosis, leading to venous infarcts (see following discussion) or, among patients with cardiac septal defects, arterial emboli.

Vasospasm is thought to be the main mechanism by which migraine causes occasional stroke; platelet aggregation may also be a triggering event. Migrainous infarction is a rare complication of a common condition and is more likely to occur in those with focal neurologic symptoms as a component of their usual migraine.[15] Vasospasm can also occur as a complication of angiography; patients with migraine may have a higher risk. Branches of the PCA are most often affected. Systemic or cerebral vasculitis is another potential cause of vasospasm and is due to autoimmune disease or drug abuse, particularly of cocaine.[15] Inflammation of the arterial walls can also cause hemorrhage, although this is more common with inflammation caused by infections.

Nearly any kind of ischemic process, if rapidly reversible, can result in temporary dysfunction without permanent damage, manifested as a TIA. As noted previously, magnetic resonance imaging (MRI) has demonstrated that permanent structural changes (i.e., infarcts) can occur, with TIAs lasting well under 24 hours, although the clinical deficits appear to resolve completely.[7] Therefore, not just acute symptomatic seizures but also epilepsy can result from a clinical TIA.

Hemorrhagic conversion of ischemic infarcts occurs when the vessel wall itself is sufficiently damaged to disturb its integrity. Clinically, this is more likely to occur with embolic infarcts than with other types. Furthermore, because current means of treating or preventing ischemic infarcts interfere with clot formation or maintenance, these therapeutic measures also pose a risk of hemorrhage. This risk is low for antiplatelet agents and moderate for anticoagulants and thrombolytic agents.

Hemorrhagic strokes share with ischemic processes a more or less sudden onset but cause cerebral damage in different ways. An arterial leak results in a concussive insult to nearby neurons and axons, leading to neuronal dysfunction and, if sufficiently severe, neuronal death. If the leak is not quickly sealed, then intracranial pressure rises, ultimately to the level of arterial pressure, and cerebral perfusion is precluded until communication between the arterial and extra-arterial cerebral space is ended. This elimination of perfusion pressure can result in global, multifocal, or localized ischemia. Locally, a blood clot constitutes a mass lesion that exerts pressure on nearby neural and vascular structures and sometimes sufficiently interferes with arterial or venous blood flow to cause an infarct. After intracerebral hemorrhage, as with ischemic infarcts, the inflammatory system is activated to dispose of cellular and hematologic debris, and this can cause vasospasm. Furthermore, blood products result in chronic exposure of neurons to iron-containing compounds, which may lead to peroxidation of lipid membranes and promote excitatory ionic currents.[8]

Congenital vascular malformations are a common cause of intracerebral hemorrhage, especially in younger people. These are usually divided into three types. Arteriovenous malformations (AVMs) have a direct arterial-to-venous connection without an intervening capillary bed. Most eventually become symptomatic, with the most common presentation being hemorrhage (40–50%) and the next most common being seizures (17–40%), especially in younger people and perhaps in those with larger malformations.[4,16] AVMs may also produce progressive, and at times transient, ischemic deficits via a steal phenomenon from surrounding normal tissue. Cavernous angiomas consist of vascular channels lined by endothelium without intervening neural tissue. Seizures are the most common presentation, occurring in at least 40–70% of patients.[16] A sizable proportion, however, are incidental findings on MRI and are estimated to occur in 0.5% of the general population[17]; diagnosis is usually dependent on a characteristic heterogeneous pattern with evidence of surrounding blood products, implying at least minor hemorrhage. Venous angiomas are aberrant venous channels that communicate with the normal venous system. Symptoms are uncommon, but of those venous angiomas that become symptomatic, most present with seizures, except those located in the cerebellum, which are the most likely ones to hemorrhage. A fourth type of vascular malformation, capillary telangiectasias, consists of dilated capillary structures with intervening neural tissue; these are most often located in the pons and are rarely symptomatic.

Subarachnoid hemorrhage may result from AVMs or from coagulation or platelet defects, but the most common cause by far is rupture of a saccular aneurysm, thought to result from an area of congenital weakness in the arterial wall, usually located at branch points near the circle of Willis. The most common locations of these aneurysms are the junction of the posterior communicating artery and ICA and the anterior communicating artery; the next most common are the proximal MCA and then the posterior circulation.[7] Although thought to be congenital, they are present in perhaps 5% of the population, and their likelihood of rupture increases markedly with advancing age, as well as with hypertension and smoking. Approximately one-third of ruptures are immediately fatal, another one-third result in significant disability, and another one-third of patients recover without major disability. The major risks after the initial bleed are rebleeding, which may be prevented by surgery to occlude the aneurysmal neck, and vasospasm causing focal or multifocal cerebral ischemia, which may in some cases be prevented by increasing perfusion pressure (unsafe unless the aneurysm has been secured). There is also a risk of hydrocephalus, which may develop early or late. Acute symptomatic seizures may occur at the time of the initial bleed, when they may be confused with syncope resulting from transient cessation of cerebral perfusion, as a result of the acute rise in intracranial pressure to equal that of systemic pressure. Epilepsy and acute symptomatic seizures may be related to hemorrhages that occur parenchymally, as well as in the subarachnoid space; intracerebral extension of the hemorrhage is often associated with rupture of aneurysms that involve the anterior communicating artery and damage the orbitofrontal cortex. Subarachnoid and subdural bleeding can result from another type of anomaly, dural arteriovenous fistulas, which may be acquired as a result of trauma or other insult; these can also cause seizures and epilepsy, although chronic headaches are the usual presentation.[18]

Intracerebral hemorrhages are most commonly due to acute and chronic hypertension, in which case most are located in the basal ganglia, especially the putamen. Although lobar hemorrhages are more likely to produce seizures and epilepsy, some deep hemorrhages, especially those involving the caudate,[19] may also lead to seizures. A substantial proportion of lobar hemorrhages may in fact be due to a different source of vascular damage than that produced by hypertension. The terms *cerebral amyloid angiopathy (CAA), cerebral congophilic angiopathy*, and *cerebrovascular amyloidosis* refer to a clinicopathologic entity characterized by hyaline eosinophilic staining properties.[20] CAA is implicated as the cause of primary nontraumatic intracerebral hemorrhage in as many as 10–15% of patients over the age of 60 years and in nearly 20% of patients over the age of 70 years.[21] This pathology may also produce seizures in the absence of gross hemorrhage; petechial hemorrhage is suspected.[22] Other causes of intracerebral hemorrhage include coagulopathies, either congenital, such as the hemophilias, or acquired, often as a result of treatment with anticoagulants or thrombolytic agents.

The term *hypertensive encephalopathy* refers to an acute cerebrovascular syndrome precipitated by sudden, severe hypertension.[11] When systemic blood pressure is raised suddenly, there is a loss of cerebral autoregulation from forced dilatation of cerebral resistance vessels. Pathologically, these vessels show abnormal permeability to protein, and the surrounding brain shows swelling of astrocytes, primarily of cortical layers 2 and 3.[10] This process results in localized cerebral edema, often affecting the parieto-occipital regions and causing focal deficits and often acute symptomatic seizures.[23,24] Patients usually make a good recovery, and although petechial hemorrhage is common, epilepsy rarely follows these insults. It is important to realize that the degree of hypertension need not be extreme, as long as it is unusually high for a given patient. A clinically and radiographically similar process occurs among patients on immunosuppressant therapy, even in those with only minor elevations of blood pressure; apparently, the immunosuppressant itself can directly affect vessel wall permeability. Eclampsia may result from a similar pathophysiologic process.[25] Again, acute symptomatic seizures are common, but epilepsy is rare. Treatment with magnesium, as discussed in the following sections, is recommended; although magnesium can block the N-methyl-D-aspartate subtype of excitatory glutamate receptors, it is not clear that systemic administration has such an effect across the blood-brain barrier, and its use in this syndrome may suc ceed because of its effects on the underlying vascular pathophysiology.[25,26]

A special situation that is closely related to the processes previously discussed is that of postendarterectomy hyperperfusion syndrome. This occurs usually a day or two after successful carotid endarterectomy and is characterized by acute headache, hemispheric edema ipsilateral to the surgery, and acute symptomatic seizures.[27] Pathophysiology is thought to be rapid restoration of perfusion pressure in a distal circulation that has been accustomed to much lower perfusion and results in a loss of autoregulation and associated dysfunction. Lowering blood pressure is the mainstay of treatment. Antiepileptic drug (AED) therapy, however, is also important to prevent further localized blood flow increases that are associated with focal seizures.

Cerebral venous occlusions may occur spontaneously in patients with a hypercoagulable state (including pregnancy or recent parturition) or in those with intracranial infections, especially in parameningeal locations, such as the mastoid. These occlusions diminish local blood flow and typically produce hemorrhagic infarctions that do not conform to the usual arterial territories. Cortical vein thrombosis commonly produces acute symptomatic seizures, but epilepsy is a much less common sequela.[28–30]

Within each stroke category, cortical involvement increases the likelihood of seizures. This is not surprising in view of the well-established conception of seizures as cortical events. In addition, larger lesions and more severe deficits are associated with a higher risk of seizures and epilepsy in most, but not all, circumstances.

Frequencies

Epidemiology of Stroke

Although the incidence and mortality of stroke have been declining since the 1960s, stroke remains the third most common cause of death, after heart disease and cancers. This decline is likely related to reductions in risk factors, mainly cessation of smoking and treatment of hypertension. Because of population increases, especially among the elderly, absolute numbers of strokes and stroke-related

deaths have nevertheless increased. An estimated 750,000 people in the United States experience stroke each year (recurrent in approximately 10%), and more than seven times that figure, approximately 4.4 million, have experienced stroke before and are at varying risk of developing epilepsy. Stroke incidence and mortality are similar among men and women, but because of differences in age distribution, 60% of stroke deaths occur in women. Incidence and mortality are also higher among African-Americans than European-Americans, with only approximately two-thirds of this difference accountable by differences in cardiovascular and socioeconomic risk factors. Age-adjusted mortality per 100,000 people is 61.5% for white men, 57.9% for white women, 88.5% for black men, and 76.1% for black women.[31,32] There are also regional differences in stroke incidence, which is highest in the southeastern United States (the "Stroke Belt") and lowest in the southwestern and highly populated northeastern states. Worldwide, there are large variations in incidence and mortality, with several countries of Eastern Europe having the highest rates. Among Asians, including Asian-Americans, stroke incidence is high, especially in relation to relatively lower cardiovascular morbidity and mortality; this group also includes a higher proportion (approximately one-third) of hemorrhagic strokes relative to ischemic strokes. Also, large artery stenosis more commonly involves intracranial rather than extracranial vessels in Asian- and African-Americans than in European-Americans.

In addition to age, hypertension (systolic and diastolic), smoking (for hemorrhage, as well as ischemia), and ethnic and regional differences, risk factors for ischemic stroke include previous stroke, heart disease, and diabetes.[31] Evidence for hypercholesterolemia as a risk factor is mixed, although recent studies suggest a benefit of "statin" type cholesterol-lowering agents; these may have other effects in addition to lowering cholesterol, such as altering endothelial surfaces. Interestingly, low cholesterol has been associated with an increased incidence of hemorrhagic strokes, especially when combined with hypertension. Obesity is associated with several other risk factors, and any independent effect is likely to be small. Cancer, especially adenocarcinoma, predisposes to hypercoagulable states. Family history may elevate risk by approximately 50%, apart from other risk factors, and may be decisive in a minority of individuals with intracranial aneurysms and vascular malformations or inborn coagulation anomalies predisposing to bleeding or clotting. Risk of ischemic stroke also increases with blood levels of fibrinogen, homocysteine, and hematocrit, even within the normal range. Lack of exercise also increases risk of ischemic stroke, in addition to being linked to other risk factors, such as heart disease. Moderate alcohol use may be somewhat protective against ischemic stroke, but heavy use definitely increases the risk of hemorrhage. Among women, high-dose oral contraceptives increase risk of ischemia, especially when combined with smoking and older age; this combination is also associated with subarachnoid hemorrhage.[31] Heart disease is a marker for atherosclerosis' predisposing to stroke and is an independent risk factor for embolic disease. Atrial fibrillation constitutes a now widely recognized risk, but myocardial infarction, especially of the anterior wall; congestive heart failure; left ventricular hypertrophy; and patent foramen ovale also are significant.

Frequencies and Risk Factors: Seizures, Epilepsy, and Stroke

Until the 1950s, studies of seizures after stroke were largely confined to necropsy studies.[33] The advent of computed tomography (CT) in the 1970s and MRI a decade later markedly increased the accuracy of clinical diagnosis of stroke mechanisms, particularly with respect to distinguishing between ischemic and hemorrhagic infarcts. Nevertheless, comparison among different studies has been difficult because of different inclusion and exclusion criteria; some have examined only ischemic stroke, others have combined ischemic and hemorrhagic stroke, and some of the latter have excluded subarachnoid hemorrhage or vascular malformations.[4] Fortunately, there have been several recent prospective studies of early,[34–36] or both early and late,[37,38] seizures that have followed large populations (more than 500 patients) for an adequate period of time to draw valid conclusions and have attempted to separately analyze clinically important subgroups. The smaller prospective or case-control studies,[33,39–48] although less valid as sources of incidence data, still provide useful information about risk factors and clinical characteristics. Separate series of patients with intracerebral[19,49–51] or subarachnoid[52–57] hemorrhage or specific vascular malformations[58–62] have provided important data about these subgroups.

Prospective analyses of combined groups have found higher overall seizure rates after hemorrhagic stroke than ischemic stroke. Bladin et al.,[37] for example, found that 10.6% of 265 patients with hemorrhagic stroke and 8.6% of 1,632 patients with ischemic stroke had seizures; because of higher mortality in the former group, survival analysis revealed an almost twofold increased risk. Among those with ischemic stroke, 4.8% occurred within the first 2 weeks (early), including 3.4% within 24 hours ("onset"); corresponding figures for hemorrhagic stroke were 7.9% early and 6.0% at onset. Late seizures occurred in 3.8% of ischemic strokes and 2.6% of hemorrhagic strokes and were more likely to recur than early seizures, a finding verified in nearly all earlier studies. In multivariate analysis, cortical location was the only risk factor for seizures after either type of stroke; increased disability predicted seizures among the ischemic group. Hemorrhagic transformation conferred greater risk on univariate analysis, but a high likelihood of embolism did not, a finding confirmed by a large cohort in the National Institute of Neurological Disorders and Stroke's Stroke Registry,[63] despite conflicting results in earlier studies[45,64] and in one large retrospective study.[34] Lacunar infarction was associated with seizures in 2.6% of cases, although further analysis questioned this relationship. However, risk factors for lacunar disease, including hypertension, serum cholesterol, and left ventricular hypertrophy[65–67] have been associated with the development of seizures or epilepsy, even in those without overt stroke.

Kilpatrick et al.[35] found early seizures in 24 (4%) of 604 patients with ischemic stroke or 4.4%, excluding brain stem and cerebellar strokes, as did Bladin et al.[37]; all 24 patients had cortical infarcts of the anterior circulation, although again embolism was not a risk factor. So et al.[38] found 4.7% onset and 6.2% early (1 week) seizures among those with infarction; initial late seizures occurred in an additional 5% of patients, and epilepsy in 3.3%. Early seizures were a significant risk factor for late seizures and epilepsy. The cumulative risk for initial late seizures was 7.4% by 5 years and 8.9% by 10 years. A British prospective study of

675 patients with a first stroke, 545 of whom had infarction, found a 5-year actuarial risk of 11.5%.[40] Such population-based studies have found seizure risk relative to the general population to be elevated by factors of 20–40. Early (2 weeks) seizures in a Danish cohort of 1,197 patients with ischemic infarct occurred in 4.2% of patients, 2.8% within 24 hours.[36] Stroke severity was the only risk factor in a multivariate analysis. Seizures have been attributed to TIA in 1–4% of patients,[34,35] and in some earlier studies,[48,68] the possibility of seizures heralding TIA or stroke has been advanced, although this relationship is tenuous.

Smaller studies examining occurrence of late seizures or epilepsy[39,47] confirm the importance of large cortical infarcts and suggest a role for apparently preserved cerebral tissue within the infarcted area.[39] Extensive white matter disease in combination with cortical infarction is also important.

No specific incidence figures have been published for border zone infarcts. One would expect that when these infarcts extend to the cortex, there would be risk similar to that of thrombotic lesions. However, the common electroencephalogram (EEG) occurrence of periodic lateralizing epileptiform discharges (PLEDs) after border zone infarcts[69] argues for a possibly higher frequency of seizures and, perhaps, of epilepsia partialis continua or other forms of partial SE. Among less common stroke mechanisms, such as vasospasm as a result of migraine or vasculitis, there is no data concerning seizures. There is only limited evidence linking seizures to specific cortical locations. An excess of anterior rather than posterior circulation strokes may relate to a higher likelihood of cortical involvement. Within a given vascular territory, the probability of seizures or epilepsy may also relate to the intrinsic epileptogenesis of specific cortical regions; limited evidence parallels that for brain tumors[70] or unselected patients[71] and suggests the highest probability associated with perirolandic cortex, followed by the temporal lobe, then prefrontal, parietal, and occipital regions.

Specific studies of intracerebral hemorrhages confirm that early seizures are common, occurring in 4.6–17.0%,[50,51] with all studies showing the highest rates for lobar hemorrhages as 15–24% or more.[19,35,50,72] Most of these patients had hypertension. Among those with deep hemorrhages, the rate of early seizures ranges from 0% to 11%[19]; the cau-

date and perhaps putamen are most often involved, the thalamus least involved. As in infarctions, the majority of early seizures occur within the first day or two, and in approximately one-half, one or more seizures are the first symptom. Late seizures and epilepsy are much less common, even in those with early seizures; between 2 and 5 years, only 6.5% of survivors had any seizures, in contrast to an observed cumulative incidence of 32%.[19] Furthermore, life-table analysis in the same study suggested a cumulative prevalence of seizures to be 50% had all patients survived to 5 years.

Many patients with lobar hemorrhage in early studies may have had CAA, although specific data for seizure risk in this syndrome are not available. Figures are not available specifically for hemorrhage caused by coagulopathies, but location probably plays an important role here also. In a retrospective study to evaluate the incidence of seizures in chronic subdural hematomas, some of which could result from coagulopathies, the rate of occurrence was less than 2%.[73] Five percent of patients presented with a generalized seizure after hemorrhage from dural arteriovenous fistulas.[18]

In general, the incidence of epilepsy as a late sequela of stroke has been estimated at 3–10%, with those who have a late-onset seizure at higher risk (a second unprovoked, late-onset seizure by definition constituting epilepsy). Late seizures may occur earlier after hemorrhage than after infarction.[45] The timing of the initial late seizure (after 1–2 weeks) does not predict later recurrence.[74] SE can occur; in one large study involving 31% of stroke patients with seizures, SE was the initial seizure type in more than half.[75]

With respect to hemorrhagic infarcts due to vascular malformations, AVMs commonly (17–40%) present with seizures.[58,61,62] Presentation with a seizure alone is more common in younger patients. The cumulative risk of epilepsy in untreated patients is estimated at 1% per year, relative to a 2–4% risk of hemorrhage. Cavernous angiomas are commonly undiagnosed until a seizure occurs, with 40–70% presenting with seizures, usually in midlife; epilepsy is typical if the lesion is untreated.[59,60] Venous angiomas rarely bleed and are usually incidental findings; when hemorrhage occurs, seizures are common.

Subarachnoid hemorrhage presents with a seizure in a sizable minority of patients, 6.3–18.0%[55,56];

in one study, thickness of the cisternal clot is the only predictive factor. Another 7% may have presenting seizures; of note is that loss of consciousness at the time of aneurysm rupture more commonly reflects temporary cessation of cerebral perfusion secondary to an acute rise in intracranial pressure. Acute symptomatic seizures may occur in 24–26%, and epilepsy can later develop in 25%, with a higher risk if there are neurologic sequelae and if acute seizures occurred.[57,76] In a small retrospectively studied cohort with unruptured intracranial aneurysms, the overall risk of postoperative seizures in initially seizure-free patients was 15.7%.[77] With cerebral venous thrombosis, seizures have been described in 40% of cases,[28] but subsequent epilepsy appears rare, despite the high incidence of hemorrhage.

Acute symptomatic seizures are one of the hallmarks of hypertensive encephalopathy and related conditions (e.g., eclampsia, hyperperfusion syndrome), occurring in the majority, although later epilepsy is rare, and paralleling the resolution of the often posterior white matter and cortical lesions typically seen on MRI.[23,24]

In the United States, migraine occurs in 18% of women and 6% of men.[78] The prevalence of migraine with aura (which includes hemiplegic migraine) is lower, around 4%,[79] and only a tiny fraction of patients ever experiences the neuroimaging changes or persistence of symptoms for more than 1 week that defines migrainous infarction. No data are available on the frequency of seizures or epilepsy as a complication of this cause of stroke.

Phenomenology

In one study, simple partial seizures, most commonly with motor manifestations with or without secondary generalization accounted for 80% of the classifiable seizures, but it was not possible to determine the seizure type in half of the cases.[39] Most of the remaining classifiable patients had what are considered to be generalized convulsions, although in the presence of a known focal lesion, often involving cortex, the likelihood of partial onset is very high, regardless of whether it is observed. One would expect complex partial seizures, characterized by altered awareness with or without automatisms, to occur particularly with temporal and prefrontal lesions, although studies have not presented sufficient information to confirm this. Simple partial somatosensory or special sensory seizures are also likely to occur but can be difficult to diagnose unless the suspicion is high or a seizure later generalizes.

Any seizure type may present with SE, and 8–17% of stroke patients with seizures have SE, often early in their course.[75] Convulsive SE, although usually clinically obvious, can be subtle in a deeply comatose person after prolonged seizures and include only minor rhythmic face, limb, or eye movements.[80] Nonconvulsive SE is difficult to diagnose and requires a high level of suspicion, especially in those who have not been known previously to have seizures.[81–84] Diagnosis is easiest when there are recurrent, stereotyped complex partial seizures, characterized by unresponsiveness and automatisms and separated by incomplete recovery from the postictal state. More difficult are patients in a continuous "twilight state," classically associated with nonconvulsive generalized SE in those with idiopathic generalized epilepsy, but increasingly recognized as occurring de novo in elderly patients as a result of partial SE, often of frontal lobe origin.[84] The diagnostic dilemma is particularly challenging in those with lesions of vascular or other origin that may in themselves impair cognition and awareness. If recovery does not occur as expected after a witnessed seizure, it is imperative to rule out nonconvulsive SE.[85]

Probably the most common form of simple partial SE after stroke is SE with focal motor manifestations. This can take the form of repeated brief tonic or clonic activity, or both, contralateral to the lesion, or sustained, somewhat irregularly repetitive movements, often confined to a very limited area, such as the hand or the thumb, termed *epilepsia partialis continua*. This condition is notoriously difficult to treat and may persist for days or weeks. Newer drugs that act on the glutamate excitatory system, such as felbamate, may more effectively terminate this form of SE. Use of conventional AEDs is still important, however, to prevent spread of the activity to involve wider areas of cortex and the corresponding hemibody or to produce complex partial or secondarily generalized seizures.

No convincing evidence associates specific seizure types with stroke mechanisms, although location is clearly important. The semiology of late seizures usually parallels that of the early seizures,[43] except that late seizures may be more likely to generalize.[86] However, because of PCA involvement, seizures resulting from posterior leukoencephalopathy due to hypertension, immunosuppressants, or eclampsia are often characterized by visual phenomena, including formed or unformed hallucinations or amaurosis, and seizures are often multiple.[23]

Assessment

As is typical in seizure diagnoses, the most important data derive from the history, which usually must be provided by observers, as well as the patient. Aside from description of the seizure phenomena, important historical features include previous seizures, stroke or other epilepsy risk factors, other medical conditions, and current medications, especially those that could predispose to seizures via either intoxication (e.g., stimulants and many other drugs) or withdrawal (e.g., benzodiazepines, alcohol, and other sedatives). The neurologic examination typically reflects the location and severity of the stroke, although an examination performed shortly after a seizure usually shows a more severe deficit. Such a postictal or Todd's paralysis, in fact, may persist for hours or days if a large stroke or other structural lesion is present.

Neuroimaging abnormalities correspond primarily to the stroke itself, although after seizures and, particularly, after SE, a variety of imaging changes may occur and sometimes persist for days or weeks.[87] These usually affect cortex, as well as white matter, and include hypodensity on CT, T2 hyperintensity on MRI, blurring of gray-white junction (localized edema), or, at least in some cases, hyperintensity on diffusion-weighted imaging. These changes may be more confusing than enlightening in trying to determine whether seizures have occurred, but serial imaging correlated with the changing neurologic exam can be crucial to understanding the clinical process. Perfusion imaging with MRI or single photon emission computerized tomography is also abnormal after stroke, showing hypoperfusion sometimes followed, after a week or more, by surrounding hyperperfusion. Perfusion images in SE, by contrast, show an increase ictally, usually a decrease postictally for minutes or

longer, and then normalization (or return to the abnormal baseline in the case of a stroke). Similar changes can occur even after single seizures, but ictal single-photon emission computed tomography injection in non-SE cases is seldom available outside the epilepsy monitoring unit.

Despite controversies about predictive value, the EEG remains the fundamental investigation for patients with seizures. The main EEG manifestation after stroke is focal slowing. The development of a seizure focus may be accompanied by the appearance of epileptiform discharges (e.g., sharp waves, spikes, or PLEDS). Studies suggest that interictal epileptiform discharges are less commonly seen in older patients than in younger patients with established epilepsy[88]; similar data are not available for acute seizures. On the other hand, sharp waves may occur even in studies of patients who do not have seizures. Well-defined spike foci may have higher predictive value than sharp waves, although detailed evidence is lacking. Most studies, however, suggest that PLEDS are a strong predictor of acute seizures.[57,64,89,90] Focal slowing alone may also be somewhat predictive.[47,86,91] EEG interpretation in the elderly must take into account that normal variants, particularly sharply contoured, alpha-frequency "wickets" in the temporal regions, are not indicators of a seizure tendency.

EEG manifestations of nonconvulsive SE require particular attention. The easiest pattern to diagnose, electrographically as well as clinically, is that of repeated individual seizures with incomplete recovery between episodes. More difficult are those that show continuous rhythmic activity, at times without well-defined spikes or sharp waves.[82,83] This must be distinguished from other causes of more or less rhythmic slowing, especially those associated with metabolic disturbances. The triphasic wave pattern, classically and most commonly seen with hepatic encephalopathy but also associated with uremia, anoxia, and other conditions, is a particular source of confusion. A trial of intravenous benzodiazepines can sometimes clarify the situation if the EEG and patient improve, but one must keep in mind that the triphasic pattern usually disappears in sleep.

Long-term video-EEG monitoring is probably underused in elderly patients in general[88] and in stroke patients in particular. This should be considered when any patient has relatively frequent events that could represent seizures or that have been treated as seizures with inadequate response. Concurrent monitoring of ECG and other physiologic parameters, such as respiratory effort and oxygen saturation, may sometimes suggest alternative diagnoses, as discussed in the following section. Laboratory evaluation is aimed at ruling out metabolic factors that could predispose to seizures.[81] Serum chemistries, particularly sodium, calcium, magnesium, glucose, and renal indices, should be measured. Levels of potentially offending drugs, such as theophylline or the normeperidine metabolite of meperidine, can at times be obtained rapidly enough to be useful. Blood and urine toxic screens can be helpful in assessing the possibility of illicit drug use, particularly in younger patients with stroke and seizures; cocaine is of particular importance. Lumbar puncture is rarely a consideration in stroke patients, except when subarachnoid hemorrhage is considered, and CT is negative for blood, or when the situation suggests that stroke could have resulted from an infectious vasculitis secondary to meningitis. In immunocompromised patients, for example, central nervous system aspergillosis is frequently accompanied by hemorrhage, as a result of fungal invasion through the vessel wall.

Differential Diagnosis

The differential diagnosis of transient neurologic dysfunction is broad, and the elderly population that is at highest risk of stroke is also at risk of many conditions that can mimic seizures.[3] Syncope, for example, may not be benign in this population and may be caused by hypovolemia (e.g., blood loss, diuretics), decreased arterial or venous tone (e.g., vasodilators, autonomic dysfunction), limited cardiac output (e.g., aortic stenosis, arrhythmias), and inappropriate baroreceptor reflexes (e.g., emotional situations, Valsalva maneuver).[92] Upright posture at onset and a typical warning of lightheadedness, nausea, warmth, and fading vision and hearing are common but not universal; in addition, stroke patients may have difficulty reporting these sensations. Cardiac arrhythmias, some potentially fatal, may lead to sudden loss of consciousness, even in the supine position; palpitations may be noted if onset is not sudden or at other times. A few myoclonic jerks commonly accompany syncope, and tonic stiffen-

ing, as well as more complex movements, may also occur, especially if the head is kept upright. The pathophysiology of such convulsive syncope is release of brain stem activity from cortical influence rather than an electrocortical seizure. In addition, syncope can rarely occur as a vertebrobasilar TIA, especially when flow through one or both carotids is severely compromised.

Migraine is an episodic headache that is unilateral or bilateral in location, pulsating in quality, and moderate to severe in intensity and is exacerbated by physical activity. Migraine with aura includes a period of 5–60 minutes of cortical or brain stem dysfunction.[93] Migraine auras are distinguished from seizures by their more gradual, often visual, warning and longer duration. Associated symptoms include nausea or vomiting, photophobia, and phonophobia. Headache usually, but not always, follows; "migraine equivalents" without headache are more common in the elderly and are occasional causes of TIA-like symptoms or of actual TIAs.[15] Loss of consciousness is rare but may occur with so-called basilar migraine. It must be recognized that migraine and epilepsy can coexist, that headaches often follow epileptic seizures, and that a migraine attack can, rarely, precipitate a seizure.[93]

TIAs themselves can be confused with seizures, although they have characteristic symptoms and (if prolonged enough to persist to the time of evaluation) signs consistent with known vascular territories. They typically evolve over minutes and last minutes to hours. As first pointed out by Jackson, unlike seizures, which generally manifest "positive" symptoms, such as stiffening or shaking in the motor system or hallucinations in the special sensory modalities, ischemic symptoms are usually "negative" (e.g., weakness, sensory loss). Exceptions to this rule include ischemic paresthesias, rare motor inhibitory seizures,[94] and "limb-shaking" TIAs.[95] The latter are rare manifestations of severe carotid stenosis and are distinguishable from motor seizures mainly by (1) their consistently postural character, usually occurring promptly on standing, and (2) their involvement of arm or leg, or both, sparing facial muscles and cognition. On the other hand, rare seizure types, such as ictal amaurosis (total or hemianopic, not monocular) or aphasic SE,[96] require EEG to be distinguished from TIAs. Also, patients with CAA have been noted to have transient events for which the underlying pathophysiology has not been established; no evidence of microscopic bleeding, transient ischemia, or epilepsy has been discovered, although duration is more similar to that of TIAs than of the other potential etiologies.[22]

Movement disorders can usually be readily distinguished from seizures; they are typically long lasting and associated with preserved consciousness. Although usually bilateral, they may be unilateral after infarction, particularly that of the basal ganglia, thalamus, or subthalamus. In patients with depressed mental status, toxic or metabolic processes may at times produce movement disorders, such as extrapyramidal reactions to neuroleptics or multifocal myoclonus in uremia. Although the multifocality is not typical of seizures, and the movements are not time locked to epileptiform discharges on EEG, such discharges are often present and imply "cortical irritability" that may later be manifest as clear-cut seizures. Asterixis, an abrupt, repetitive loss of muscle tone during maintenance of certain postures, often occurs in patients with depressed mental status due to hepatic or other encephalopathies. After cerebral or brain stem stroke, it can occur unilaterally, contralateral to the lesion. Its positional nature usually distinguishes it from motor seizures, although rare cases of epileptic asterixis have been reported. Finally, AEDs, especially at toxic levels, can produce involuntary movements, such as dystonia with phenytoin or tremor with valproate.

Sleep disorders may result in microsleeps or more prolonged sleep attacks due to any cause of hypersomnolence, most commonly disrupted sleep from obstructive sleep apnea. This condition, like stroke, is common among patients with hypertension, atherosclerosis, and obesity. Furthermore, many thrombotic strokes, in particular, occur during sleep and are characterized by patients' awakening with a new deficit. Sleep attacks may also occur when patients are sleep deprived for any reason; after sleep apnea, the most common medical reason for this is the movement disorder termed *periodic limb movements in sleep*.[97] These movements usually involve one or both lower limbs, with dorsiflexion of the ankle and flexion of the knee and hip, and are sustained for 1–2 seconds and repeated approximately every one-half minute. This condition is associated with restless legs syndrome, a need to walk around or otherwise move the legs, often in response to a crawling sensation that is felt when lying in bed or otherwise at rest. Narcolepsy is a more dramatic but much less common cause of hypersomnolence. Associated symptoms of hypnagogic or hypnopompic hallucinations, sleep paralysis, and especially cataplexy are usually present.[97] Onset is rare after early adulthood, although symptomatic cases related to brain stem trauma, demyelination, and, rarely, infarction have been reported. Although microsleeps may occur without warning, more prolonged sleep attacks are usually preceded by a subjective feeling of sleepiness; in contrast to patients having complex partial seizures, the eyes are usually closed, and the patient may be awakened with stimulation.

Parasomnias can be difficult to distinguish from nocturnal seizures. The classic parasomnias of slow-wave sleep, sleepwalking, and night terrors are conditions of childhood, although the former sometimes persists into adulthood; there is no association with stroke. In the population at risk for stroke, nocturnal wandering is more likely to occur after a complex partial seizure, and patients usually return to normal awareness rapidly, if stimulated. A parasomnia of rapid eye movement (REM) sleep, REM behavior disorder, by contrast, typically begins late in life and may be associated with extrapyramidal syndromes such as Parkinson's disease; cases in patients with stroke may be coincidental, given the typical ages for both disorders. These attacks consist of partial arousals from REM with a loss of the usual muscle atonia, resulting in "acting out" of dreams, often in a violent manner that may reflect defensive behavior prompted by a frightening dream.[97] The timing of the spells later in the night, when REM periods are longer, can be a useful clue. Polysomnography with additional EEG electrodes may be necessary to distinguish this disorder from nocturnal partial seizures.

Altered behavior due to toxic-metabolic disturbances usually lasts much longer than changes due to seizures. The possibility of certain causes of encephalopathy (e.g., hyper- or hypoglycemia, hyponatremia, hypocalcemia, hypomagnesemia) precipitating acute symptomatic seizures can further confuse the picture. The EEG, although typically showing diffuse slowing, can, at times, display multifocal sharp waves or the triphasic wave pattern, which as previously discussed may be difficult to distinguish from the generalized sharp-slow complexes of nonconvulsive generalized SE.

Distinguishing psychogenic nonepileptic seizures (NESs; e.g., pseudoseizures, psychogenic seizures) from epileptic seizures is a major undertaking of epilepsy monitoring units. Evidence suggests that this phenomenon is most common in young adults, especially women, but there are few data on the frequency and manifestations in elderly patients, and it may be underdiagnosed. Patients with a previous psychiatric history are likely to be at higher risk, as may be those with depression or other psychiatric complications of stroke, but data are unavailable. In general, compared to epileptic seizures, psychogenic NESs display less stereotypy, longer duration, a more waxing and waning nature, and nonphysiologic progression.[98] Eyes tend much more often to be closed during unresponsive periods. Environmental precipitants are more likely and injuries less likely, although there are many exceptions. Unlike epileptic seizures, NES do not arise from sleep, although they may arise from "pseudosleep," and video-EEG monitoring may be required.

Finally, transient increases in intracranial pressure can result in temporary alteration in awareness or, less often, focal neurologic dysfunction. Although the classic situations are those of a third ventricular tumor's intermittently obstructing ventricular flow or a posterior fossa mass, acute hydrocephalus can occur in patients after subarachnoid hemorrhage[99] or after ischemic or hemorrhagic stroke in the cerebellum. Patients with cerebral edema, as a result of hemispheric infarction, are likely to show catastrophic focal deficits followed by progressive obtundation. Headache is common in all of these scenarios, if the patient is alert and articulate enough to report it.

Treatment

The mainstay of treating seizures associated with acute or chronic stroke, after identification and elimination of toxic or metabolic disturbances lowering the seizure threshold, is the use of AEDs. Whether other therapies such as antioxidants or neuroprotective agents can, if given shortly after the insult, prevent the later development of epilepsy is an area of active research, but as yet no clear recommendations have emerged.

Of approximately 30 drugs approved in the United States for the treatment of epilepsy, fewer than a dozen are in widespread use; these include several that have been developed and approved in the 1990s.[100] There are few comparative studies; they do not suggest major differences in efficacy. There is wider variation with respect to common adverse effects, available routes of administration, recommended dosing interval, interactions, and cost. These differences may be of particular importance in stroke patients.

The first step in treatment is to verify whether the episode was a seizure, as opposed to another type of transient event discussed in the previous section. Once that condition is satisfied, the decision to treat depends on the likelihood and potential morbidity of another seizure versus risks of treatment. In reported studies, relatively few patients have multiple acute seizures; the fact that most of such patients are given AEDs may account for this. Although there are no data on the treatment efficacy of acute seizures specifically in the setting of stroke, it may be reasonable to extrapolate from the widely cited study by Temkin et al. of patients with moderate and severe head trauma[101]: In these patients, phenytoin was effective in preventing seizures within the first week, but it did not decrease the incidence of a first late seizure in patients followed for approximately 1 year.

Potential morbidity of acute poststroke seizures includes increase in blood flow to an already edematous cerebrum, elevation of blood pressure, and danger of aspiration. Although seizures and SE are uncommon causes for deterioration,[34,43] there are cases reported that involve permanent worsening after a seizure, despite lack of evidence of any additional stroke.[102] On balance, it is reasonable to treat for a limited period of time any patient with a stroke, especially a large stroke, who has an acute seizure that does not have an obvious toxic or metabolic precipitant. The duration of such treatment should be at least a week, and perhaps a month or longer. In the case of a single late seizure, the majority, although not all, go on to develop epilepsy, and treatment at this time is justified for a longer period, perhaps for 1–2 years. When epilepsy has developed (i.e., after two late seizures), longer treatment of at least 2 years, as in other cases of epilepsy, is indicated. The use of EEG findings in deciding when to stop treatment has been questioned, although unequivocal epileptiform discharges and PLEDS in the acute or subacute setting would argue for continued treatment. A history of SE of any type would also suggest longer treatment duration, because, in adults, unlike in children, the occurrence of SE as the first seizure carries a higher risk of seizure recurrence.[6]

One potential consideration concerns whether many AEDs, including phenytoin, phenobarbital, and benzodiazepines, perhaps by virtue of their ability to dampen sustained repetitive neuronal firing, may inhibit recovery from stroke.[103] There is moderate laboratory and sparse clinical evidence that this is true. Because of the very real risk of morbidity posed by seizures in many situations, this possibility should not argue against treatment after a seizure has occurred, but it may be a consideration in cases in which prophylaxis is considered (e.g., large hemispheric lesions with edema) and may affect AED selection when there is more information available.

In subarachnoid hemorrhage, most seizures occur with rerupture of the aneurysm.[53] Currently, no data are available to specifically justify prophylactic anticonvulsant agents in the presentation of a ruptured subarachnoid hemorrhage, but awareness of the morbidity risk of a seizure in this setting and the extrapolation of the Temkin et al. data for head trauma[101] would favor treatment. In lobar hemorrhages, owing to the prevalence of generalized seizures, one can argue that prophylaxis is justified.[19,35,49,50] Also, the theoretical risk of impeding recovery from infarction would not apply. In cerebral venous thrombosis, prophylactic administration of antiepileptic medication is not justified if it has not presented with a seizure.

As mentioned, choice of AED depends on potential routes of administration, interactions with other medications, and specific metabolic conditions, such as renal or hepatic impairment. Because of its relative lack of sedation and ease of loading by a parenteral route, the mainstay of acute seizure treatment in the United States remains phenytoin, although it is not clearly efficacious in all circumstances (e.g., hypoglycemia or alcohol withdrawal). The recent availability of fosphenytoin provides more flexibility, mainly by allowing intramuscular administration to those without adequate intravenous access. Although fosphenytoin can be

given more quickly intravenously than phenytoin, because of the time taken to dephosphorylate the molecule, adequate brain phenytoin levels may not be achieved significantly more quickly. Fosphenytoin is dosed in phenytoin equivalents, rather than in actual quantities of fosphenytoin itself. In the inpatient setting, typically some or all of the loading dose is given parenterally. Although the familiar "gram of phenytoin" is adequate for loading in a patient who has had a single seizure, in treating convulsive SE, the target level should be in the range of 20–25 mg/liter, and so a loading dose of 18–20 mg/kg (keeping in mind that volume of distribution in adults is 0.8 mg/liter) should be given at the maximal rate of 50 mg per minute of phenytoin or 150 mg of fosphenytoin (in phenytoin equivalents) per minute.[101] Because of the possibility of decreases in pulse rate and blood pressure, cardiovascular monitoring is mandatory, sometimes necessitating a slower rate of infusion, administration of fluids, or, less commonly, pressors. Monitoring of vital signs is particularly important in stroke patients, who are usually elderly and often have cardiac disease. Because of the slow absorption of phenytoin 100-mg or 30-mg extended-release capsules, oral loading is affected by metabolism, so that the dose to obtain a given peak level must be higher, approximately 1 mg/kg for each desired 1 mg/liter rise in level. Peak oral level is reached more quickly if the 50-mg chewable tablet is used; of note is that this preparation, which contains the acid form rather than the sodium salt, has a slightly higher amount of phenytoin than does the equivalent dose of phenytoin sodium capsules. The 125 mg/5 ml suspension also contains the acid form. Although this may be convenient to use in patients receiving tube feedings, unless this preparation is vigorously shaken, the phenytoin may precipitate in the bottom of the bottle, yielding doses that are lower (if from the full bottle) or higher (if from the bottom of the bottle) than intended.

Important interactions with other drugs follow from two characteristics of phenytoin. First, as noted, it is highly protein bound, so that mutual displacement from binding sites occurs with several other drugs, most notably aspirin. Second, phenytoin is, like carbamazepine and phenobarbital, a potent inducer of the P-450 mixed-function oxidase hepatic enzyme system that is responsible for the metabolism of many important drugs; in stroke patients, the most important of these drugs is warfarin. When phenytoin is added to these drugs, their doses typically must be increased if the therapeutic effect is to remain constant; careful monitoring is needed of levels or therapeutic effects, or both (e.g., prothrombin time). This interaction takes several days to develop fully. Conversely, when phenytoin is withdrawn, the warfarin dose must be reduced and prothrombin times followed closely. Other drugs frequently used in stroke patients whose metabolism is induced by phenytoin, phenobarbital, and carbamazepine include digoxin, many anti-arrhythmic agents, and beta-blockers.

The situation most commonly necessitating phenytoin discontinuation is the development of a rash, which occurs in 5–10% of patients or less common idiosyncratic reactions, such as fever, lymphadenopathy, or hepatic dysfunction, or a combination of these. Although the rash may resolve even without discontinuation, most clinicians elect not to continue treatment. One must recognize, however, that in elderly patients, who often take a number of medications, many other drugs, particularly antibiotics, can also cause rash. There is no evidence that sudden discontinuation of phenytoin causes withdrawal seizures, but if it is needed for seizure control, prudence dictates coverage with adequate doses of an alternative AED when phenytoin is withdrawn. It must be recognized that the two most commonly used alternatives, phenobarbital and carbamazepine, may cause cross-reactivity allergic reactions as often as 20% of the time. If the reaction is not severe, this risk may be reasonable. Dose-related side effects primarily include dizziness and ataxia; chronic effects include gum hyperplasia, more common in children, and osteopenia, mediated largely but not completely through interference with vitamin D metabolism. This is a particular concern in older women, who, if long-term treatment is anticipated, should be considered for bone density screening, vitamin D supplementation, and other medical therapy.

Phenobarbital offers the advantage of parenteral (intravenous or intramuscular) administration. As with phenytoin, loading doses may be given, but they increase the chance of sedation depending on dose, rate, and route. Many laboratories consider the therapeutic range to be 15–40 µg/ml, although levels of 10–15 µg/ml or less may be enough to control seizures in many patients. The target level depends on the perceived risk of adverse effects, principally sedation, versus the risk and potential morbidity of another seizure. Because the volume of distribution in adults is approximately 0.5 liter/kg, a loading dose of 2 mg/kg is needed to raise the level by 1 µg/ml. In SE, 10–20 mg/kg can be given at up to 100 mg per minute, but again, cardiovascular depression is a significant risk, especially in the elderly. Respiratory suppression in this setting is virtually universal, particularly if benzodiazepines have been given first. At more modest doses, sedation is the most common adverse effect, although patients with neurologic impairments can sometimes have "paradoxic" agitation, probably resulting from disinhibition of behavioral control or exacerbation of pre-existing focal or global neurologic deficits.

Discontinuation of phenobarbital, at least in patients on chronic treatment, has been linked to withdrawal seizures. Like phenytoin and carbamazepine, phenobarbital is a potent inducer of the hepatic P-450 enzyme system and has similar effects on the metabolism of warfarin and other drugs and on bone density. Dose-related effects include sedation, depression, and cognitive slowing, as well as dizziness and ataxia. Chronic effects on connective tissue, such as frozen shoulder, have also been reported.

Carbamazepine is considered, along with phenytoin, to be a first-choice drug for chronic treatment of partial or secondarily generalized seizures. There is no parenteral formulation, however, and oral loading doses or even an average maintenance dose, such as 800 mg per day in an adult, are poorly tolerated when therapy is initiated, leading to dizziness, diplopia, and malaise. On the other hand, because of slow metabolism before autoinduction of appropriate hepatic enzymes in 2–6 weeks, even a typically well-tolerated starting dose of 100 mg twice a day (b.i.d.) may produce levels in the therapeutic range of 4–12 µg/ml, providing some protection against seizure recurrence. Titration schedule is variable, but increases of 100–200 mg per day can be made every 2–4 days, aiming for an initial target dose of 400–800 mg per day. The recent development of slow-release preparations suitable for b.i.d. administration has simplified carbamazepine administration. The liquid form may not produce sufficiently reliable absorption, but pharmacies can formulate suppositories for rectal administration. Important considerations in the elderly patient, in addition to drug interactions, such as those described previously for phenytoin and phenobarbital, are of the possibilities, especially at high levels, of bradyarrhythmias due to slowed conduction at the atrioventricular node and of hyponatremia as a result of renal insensitivity to antidiuretic hormone. The most common dose-related adverse effects are dizziness and diplopia. Carbamazepine metabolism is sensitive to many other enzyme inducers and inhibitors; among the latter, which can produce major carbamazepine toxicity, are such commonly used drugs as erythromycin, cimetidine, and verapamil.

Valproate or the dimeric form, divalproex, offers a useful alternative to the previous drugs, especially with the intravenous formulation that became available in the mid-1990s. It is effective against tonic-clonic, including secondarily generalized, seizures, as well as absence, myoclonic, and simple and complex partial seizures, although carbamazepine may have slight advantages for patients whose partial seizures do not secondarily generalize. Because of its short half-life (12–16 hours without concomitant administration of P-450–inducing drugs, 5–10 hours with such administration), a steady state is reached rapidly at the maintenance dose of 15–30 mg/kg; higher loading doses may also be used, although gastrointestinal upset can occur. A liquid form is also available, at 250 mg/5 ml. It should be recognized that the enteric-coated divalproex preparation, although less likely to produce gastrointestinal upset, has delayed absorption, resulting in peak levels 4–6 hours after administration. The intravenous formulation offers an option when gastrointestinal administration is unavailable, such as postoperatively or with impaired swallowing and no nasogastric access. It also has been used successfully off label in treating SE, often at administration rates much faster than the recommended 20 mg/kg per hour.

One advantage of valproate is its lack of cross-reactivity with phenytoin, phenobarbital, and carbamazepine; rashes and other overt allergic reactions are uncommon. Although idiosyncratic hepatic dysfunction and pancreatitis are the most feared adverse reactions, these are extremely rare after infancy in the absence of pre-existing organ dysfunction. A potentially more important risk in an ill, elderly patient is the possibility of thrombocytopenia or thrombocytopathy. Although idiosyncratic, this is more common at high doses and levels. Bleeding time is not always abnormal, and aspirin can potentiate this effect. There have been no studies of whether this antiplatelet effect can be beneficial in patients with vascular disease. Aspirin also potentiates the therapeutic effects of valproate by displacing it from binding sites, thereby elevating free levels; the total level may be unchanged or even decline slightly because of increased free drug as a substrate for metabolism. Among other potential adverse effects, tremor is most common at high doses and levels, and weight gain with chronic use occurs in approximately 30% of patients.

With respect to relative cognitive effects of the older AEDs, no major differences have been found among phenytoin, carbamazepine, and valproate, although phenobarbital is likely to have more detrimental effects, on average.[104,105] Further studies are needed to establish whether the newer drugs have less effect on cognition than the older AEDs.

Among the AEDs approved since 1993 in the United States, gabapentin is one of the most widely used to treat seizures and other conditions, especially chronic pain. Although it has not been approved as monotherapy, and there is no evidence that it is any more effective or even as effective as the previously discussed drugs when used alone, it has several advantages. It is usually well tolerated, even when rapidly titrated upward; it bypasses hepatic metabolism, being almost completely renally excreted unchanged; and it lacks pharmacokinetic interactions with other drugs. Although there is no parenteral form, the capsules or their contents may be administered through feeding tubes. Its spectrum of action, encompassing partial seizures, including those with secondary generalization, is appropriate for most stroke patients with new-onset seizures. In patients with refractory epilepsy and no renal impairment, there is a dose-related improvement in seizure control between 900 mg per day and at least 1,800 mg per day; higher doses of up to 3,600 mg per day or more have led to improved control in some patients. For the hospitalized patient with a first seizure, initiation with 300 mg 3 times a day (t.i.d.) is reasonable and, if tolerated and necessary, this can be increased over 1–3 days to 600 mg t.i.d.; in patients with impaired renal function, these doses should be scaled back in proportion to creatinine clearance. A slower titration in less acute settings is 300 mg per hour, adding an additional 300-mg dose every 1–3 days. Side effects are usually transient and mild and include fatigue, dizziness, and sedation; hypotension may occur rarely.

Lamotrigine has been approved as an adjunct and a monotherapy agent for treating partial or tonic-clonic seizures. However, the slow titration regimen required to minimize the chance of an allergic reaction, particularly rash, limits its use in hospitalized patients. It is a good alternative for patients who have not responded well to one of the enzyme-inducing drugs; if the response to the combination is favorable, then the initial drug may be cautiously withdrawn over several weeks. When added to a regimen including valproate, which markedly inhibits the metabolism of lamotrigine, the titration rate must be still slower, starting in adults at 25 mg every other day, rather than 50 mg per day. The approved guidelines for using this drug do not encompass initiating it in patients not taking AEDs or in patients taking valproate without an enzyme-inducing drug. Experience suggests, however, that a reasonable approach in the first case is to start at 25 mg every other day and, in the latter case, at 12.5 mg every other day.

Topiramate is another relatively new AED that needs to be slowly titrated to avoid primarily cognitive side effects. A starting dose of 25 mg per day, increasing weekly by 25 mg to a target of 200–400 mg per day, is recommended. Of note is a 1–2% risk of renal stones, suggesting avoidance or at least careful attention to hydration in patients prone to this condition.

Oxcarbazepine, a newly approved drug in the United States, although it has been in widespread use in Europe for several years, is closely related to carbamazepine but has a different metabolic profile and less impact on hepatic enzymes; no effect on warfarin metabolism, for example, has been found. It is approved as monotherapy, and the starting dose, 300 mg b.i.d., is considered to be therapeutic. It can be increased at a rate of 300 mg b.i.d. every week to a maximum of 1,200 mg b.i.d., although slower rates probably minimize side effects. Adverse effects are similar to those of carbamazepine, consisting mainly of dizziness and diplo-

pia at high doses, hyponatremia, and an allergic rash; cross-reactivity with carbamazepine is estimated at 25–30%. Oxcarbazepine metabolism is accelerated by enzyme-inducing AEDs, and oxcarbazepine itself may decrease phenytoin levels by approximately 30%.

Another new AED worthy of consideration is levetiracetam, which is relatively well tolerated, free of pharmacokinetic interactions, and efficacious. Currently approved only for adjunctive use, it can be started at a low therapeutic dose of 500 mg b.i.d. and increased by a similar amount every 2 weeks to a target dose of 1,500 b.i.d., but slower titration rates may be better tolerated in elderly patients or others with reduced renal function. Zonisamide and tiagabine are other new AEDs, both approved as adjunctive therapy for partial seizures, that need to be titrated slowly to avoid primarily cognitive side effects. Zonisamide cross reacts with sulfa drugs and should be avoided in those with sulfa allergies.

Benzodiazepines have a limited but important role in the treatment of seizures in patients with stroke or other serious illnesses. Parenteral administration allows onset of activity within minutes, which is useful especially in the treatment of SE. However, duration of action is limited, particularly for diazepam, which is redistributed out of the brain into other fatty tissues within 15–20 minutes. Lorazepam, by contrast, may remain active for 4–12 hours. Clonazepam has an even longer half-life but is not usually used intravenously in the United States. Other routes of administration are worthy of consideration for conditions milder than generalized convulsive SE, such as clusters of seizures with recovery between them or simple or complex partial SE without secondary generalization. In the first case, rectal diazepam gel is an approved safe and effective method; dosing depends on patient weight but ranges between 10 and 20 mg for adults. Alternatives include sublingual lorazepam, 0.5–2.0 mg, or buccal midazolam, 2–4 mg, both resulting in more rapid absorption than oral administration; both require patient cooperation.

The urgency of treating partial SE, especially complex partial SE, is controversial; options include full intravenous treatment identical to that for generalized convulsive SE; sublingual or buccal benzodiazepines, along with intravenous phenytoin, phenobarbital, or valproate; and oral boluses of AEDs. For refractory tonic-clonic SE, intravenous propofol, midazolam, or pentobarbital have been used.[106] The first two agents are preferable to the third in most stroke patients, who are more prone to hypotensive effects because of age and comorbidity. Drug-induced coma with these agents is also a consideration in refractory complex partial SE.

For acute symptomatic seizures due to eclampsia, phenytoin and benzodiazepines may have a role, but recent studies suggest that intravenous magnesium is the mainstay of treatment.[25,26] One regimen is a 4-g load, followed by continuous infusion of 2–4 g per hour, to maintain a level of 4–8 mg/dl without losing deep tendon reflexes and muscle strength. Whether this regimen should also be used in hypertensive or immunosuppressant-related posterior leukoencephalopathy is not known. When hypertension is clearly a causal factor, rapid control of blood pressure using labetalol or nitroprusside is recommended.

Stroke treatments sometimes need to be modified because of the coexistence of seizures or AED use. As mentioned, the use of the enzyme-inducing AEDs phenytoin, carbamazepine, or phenobarbital produces major increases in warfarin metabolism, and warfarin doses must be adjusted when these AEDs are initiated or withdrawn, or when major dose changes are made. Furthermore, if seizures are not completely controlled and sometimes result in falls, warfarin may be contraindicated. This is a concern mainly in patients with atrial fibrillation, the best supported indication for anticoagulation. It is likely that alternative treatments, such as adjusted subcutaneous heparin or low-molecular-weight heparin preparations, pose similar risk of serious bleeding in those at risk of falls or other trauma. Antiplatelet agents have lower risk but also lower efficacy in stroke prevention for those with atrial fibrillation. Antiplatelet agents, as discussed previously, must be used with caution in patients on valproate.

For those undergoing surgery, including endarterectomies, aneurysm clipping, or resection of a vascular malformation, postoperative changes in absorption and metabolism of AEDs must be considered. Medications with intravenous formulations do not pose a problem, as doses are equivalent to the oral forms. Medications without parenteral forms generally can be given via a nasogastric tube, but only if the gastrointestinal tract is functional. Pharmacies can prepare suppositories for rectal administration in some cases, as for carbamazepine. An alternative is temporary administration of an alternative drug intravenously; for example, lorazepam 1 mg b.i.d. or t.i.d. can provide adequate antiseizure coverage in many cases for 1 or 2 days. If longer parenteral administration is required, phenytoin is a reasonable alternative. Regarding postoperative metabolic changes, phenytoin levels fall after general anesthesia, and carefully following levels and giving boluses as needed can prevent seizures in this setting. Carbamazepine levels may fall initially, either as a result of missing oral doses or of decreased absorption, but on the next day may sometimes rise significantly; clinical toxicity often does not occur, however, because the increase may be due to diminished conversion to the somewhat more toxic epoxide metabolite.

Another potential issue is the recent observation that many AEDs not only decrease folic acid levels, but also increase homocysteine levels, a recently identified risk factor for stroke.[107] Although numbers of patients on newer medications were small, a surprising finding was that this effect was not limited to the enzyme-inducing AEDs that are known to increase folate metabolism. Effects were larger in older individuals and in men. Although most patients had folate and homocysteine levels in the normal range, there may still be implications for stroke risk.

A final consideration in modifying stroke treatment when patients have seizures concerns the unusual condition of vasculitis. The immunosuppressant drugs used to treat these conditions, including cyclosporine A and corticosteroids, are metabolized by hepatic enzymes, and doses may need to be increased when inducing AEDs are added. Furthermore, cyclosporine A can lower the seizure threshold and must be used with caution in seizure patients.

Prognosis

Most studies have not shown an effect of seizures per se on stroke morbidity or mortality,[35,37] although this is confounded, especially in hemorrhagic stroke, by mortality in the most severely affected patients before development of seizures.[19] In addition, there are rare cases of deficits seeming to worsen permanently after a seizure or series of seizures.[102] The prognosis of epilepsy caused by stroke is not clearly different from epilepsy due to other causes, although as a group, elderly patients tend to have better seizure control than younger patients.[3] Most series that address this issue indicate that seizures are readily controlled with AEDs.[34,35,84] Whether this differs for ischemic or hemorrhagic stroke is unclear. The occurrence of seizures in 15% of stroke rehabilitation patients did not affect functional outcome.[108]

Poststroke epilepsy usually responds well to adequate doses of a single agent. If seizures are completely controlled, AED withdrawal can be considered after 2 years, but recurrence risk is probably higher among patients with structural lesions and an abnormal examination than those without (particularly if there were also acute symptomatic seizures).[109,110] The potential consequences of a recurrent seizure are highly variable, depending on activities such as driving or medications such as anticoagulants. Just as in deciding whether to start AEDs, the decision to withdraw must be individualized.

References

1. Jackson JH. On the Scientific and Empirical Investigation of the Epilepsies. In J Taylor (ed), Selected Writings of John Hughlings Jackson. London: Hodder and Stoughton, 1931;233. Referenced in: Lesser RP, Luders H, Dinner DS, Morris HH. Epileptic seizures due to thrombotic and embolic cerebrovascular disease in older patients. Epilepsia 1985;26:622–630.
2. Gowers WR. Epilepsy and Other Chronic Convulsive Disorders. New York: Dover, 1964;106. Referenced in: Lesser RP, Luders H, Dinner DS, Morris HH. Epileptic seizures due to thrombotic and embolic cerebrovascular disease in older patients. Epilepsia 1985;26:622–630.
3. Bromfield EB. Seizure Disorders in the Elderly. In SC Schachter, D Schomer (eds), The Comprehensive Evaluation and Treatment of Epilepsy: a Practical Guide. San Diego: Academic, 1997;233–254.
4. Ettinger AE. Structural causes of epilepsy. Neurol Clin 1994;12:41–56.
5. Thomas SV, Pradeep KS, Rajmohan SJ. First ever seizures in the elderly: a seven-year follow-up study. Seizure 1997;6:107–110.
6. Hesdorffer DC, Lograscino G, Cascino G, et al. Risk of unprovoked seizure after acute symptomatic seizure or status epilepticus. Ann Neurol 1998;44:908–912.
7. Sigurdsson AP, Feldmann E. Stroke. In MA Samuels (ed), Hospitalist Neurology. Boston: Butterworth–Heinemann, 1999;133–158.
8. Suzer T, Coskun E, Demir S, Tahta K. Lipid peroxidation and glutathione levels after cortical injection of ferric chloride in rats: effects of trimetazidine and deferoxamine. Res Exp Med 2000;199:223–229.
9. Willmore LJ, Sypert GW, Munson JB. Recurrent seizures induced by cortical iron injection: a model of posttraumatic epilepsy. Ann Neurol 1978;4:329–336.
10. Nag S, Robertson DM, Dinsdale HB. Cerebral cortical changes in acute experimental hypertension: an ultrastructural study. Lab Invest 1977;36:150–161.
11. Oppenheimer BS, Fishberg AM, Hypertensive encephalopathy. Arch Intern Med 1928;41:264.
12. Caplan LR. Basic Pathology, Anatomy, and Pathophysiology of Stroke. In LR Caplan (ed), Stroke: A Clinical Approach. Boston: Butterworth–Heinemann, 1993;23–66.
13. Caplan LR. Brain Embolism. In LR Caplan (ed), Stroke: A Clinical Approach. Boston: Butterworth–Heinemann, 1993;349–375.
14. Wijdicks EF, Parisi JE, Sharbrough FW. Prognostic value of myoclonus status in survivors of cardiac arrest. Ann Neurol 1994;35:239–243.
15. Caplan LR. Nonatherosclerotic Ischemia. In LR Caplan (ed), Stroke: A Clinical Approach. Boston: Butterworth–Heinemann, 1993;319–348.
16. O'Brien TJ, Kazemi J, Cascino GD. Localization-Related Epilepsies Due to Specific Lesions. In J Engel Jr, TA Pedley (eds), Epilepsy: A Comprehensive Textbook. Philadelphia: Lippincott–Raven, 1997;2433–2445.
17. Robinson JR, Awad IA, Little JR. Natural history of the cavernous angioma. J Neurosurg 1991;75:709–714.
18. Daffau H, Lopes M, Janosevic V, et al. Early rebleeding from intracranial dural arteriovenous fistulas: report of 20 cases and review of the literature. J Neurosurg 1999;90:78–84.
19. Faught E, Peters D, Bartolucci A, et al. Seizures after primary intracerebral hemorrhage. Neurology 1989;39:1089–1093.
20. Coria F, Rubio I. Cerebral amyloid angiopathies. Neuropathol Appl Neurobiol 1996;22:216–227.
21. Gilbert JJ, Vinters HV. Cerebral amyloid angiopathy; incidence and complications in the aging brain. Cerebral hemorrhage. Stroke 1983;14:915–923.
22. Greenberg SM, Vonsattel JP, Stakes JW, et al. The clinical spectrum of cerebral amyloid angiopathy. Neurology 1993;43:2073–2079.
23. Hinchey J, Chaves C, Appignani B, et al. A reversible posterior leukoencephalopathy syndrome. N Engl J Med 1996;334:494–500.
24. Schwartz RB, Jones KM, Kalina P, et al. Hypertensive encephalopathy: findings on CT, MR imaging, and

SPECT imaging in 14 cases. AJR Am J Roentgenol 1992;159:279–383.

25. Cunningham FG, MacDonald PC, Gant NF, et al. Hypertensive Disorders in Pregnancy. In: Williams Obstetrics (20th ed). Stamford, CT: Appleton & Lange, 1997;693–744.

26. Chien PF, Khan KS, Arnott N. Magnesium sulphate in the treatment of eclampsia and pre-eclampsia: an overview of the evidence from randomised trials. J Obstet Gynaecol 1996;103:1085–1091

27. Reigel MM, Hollier LH, Sundt T, et al. Cerebral hyperperfusion syndrome: a cause of neurologic dysfunction after carotid endarterectomy. J Vasc Surg 1987;5:628–634.

28. Bousser MG, Barnett HJ. Cerebral Venous Thrombosis. In Barnett HJ, Mohr JP, Stein BM, Yatsu FM (eds), Stroke (3rd ed). New York: Churchill Livingstone, 1998;623–648.

29. Partziguian T, Camerlingo M, Castro L, et al. Cerebral venous thrombosis in young adults: experience in a stroke unit, 1988–1994. J Neurol Sci 1996;17:419–422.

30. Preter M, Tzourio C, Ameri A, Bousser MG. Long-term prognosis in cerebral venous thrombosis: follow-up of 77 patients. Stroke 1996;27:243–246.

31. Wolf, PA. Epidemiology and Stroke Risk Factors. In MA Samuels, S Feske (eds), Office Practice of Neurology. New York: Churchill Livingstone, 1996;224–236.

32. http://www.americanheart.org/ Heart_and_Stroke_A_Z_Guide/strokes.html. Accessed 2001.

33. Richardson EP, Dodge PR. Epilepsy in cerebral vascular disease. A study of the incidence and nature of seizures in 104 consecutive autopsy-proven cases of cerebral infarction and hemorrhage. Epilepsia 1954;3:49–65.

34. Giroud M, Gras P, Fayolle H, et al. Early seizures after acute stroke: a study of 1640 cases. Epilepsia 1994;35:959–964.

35. Kilpatrick CJ, Davis SM, Tress BM, et al. Epileptic seizures in acute stroke. Arch Neurol 1990;47:157–160.

36. Reith J, Jorgensen HS, Nakayama H, et al. Seizures in acute stroke: predictors and prognostic significance. The Copenhagen Stroke Study. Stroke 1997;28:1585–1589.

37. Bladin CF, Alexandrov AV, Bellavance A, et al. Seizures after stroke: a prospective multicenter study. Arch Neurol 2000;57:1617–1622.

38. So EL, Annegers JF, Hauser WA, et al. Population-based study of seizure disorders after cerebral infarction. Neurology 1996;42:350–355.

39. Awada, AM, Omojola MF, Obeid T. Late epileptic seizures after cerebral infarction, Acta Neurol Scand 1999;99:265–268.

40. Burn J, Dennis M, Bamford J, et al. Epileptic seizures after a first stroke: the Oxfordshire Community Stroke Project. BMJ 1997;315:1582–1587.

41. Cocito L, Favale E, Reni L. Epileptic seizures in cerebral arterial occlusive disease. Stroke 1982;13:189–195.

42. Daniele O, Mattaliano A, Tassinari CA, Natale E. Epileptic seizures and cerebrovascular disease. Acta Neurol Scand 1989;80:17–22.

43. Kilpatrick CJ, Davis SM, Hopper JL, Rossiter SC. Early seizures after stroke: risk of late seizures. Arch Neurol 1992;49:509–511.

44. Lancman ME, Golimstok A, Norscini J, et al. Risk factors for developing seizures after a stroke. Epilepsia 1994;34:141–143.

45. Lesser RP, Luders H, Dinner DS, Morris HH. Epileptic seizures due to thrombotic and embolic cerebrovascular disease in older patients. Epilepsia 1985;26:622–630.

46. Louis S, McDowell F. Epileptic seizures in non-embolic cerebral infarction. Arch Neurol 1967;17:414–418.

47. Olsen TS, Hagenhaven H, Thage O. Epilepsy after stroke. Neurology 1987;37:1209–1212.

48. Shinton RA, Gill JS, Melnick AK. The frequency, characteristics, and prognosis of epileptic seizures at the onset of stroke. J Neurol Neurosurg Psychiatry 1988;51:273–276.

49. Weisberg LA, Shamsnia M, Elliott D. Seizures caused by nontraumatic parenchymal brain hemorrhages. Neurology 1991;41:1197–1199.

50. Berger AR, Lipton RB, Lesser ML, et al. Early seizures following intracerebral hemorrhage: Implications for therapy. Neurology 1988;38:1363–1365.

51. Sung CY, Chu NS. Epileptic seizures in intracerebral hemorrhage. J Neurol Neurosurg Psychiatry 1989;52:1273–1276.

52. Butzkueven H, Evans AH, Pitman A, et al. Onset seizures independently predict poor outcome after subarachnoid hemorrhage. Neurology 2000;55:1315–1320.

53. Hasan D, Schonck RS, Avezaat CJ, et al. Epileptic seizures after subarachnoid hemorrhage. Ann Neurol 1993;33:286–291.

54. Olafsson E, Gudmundsson G, Hauser WA. Risk of epilepsy in long-term survivors of surgery for aneurysmal subarachnoid hemorrhage: a population-based study in Iceland. Epilepsia 2000;41:1201–1205.

55. Pinto AN, Canhao P, Ferro JM. Seizures at the onset of subarachnoid haemorrhage. J Neurol 1996;243:161–164.

56. Rhoney DH, Tipps LB, Murry KR, et al. Anticonvulsant prophylaxis and timing of seizures after aneurysmal subarachnoid hemorrhage. Neurology 2000;55:258–265.

57. Sundaram MB, Chow F. Seizures associated with spontaneous subarachnoid hemorrhage. Can J Neurol Sci 1986;13:229–231.

58. Del Curling O, Kelly DL, Elster AD, Craven TE. An analysis of the natural history of cavernous angiomas. J Neurosurg 1991;75:702–708.

59. Farmer JP, Cosgrove GR, Villemure JG, et al. Intracerebral cavernous angiomas. Neurology 1988;38:1699–1704.

60. Fults D, Kelly DL. Natural history of arteriovenous malformations of the brain: a clinical study. Neurosurgery 1984;15:658–662.

61. Hofmeister C, Stapf C, Hartmann A, et al. Demographic, morphological, and clinical characteristics of 1289 patients with brain arteriovenous malformations. Stroke 2000;31:1307–1310.

62. Piepgras DG, Sundt TM, Ragoowansi AT, Stevens L. Seizure outcome in patients with surgically treated cerebral arteriovenous malformations. J Neurosurg 1991;78:5–11.

63. Kittner SJ, Sharkness CM, Price TR, et al. Infarcts with a cardiac source of embolism in the NINCDS Stroke Data Bank: historical features. Neurology 1990;40:281–284.

64. Holmes GL. The electroencephalogram as a predictor of seizures following cerebral infarction. Clin Electroencephalogr 1980;11:83–86.

65. Li X, Breteler MM, deBruyne MC, et al. Vascular determinants of epilepsy: the Rotterdam study. Epilepsia 1997;38:1216–1220.

66. Ng SK, Hauser WA, Brust, JC, et al. Hypertension and the risk of new-onset unprovoked seizures. Neurology 1993;43:425–428.

67. Hesdorffer DC, Hauser WA, Annegers JF, Rocca WA. Severe, uncontrolled hypertension and adult-onset seizures: a case-control study in Rochester, Minnesota. Epilepsia 1996;37:736–741.

68. Cocito L, Favale E, Reni L. The frequency, characteristics, and prognosis of epileptic seizures at the onset of stroke. J Neurol Neurosurg Psychiatry 1989;52:292.

69. Franck G. Borderzone ("watershed") cerebral ischemia. Electroencephalogr Clin Neurophysiol 1982;35[Suppl]: 297–306.

70. Ketz E. Brain Tumors and Epilepsy. In PJ Vinken, GW Bruyn (eds), Handbook of Clinical Neurology. Amsterdam: North Holland Publishing, 1974;254–269.

71. Manford M, Hart YM, Sander JW, Shorvon SD. National general practice study of epilepsy (NGPSE): partial seizure patterns in a general population. Neurology 1992;42:1911–1917.

72. Sing CY, Chu NS. Epileptic seizures in intracerebral haemorrhage. J Neurol Neurosurg Psychiatry 1989;52: 1273–1276.

73. Ohno K, Maehara T, Ichimura K, et al. Low incidence of seizures in patients with chronic subdural haematoma. J Neurol Neurosurg Psychiatry 1993;56:1231–1233.

74. Asconape JJ, Penry JK. Poststroke seizures in the elderly. Clin Geriatr Med 1991;7:483–492.

75. Rumbach L, Sablot D, Berger E, et al. Status epilepticus in stroke: report on a hospital-based cohort. Neurology 2000;54:350–354.

76. Hart RG, Byer JA, Slaughter JR, et al. Occurrence and implications of seizures in subarachnoid hemorrhage due to ruptured intracranial aneurysms. Neurosurgery 1981;8:417–421.

77. Rabinowicz AL, Ginsburg DL, DeGiorgio CM, et al. Unruptured intracranial aneurysms: seizures and antiepileptic drug treatment following surgery. J Neurosurg 1991;75:371–373.

78. Adams HP Jr, Putman SF, Corbett JJ, et al. Amaurosis fugax; the results of arteriography in 59 patients. Stroke 1983;14:742–744.

79. Rasmussen BK, Olesen J. Migraine with aura and migraine without aura; an epidemiological study. Cephalalgia 1992;12:221–228.

80. Drislane FW, Schomer DL. Clinical implications of generalized electrographic status epilepticus. Epilepsy Res 1994; 19:111–122.

81. Bromfield EB. Seizures. In MA Samuels (ed), Hospitalist Neurology. Boston: Butterworth–Heinemann, 1999;79–108.

82. Jordan KG. Continuous EEG and evoked potential monitoring in the neuroscience intensive care unit. J Clin Neurophysiol 1993;10:445–475.

83. Privitera M, Hoffman M, Moore JL, Jester D. EEG detection of non–tonic-clonic status epilepticus in patients with altered consciousness. Epilepsy Research 1994;18:155–166.

84. Tomson T, Svanborg E, Wedlund JE. Nonconvulsive status epilepticus: high incidence of complex partial status. Epilepsia 1986;27:276–285.

85. Fagan KJ, Lee SI. Prolonged confusion following convulsions due to generalized nonconvulsive status epilepticus. Neurology 1990;40:1689–1694.

86. Gupta SR, Neheedy MH, Elias D, et al. Postinfarction seizures: a clinical study. Stroke 1988;19:1477–1481.

87. Yaffe K, Ferriero D, Barkovich AJ, Rowley H. Reversible MRI abnormalities following seizures. Neurology 1995;45:104–108.

88. Drury I. Diagnostic Assessment of Seizures in the Elderly. In LJ Willmore (ed), Epilepsy in the Elderly. West Hartford, CT: American Epilepsy Society, 1998;17–28.

89. Charlin C, Tiberge M, Calvet U, et al. The clinical significance of periodic lateralized epileptiform discharges in acute ischemic stroke. J Stroke Cerebrovasc Dis 2000;9:298–302.

90. Pohlmann-Eden B, Hoch DB, Cochius JI, Chiappa KH. Periodic lateralized epileptiform discharges—a critical review. J Clin Neurophysiol 1996;13:519–530.

91. Hughes JR, Zialcita ML. EEG in the elderly: seizures vs. syncope. Clin Electroencephalogr 2000;31:131–137.

92. Linzer M, Grubb B, Ho S, et al. Cardiovascular causes of loss of consciousness in patients with presumed epilepsy. Am J Med 1994;96:146–154.

93. Ehrenberg BL. Unusual manifestations of migraine and "the borderland of epilepsy"—re-explored. Semin Neurol 1991;11:118–127.

94. Lee H, Lerner A. Transient inhibitory seizures mimicking crescendo TIAs. Neurology 1990;40:165–166.

95. Baquis GD, Pessin MP, Scott M. Limb shaking—a carotid TIA. Stroke 1985;16:444–448.

96. Grimes DA, Guberman A. De novo aphasic status epilepticus. Epilepsia 1997;38:945–949.

97. Labar DR. Sleep disorders and epilepsy: differential diagnosis. Semin Neurol 1991;11:128–134.

98. Devinsky O. Nonepileptic psychogenic seizures: quagmires of pathophysiology, diagnosis, and treatment. Epilepsia 1998;39:458–462.

99. Hasan D, Vermeulen M, Wijdicks EF, et al. Management problems in acute hydrocephalus after subarachnoid hemorrhage. Stroke 1989;20:747–753.

100. Brodie MJ, Dichter MA. Antiepileptic drugs. N Engl J Med 1996;334:168–175.

101. Temkin NR, Dikmen SS, Wilensky AJ, et al. A randomized, double-blind study of phenytoin for the prevention of post-traumatic seizures. N Engl J Med 1990;323:497–502.

102. Bougousslavsky J, Martin R, Regli F, et al. Persistent worsening of stroke sequelae after delayed seizures. Arch Neurol 1992;49:385–388.

103. Goldstein LB. Common drugs may influence motor recovery after stroke. The Sygen In Acute Stroke Study Investigators. Neurology 1995;45:865–871.

104. Dodrill CB, Troupin AS. Neuropsychological effects of carbamazepine and phenytoin; a reanalysis. Neurology 1991;41:141–143.

105. Meador KJ, Loring DW, Huh K, et al. Comparative cognitive effects of anticonvulsants. Neurology 1990;40:391–394.

106. Lowenstein DH, Alldredge BK. Current concepts: status epilepticus. N Engl J Med 1998;338:970–976.

107. Ali I, Khuder S, Pirzada N, et al. Folate and plasma homocysteine in patients on long term antiepileptic drug therapy. Epilepsia 2000;41[Suppl 41]:203(abst).

108. Paolucci S, Silvestri G, Lubich S, et al. Poststroke late seizures and their role in rehabilitation of inpatients. Epilepsia 1997;38:266–270.

109. Berges S, Moulin T, Berger E, et al. Seizures and epilepsy following stroke: recurrence factors. Eur Neurol 2000;43:3–8.

110. Annegers JF, Hauser WA, Elveback LR. Remission of seizures and relapse in patients with epilepsy. Epilepsia 1979;20:729–737.

Section C

Sexuality and Pregnancy in Epilepsy

Chapter 16

Sexuality Issues in Epilepsy

Susan Duncan

The notion that patients with epilepsy have an increased risk for sexual dysfunction is controversial. Although Chapter 17 provides evidence to support this idea, this discussion provides an alternative viewpoint and raises important questions about this commonly accepted conclusion.

Sexuality and epilepsy have been intimately linked in the minds of physicians and laymen since ancient times. The oldest written system of medicine in the world, the Ayurveda of India, opined that epilepsy could be caused by sexual excess.[1] Hippocrates wrote that complete abstinence from and excessive indulgence in intercourse could cause epilepsy and described the orgasm as a form of seizure.[2] Galen stated that seizures often occurred in girls who had intercourse at too early an age,[2] a particularly interesting observation in the light of modern evidence linking sexual abuse with nonepileptic seizures.[3–5]

In 1892, von Krafft-Ebing[6] wrote

> Moreover, in many epileptics the sexual instinct is very intense. For the most part, it is satisfied by masturbation, now and then by attacks on children and by pederasty. Perversion of the instinct with perverse sexual acts seems to be infrequent.

The belief that people with epilepsy were possessed of unbridled sexual desire was the rationale behind the introduction of bromides in the second half of the nineteenth century. These compounds had been noted to cause impotence, and it was reasoned that a reduction in the libido would lead to a diminution in the number of seizures.[7,8] Other members of the profession, convinced that masturbation was the root of all epilepsy, advocated castration and cliterectomy.[7]

In the 1950s, however, the medical profession did a volt face with the publication of Gastaut and Collomb's paper, *Etude du Comportement Sexuel chez les Epileptiques Psychomoteurs*.[9] This study reported an apparent lack of interest in sexual activity in individuals with complex partial seizures and heralded the beginning of a new orthodoxy in medical opinion.

Human sexual response requires the interaction of both psychological and physical processes (Figure 16-1).[10] Cognitive processes, in turn, influence the limbic system with its rich connections with the hypothalamus and pituitary. This influences the periphery via the spinal reflexes that, via somatic and autonomic systems, mediate the genital and cardiovascular responses to sexual stimulation. Perception and an interpretation of these changes as being sexual and pleasurable complete the circle. This circle of activity leads to the orgasm, the underlying neurophysiologic mechanism of which remains enigmatic. Given the complexity of the process, it can be easily appreciated that disruption of any one of the stations on the circle can lead to sexual dysfunction.

Increased sexual dysfunction in people with epilepsy is uncritically accepted by many authorities, because many supportive studies were done in institutions,[11] "epilepsy colonies," or individuals awaiting surgical treatment.[12] Few studies have involved those patients whose seizures were suffi-

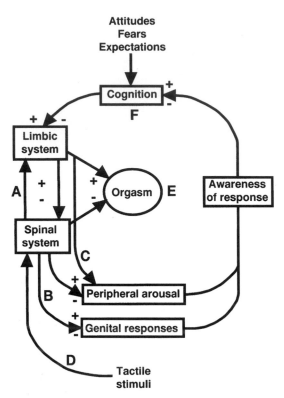

Figure 16-1. The psychosomatic circle of sex. (Reprinted with permission from J Bancroft. Human Sexuality and Its Problems. New York: Churchill Livingstone, 1989;323.)

Although several authors have written about sexual dysfunction in people with epilepsy, few, if any, have included the incidence of sexual dysfunction in the population at large. A Dutch study[15] from the late 1970s, which aimed at recruiting as representative a population as possible, showed that 12% of men and 9% of women avoided sexual activity. In total, 26% of men and 43% of the women in this study reported difficulties with arousal and enjoyment. In a Danish study of women[16] aged 40 years, 15% said they had no motivation for sexual activity. In a large study[17] from the United Kingdom, 22% of women and 15% of men reported low sexual interest. In another study,[18] again from the United Kingdom, 30 men and 30 women attending their general practitioner for nonsexual problems were interviewed; 20% of the women and 10% of the men reported difficulty in becoming sexually aroused, 7% of the men reporting some form of frequent erectile failure.

There are several possible mechanisms for reduced sexual interest in people with epilepsy. They can be grouped under three main categories:

- Psychosocial effects of epilepsy

- Intrinsic disorders of brain function that cause epilepsy and interrupt those processes necessary for sexual interest

- Effects of antiepileptic drugs (AEDs) on sex hormone levels or cognitive or limbic functions

Psychosocial Effects of Epilepsy

In the nineteenth century, the French physician Billod (1843) summed up the lot of the "epileptic"[19]:

> Usually the epileptic is avoided; on all faces he reads his sentence to isolation. Everywhere he goes, menacing and insurmountable obstacles arise to his obtaining a position, to his establishing himself, to his relationships and to his very livelihood: he has to say goodbye to his dreams of success for the masters even refuse him work in shops, goodbye to his dreams of marriage and fatherhood, goodbye to the joys of the domestic hearth. This is death to the spirit.

Epilepsy is regarded as unique in its capacity for causing social embarrassment. Adults developing

ciently well controlled to enable them to live independent lives in the community. Rarely is the social background of the country or the time at which the studies were conducted taken into account. In one paper from the Indian subcontinent,[13] the authors, and presumably their society, define normal sexual behavior differently from a Western Hemisphere country. Indeed, one of the most interesting aspects of the whole body of literature pertaining to sexual dysfunction and epilepsy can be found in the usually single case studies of abnormal sexual behavior published in the 1950s and 1960s. In these studies, it is confidently asserted that homosexuality[12,14] is more frequent among epileptics. There are no papers alluding to this association in medical journals published in the United Kingdom after 1967, the year in which sexual activity between consenting adults of the same sex was legalized. This example reminds us of the unconscious values all investigators bring to this area of research.

epilepsy face numerous problems: loss of their driving license, curtailment of employment opportunities or career progression, the side effects of medication, and unwitting prejudice of the public. A survey of attitudes to people with epilepsy in the United States in 1979[20] showed that 3% of the population thought epilepsy a form of insanity, 6% did not want their child to play with a child with epilepsy, and 18% said they would object to their child's marrying a person with epilepsy. Two surveys carried out in Australia found physicians believed people with epilepsy were more likely to lose time from work and be less reliable than their peers.[21,22] Hansson et al.[23] asked a group of American college students to examine a series of photographs of individuals of the opposite gender and to identify from purely facial characteristics whom they considered to be experiencing epilepsy. Students of both genders consistently chose a physically unattractive person. When challenged about his choice, one student replied that he had worked with epileptics, and he could identify them by the look in their eyes. Although such statements may seem risible, prior medical literature describes the "epileptic personality," usually ascribed to individuals with temporal lobe epilepsy. It comprises a constellation of unattractive traits. They are said to be "viscous"—a term much used but never defined.[24,25] Other descriptions include meticulous in attention to minor and often irrelevant detail,[26] excessively religious, and prone to aggression and psychosis.[27,28] Tizard[29] argued against the existence of an "epileptic personality," noting that much of this literature was derived from severely afflicted individuals, a different population than those who lived and worked in the community.

One condition that does approach epilepsy in its potential for social embarrassment is narcolepsy or cataplexy. Broughton et al.[30] studied three groups of men and women: a control group, a group with narcolepsy or cataplexy, and a group with epilepsy. The men in the epilepsy and narcolepsy groups reported higher incidences of impotence than the controls, but there was no difference in the occurrence of impotence between the epilepsy and narcolepsy groups. No inquiries were made of the women's sexual lives. Narcolepsy or cataplexy may also affect sexuality by intrinsic brain dysfunction related to the disorder, as well as effects of central nervous system stimulants, tricyclics, and other drugs.

Given that the seeds of our future emotional development are sewn in childhood, there is ample evidence pointing to the deleterious effect epilepsy can have on the young and their families. In 1972,[31] Hartlage et al. compared dependency rates in three sets of children younger than age 12 years. One group experienced seizures, a second experienced cystic fibrosis, and the third was an essentially healthy group undergoing tonsillectomy. No significant differences in parental attitudes were found between the three groups, but the children with epilepsy exhibited a higher degree of emotional dependency, as assessed by validated questionnaires, than the children in the other two groups. Seizure type and AED therapy had no effect on these results. There was a tendency among the parents of children with epilepsy to try and suppress expressions of anger, aggression, and sexuality by the affected child. Long et al.[32] interviewed parents of children with epilepsy, finding that the majority expected the child to underachieve at school, play fewer sports, be higher strung, and enjoy a limited choice of occupation in adulthood in comparison to their other children. Lechtenburg[33] noted that, in families with a child with epilepsy, the mother appeared to be dominant, with her decisions on what activities were safe for the child over-ruling those of her husband. In addition, he described different strategies adopted by different families to cope with the problem. In some, the mother encouraged emotional dependency in the child, and in others there was a denial of the disorder, preventing the child and his or her brothers and sisters from articulating their fears or curiosities about the condition.

Matthews et al.[34] studied 15 children with seizures, comparing them to age-matched healthy controls and children with diabetes. The children with seizures, perhaps not surprisingly, attributed control over their lives to outside agencies—parents, teachers, God—and considered any successes they achieved to be due to this external force. They had lower self-esteems, with some reporting they were last to be picked for team games, and exhibited greater anxiety about everyday social situations. Children with epilepsy usually have been seen as prone to antisocial behavior and violence.[29] More recent work, however, suggests that epileptic children are more anxious and fearful and have fewer friends than their peers.[35–37] Stores[35] noted that boys with seizures were more likely to exhibit these traits, along with a greater need for reassurance, often from their mothers, and physical affection, than were girls with epilepsy. In contrast, Hoare[36] found the same level of dependency in both genders. Hoare et al.[37] subsequently compared the relationship between self-esteem and behavioral adjustment in a group of children with epilepsy, as compared to children with diabetes. Children with epilepsy had lower self-esteems and were more behaviorally disturbed than those children with diabetes. These studies suggest that emotional development in children with seizure disorders is affected; they also point to the difficulties these children may have in acquiring the social skills necessary to build a network of friends and acquaintances from which they may ultimately find a partner.

Temporal Lobe Pathology

Mesial temporal sclerosis with loss of neurones in the hippocampus and amygdala is the most common finding in people undergoing temporal lobe resection for intractable complex partial seizures.[38,39] Complex partial epilepsy is most commonly associated with hyposexuality. These structures appear to be of fundamental importance in motivational behavior, such as feeding, reproduction, and social interaction in nonhuman primates and lower mammals.[40]

In 1939, Klüver and Bucy[41] performed bilateral temporal lobectomy on rhesus monkeys and observed a profound change in the cage-bound behavior of these animals. They developed "psychic blindness" or visual agnosia, approaching objects and individuals from which they had previously fled. They ceased to display the vocal and motor reactions usually associated with fear and anger and showed a marked tendency to investigate every object encountered orally. In addition, there was a striking increase in sexual activity, with animals making indiscriminate attempts at copulation. None of these changes followed unilateral temporal lobectomy. These behavioral changes occurred when the greater part of the hippocampus and amygdala was removed bilaterally. Resection of the temporal neocortex and severance of the frontotemporal and occipital-temporal pathways did not induce the syndrome.

Monkeys with bilateral amygdalar lesions rather than complete temporal lobectomies exhibited the same behavioral changes.[42,43] However, the changes in sexual activity described by Klüver and Bucy only occurred when the animals were caged, especially if confined with another animal who had undergone similar surgery. When these monkeys were released into the wild, they tended to become social isolates, ceasing to indulge in mutual grooming, the staple social interaction in primate society, and losing their position in the social hierarchy.[42,43] This loss in rank reduced the male monkeys' access to female monkeys. In addition, the operated animals displayed fear in the face of friendly approach by other monkeys, and, in the case of one female monkey, a very marked disinclination to indulge in social foreplay before mating with an unoperated male monkey.[42]

Behavioral changes similar to those seen in the Klüver-Bucy monkeys have been reported in humans. After bilateral temporal lobectomy for intractable seizures, a 19-year-old man exhibited a flat affect, voracious appetite, and impaired memory, made persistent sexual overtures to male members of staff that were easily rebuffed, and masturbated openly.[44] He failed to recognize even close relatives and did not display any form of emotion toward them, despite having a warm and affectionate relationship with his mother before the operation. His condition remained unchanged at follow-up 2 years later. Lilly et al.[45] reported 12 cases of Klüver-Bucy syndrome caused by herpes encephalitis, Niemann-Pick disease, Alzheimer's disease, and trauma. Hypersexuality and sensory agnosias were less common, whereas placidity and exaggerated oral activities were the most frequent partial syndromes.

Unilateral anterior temporal lobe damage, by contrast, can decrease sexual activity. Hierons et al.[46] reported the cases of 15 men, eight of whom had neoplastic or traumatic lesions of one temporal lobe, and reported that, although libido was retained, the men became impotent.

Visual agnosia, a feature of Klüver-Bucy syndrome, may contribute to sexual disorders in patients with temporal lobe epilepsy. Visual perception of objects and their significance is a function of the inferior temporal neocortex,[40,41] which has connections with the amygdala and hippocampus.[40] Motivational behavior in human and nonhuman primates is guided by visual stimuli,[40] and any interruption in their processing at amygdalar level could compromise the individual's capacity for social interaction.[42,43]

The temporal lobes in humans contain areas involved in visual and auditory perception, including language. Closely allied to these areas are the amygdala and hippocampus, which, in turn, are linked to the hypothalamus that mediates basic drive mechanisms.[40] Damage to the amygdala and hippocampus at an early stage in life may prevent the integration of those higher functions, such as language, that are situated in the neocortex, with basic drives leaving the affected individual unable to recognize or be moved by social cues used by the other gender to encourage intimacy.

Effects of Antiepileptic Drugs on Androgens

Androgen Physiology in Men

Testosterone, the most abundant androgen in men, is produced in the Leydig[47] cells of the testes. It can act directly on target tissues, but it can also be converted to dihydrotestosterone by the enzyme 5-α-reductase or to estradiol by the aromatase enzyme complex. The role of these two metabolites on various aspects of sexual behavior remain to be elucidated.[47] In some species, aromatization of testosterone to estradiol is important in stimulating sexual behavior. Studies in men, however, so far suggest that estradiol may play little role in sexual interest.[48] Approximately 43% of testosterone is bound to sex hormone–binding globulin (SHBG), 55% is bound to albumin, and 2% is free.[47] This combination of free and albumin-bound testosterone is physiologically active. In men, 44% of binding sites for testosterone on SHBG are free, and this, in tandem with albumin's large binding capacity, means that increases in total hormone concentrations do not cause changes in the free-hormone fraction. Conversely, changes in SHBG concentrations can produce marked changes in free and albumin-bound levels of testosterone.[49]

Androgen-deficient men report reduced libido and erectile dysfunction. Androgen replacement therapy increases sexual interest and the quality and quantity of nocturnal erections.[50] However,

androgens may not be important in erectile responses to erotic stimuli, but rather in behavior directly related to the libido.[51] Bagatell et al.[48] suppressed androgen in a group of healthy men by administering a gonadotropin-releasing hormone antagonist. At the end of the 6-week period of study, men reported significantly reduced sexual desire, fewer sexual fantasies, fewer spontaneous erections, and decreased frequency of intercourse and masturbation. The ability to maintain an erection or achieve orgasm was not, however, significantly altered. There is a nonlinear relationship between testosterone levels and sexual function, with the level of testosterone required to maintain sexual function varying considerably between individual men. A testosterone level in the low-normal range (5–11 nmol/liter of total testosterone) appears necessary in men to maintain sexual interest.[52] Increasing testosterone beyond that threshold does not result in a concomitant increase in sexual interest. Suppressing testosterone levels to half the baseline levels[53] does not impair sexual function. This concept of an "androgen threshold" above which testosterone levels do not appear to influence sexual activity is an important one, given the prevailing belief that the reductions in free testosterone (FT) caused by AEDs may contribute to sexual dysfunction in men with epilepsy.

The difficulty in measuring FT has led to various formulas to ascertain androgen status. The most frequently used is the free androgen index (FAI)[54]:

$$\text{Total testosterone} \div \text{SHBG} \times 100$$

Originally developed to assess androgen status in hirsute women, it may not be valid in men. One study demonstrated a correlation coefficient (r) of 0.86 between the FAI and directly measured FT in women, but in men the correlation was only $r = 0.43$.[55]

Enzyme-inducing AEDs, such as phenytoin, phenobarbitone, and carbamazepine, cause an increase in SHBG[56,57] concentrations, which decreases the FAI. This has led to the assumption that hyposexuality in men with epilepsy can at least in part be explained by changes in testosterone levels. This assumption may be flawed for two reasons. First, the FAI may not be accurate in men. Second, there is not a linear relationship between sexual interest and testosterone levels, with men being able to withstand reductions in testosterone levels to the lower end of the male range without compromising their libido.

Numerous studies of testosterone levels in men taking AEDs have used different methods to measure or calculate FT with varied results (Table 16-1).[11,58–65] Four of these studies correlated sexual function with hormonal results. Toone et al.[58] studied three groups of men with epilepsy: (1) those in a residential institution, (2) those in a university hospital clinic, and (3) those treated by a general practitioner. One-third of those men in the institution exhibited a lack of sexual interest, as did one-third of those men attending the hospital-based outpatient clinic. Men attending their general practitioner also reported hyposexuality. These men's FT levels were significantly lower than those of a control group drawn from hospital employees. However, the mean FT in the epilepsy group was within the normal range. The method by which FT was determined was not stated in the study. Jensen et al.[62] compared 38 men with epilepsy to healthy controls and men with diabetes. Sexual function was assessed by a validated questionnaire. Eight percent of the men with epilepsy had significant sexual dysfunction, compared to 13% of the control group and 44% of the diabetics. FT levels by radioimmunoassay for all three groups were within normal range, and there were no significant differences between the three groups. Duncan et al.[63] compared 150 men with epilepsy taking monotherapy, polytherapy, and no treatment to healthy controls. These men lived independent lives in the community and were not medically refractory. There were no significant differences in frequency or enjoyment of intercourse or spontaneous erections between the groups. The FT coefficient was $r = 0.84$; there was no significant difference in FT levels between the groups. Rodin et al.[64] studied men with sexual dysfunction on the Bear Fedio Inventory and found that, overall, these men did not have significantly lower total testosterone levels than controls.

In a more recent study,[66] Rattya and colleagues examined the effects of carbamazepine, sodium valproate, and oxecarbazepine in sexual function and hormone levels in men. There were no significant differences in sexual interest between the three treatment groups and a control group; neither were there any differences between the groups and total or free testosterone levels. Free testosterone in this study being ascertained by radioimmunoassay (see Table 16-1). Disappointingly, given the unsuit-ability of the FAI in men, this ratio is used in this study and is invoked as the reason behind reduced libido in 7 out of 40 men taking carbamazepine.

Stoffel-Wagner et al.[65] studied 26 men awaiting temporal lobectomy, using radioimmunoassay to measure FT, and found that those men with epilepsy had significantly lower FT than controls. Fifty-eight percent of the men with epilepsy had FT levels below the fifth centile of the healthy men, 15% complained of difficulty in getting or maintaining an erection, 27% complained of never experiencing erections on waking, and 27% denied any sexual drive. In this study of androgen metabolism, the German group used identical methods to ascertain FT as Isojarvi's[59,60] group, yet Isojarvi reported no difference in FT between study and control groups. Thus, low testosterone does not inevitably lead to sexual dysfunction. Isojarvi's[59,60] and Duncan's[63,67] studies were based on men living in the community; they are a different population from Stoffel-Wagner's. It serves to remind us of the role primary temporal lobe pathology may play and of the difficulties in disentangling the effects of the social disruption caused by uncontrolled epilepsy.

Other studies have concentrated purely on the effects of AEDs on hormone levels without seeking to correlate them with behavior. Few are prospective. In two studies, Isojarvi et al.[59,60] found elevated SHBG in men taking enzyme-inducing AEDs but no significant differences in FT. A small prospective study[68] on healthy volunteers taking carbamazepine found an initial fall in total testosterone and FAI, with these parameters returning to normal toward the end of the 3-week study period. Macphee et al,[61] using the same methods as Duncan,[63] found that men taking carbamazepine or more than one AED had a significantly lower calculated FT than controls.

Estradiol has been invoked as a possible cause of sexual dysfunction in men.[69] There are no compelling data in human reproductive science to support this hypothesis, and other investigators have not found raised estradiol.[59,62,63] Herzog's group measured non–SHBG-bound as well as total estradiol levels. Other groups have only measured total estradiol levels. Claims that treatment of men with raised estradiol with testosterone and testolactone, an aromatase inhibitor, produces improved sexual function should be considered as preliminary, because the study was open.

Table 16-1. Methods Used to Measure Free Testosterone

Authors	Method of Measuring Free Testosterone (FT)	Method of Inquiry of Patients' Sexual Function	Results
Fenwick et al. (1985)	Free androgen index (FAI)	Structured interview.	Men in a residential institution studied. Reduced FAI and libido found in a significant number of men.
Taylor (1969)		Structured interview.	Men awaiting temporal lobectomy. Taylor found reduced sexual interest in majority.
Shukla and Srinvastava (1979)	No hormonal parameters measured	Interview.	63% of men considered hyposexual compared to controls. Controls not matched for age, educational level or social class.
Toone et al. (1980)	FT calculated by method of Nanjee and Wheeler	Structured interview.	Three groups of men drawn from a residential home, hospital clinic, and general practitioner (GP) practice were studied. All were considered hyposexual, but the men attending their GP were less so than the other two groups.
Isojarvi et al. (1988)	Radioimmunoassay (Diagnostic Products, Los Angeles)	None.	No difference in FT between antiepileptic drug (AED)–treated men and controls.
Isojarvi et al. (1990)	Radioimmunoassay (Diagnostic Products)	None.	No difference in FT between AED-treated men and controls.
Macphee et al. (1988)	FT calculated by method of Nanjee and Wheeler	None.	Men receiving more than one AED or carbamazepine monotherapy had significantly lower FT than controls.
Rodin et al. (1984)	Total testosterone only measured	Bear-Fedio Questionnaire.	Men who reported reduced arousal on Bear-Fedio inventory had significantly lower total testosterone than those who did not report arousal and controls.
Stoffel-Wagner et al.	Radioimmunoassay (Diagnostic Products)	Interview.	Men under consideration for temporal lobectomy were studied. FT significantly lower than control group. 15% had erectile difficulties.
Duncan et al. (1999)	FT calculated by method of Nanjee and Wheeler	Validated questionnaire aimed at exploring various domains of sexual function.	No significant differences in FT between men taking AEDs and controls. No evidence of sexual dysfunction in men with epilepsy.
Jensen et al. (1990)	Radioimmunoassay	Validated questionnaire aimed at exploring various domains of sexual function. Also, Brief Symptom Inventory and Disease Acceptance questionnaire administered.	No difference between the men or women with epilepsy, when compared with controls, in terms of sexual function or FT levels.

Androgen Physiology in Women

Women produce only one-tenth of the amount of testosterone as men. Twenty-five percent of circulating testosterone comes from the ovaries, another 25% from the adrenals, and the rest from peripheral conversion of precursor hormones.[47]

Some studies have found a positive correlation between androgen levels and sexual activity in premenopausal women; others have not. Bancroft[70] found no correlation between testosterone levels and sexual intercourse, thoughts, or feelings. He did, however, find a strong correlation between testosterone levels and masturbation frequency. Others found a correlation between testosterone levels and vaginal response to erotic stimuli but not between androgen concentration and other sexual behavior. As with men, reduced sexual interest does not necessarily mean a low serum testosterone,[71] and like men, administering testosterone to women with normal testosterone levels does not enhance sexual interest.

Studies on the effects of AEDs on female sexual function have used the FAI to determine FT status. It would appear that in women this is fairly accurate.

Studies of sexual function in women with epilepsy are rarer than in those of men. Studies in which sex hormone levels and sexual function have been ascertained at the same time in the same study population are even rarer. Demedash et al.[72] studied a group of 700 Egyptian women with epilepsy and found an incidence of sexual dysfunction in 18%. A significant proportion of these women reported exhibitionism, fetishes, and transvestism, behaviors more common in men, and none admitted to homosexuality or masturbation. Sex hormones were not measured during this study. As with other studies, we are told little about the control group that was recruited from another clinic. Jensen et al.[62] studied 38 women with epilepsy, comparing them with a group of women with diabetes and a control group. As with the male part of this group's study, a validated questionnaire was used to ascertain sexual function. Twenty-nine percent of the women with epilepsy reported sexual dysfunction, compared to 28% of those with diabetes and 25% of the control group. There were no differences between the groups in FT or other hormonal parameters. Duncan et al.[67] studied 195 women with epilepsy attending a hospital based clinic and found that those women with epilepsy appeared to have a less permissive attitude to sexual behavior than controls, but those with partners had intercourse as frequently as controls and reported similar levels of enjoyment. There were no significant differences in FT levels between women taking AEDs and controls. Stoffel-Wagner[66] studied 22 women under consideration for temporal lobectomy. There were no differences between mean FT levels of the study group compared with the controls.

Ndegwa et al.[73] studied 30 women with epilepsy attending their general practitioner and 30 randomly selected controls from the same practice. Using a validated questionnaire, they could find no differences between the two groups in terms of orgasm achievement, dissatisfaction with their sexual relationship, or feelings of nonsensuality. The women with epilepsy, however, had intercourse less frequently than the controls and reported a higher incidence of vaginismus. Using similar methods, Bergen[74] looked at a group of women attending an outpatient clinic and found no difference overall between women with epilepsy and controls. There was a small subgroup of women, however, who reported never experiencing sexual desire or intercourse. Neither of these studies measured sex hormone levels. Morrell et al.[75] studied genital blood flow in women with epilepsy during exposure to erotic material and found that genital blood flow did not increase to the same degree in these women as compared to controls, suggesting that there may be failure of arousal owing to central mechanisms.

Two studies[76,77] of the effects of AEDs on androgen levels in women have shown a fall in the FAI but the FT within normal range. This may reflect the fact that FT is maintained in the face of raised SHBG by some other mechanism, or it may represent the fact that the methods used to measure FT in these women are prone to error.

Conclusion

From the point of view of this author, the case for sexual dysfunction in people with epilepsy remains unproven. It is interesting that those studies conducted in recent times using sexologic methods have failed to show hyposexuality in either gender. This does not mean that sexual dysfunction does not occur, but it may not be any more common than in individuals with other chronic conditions. Disentangling the psychosocial effects of epilepsy, especially in those who developed the condition at a young age, may prove impossible, but it should always be borne in mind when reading the literature on this topic. The belief that those changes wrought in SHBG and FT levels by AEDs are a cause of sexual dysfunction are, as we have seen, based on a misconception as to the levels of testosterone required to maintain sexual interest. The variety of methods used throughout the literature to ascertain FT complicates matters.

Future research should be prospective and use validated questionnaires or standard interviews. In addition, the selection of controls must be more rigorous than it has been in the majority of the studies cited, with not only age and marital status, but also level of education, religious values, and sibling status, taken into account, as all of these factors are known to affect attitudes to sexual activity.

References

1. Manyam BV. Epilepsy in ancient India. Epilepsia 1992;33:473–475.
2. Temkin O. The Falling Sickness. A History of Epilepsy from the Greeks to the Beginnings of Modern Neurology (2nd ed). Baltimore: Johns Hopkins University Press, 1971.
3. Liske E, Forster FM. Pseudoseizures: a problem in the diagnosis and management of epileptic patients. Neurology 1964;8:41–49.
4. Standage DF. Etiology of hysterical seizures. Can Psychiatr Assoc J 1975;20:67–73.
5. Desai BT, Porter RJ, Penry K. Psychogenic seizures: a study of 42 attacks in six patients with intensive monitoring. Arch Neurol 1982;39:202–209.
6. von Krafft-Ebing R. Psychopathia Sexualis. Authorized Translation of the 7th Enlarged and Revised German Edition by Charles G. Chaddock. Philadelphia: FA Davis Co, 1892.
7. Sieveking EH. Analysis of 52 cases of epilepsy observed by the author. Lancet 1857;1:527–528.
8. Gowers WR. Epilepsy and Other Chronic Convulsive Diseases. Their Causes, Symptoms and Treatment. New York: William Wood, 1885;225.
9. Gastaut H, Collomb H. Etude du comportement sexuel chez les epileptiques psychomoteurs. Ann Med Psychol 1954;112:657–696.
10. Bancroft J. Human Sexuality and Its Problems. New York: Churchill Livingstone, 1989.
11. Fenwick PB, Toone BK, Wheeler MJ, et al. Sexual behavior in a centre for epilepsy. Acta Neurol Scand 1985;71:428–435.
12. Taylor DC. Sexual behavior and temporal lobe epilepsy. Arch Neurol 1969;21:510–516.
13. Shukla GD, Srinvastava ON, Katiyar BC. Sexual disturbances in temporal lobe epilepsy: a controlled study. Br J Psychiatry 1979;134:288–292.
14. Kolinarsky A, Freund K, Machek J, Polak O. Male sexual deviation. Arch Gen Psychiatry 1967;17:735–743.
15. Frenken J. Afkeer van sexualiteit [English summary]. Deventer, Netherlands: Van Loghum Slaterus, 1976;219–225.
16. Garde K, Lunde I. Female sexual behavior. A study in a random sample of 40 year old women. Maturitas 1980;2:225–240.
17. Saunders D. The Woman Book on Love and Sex. London: Joseph, 1985.
18. Golombok S, Rust J, Pickard C. Sexual problems encountered in general practise. Br J Sex Med 1985;11:171–175.
19. Billod. Recherches et considerations relatives a la symtomatologie de l'epilepsie. Ann Med Psychol 1843;381–423.
20. Caveness WF, Gallup GH. A survey of public attitudes towards epilepsy in 1979 with an indication of trends over the past thirty years. Epilepsia 1980;21:509–518.
21. Beran RG, Jennings VR, Read T. Doctors perspectives of epilepsy. Epilepsia 1981;22:397–406.
22. Beran RG, Read T. A survey of doctors in Sydney, Australia: perspectives and practices regarding epilepsy and those affected by it. Epilepsia 1983;24:79–104.
23. Hansson RO, Duffield BJ. Physical attractiveness and the attribution of epilepsy. J Soc Psychol 1976;99:233–240.
24. Small JG, Milstein V, Stevens JR. Are psychomotor epileptics different? Arch Neurol 1962;7:188–194.
25. Bear D, Levin K, Blumer D, et al. Interictal behavior in hospitalised temporal lobe epileptics: relationship to idiopathic psychiatric syndromes. J Neurol Neurosurg Psychiatry 1982;45:481–488.
26. Waxman SG, Geschwind N. The interictal behavior syndrome of temporal lobe epilepsy. Arch Gen Psychiatry 1975;32:1580–1586.
27. Flor-Henry P. Psychosis and temporal lobe epilepsy; a controlled investigation. Epilepsia 1969;10:363–395.
28. Dewhurst K, Beard AW. Sudden religious conversion in temporal lobe epilepsy. Br J Psychiatry 1970;117:497–507.
29. Tizard B. The personality of epileptics: a discussion of the evidence. Psychol Bull 1962;3:196–210.
30. Broughton RJ, Guberman A, Roberts J. Comparison of the psychosocial effects of epilepsy and narcolepsy/cataplexy: a controlled study. Epilepsia 1984;25:423–433.
31. Hartlage LC, Green JB, Offutt L. Dependency in epileptic children. Epilepsia 1972;13:27–30.

32. Long CG, Moore JR. Parental expectation for their epileptic children. J Child Psychol Psychiatry 1979;20:299–312.

33. Lechtenberg R. Epilepsy and the Family. Cambridge, MA: Harvard University Press, 1984.

34. Matthews WS, Barabal G, Ferrari M. Emotional concomitants of childhood epilepsy. Epilepsia 1982;23:671–681.

35. Stores G. School children with epilepsy at risk for learning and behavior problems. Dev Med Child Neurol 1978;20:502–508.

36. Hoare P. Psychiatric disturbance in the families of epileptic children. Dev Med Child Neurol 1984;26:14–19.

37. Hoare P, Kerley S. Psychosocial adjustment of children with chronic epilepsy and their families. Dev Med Child Neurol 1991;33:201–215.

38. Falconer MF, Taylor DC. Surgical treatment of drug-resistant epilepsy due to mesial temporal sclerosis. Arch Neurol 1969;19:353–360.

39. Bruton CJ. The Neuropathology of Temporal Lobe Epilepsy. New York: Oxford University Press, 1988.

40. Gloor P. Temporal Lobe Epilepsy: Its Possible Contribution to the Understanding of the Functional Significance of the Amygdala and of Its Interaction with Neocortical-Temporal Mechanisms. In BE Eleftheriou (ed). Neurobiology of the Amygdala; the Proceedings of a Symposium on the Neurobiology of the Amygdala, Bar Harbor, Maine, June 6–17, 1971. New York: Plenum, 1972.

41. Klüver H, Bucy PC. Preliminary analysis of functions of the temporal lobes in monkeys. Arch Neurol Psychiatry 1939;42:979–1000.

42. Dicks D, Myers RE, Kling A. Uncus and amygdala lesions: effects on social behavior in the free-ranging rhesus monkey. Science 1968;165:69–71.

43. Kling A. Effects of Amygdalectomy on Social-Affective Behavior in Non-Human Primates. In BE Eleftheriou (ed), Neurobiology of the Amygdala; the Proceedings of a Symposium on the Neurobiology of the Amygdala, Bar Harbor, Maine, June 6–17, 1971. New York: Plenum, 1972.

44. Terzian H, Ore GD. Syndrome of Klüver and Bucy reproduced in man by bilateral removal of temporal lobes. Neurology 1953;5:373–380.

45. Lilly R, Cummings JL, Benson F, Frankel M. The human Klüver-Bucy syndrome. Neurology 1983;33:1141–1145.

46. Hierons R Saunders M. Impotence in patients with temporal lobe lesions. Lancet 1966;2:761–764.

47. Bagatell CJ, Bremner WJ. Androgens and behavior in men and women. Endocrinologist. 1997;7:97–102.

48. Bagatell CJ, Heiman JR, Rivier JE, Bremner WJ. Effects of endogenous testosterone and estradiol on sexual behavior in normal young men. J Clin Endocrinol Metab 1994;77:711–716.

49. Selby C. Sex hormone binding globulin: origin, function, and clinical significance. Ann Clin Biochem 1990;27:532–541.

50. Kwan M, Greenleaf WJ, Mann J, et al. The nature of androgen action in male sexuality: a combined laboratory self report study on hypogonadal men. J Clin Endocrinol Metab 1983;57:557–563.

51. Bancroft J, Wu FC. Changes in erectile responsiveness during androgen replacement therapy. Arch Sex Behav 1983;12:59–66.

52. Gooren LJ. Androgen levels and sex functions in testosterone treated hypogonadal men. Arch Sex Behav 1987;6:463–473.

53. Buena F, Swerdloff RS, Steiner BS, et al. Sexual function does not change when serum testosterone levels are pharmacologically varied within the normal range. Fertil Steril 1993;59:1118–1123.

54. Nanjee MB, Wheeler MJ. Plasma free testosterone—is an index sufficient? Ann Clin Biochem 1985;22:387–390.

55. Kapoor P, Luttrell BM, Williams D. The free androgen index is not valid for adult males. J Steroid Biochem Mol Biol 1993;4:325–326.

56. Barragry JM, Makin HL, Trafford DJ, Scott DF. Effect of anticonvulsants on plasma testosterone and sex hormone binding globulin levels. J Neurol Neurosurg Psychiatry 1978;41:913–941.

57. Victor A, Lundberg PO, Johansson ED. Induction of sex-hormone-binding-globulin by phenytoin. BMJ 1977;2:934–935.

58. Toone BK, Wheeler M, Fenwick PB. Sex hormone changes in male epileptic patients. Clin Endocrinol 1980;12:391–395.

59. Isojarvi JI, Pakarinen A, Ylipalosaari PK, Myllyla VV. Serum hormones in male epileptic patients receiving anticonvulsant medication. Arch Neurol 1990;47:670–676.

60. Isojarvi JI, Pakarinen A, Myllya VV. Effects of carbamazepine therapy on serum sex hormone levels in male patients with epilepsy. Epilepsia 1988;29:781–786.

61. Macphee GJ, Larkin JG, Butler E, et al. Circulating hormones and pituitary responsiveness in young epileptic men receiving long-term antiepileptic medication. Epilepsia 1988;29:468–475.

62. Jensen P, Jensen SB, Sorensen PS, et al. Sexual dysfunction in male and female patients with epilepsy: a study of 86 outpatients. Arch Sex Behav 1990;19:1–14.

63. Duncan S, Blacklaw J, Beastall GH, Brodie MJ. Sexual function in men with epilepsy. Epilepsia 1999;40:197–204.

64. Rodin E, Subramanian MG, Gilroy J. Investigation of sex hormones in male epileptic patients. Epilepsia 1984;25:690–694.

65. Rattya J, Turkka J, Pakarinen AJ, et al. Reproductive effects of valproate, carbamazepine, and oxecarbazepine in men with epilepsy. Neurology 2001;56(1):31–41.

66. Stoffel-Wagner B, Bauer J, Flugel D, et al. Serum sex hormones are altered in patients with chronic temporal lobe epilepsy receiving anticonvulsant medication. Epilepsia 1998;39:1164–1173.

67. Duncan S, Blacklaw J, Beastall GH, Brodie MJ. Sexual function in women with epilepsy. Epilepsia 1997;38:1074–1081.

68. Connell JM, Rapeport WG, Beastall GH, Brodie MJ. Changes in circulating androgens during short term androgen therapy. Br J Clin Pharmacol 1984;17:347–351.

69. Herzog AG, Klein P, Jacobs AR. Testosterone versus testosterone and testolactone in treating reproductive and sexual dysfunction in men with epilepsy and hypogonadism. Neurology 1998;50:782–784.

70. Bancroft J, Sherwin BB, Alexander GM, et al. Oral contraceptives, androgens, and the sexuality of young women. II, the role of androgens. Arch Sex Behav 1991;20:121–135.

71. Schreiner-Engel P, Shiavi RC, White D, Ghizzani A. Low sexual desire in women; the role of reproductive hormones. Horm Behav 1989;23:221–234.

72. Demerdash A, Shaalon M, Midori A. Sexual behavior of a sample of females with epilepsy. Epilepsia 1991;32:82–85.

73. Ndegwa D, Rust J, Golombok S, Fenwick P. Sexual problems in epileptic women. Sex Marital Ther 1986;1:175–177.

74. Bergen D, Daugherty S, Eckenfels E. Reduction of sexual activities in females taking antiepileptic drugs. Psychopathology 1992;25:1–4.

75. Morrell MJ, Sperling MR, Stecker M, Dichter MA. Sexual dysfunction in partial epilepsy: a deficit in physiologic sexual arousal. Neurology 1994;44:243–247.

76. Backstrom T, Sodergard R. Testosterone-estradiol binding globulin, unbound and total estradiol and testosterone, and total progesterone during the menstrual cycle in women with epilepsy taking antiepileptic drugs, J Endocrinol Invest 1979;2:359–366.

77. Isojarvi JI, Pakarinen AJ, Myllyla VV. A prospective study of serum sex hormones during carbamazepine therapy. Epilepsy Res 1991;9:139–144.

Chapter 17

Epilepsy and Disorders of Reproduction

Mark N. Friedman and Andrew G. Herzog

Hormones affect seizures, and seizures affect hormonal regulation and secretion. It is important to understand how different hormones may improve or exacerbate seizures in an effort to further optimize the care of patients with epilepsy. This includes an understanding of the role of adjunctive hormonal therapy in treating seizures. Reproductive dysfunction is unusually common among women and men who have epilepsy,[1] specifically localization-related epilepsy of temporal lobe origin (temporal lobe epilepsy [TLE]),[2,3] and particularly more so with medial rather than lateral temporal lobe involvement.[4] This may result from the effects of epilepsy itself or from the use of antiepileptic drugs (AEDs),[1] both of which can adversely affect reproductive hormone secretion.

The reproductive neuroendocrine system consists of the limbic system, hypothalamus, pituitary, peripheral endocrine glands, liver, and adipose tissue. Reproductive endocrine disorders can lead to reproductive dysfunction and an exacerbation of epilepsy.[1] Dysfunction of reproduction in women can manifest as infertility and menstrual disorders (e.g., amenorrhea, oligomenorrhea, abnormally prolonged or shortened cycle intervals, and menometrorrhagia). It can also manifest as hirsutism and galactorrhea.[5–8] Evidence suggests that anovulatory cycles are more common in association with TLE than with primary generalized epilepsy.[2] Women with idiopathic epilepsy are only 37% as likely as unaffected female siblings to become pregnant.[9] This finding is not attributable to marital rate, seizure type, age of seizure onset, or family history of epilepsy.[9]

In men, reproductive dysfunction manifests as diminished potency and abnormal sperm structure and function.[1] Although AED use is a factor, evidence suggests that untreated men are also commonly affected.[10] Men with idiopathic epilepsy are only 36% as likely as male unaffected siblings to ever father a pregnancy.[9] Factors that influence this low rate of reproduction include partial onset seizures, onset before 20 years of age, absence of a family history of epilepsy, and reduced marital rates in men with epilepsy.[9] Among married men with epilepsy, reproductive disadvantage was confined to those with onset before 10 years of age.[9]

Reproductive Physiology

Ovulation is controlled by the pituitary hormones, luteinizing hormone (LH) and follicle-stimulating hormone (FSH). These hormones are regulated by luteinizing hormone–releasing hormone (LHRH), which is secreted by a widely distributed system of hypothalamic LHRH-containing neurons. The LHRH neurons release LHRH in a pulsatile manner into the portal hypophyseal circulation, which then carries it to the anterior pituitary gland. It is here that LHRH stimulates LH and FSH release into the systemic circulation, also in a pulsatile manner. FSH stimulates the maturation of the follicle within the ovaries. This leads to the production of estrogen by the ovary during the follicular phase of the menstrual cycle. When the follicle reaches maturity, a surge of estrogen production stimulates a surge in LH secretion from the pituitary through a positive feedback mechanism. What follows is the release of the ovum from the follicle (i.e., ovulation). The remaining follicle subsequently becomes transformed into the corpus luteum, which secretes progesterone and estrogen during the luteal half of the menstrual cycle. At the end of this phase, the production of estrogen and progesterone declines, and menstruation follows.

In women with epilepsy, neuroendocrine issues of importance include the following: (1) the effects of hormones on epilepsy, (2) the effects of epilepsy on hormones throughout reproductive life (e.g., menarche, menstruation, pregnancy, and menopause), and (3) the therapeutic potential of reproductive hormones, metabolites, or synthetic analogs.

Hormonal Effects on Epilepsy

Changes in reproductive hormonal status associated with menarche, menstruation, pregnancy, and menopause may affect clinical manifestations of seizures. As a result of puberty, late childhood and early adolescence are times of great change in the reproductive steroid milieu. This stage of reproductive development forms a temporal continuum of various neuroactive steroids that originate from the adrenal glands and gonads. These hormones may benefit or exacerbate various forms of epilepsy. In fact, puberty may be associated with the resolution of some forms of epilepsy and the exacerbation of others. For example, some of the primary partial epilepsies may resolve almost invariably by 16 years of age (e.g., benign rolandic epilepsy of childhood and benign occipital epilepsy of childhood with occipital paroxysms).[11,12] The mechanism for such improvement may involve changes not only in gonadal steroids, but also in adrenal neuroactive steroids that are associated with puberty and adrenarche. On the other hand, secondary partial seizures (e.g., idiopathic or lesional seizure) may show an exacerbation during menarche. In general, late childhood and adolescence are peak periods for the first manifestation of epilepsy.[13,14] This is particularly true among women with catamenial epilepsy, two-thirds of whom may experience the onset of seizures within 3 years of menarche.[14,15] Pre-existing complex partial seizures in women

may also increase in frequency at the time of menarche.[16] This may relate to increased neuronal excitability associated with the elevation of estrogens at the time of menarche. In animal studies, this is suggested by the finding that oophorectomy in rats before sexual maturation decreases their susceptibility to seizures in adulthood.[17]

During the menstrual cycle, seizure frequency may increase during conditions in which there is an elevated serum estrogen to progesterone (E-P) ratio. This normally occurs during the ovulatory and premenstrual phases. Premenstrual exacerbation of seizures may also be related to a decline in anticonvulsant medication levels. Hepatic microsomal enzymes metabolize gonadal steroids and several anticonvulsants (e.g., phenytoin and carbamazepine), with competition between the two. The premenstrual decline in gonadal steroid secretion may therefore permit increased metabolism of AEDs, resulting in lower serum levels of these medications and an exacerbation of seizures. Not all AEDs are affected in this manner (e.g., phe-nobarbital), and the catamenial effects of most of the newer AEDs have yet to be adequately studied.

Pregnancy can have variable effects on epilepsy. For example, seizure frequency decreases in approximately one-sixth of women, possibly because of increased medication compliance.[18,19] On the other hand, women can experience seizures for the first time during pregnancy and have seizures only during pregnancy. For those with an established history of seizures, approximately one-third of these women may have worsening seizures during pregnancy. This may relate to decreased serum levels of AEDs, AED protein-binding changes, and a higher rate of hepatic renal metabolism of these medications.[18,19] Total concentrations of all first-line AEDs (e.g., carbamazepine, phenytoin, phenobarbital, and valproic acid) fall significantly during pregnancy compared to baseline. Free or unbound drug concentrations, however, fall significantly only for phenobarbital yet can increase for valproic acid by 25% by the time of delivery. On the other hand, women taking carbamazepine, phenytoin, or valproate may be relatively protected by adequate free concentrations of these compounds throughout pregnancy.[20] Therefore, proper management of epilepsy in pregnant women should include measuring free AED concentrations so that proper dose adjustments can be achieved to maintain the therapeutic range of these medications.

Similarly, the effect of menopause on epilepsy is also variable. In some patients, seizures may cease at the time of menopause, whereas in other patients, seizures may worsen. This change and variability in seizure expression may have a reproductive hormonal contribution. During menopause, the effects of this process may differ significantly from person to person, particularly with regard to seizure expression. For example, although estrogen levels decline as ovarian function diminishes, progesterone typically declines more substantially, resulting in an elevated E-P serum ratio. Thus, perimenopausally, anovulatory cycles may develop and lead to an increased E-P ratio that would be expected to promote the occurrence of seizures.[21] However, as menopause progresses and reaches its final stages, ovarian estrogen production may become essentially undetectable and may potentially improve seizure control.

Seizures may also become exacerbated or occur for the first time in menopausal women who take hormone replacement therapy. Specifically, an exacerbation of seizures may occur with the initiation of estrogen replacement therapy. However, this effect may occur even if a woman is also taking the synthetic form of progesterone replacement therapy, which has minimal anticonvulsant properties. Menopausal women with epilepsy may, in fact, be at risk for an increase in seizure rate when they use hormone replacement therapy consisting of synthetic estrogen or progesterone replacement.[22]

Pharmacologic Effects on Hormones and Seizures

The effects of specific medications may potentially affect seizures. For example, the rate of oral contraceptive failure is notably greater in women with epilepsy who take AEDs (estimated to be 3.1 per 100.0 woman-years using the regular pill formulation: 80 μg estrogen plus 1 mg progestin) than in untreated epileptic women and women in the general population (0.7 per 100.0 woman-years).[23] This rate of failure may be considerably higher in the currently popular lower-formulation (35.0 μg estrogen plus 0.5 mg progestin) minipills, particularly because of

how these medications are metabolized by enzyme-inducing AEDs (e.g., barbiturates, phenytoin, and carbamazepine).[24] This category of AEDs is thought to induce microsomal enzymes that increase the catabolism of sex steroids (including those found in oral contraceptives) by the liver and that increase the conjugation of sex steroids in the gut.[24] Serum levels of the estrogen and progestin components vary considerably but, in some, may drop three- to four-fold.[25,26] AEDs also induce increased sex hormone–binding globulin (SHBG) synthesis by the liver, thereby decreasing the biologically active portion of the steroid.[24] However, these effects do not appear to be the case for non–enzyme-inducing AEDs, such as valproate and benzodiazepines and, possibly, felbamate and gabapentin.[24] So, for women with epilepsy who take enzyme-inducing AEDs, higher-dose, rather than minipill formulation, birth control pills are recommended, especially if those women experience irregular cycles and breakthrough bleeding.[24] These hormonal relationships are important to consider in the setting of birth control and also in women with epilepsy who take hormones for other reasons, such as for the treatment of menstrual disorders and endometriosis.

Reproductive Endocrine Disorder Effects on Seizures

Reproductive endocrine disorders may favor the development of TLE in women. These disorders are characterized by anovulatory cycles, which consequently lead to a chronically elevated E-P ratio and the promotion of increased neuronal excitability. When this occurs, the frequency of seizures may increase as a result of the constant exposure of temporal lobe structures to estrogen without the balance of normal luteal levels of progesterone. There is also evidence to suggest that progesterone therapy may lessen the frequency of interictal discharges in some women with partial seizures and anovulatory cycles or amenorrhea.[27]

Catamenial epilepsy refers to seizure exacerbation in relation to specific phases of the menstrual cycle. This may occur during the time of menstruation (perimenstrually, type I), before ovulation (type II), or throughout the entire second half of the menstrual cycle (luteal phase, type III; Figure 17-1).[28] To establish a causal relationship between

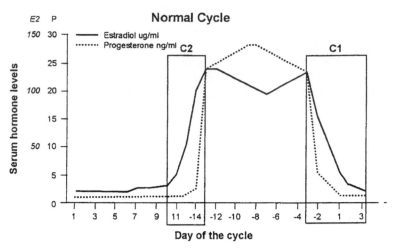

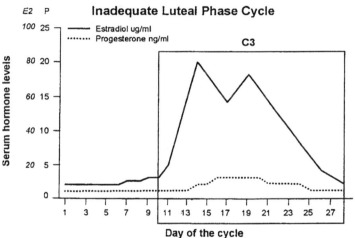

Figure 17-1. Three proposed patterns of catamenial epilepsy: perimenstrual (C1) and periovulatory (C2) exacerbations during normal cycles and entire second half of the cycle (C3) exacerbation during inadequate luteal phase cycles. (E2 = estradiol; P = progesterone.)

seizures in a woman and specific phases of her menstrual cycle, it is helpful for her to keep a careful seizure diary (using the first day of menstrual bleeding as the first day of the cycle). The menstrual cycle is divided into four phases: (1) menstrual, counting days −3 to +3; (2) follicular, days +4 to +9; (3) ovulatory, days +10 to +16; and (4) luteal, days +17 to −4. The number of seizures in each phase is counted, and the average daily number of seizures for each menstrual phase is then analyzed to see whether a pattern of exacerbation or remission at certain phases of the menstrual cycle is present. We define catamenial seizure exacerbation as a twofold or greater increase in average daily seizure frequency (during the affected part of the menstrual cycle) compared to the remainder of the cycle. Catamenial epilepsy types I and II occur in women with normal menstrual cycles. Type III is the most difficult one to distin-

guish, because the time of seizure exacerbation is prolonged rather than focused and occurs in women with abnormal menstrual cycles. Such women have anovulatory cycles and inadequate luteal phase syndrome. Because they do not ovulate, no corpus luteum is formed during the second (luteal) half of the menstrual cycle, and no progesterone is secreted.[29]

The menstrual cycle–related hormonal fluctuations in estrogen and progesterone underlie the different patterns of catamenial seizures. As mentioned previously, the estrogens, particularly estradiol, have potent proconvulsant properties and exert an excitatory effect on neurons by potentiating excitatory conduction that is mediated by N-methyl-D-aspartate–type glutamate receptors.[30] In several animal seizure models, estrogens can precipitate seizures, even status epilepticus, when they are administered intraperitoneally, intravenously, or topically to the brain surface.[17,31–33] In contrast, the natural form of progesteronc has anticonvulsant properties in many models of epilepsy. One of its natural endogenous metabolites, allopregnanolone, acts as an agonist at the γ-aminobutyric acid (GABA) alpha receptor, with a potency that is almost 1,000-fold greater than that of pentobarbital and the most potent benzodiazepine, flunitrazepam.[34,35] In animal seizure models, progesterone lessens epileptiform discharges, inhibits pre-existing seizures,[17,36] and protects against the development of seizures.[33]

Concerning the management of catamenial epilepsy, we suggest the following guidelines[28]:

1. Establish the presence of a catamenial pattern of seizure exacerbation using a careful seizure and menstrual diary, as previously outlined.
2. Establish the clinical menstrual pattern (i.e., normal or abnormal menstrual cycles).
3. Check midluteal serum progesterone levels (e.g., on day 22 of a 28-day menstrual cycle) to determine whether an inadequate luteal phase is present.
4. If type I (perimenstrual) catamenial seizure exacerbation is present, check trough AED levels on days 22 (i.e., when estradiol and progesterone levels are high, and the AED level should be in the therapeutic range) and 1 (i.e., menstrual, when estradiol and progesterone levels are low) to determine whether the level is low at this time and could be the cause of perimenstrual seizure exacerbation.

Epilepsy Effects on Hormones

Persistent Interictal Effects on Reproductive Hormones

Altered function of temporal lobe structures, a factor common to all patients with TLE who have reproductive dysfunction, may contribute to reproductive and sexual changes.[1] TLE most often originates from, or involves to a major degree, limbic portions of the temporal lobe.[37] Partial seizures of temporal lobe origin (TLE) may promote the development of polycystic ovarian syndrome (PCOS) and hypothalamic amenorrhea (i.e., hypogonadotropic hypogonadism [HH]), two of the conditions associated with inadequate luteal phase syndrome.[6] TLE may also be associated with premature menopause. As mentioned, reproductive dysfunction and endocrine disorders are unusually common among women with epilepsy. Fertility is reduced by 15–30% of the expected number of offspring among married epileptic women, although the reduction may affect only women whose seizures began before the age of 10 years.[38] Thirty-five percent of cycles in women with partial seizures of temporal lobe origin may be anovulatory.[2] In addition, approximately one-half of women with TLE may have menstrual cycle abnormalities (e.g., amenorrhea, oligomenorrhea, or abnormally long [>32 days] or short [<26 days] menstrual cycle intervals).[6]

These menstrual cycle abnormalities are often associated with distinct reproductive endocrine disorders. For example, PCOS and HH are present in 20% and 12%, respectively, of women with TLE, as compared to 5.0% and 1.5% of women in the general population. Premature menopause and functional hyperprolactinemia are present in 4% and 2%, respectively, of women with TLE, as compared with fewer than 1% (for either condition) of women in the general population.[6] The pathogenic mechanism of these disorders has not been firmly established, but several possibilities exist:

1. The effect of temporal lobe seizures or interictal epileptiform discharges on the functioning of the hypothalamic-pituitary–gonadal hormonal axis may be one pathogenic mechanism. These types of seizures or discharges are more common in untreated than treated women with epilepsy. Abnormal serum levels of gonadotropins and prolactin and altered LH response to gonadotropin-releasing hormone (GnRH) in women with epilepsy suggest altered function of the hypothalamic-pituitary axis.[6,39] With regard to gonadotropins, the amygdala has extensive, direct anatomic connections with the arcuate and preoptic hypothalamic nuclei, which are involved in the regulation, production, and secretion of GnRH.[40] Alterations in the physiologic frequency or concentration of pulsatile GnRH secretion can subsequently induce changes in serum LH and FSH. These changes may resemble patterns found in reproductive endocrine disorders (e.g., PCOS and HH).[41]

2. The pathogenetic mechanism of the co-occurrence of reproductive endocrine disorders and epilepsy may relate to possible parallel effects of prenatal factors that are common to the development of the brain and the reproductive system.[6] For

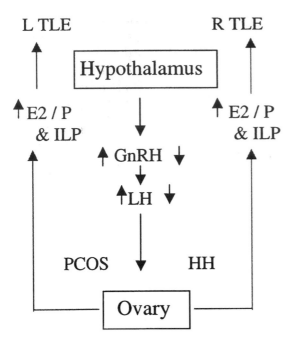

L TLE   R TLE

Figure 17-2. Effects of lateralized cerebral influences on reproductive endocrine function. (E2 = estradiol; GnRH = gonadotropin-releasing hormone; HH = hypogonadotropic hypogonadism; ILP = inadequate luteal phase; L = left; LH = luteinizing hormone; P = progesterone; PCOS = polycystic ovarian syndrome; R = right; TLE = temporal lobe epilepsy.)

example, each of these categories of disorders (i.e., TLE, PCOS, and HH) has a tendency to be familial, and each has recently been shown to have a genetic basis. Therefore, the possibility of genetic linkage exists. The inheritance of polycystic ovaries has an autosomal-dominant pattern of inheritance.[42] GnRH deficiency (HH) may be inherited via autosomal-dominant, autosomal-recessive, and x-linked modes of inheritance.[43] In 1997, four autosomal-dominant partial epilepsies were described,[44] one of which includes a form of TLE (familial TLE). This TLE subtype was associated with linkage to chromosome 10q in one family, but the genetic defect is unknown.

A role for altered temporolimbic electroencephalogram (EEG) activity in the development of some reproductive endocrine disorders among women with epilepsy is supported by the finding of a significant difference between the EEG laterality distributions associated with PCOS and HH.[45] Among 30 women who had reproductive endo-

crine disorders and complex partial seizures with unilateral temporal lobe interictal epileptiform discharges, there was a strong predominance of left-sided discharges (15 versus 1) with PCOS, and right-sided discharges (12 versus 2) with HH. Each distribution differed significantly from that of 30 women with epilepsy who had no reproductive endocrine disorder (left/right was 17/13). Moreover, among women with PCOS who had unilateral non–temporal lobe foci, six of seven had right-sided epileptiform discharges. This represents a significant difference from the EEG laterality distribution of women with PCOS who had temporal foci. These findings suggest that the pattern of reproductive hormonal secretion in women with epilepsy is influenced by the laterality and focality of the epilepsy (Figure 17-2).

The control of the pulsatile release of LHRH by hypothalamic neurons is subject to modulatory influences from forebrain and extrahypothalamic brain stem regions.[46] The most notable forebrain influence is from the amygdala, which has massive, direct anatomic connections to the preoptic area and the mediobasal hypothalamus, the principal locations of the LHRH-containing neurons.[40,47] The amygdala can be divided, anatomically and functionally, into two distinct parts: the corticomedial and the basolateral divisions. The basolateral amygdala exerts an inhibitory influence on gonadotropin function and ovulation, whereas the corticomedial amygdala stimulates hypothalamic gona- dotropin function and ovulation. Thus, involvement of temporal lobe structures, namely the amygdala, by ictal or interictal epileptiform discharges may disrupt normal limbic modulation of reproductive endocrine secretion. This disruption is reflected at the hypothalamic, pituitary, and peripheral gland levels. For example, discharges involving the left amygdala are associated with increased hypothalamic LHRH pulse frequency, which leads to the preferential secretion of LH over FSH by the pituitary gonadotrope.[45] This pattern of gonadotrope release then leads to a failure of ovarian follicular development and to the accumulation of small ovarian cysts. The immature follicles lack aromatase, which converts testosterone to estradiol, and hence leads to androgenization. Hyperandrogenic chronic anovulation can be viewed as a form of PCOS. Conversely, discharges involving the right amygdala may lead to reduced LHRH pulse frequency and the development of hypothalamic amenorrhea, formerly known as HH.[45,48]

In men, the disruption of normal temporolimbic modulation of hypothalamic-pituitary function by epileptiform discharges may promote the development of reproductive endocrine disorders as well.[1] Hypogonadism is unusually common among men with epilepsy. In our own series of 20 men with partial seizures of temporal lobe origin (TLE), 11 (55%) had reproductive dysfunction or hyposexuality.[6] Nine of these 11 men (45% overall) had reproductive endocrine disorders, including HH in 25%, hypergonadotropic hypogonadism in 10%, and functional hyperprolactinemia in 10%. Hypogonadism and abnormal semen analysis may possibly be as common among untreated as among treated men with epilepsy.[10] Serum estradiol levels are also significantly more variable in untreated men with TLE than in healthy controls. Lateralized cerebral and hypothalamic asymmetries, moreover, may be responsible for the association of different patterns of reproductive endocrine secretion with left and right TLE.[49,50]

Interactions between Reproductive Hormones and Antiepileptic Drugs

AEDs affect serum reproductive hormone levels. For example, AED use is associated with a diminished bioactive to total testosterone ratio in the serum.[51] The biologically active portion of testosterone includes the large fraction (53–55%) of albumin-bound as well as the small fraction (2–3%) of entirely free testosterone. There are data to suggest an association between AED use and markedly diminished serum levels of the adrenal androgen metabolite dehydroepiandrosterone sulfate.[6,52] AEDs, such as barbiturates, phenytoin, and carbamazepine, induce hepatic enzymes to increase the rate of steroid metabolism and thereby lower biologically active androgen levels, whereas sodium valproate does not have this effect.

With regard to PCOS, there is a difference in incidence between valproate-treated women and women treated with other AEDs. On the one hand, valproate may promote PCOS development by inducing weight gain and insulin resistance.[53] An additional consideration is that this may be related to a beneficiary effect on PCOS by hepatic-inducing AEDs, such as barbiturates, phenytoin, and carbamazepine.[54] Thus, PCOS is

less common in treated women (13%) than in untreated women (30%) with TLE, when treatment does not include sodium valproate.[6] On the other hand, hepatic enzyme-inducing AEDs lower biological androgen levels, whereas valproate does not. AEDs other than valproate, therefore, may treat epilepsy-related hyperandrogenism and thus PCOS, whereas valproate therapy may not and may actually exacerbate the disorder.[54]

In men, AEDs may reduce biologically active testosterone by direct inhibition of synthesis and the induction of binding globulin. They act at various levels of the gonadal testosterone synthesis cascade to inhibit testosterone production.[55] In an in vitro, rat Leydig cell model, carbamazepine exhibited potent inhibitory effects at therapeutic range concentrations. Phenytoin required higher concentrations. Valproate effects were the smallest at therapeutic concentrations. In an investigation comparing serum reproductive steroid levels among 20 men who were treated with phenytoin for complex partial seizures, 21 untreated men with complex partial seizures, and 20 age-matched healthy controls, total and non–SHBG-bound estradiol levels were significantly higher in the phenytoin group than in either the untreated or healthy control groups.[56] Carbamazepine and barbiturates appear to have similar effects. These findings suggest that some AEDs may lower free testosterone not only by the induction of SHBG synthetase, but perhaps also by the induction of aromatase, which converts free testosterone to estradiol. Although comprising only approximately 1% of the total gonadal steroids in men, estradiol exerts a potent inhibitory influence on LH secretion and may play a major role in negative feedback in men as well as women.[57,58] Suppression of LH secretion results in HH. Chronically low free testosterone leads to testicular failure and hypergonadotropic hypogonadism. This may explain the frequent occurrence of both of these reproductive endocrine disorders in men with epilepsy.[6] Finally, estradiol can produce premature aging of the hypothalamic arcuate nucleus, which secretes GnRH.[59,60]

Therapeutic Potential of Reproductive Hormones in Epilepsy

Hormonal treatment of epilepsy focuses on the enhancement of the inhibitory GABA-ergic activity of progesterone and the suppression of the excitatory glutamatergic effects of estrogen. Investigational treatments include the use of natural progesterone, estrogen antagonists, GnRH analogs that suppress the pituitary-gonadal axis, and medications that suppress the activity of the hypothalamic-pituitary–adrenal axis. These therapies may be considered in particular for individuals with refractory seizures that occur in patterns and suggest a hormonal contribution (e.g., catamenial epilepsy). As mentioned previously, one of the bioactive metabolites of natural progesterone, allopregnanolone, has potent anticonvulsant, GABA-ergic effects, whereas the synthetic progestins are not readily metabolized in this manner. The oral use of synthetic progestin therapy has minimal, if any, anticonvulsant benefits. In a study of women with refractory partial seizures and normal ovulatory cycles, a medroxyprogesterone dose large enough to induce amenorrhea (i.e., 120–150 mg every 6–12 weeks intramuscularly or 20–40 mg orally daily) resulted in a 40% average seizure reduction.[61] We have found weekly doses of 400 mg of intramuscular depo medroxyprogesterone to be remarkably effective in some exceptional cases. Potential side effects of progesterone therapy include depression, sedation, breakthrough vaginal bleeding, and delay in the return of regular menstrual cycles. However, this last side effect is seen more with the depo form of medroxyprogesterone.

Natural progesterone therapy may be beneficial in women who have catamenial seizure exacerbation.[62] In a study of 25 women with a catamenial pattern of complex partial seizure exacerbation of temporal lobe origin (14 with inadequate luteal phase or anovulatory cycles and 11 with normal cycles and perimenstrual seizure exacerbation), 72% of the women improved. There was a 55% decline in average seizure frequency.[62] Progesterone was administered as lozenges, 200 mg three times daily on days 23 through 25 of each menstrual cycle, for perimenstrual exacerbation and on days 15 through 25 of each menstrual cycle, with a tapering dose over days 26 through 28, for exacerbations lasting through the entire luteal phase.

Natural progesterone is available as a plant extract in lozenge, micronized capsule, cream, and suppository form. The usual daily regimen to achieve physiologic luteal range serum levels is generally 100–200 mg 3 times daily.[62] Potential side effects may include sedation, depression, weight gain, breast tenderness, and breakthrough vaginal bleeding, all of which are readily reversible with discontinuation of the hormone or by lowering the dose.

Clomiphene citrate is an estrogen analog with estrogenic and antiestrogenic effects that are dose dependent. Clinically, it acts primarily as an antiestrogen at the hypothalamic and pituitary level to stimulate gonadotropin secretion, ovulation, and fertility. In rats, it exerts an anticonvulsant effect in a dose-related manner.[33] A remarkable reduction in seizure frequency was reported in a number of isolated cases in men and women.[63–65] In one series of 12 women who had complex partial seizures and severe menstrual disorders (i.e., in the setting of PCOS or inadequate luteal phase cycles of uncertain etiology) and who were given clomiphene, 10 significantly improved with an 87% average decline in seizure frequency.[65] The improvement in seizure frequency was also associated with normalization of the menstrual cycle and of luteal progesterone secretion. The only two women who did not improve continued to have menstrual abnormalities. Side effects included one unwanted pregnancy, two cases of ovarian cysts, and three cases of transient breast tenderness and pelvic cramps. Hence, clomiphene may be a useful adjunctive antiepileptic treatment in women with refractory seizures and severe menstrual disorders. Recommended doses range from 25 to 100 mg daily on days 5–9 of each menstrual cycle. Side effects can be substantial and include ovarian overstimulation syndrome, an increased seizure frequency during the enhanced preovulatory rise in serum estradiol levels, and the potential for unwanted pregnancy. Therefore, clomiphene should not be administered in the absence of adequate birth control measures, unless it is used in conjunction with a gynecologic consultation as part of a fertility program. It should also not be used in cases of suspected pregnancy. Clomiphene should be discontinued if visual disturbances, especially palinopsia, develop. Clomiphene use does carry the potential for seizure exacerbation in the late follicular phase, in relation to the enhancement of preovulatory estrogen secretion. Therefore, seizure frequency should be monitored carefully, especially during this phase. Additional studies are needed in establishing the role of clomiphene in the treatment of epilepsy.

In men, manipulation of testosterone and estradiol levels may also have some potential in the management of refractory seizures in those with reproductive dysfunction and hypogonadism. Testolactone is an inhibitor of the enzyme aromatase, which catalyzes the conversion of testosterone to estradiol. Combined treatment using testosterone and testolactone may be more effective than testosterone replacement alone in managing men with epilepsy who have hyposexuality or reproductive dysfunction.[66] A concomitant reduction in seizure frequency has been associated with combined but not lone therapy. This decline in seizure frequency may be related to a reduction in the proconvulsant effects of estrogen.

In summary, highly epileptogenic regions of the brain, most notably temporolimbic structures, such as the amygdala and hippocampus, are sites of origin or at least involvement in most adult cases of epilepsy and also serve as centers that modulate endocrine secretion and feedback. Disruption of this endocrine modulatory role by epileptiform discharges alters reproductive endocrine secretion and promotes the development of reproductive endocrine disorders and reproductive dysfunction. Because many reproductive steroids have highly neuroactive properties, and temporolimbic structures show exquisitely sensitive neurophysiologic responses to steroid hormonal input, changes in the hormonal environment, whether physiologic, pathologic, or pharmacologic, may alter the frequency, severity, and temporal pattern of seizure occurrence. AED actions at limbic, hypothalamic-pituitary, peripheral gland, hepatic, and adipose tissue sites must be considered under the category of pharmacologic influences. A better understanding of the reciprocal relationships between epilepsy and hormones is important not only to our understanding of the pathophysiology of epilepsy, but also to comprehensive management.

References

1. Herzog AG. A hypothesis to integrate partial seizures of temporal lobe origin and reproductive disorders. Epilepsy Res 1989;3:151–159.
2. Cummings LN, Morrell MJ, Giudice L. Ovulatory function in epilepsy. Epilepsia 1995;36:353–357.
3. Gastaut H, Collomb H. Etude du comportement sexuel chez les epileptiques psychomoteurs. Ann Med Psychol 1954;112:657–696.
4. Pritchard PB, Wannamaker BB, Sagel J, DeVillier C. Endocrine dysfunction in temporal lobe epilepsy. Arch Neurol 1982;39:786–787.
5. Cogen PH, Antunes JL, Correl JW. Reproductive function in temporal lobe epilepsy: the effect of temporal lobectomy. Surg Neurol 1979;12:243–246.
6. Herzog AG, Seibel MM, Schomer DL, et al. Reproductive endocrine disorders in women with partial seizures of temporal lobe origin. Arch Neurol 1986;43:341–346.
7. Jensen I, Vaernet K. Temporal lobe epilepsy: follow-up investigation of 74 temporal lobe resected patients. Acta Neurochir 1977;37:173–200.
8. Trampuz V, Dimitrijevic M, Kryanovski J. Ulga epilepsije u patogenezi disfunkeije ovarija. Neuropsihijatrija 1975;23:179–183.
9. Schupf N, Ottman R. Likelihood of pregnancy in individuals with idiopathic/cryptogenic epilepsy: social and biologic influences. Epilepsia 1994;35:750–756.
10. Taneja N, Kucheria K, Jain S, Maheshwari MC. Effect of phenytoin on semen. Epilepsia 1994;35:136–140.
11. Beaussart M, Faou R. Evolution of epilepsy with rolandic (centrotemporal) paroxysmal foci. Epilepsia 1978;19:337–342.
12. Panayiotopoulos CP. Benign childhood epilepsy with occipital paroxysms: a 15-year prospective study. Ann Neurol 1989;26:51–56.
13. Lennox WG, Cobb S. Epilepsy. Medicine 1928;27:105–290.
14. Longo LP, Saldana LEG. Hormones and their influences in epilepsy. Acta Neurol Latinoam 1966;12:29–47.
15. Logothetis J, Harner R, Morrell F, et al. The role of estrogens in catamenial exacerbation of epilepsy. Neurology 1959;9:35–36.
16. Rosciszewska D. The course of epilepsy at the age of puberty in girls. Neurol Neurochir Pol 1975;9:597–602.
17. Woolley DE, Timiras PS. The gonad-brain relationship: effects of female sex hormones on electroshock convulsions in the rat. Endocrinology 1962;70:196–209.
18. Knight AH, Rhind EG. Epilepsy and pregnancy: a study of 153 pregnancies in 59 patients. Epilepsia 1975;16:99–110.
19. Schmidt D, Canger R, Avanzini G. Change in seizure frequency in pregnant epileptic women. J Neurol Neurosurg Psychiatry 1985;46:751–755.
20. Yerby MS, Friel PN, McCormick K. Antiepileptic drug disposition during pregnancy. Neurology 1992;42[Suppl 5]:12–16.
21. Backstrom T. Epileptic seizures in women related to plasma estrogen and progesterone during the menstrual cycle. Acta Neurol Scand 1976;54:321–347.
22. Harden CL, Pulver MC, Ravdin L, Jacobs AR. The effect of menopause and perimenopause on the course of epilepsy. Epilepsia 1999;40:1402–1407.
23. Coulam CB, Annegers JF. Do anticonvulsants reduce the efficacy of oral contraceptives? Epilepsia 1979;20:519–526.

24. Mattson RH, Cramer JA, Darney PD, Naftolin F. Use of oral contraceptives by women with epilepsy. JAMA 1986;256:238–240.

25. Back DJ, Bates M, Bowden A, et al. The interaction of phenobarbital and other anticonvulsants with oral contraceptive steroid therapy. Contraception 1980;22:495–503.

26. Orme MU. The clinical pharmacology of oral contraceptive steroids. Br J Clin Pharmacol 1982;14:31–42.

27. Backstrom T, Zetterlund B, Blom S, et al. Effects of intravenous progesterone infusions on the epileptic discharge frequency in women with partial epilepsy. Acta Neurol Scand 1984;69:240–248.

28. Herzog AG, Klein P, Ransil BJ. Three patterns of catamenial epilepsy. Epilepsia 1997;38:1082–1088.

29. Klein P, Herzog AG. Endocrine Aspects of Partial Seizures. In SC Schachter, DL Schomer (eds), The Comprehensive Evaluation and Treatment of Epilepsy: a Practical Guide. San Diego: Academic, 1997;207–232.

30. Smith SS. Estrogen administration increases neuronal responses to excitatory amino acids as a long-term effect. Brain Res 1989;503:354–357.

31. Hom AC, Buterbaugh GG. Estrogen alters the acquisition of seizures kindled by repeated amygdala stimulation or pentylenetetrazol administration in ovariectomized female rats. Epilepsia 1986;27:103–108.

32. Logothetis J, Harner R. Electrocortical activation by estrogens. Arch Neurol 1960;3:290–297.

33. Nicoletti F, Speciale C, Sortino MA, et al. Comparative effects of estradiol benzoate, the antiestrogen clomiphene citrate, and the progestin medroxyprogesterone acetate on kainic acid-induced seizures in male and female rats. Epilepsia 1985;26:252–257.

34. Majewska MD, Harrison NL, Schwartz RD, et al. Steroid hormone metabolites are barbiturate-like modulators of the GABA receptor. Science 1986;232:1004–1007.

35. Paul SM, Purdy RH. Neuroactive steroids. FASEB J 1992;6:2311–2322.

36. Landgren S, Backstrom T, Kalistratov G. The effect of progesterone on the spontaneous interictal spike evoked by the application of penicillin to the cat's cerebral cortex. J Neurol Sci 1978;36:119–133.

37. Falconer MA, Serafetinides EA, Corsellis JA. Etiology and pathogenesis of temporal lobe epilepsy. Arch Neurol 1964;10:233–248.

38. Dansky LV, Andermann E, Andermann F. Marriage and fertility in epileptic patients. Epilepsia 1980;21:261–271.

39. Herzog AG, Russell V Vaitukaitis JL, et al. Neuroendocrine dysfunction in temporal lobe epilepsy. Arch Neurol 1982;39:133–135.

40. Renaud LP. Influence of amygdala stimulation on the activity of identified tuberoinfundibular neurones in the rat hypothalamus. J Physiol 1976;260:237–252.

41. Gnobil E. The neuroendocrine control of the menstrual cycle. Recent Prog Horm Res 1980;36:53–80.

42. Govind A, Obhrai MS, Clayton RN. Polycystic ovaries are inherited as an autosomal dominant trait: analysis of 29 polycystic ovary syndrome and 10 control families. J Clin Endocrinol Metab 1999;84:38–43.

43. Hall JE. Physiologic and genetic insights into the pathophysiology and management of hypogonadotropic hypogonadism. Ann Endocrinol (Paris) 1999;60:93–101.

44. Berkovic SF, Scheffer IE. Epilepsies with single gene inheritance. Brain Dev 1997;19:13–18.

45. Herzog AG. A relationship between particular reproductive endocrine disorders and the laterality of epileptiform discharges in women with epilepsy. Neurology 1993;43:1907–1910.

46. Maeda K, Tsukamura H, Okhura S, et al. The LHRH pulse generator: a mediobasal hypothalamic location. Neurosci Biobehav Rev 1995;19:427–437.

47. Canteras NS, Simerly RB, Swanson LW. Organization of projections from the medial nucleus of the amygdala: a PHAL study in the rat. J Comp Neurol 1995;360:213–245.

48. Drislane FW, Coleman AE, Schomer DL, et al. Altered pulsatile secretion of luteinizing hormone in women with epilepsy. Neurology 1994;44:306–310.

49. Herzog AG, Coleman AE, Drislane FW, et al. Lateralized asymmetry in the temporolimbic regulation of luteinizing hormone secretion. Paper presented at the 3rd International Congress of Neuroendocrinology, July, Budapest, 1994.

50. Herzog AG, Drislane FW, Schomer DL, et al. Abnormal pulsatile secretion of luteinizing hormone in men with epilepsy: relationship to laterality and nature of paroxysmal discharges. Neurology 1990;40:1557–1561.

51. Herzog AG. Hormonal changes in epilepsy. Epilepsia 1995;36:323–326.

52. Levesque LA, Herzog AG, Seibel MM. The effect of phenytoin and carbamazepine on serum dehydroepiandrosterone sulfate in men and women who have partial seizures with temporal lobe involvement. J Clin Endocrinol Metab 1986;63:243–245.

53. Isojarvi JIT, Laatikainen TJ, Knip M, et al. Obesity and endocrine disorders in women taking valproate for epilepsy. Ann Neurol 1996;39:579–585.

54. Herzog AG. Polycystic ovarian syndrome in women with epilepsy: epileptic or iatrogenic? Ann Neurol 1996;39:559–561.

55. Kuhn-Velten WN, Herzog AG, Muller MR. Acute effects of anticonvulsant drugs on gonadotropin-stimulated and precursor-supported testicular androgen production. Eur J Pharmacol 1990;181:151–155.

56. Herzog AG, Levesque LA, Drislane FW, et al. Phenytoin-induced elevation of serum estradiol and reproductive dysfunction in men with epilepsy. Epilepsia 1991;32:550–553.

57. Loriaux D, Vigersky S, Marynick S, et al. Androgen and Estrogen Effects in the Regulation of LH in Man. In P Troen, H Nankin (eds), The Testis in Normal and Infertile Men. New York: Raven Press, 1977;213.

58. Winters S, Janick J, Loriaux L, Sherins R. Studies on the role of sex steroids in the feedback control of gonadotropin concentrations in men. II. Use of the estrogen antagonist clomiphene citrate. J Clin Endocrinol Metab 1979;48:222–227.

59. Brawer J, Schipper H, Robaire B. Effects of long-term androgen and estradiol exposure on the hypothalamus. Endocrinology 1983;112:194–199.

60. Finch CE, Felicio LS, Mobbs CV, Nelson JF. Ovarian and steroidal influences on neuroendocrine aging processes in female rodents. Endocrinol Rev 1984;5:467–497.

61. Mattson RH, Cramer JA, Caldwell BV, et al. Treatment of seizures with medroxyprogesterone acetate: preliminary report. Neurology 1984;34:1255–1258.

62. Herzog AG. Progesterone therapy in women with complex partial and secondary generalized seizures. Neurology 1995;45:1660–1662.

63. Herzog AG. Seizure control with clomiphene therapy: a case report. Arch Neurol 1988;45:209–210.

64. Login IS, Dreifuss FE. Anticonvulsant activity of clomiphene. Arch Neurol 1983;40:525.

65. Herzog AG. Clomiphene therapy in epileptic women with menstrual disorders. Neurology 1988;38:432–434.

66. Herzog AG, Klein P, Jacobs AR. Testosterone versus testosterone and testolactone in treating reproductive and sexual dysfunction in men with epilepsy and hypogonadism. Neurology 1998;50:782–784.

Chapter 18

Reproductive Issues or Pregnancy and Epilepsy

Deborah T. Combs Cantrell

Women with epilepsy (WWE) are faced with many unique issues concerning reproductive health and sexuality. Structural lesions of the brain, physiologic changes in brain function, alterations of the neuroendocrine axis due to antiepileptic drugs (AEDs) and epilepsy, and endocrine effects on seizure threshold and brain function impact the reproductive health of WWE. Interest in these issues is relatively recent, and data on the subject are limited. Pregnancy in WWE has been studied for decades; however, human data are extremely limited concerning the risks versus the benefits of AEDs. Furthermore, information concerning sexual dysfunction, neuroendocrine disorders, and fertility is even less available. This chapter reviews the major issues in the reproductive health of WWE.

Elevated prolactin levels, abnormal concentrations of luteinizing hormone,[1,2] altered release of luteinizing hormone,[3,4] and alteration of pituitary response to gonadotrophin-releasing hormone have been described.[5,6] Seizure discharges can disrupt the hypothalamic-pituitary axis.[7] AEDs directly alter the neurochemical pathways of the hypothalamic-pituitary axis; moreover, AEDs affect the feedback mechanism of the gonadal steroid hormones.[8] AEDs that induce the cytochrome P-450 system of the liver increase gonadal steroid metabolism and increase binding to steroid hormones,[9] whereas AEDs that are enzyme inhibitors increase the concentration of steroid hormones.[10]

WWE have an increased frequency of menstrual irregularities, anovulatory cycles, luteal phase defi-

ciency, and polycystic ovaries.[8] Reduced fertility rates are noted after the onset of seizures in association with partial seizures and in those with seizure onset before puberty.[11] Anovulatory menstrual cycles occur in 30% of women with temporal lobe epilepsy.[12]

Duncan, Friedman, and Herzog discuss the nature and controversies of sexual dysfunction in WWE in Chapters 16 and 17. In brief, sexual dysfunction in WWE has been estimated to occur with a frequency of 14–50%.[13–16] The etiology of sexual dysfunction includes psychological and physiologic causes. Physiologic causes include epileptic discharges in the limbic structures of the brain, neuroendocrine disorders, and hormonal abnormalities induced by AEDs.[17]

An estimated 20,000 pregnancies in the United States occur in WWE.[18] Pregnancies in WWE are high risk because of seizures, increased maternal complications, and increased adverse outcomes in the newborn.

Risk of Seizures during Pregnancy

Approximately 25–50% of WWE have been reported to have a change in seizure frequency compared to their pregestational rate.[19–21] In a prospective study of 84 pregnant WWE, Cantrell et al. determined that 75% of patients had no change in their seizure frequency, 21% had an increase, and 4% had a decrease. Moreover, 62% of the patients remained seizure free. The patient's age, seizure type, number of prior pregnancies, and ethnicity did not influence seizure frequency.[21] Yerby documented that seizure type, seizure frequency in a previous pregnancy, and the duration of the seizure disorder do not correlate with seizure control.[18] An elevated seizure frequency before pregnancy is often associated with an increased frequency during pregnancy.[22,23] An increase in seizure frequency during pregnancy can be seen with increases in physical and psychological stress, sleep deprivation, and noncompliance with AEDs.[20,24,25] Cantrell et al. documented that seizure control can be obtained and maintained throughout pregnancy.[21] Seizure control should be achieved before pregnancy; preferably, WWE should be seizure free for at least 6–12 months before conception. Alterations or discontinuation of the AED regimen should occur before pregnancy, and complete seizure control should be achieved for at least 6 months before conception, after these changes have been made.

Bound and unbound serum AED concentrations decrease throughout pregnancy. Protein binding of AEDs decreases during pregnancy, resulting in an increased AED free fraction. Therefore, total serum levels of AEDs are less reliable during pregnancy. Because free levels represent the active portion of an AED, free concentration measurements are recommended in pregnancy.

Literature on the specific effect of seizures on the fetus is limited. Generalized tonic-clonic seizures can endanger the mother and the fetus owing to the risk of acidosis and hypoxia.[26] Maternal generalized tonic-clonic seizures have been associated with stillbirths,[27] fetal intraventricular hemorrhage,[28] and fetal bradycardia,[26,29] although specific incidence rates are unknown. The rate of stillbirths is significantly increased in WWE if seizures occur during the pregnancy.[30]

An acute change in fetal heart rhythm is a major indicator of fetal central nervous system dysfunction. Chronic prenatal exposure to AEDs does not appear to interfere with fetal heart rhythm.[31] However, there are documented observations of prolonged fetal heart rate deceleration occurring after a single brief generalized tonic-clonic seizure.[26,29] Yerby et al. suggest that the increased rate of neonatal hypoxia and low Apgar scores may be related to seizure occurrence during pregnancy.[32]

Ramus et al. reported a case of complex partial seizure with secondary generalization complicated by prolonged fetal bradycardia and the induction of forceful uterine contractions. They postulated that partial seizures during pregnancy endanger the fetus because of the risk of acidosis and hypoxia that result from prolonged fetal bradycardia induced by forceful uterine contractions. They also speculated that aberrant uterine contractions could account for the increased risk of miscarriage, stillbirths, and intraventricular hemorrhage occurring in pregnancies complicated by epilepsy.[33]

Teramo and Hiilesmaa reported 29 cases of status epilepticus during pregnancy, finding a 31% maternal mortality rate and a 48% infant mortality rate.[34] Therefore, pregnancy should not preclude aggressive treatment of seizure control during pregnancy.

Maternal Adverse Outcomes

WWE are at increased risk for complications during pregnancy and delivery. Bjerkedal and Bahana found a two- to threefold increase in the incidence of pregnancy-induced hypertension, cesarean delivery, and preterm delivery in WWE. They also described a 1.6-fold increase in hyperemesis gravidarum and a 1.7-fold increase in toxemia in WWE in comparison to controls.[35]

Wilhelm et al. compared outcomes in 98 pregnancies complicated by epilepsy with nonepileptic controls and found a 25% increase of seizures and an increased incidence of preeclampsia and preterm delivery.[36] In the Collaborative Perinatal Project and the Norwegian Birth Registry study, an increase in vaginal hemorrhage was noted.[35,37] A two- to threefold increase in abruptio placentae, a condition in which the placentae separates from the uterine wall, has been described.[38,39]

The need for labor induction, cesarean section, vacuum extraction, forceps, or artificial rupture of the membranes in epileptic women may be a complication of AED use.[35,39] Weak uterine contractions[40] and term breach presentation[41] have been noted with AED use.

Fetal and Neonatal Complications

Malformations and Anomalies

In 1963, Mullers-Kuppers was the first to report an association of fetal malformations with AEDs. He described mental retardation, microcephaly, intestinal malrotation, and cleft palate in a child who was exposed to mephenytoin in utero.[42] Although congenital malformations occur at a rate of 30 per 1,000 in the general population,[26] infants of WWE have a two- to threefold increase in the rate of fetal deformities.[36,42,43] Investigators have hypothesized that the increased incidence of malformations is secondary to genetic predisposition, exposure of the fetus to seizures, and in utero exposure to AEDs. However, the relative contribution of each factor is undetermined.

The following observations support the concept that malformations may be genetically linked to epilepsy: Dysmorphic features were noted in infants of epileptic mothers before the availability of AEDs[44,45]; no specific relationship has been noted between particular abnormalities and AEDs[43]; congenital malformations are more common in neonates of fathers with epilepsy[46–48]; and evidence supports a genetic predisposition to AED-induced malformations.[49,50]

Before the availability of AEDs, dysmorphic features were noted in infants of WWE.[44,45] WWE who have prior pregnancies with specific birth defects in association with a particular AED are at increased risk in subsequent pregnancies for these malformations to recur if they remain on the same AED.[51]

Janz and Hauser concluded that malformations did occur in infants of epileptic fathers and that they occurred at a rate somewhat less than that of epileptic mothers.[52,53] These observations preclude the correlation of in utero exposure to AEDs and fetal malformations.

The teratogenetic effects of certain AEDs may relate to genetic defects in the enzymatic pathways necessary for the metabolism of the AED intermediary metabolites.[49,50,54] In a prospective study of 19 pregnancies involving WWE on phenytoin monotherapy, four women had low epoxide hydrolase activity with phenytoin embryopathy apparent in their infants.[50] This suggests that epoxide hydrolase deficiencies may increase the risk of teratogenicity. Furthermore, it may be possible in the future to prenatally screen fetuses at increased risk for congenital malformations after AED exposure in utero.

Two Japanese investigations distinguished the teratogenic effect of seizure occurrence versus AEDs. A 1.1- to 1.4-fold increase in malformations occurred in infants exposed to seizures during gestation as compared to unexposed cases.[55,56] Similarly, Beck-Mannagetta et al. found a 1.2-fold increase in the malformation rate with in utero exposure to seizures.[47] Nelson et al.'s study of 54,000 pregnancies found a 2.4-fold greater risk of a low intellectual quotient (less than 70) in the offspring of mothers who experienced a seizure during pregnancy, when contrasted to those who had never had a seizure.[37] In contrast, Annegers et al. found no correlation between the occurrence of seizures during pregnancy and the risk of fetal malformations.[57]

Depending on the clinical circumstances, WWE can safely discontinue AEDs before pregnancy. All AEDs cross the placenta. In an analysis of 427 pregnancies in WWE, infants exposed to AEDs in utero had a twofold increase in congenital malformations. Infants exhibited no single anomaly but rather displayed a range of defects from dysmorphic facial features to major congenital malformations.[43] Growth retardation, mental subnormality, nail and digital hypoplasia, and craniofacial anomalies were reported in 1975 by Hanson and Smith, who referred to this constellation of findings as the *fetal hydantoin syndrome*.[58] However, since that time, various "syndromes" have been reported associated with fetal exposure to phenobarbital,[59] phenytoin,[58] carbamazepine,[60] valproic acid,[61] primidone,[62] and trimethadione.[63] Therefore, Yerby has suggested that these collections of anomalies be more appropriately termed the *fetal AED syndrome*.[18]

Although human teratogenetic effects have been documented for the standard AEDs, the teratogenetic potentials for the newly established AEDs are unknown. Therefore, if a new AED is appropriate for the seizure type, efficacious in seizure control, and well tolerated, then the same guidelines for the standard AEDs should be followed during pregnancy.[64,65]

Virtually all studies in the medical literature support an increase in fetal malformation rates after in utero AED exposure. However, there was no definitive link established between a specific AED and a particular abnormality until 1982. Bjerkedal et al. reported that infants of epileptic mothers exposed in utero to valproic acid to have a 20-fold increased risk of neural tube defects over the general population.[66] A risk of 1–2% of neural tube defects is documented for in utero exposure to valproic acid.[67] An increased risk of 0.5–1.0% for neural tube defects has been described with carbamazepine used in polytherapy.[68] Trimethadione has not been affiliated with any particular defect; however, its use during pregnancy has resulted in major malformations in up to 83% of fetuses, spontaneous abortions in 25% of the pregnancies, neonatal deaths primarily due to congenital heart defects in 35%, mental retardation, microcephaly, orofacial clefts, and a host of dysmorphic features.[69] For these reasons, trimethadione is unequivocally contraindicated in pregnancy.

The duration of AED therapy before pregnancy does not correlate with the occurrence of fetal malformations; however, the phase of gestation in which the fetus is exposed to AEDs may augment the occurrence of malformations.[70] The offspring of WWE who received AEDs during the first trimester have an increased risk of congenital malformations compared to those exposed to AEDs after the first trimester. In one study,[57] the group of offspring exposed to AEDs after the first trimester had a comparable rate of congenital malformations as offspring in the general population.[70]

Malformations are more prevalent in infants whose mothers were maintained on high serum concentrations of AEDs.[67,71] Polytherapy increases the risk of malformations.[55,56,72] Hauser and Hesdorffer's analysis of four studies[55,56,72,73] demonstrated that pregnant WWE maintained on four AEDs were 1.6–4.2 times more likely to produce an infant with malformations, compared to the offspring of those receiving only two AEDs.[53] Tanganelli et al. observed a two- to fourfold increase in congenital malformations for women who had received two or more AEDs, irrespective of plasma drug levels, during pregnancy.[74] In a study of 902 pregnancies, the percentage of infants presenting with malformations was 1.9% if the pregnant mother received no AEDs during pregnancy, 5.5% if two AEDs, 11% if three, and 23% if four.[55,56]

Specific AED combinations augment the risk of fetal malformations. An elevated teratogenic risk has been noted with the combination of phenobarbital, phenytoin, and primidone.[75] Exposure to a combination of carbamazepine, phenobarbital, and valproate, with or without phenytoin, has been associated with malformations in 58% of the infants.[75]

Several mechanisms have been proposed to explain AED-related teratogenicity. AEDs have antifolate effects by intestinal malabsorption, hepatic enzyme induction, increased urinary excretion, and impedance of folate at the enzymatic level.[76–78] Decreased preconceptual serum folate levels in WWE have been affiliated with an increase in fetal malformations and spontaneous abortions.[79] Preconceptual folate supplementation decreased the rate of malformations in offspring of mothers who received AEDs in human and animal studies.[79–81] A prospective trial suggested that folic acid supplementation of 4 mg per day in women with a prior history of offspring with neural tube defects lowered the risk of neural tube defects in subsequent offspring.[82] The United States Public Health Service recommends that all women of childbearing potential receive 0.4 mg per day of folic acid to reduce the risk of neural tube defects.[83] Therefore, the exact dosage of folate that WWE should receive is unknown.

The obligatory intermediates of AED metabolism have also been postulated to induce teratogenicity. AED metabolism through the microsomal monooxygenase system produces arene oxides or epoxides. These epoxides are detoxified by epoxide hydrolase in the cytoplasm and by conjugation with glutathione in the microsome.[84] The fetus produces arene oxides when exposed to AEDs,[85] and epoxide hydrolase activity is decreased in the fetus.[86] The highest levels of epoxides are created with AED polytherapy.[72] Decreased epoxide hydrolase activity is associated with congenital malformations and may have a genetic predisposition.[49,50]

AEDs produce free radicals that covalently bind to macromolecules.[84] Agents that lower the concentration of free radicals can reduce the risk of malformation.[87] Glutathione is thought to detoxify free radicals. The free radicals produced by the metabolism of AEDs may be an important contributor to teratogenicity.[84]

Other contemplated mechanisms of AED teratogenicity include the alternations of intracellular pH of weak acids, such as valproic acid[88]; disruption of lipid metabolism[88]; modification of zinc levels[89]; and increased concentration of fetal glucocorticoid receptors.[90]

Mortality

The rate of spontaneous abortion in WWE is comparable to rates in the general female population; however, the rate of spontaneous abortion in WWE receiving an AED is twice that of WWE off

AEDs.[91,92] Stillbirths are 2–3 times more common in WWE than in offspring from women in the general population.[37,93] Finell's literature review noted that perinatal death rates range from 1.3% to 7.8% in neonates of WWE compared to 1.0–3.9% for controls.[70]

Neonatal Hemorrhage

There may be up to a 10–30% risk of significant hemorrhage of the intracranial, intrathoracic, or intra-abdominal cavities within the first 24 hours of life in infants with in utero AED exposure. The mortality rate after hemorrhage exceeds 30%.[18] Hemorrhage is a consequence of a deficiency of vitamin K–dependent factors II, VII, IX, and X usually associated with the maternal use of phenobarbital, primidone, phenytoin, carbamazepine, diazepam, mephobarbital, amobarbital, ethosuximide, and trimethadione.[94,95] Affected infants demonstrate prolonged prothrombin and partial thromboplastin times and decreased vitamin K–dependent clotting factors, whereas the maternal clotting factors remain normal.[96–99] A precursor of prothrombin has been located in the serum of mothers receiving AEDs; therefore, prenatal screening may be available in the future.[8,100]

Prophylaxis can be achieved by the administration of 10–20 mg per day of vitamin K_1 (phytonadione) in the final month of pregnancy.[98] Umbilical cord values of the prothrombin and partial thromboplastin time should be obtained. The newborn should receive 1 mg of vitamin K_1 intramuscularly or intravenously at birth.[96,101] If a hemorrhage occurs, the only alternative is to administer intravenous fresh-frozen plasma.[96,98,101]

Neonatal Feeding Difficulties

Five to ten percent of infants with a history of intrauterine exposure to AEDs have listlessness, sedation, and nursing difficulties. This occurs more often after exposure to phenobarbital, primidone, and phenytoin.[97,102]

All AEDs enter breast milk. AEDs with a lower protein binding have a higher concentration in breast milk. Therefore, phenobarbital, primidone, ethosuximide, and diazepam reach high concentra-

tions in breast milk. Most mothers receiving AEDs can successfully breast-feed and should be encouraged to do so. Formula should be substituted if the newborn becomes sedated or continues to lose weight.

Neonatal Drug Withdrawal

Evidence of drug withdrawal has been observed in 20–65% of newborns exposed to AEDs during pregnancy.[103] Symptoms usually occur within the first 72 hours of life and may include hyperexcitability, tremors, seizures, vomiting, poor nursing, excessive crying, hyperactivity, sleep disturbance, myoclonic jerks, hypertonia, hyperreflexia, and hyperventilation.[97,104]

Management

WWE who desire to have children have increased risk of maternal and fetal complications. Their care necessitates a comprehensive approach and open communication between the patient and the patient's primary care physician. A proposed management scheme is contained in Figure 18-1.

Preconceptual Management

WWE require education on the increased risks that can occur and the management strategies that decrease the risk of adversities during pregnancy.

A 25-fold increased risk of contraceptive failure and breakthrough bleeding is associated with the co-administration of oral contraceptives and AEDs.[105] This increased risk is seen with the concomitant use of phenobarbital, primidone, phenytoin, carbamazepine, oxcarbazepine, and topiramate and an oral contraceptive. These AEDs induce the hepatic P-450 microsomal enzyme system of the liver, which, in turn, increases the metabolism of the estrogen fraction of the oral contraceptive. Alternative contraceptive methods should be proposed to women at risk for these drug interactions. The use of oral contraceptives is not associated with exacerbation of seizures.

Verification of the diagnosis of epilepsy and optimization of AED therapy for seizure control

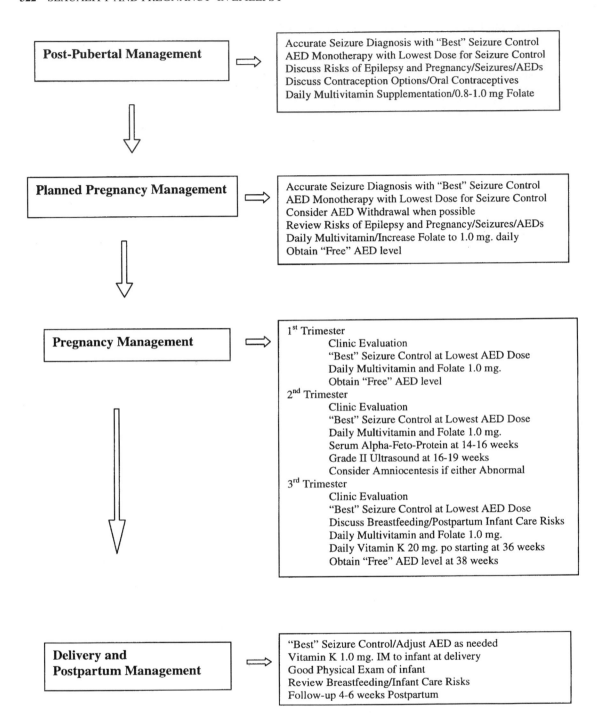

Post-Pubertal Management

Accurate Seizure Diagnosis with "Best" Seizure Control
AED Monotherapy with Lowest Dose for Seizure Control
Discuss Risks of Epilepsy and Pregnancy/Seizures/AEDs
Discuss Contraception Options/Oral Contraceptives
Daily Multivitamin Supplementation/0.8-1.0 mg Folate

Planned Pregnancy Management

Accurate Seizure Diagnosis with "Best" Seizure Control
AED Monotherapy with Lowest Dose for Seizure Control
Consider AED Withdrawal when possible
Review Risks of Epilepsy and Pregnancy/Seizures/AEDs
Daily Multivitamin/Increase Folate to 1.0 mg. daily
Obtain "Free" AED level

Pregnancy Management

1st Trimester
    Clinic Evaluation
    "Best" Seizure Control at Lowest AED Dose
    Daily Multivitamin and Folate 1.0 mg.
    Obtain "Free" AED level
2nd Trimester
    Clinic Evaluation
    "Best" Seizure Control at Lowest AED Dose
    Daily Multivitamin and Folate 1.0 mg.
    Serum Alpha-Feto-Protein at 14-16 weeks
    Grade II Ultrasound at 16-19 weeks
    Consider Amniocentesis if either Abnormal
3rd Trimester
    Clinic Evaluation
    "Best" Seizure Control at Lowest AED Dose
    Discuss Breastfeeding/Postpartum Infant Care Risks
    Daily Multivitamin and Folate 1.0 mg.
    Daily Vitamin K 20 mg. po starting at 36 weeks
    Obtain "Free" AED level at 38 weeks

Delivery and Postpartum Management

"Best" Seizure Control/Adjust AED as needed
Vitamin K 1.0 mg. IM to infant at delivery
Good Physical Exam of infant
Review Breastfeeding/Infant Care Risks
Follow-up 4-6 weeks Postpartum

Figure 18-1. Proposed management scheme for women with epilepsy. (AED = antiepileptic drug.)

should occur preconceptually. *The AED of choice is the one that is appropriate for the seizure type and provides seizure control without producing toxicity.* AEDs should be used in monotherapy and at the lowest possible dose for seizure control. Sei-

zure frequency should be followed closely. Administration of multivitamins and 1 mg of folic acid per day should commence at least 1 month before conception. If the woman has a family history of neural tube defects or a previous pregnancy complicated by a neural tube defect, then 4 mg of folic acid should be prescribed. Patients who have been seizure free for at least 2 years warrant consideration for AED discontinuation before attempting to conceive. Conception should be avoided during the first 6 months to 1 year after AED withdrawal to permit observation for potential seizure recurrence.

Prenatal Management

Major malformations occur within the first few weeks of pregnancy. Seizures during pregnancy can have deleterious effects on the maternal and fetal health. Therefore, cessation or changes in AED regimen should not be altered postconception unless clinically indicated secondary to poor seizure control or toxicity.[106] Low-dose monotherapy is favored during the period of organogenesis. Free AED levels should be obtained as a baseline before pregnancy, during the first trimester, 1–2 weeks before the delivery date, and when clinically indicated. The management of seizures during pregnancy should be a coordinated effort between the patient's neurologist and primary care physician. If a seizure occurs during pregnancy, the etiology for its occurrence should be pursued. The possibilities of noncompliance, sleep deprivation, increased stress, hyperemesis gravidum, pre-eclampsia, and concurrent infection should be considered. Increasing the AED dose or instituting an additional AED should be based on clinical necessity.

All women taking AEDs, especially valproic acid or carbamazepine in polytherapy, should undergo testing of the serum alpha-fetoprotein level at 14 weeks' gestation and a grade II abdominal ultrasound between 16 and 19 weeks of gestation. If either test is abnormal, amniocentesis should be suggested.

Adequate nutrition, multivitamin supplementation, and 1–4 mg of folic acid should be ensured each day. The expectant WWE should alert the labor and delivery staff to the following details: the diagnosis of epilepsy, the seizure type, the AED regimen, the timing of her usual AED dose, the time of the last AED dose, and any AED allergies.

The mother should receive safety guidelines for infant care that may help to avoid neonatal injuries during maternal seizures. Infant feedings should be performed in a sitting position on a padded exercise mat. Clothing or diaper changes should be performed in the same manner or, alternatively, on an infant changing table with the use of a safety belt.

During maternal ambulation with the infant, a stroller should be used. Bathing of the infant should occur in the presence of or with the knowledge of another adult. Infant bathing devices should provide elevation of the upper torso and head and a safety strap. The infant should be placed in a playpen, infant car seat, or highchair during maternal activities such as cooking.

Postpartum Management

In the postpartum period, the metabolic rate and protein levels return to pregestational status. If the AED dose is increased during pregnancy, the patient's clinical status and AED levels should be closely monitored to avoid toxicity during the first 6 weeks postpartum. In such cases, the AED requirements may drop substantially. The mother must be cautioned to avoid sleep deprivation and to seek assistance with the care of the newborn to circumvent seizure exacerbation. Breast-feeding should be encouraged. Infant care safety guidelines should continue to be emphasized.

At birth, umbilical cord levels should be obtained for prothrombin and partial thromboplastin times. The newborn should receive 1 mg of vitamin K within the first 24 hours. A detailed general physical examination should be performed, looking specifically for congenital malformations.

Conclusion

Although WWE and their progeny are at greater risk for adverse outcomes, 90% of WWE have uncomplicated pregnancies and give birth to healthy neonates. Further research and coordination of care between the patient's neurologist and primary care physician can achieve better outcomes for WWE and their children.

References

1. Gallagher BB, Marvin A, Flanigin HF, et al. Pituitary and adrenal function in epileptic patients. Epilepsia 1984;25:683–689.
2. Bonucelli U, Murialdo G, Rossi G, et al. Prolactin secretion in epileptic subjects treated with phenobarbital: sex differences and circadian periodicity. Epilepsia 1986;27:142–148.

3. Herzog AG. Reproductive endocrine considerations and hormonal therapy for women with epilepsy. Epilepsia 1991;32[Suppl 6]:S527–S533.
4. Drislane FW, Coleman AE, Scomer DL, et al. Altered pulsatile secretion of luteinizing hormone in woman with epilepsy. Neurology 1994;44:306–310.
5. Meo R, Bilo L, Nappi C, et al. Derangement of the hypothalamic GnRH pulse generator in women with epilepsy. Seizure 1993;2:241–252.
6. Dana-Haeri J, Okley J, Richens A. Pituitary responsiveness to gonadotrophin-releasing and thyrotrophin-releasing hormones in epileptic patients receiving carbamazepine or phenytoin. Clin Endocrinol (Oxf) 1984;20:163–168.
7. Morrell MJ. Effects of epilepsy on women's reproductive health. Epilepsia 1998;39[Suppl 8]:32–37.
8. Mattson RH, Cramer JA. Epilepsy, sex hormones, and antiepileptic drugs. Epilepsia 1985;26:S40–S51.
9. Dana-Haeri J, Trimble MR, Oxley J. Prolactin and gonadotrophin changes following generalized and partial seizures. J Neurol Neurosurg Psychiatry 1983;46:331–335.
10. Isojarvi JI, Laatikainen TJ, Pakarinen AJ, et al. Polycystic ovaries and hyperandrogenism in women taking valproate for epilepsy. N Engl J Med 1993;329:1383–1388.
11. Schupf N, Ottman R. Reproduction among individuals with idiopathic/cryptogenic epilepsy: risk factors for reduced fertility in marriage. Epilepsia 1996;37:833–840.
12. Cummings LN, Giudice L, Morrell MJ. Ovulatory function in epilepsy. Epilepsia 1995;36:355–359.
13. Taylor DC. Sexual behavior and temporal lobe epilepsy. Arch Neurol 1969;21:510–516.
14. Blumer D, Walker AE. Sexual behavior in temporal lobe epilepsy. Arch Neurol 1967;16:37–43.
15. Jensen P, Jensen SB, Sorensen PS, et al. Sexual dysfunction in male and female patients with epilepsy: a study of 86 outpatients. Arch Sex Behav 1990;19:1–14.
16. Morrell MJ, Guldner GT. Self-reported sexual function and sexual arousability in women with epilepsy. Epilepsia 1996;37:1204–1210.
17. Morrell MJ. Seizures and Epilepsy in Women. In PW Kaplan (ed), Neurologic Disease in Women. New York: Demos Publications, 1988:198.
18. Yerby MS. Pregnancy and epilepsy. Epilepsia 1991;32[Suppl 6]:51–59.
19. Bardy AH. Seizure Frequency in Epileptic Women during Pregnancy and Puerperium: Results of the Prospective Helsinki Study. In D Janz et al. (eds), Epilepsy, Pregnancy and the Child. New York: Raven Press, 1982:27–31.
20. Schmidt D, Canger R, Avanzini G, et al. Change of seizure frequency in pregnancy epileptic women. J Neurol Neurosurg Psychiatry 1983;46:751–755.
21. Cantrell DC, Riela SJ, Ramus R, Riela AR. Epilepsy and pregnancy: a study of seizure frequency and patient demographics. Epilepsia 1997;38[Suppl 8]:231.
22. Knight AH, Rhind EG. Epilepsy and pregnancy: a study of 153 pregnancies in 59 patients. Epilepsia 1975;6:99–110.
23. Remillard G, Dansky L, Andermann E, Andermann F. Seizure Frequency during Pregnancy and the Puerperium. In D Janz et al. (eds), Epilepsy, Pregnancy, and the Child. New York: Raven Press, 1982;15–26.
24. Schmidt D. The Effect of Pregnancy on the Natural History of Epilepsy: Review of the Literature. In D Janz et al. (eds), Epilepsy, Pregnancy, and the Child. New York: Raven Press, 1982;3–14.
25. Otani K. Risk factors for the increased seizure frequency during pregnancy and puerperium. Folia Psychiatr Neurol Jpn 1985;39:33–42.
26. Yerby MS. Problems and management of the pregnant woman with epilepsy. Epilepsia 1987;28[Suppl 3]:29–36.
27. Higgins TA, Comerford JB. Epilepsy in Pregnancy. J Ir Med Assoc 1974;67:317–329.
28. Minkoff H, Schaffer RM, Delke L, et al. Diagnosis of intracranial hemorrhage in utero after a maternal seizure. Obstet Gynecol 1985;65:S22–S24.
29. Teramo K, Hiilesmaa V, Bardy A, et al. Fetal heart rate during a maternal grand mal epileptic seizure. J Perinat Med 1979;7:3–6.
30. Nelson KB, Ellenberg JH. Maternal seizure disorder, outcome of pregnancy, and neurologic abnormalities in children. Neurology 1982;32:1247–1254.
31. Swartjes JM, Van Geijn HP, Meinardi H, Mantel R. Fetal heart rate patterns and chronic exposure to antiepileptic drugs. Epilepsia 1992;3:721–728.
32. Yerby MS, Koepsell T, Faling J. Pregnancy complications and outcomes in a cohort of women with epilepsy. Epilepsia 1985;2:631–635.
33. Ramos RM, Cantrell DC, Cunningham FG, et al. Effects of partial seizures on the infants of women with epilepsy. Epilepsia 1997;38[Suppl 8]:230.
34. Teramo K, Hiilesmaa VK. Pregnancy and Fetal Complications in Epileptic Pregnancies: Review of the Literature. In D Janz et al. (eds), Epilepsy, Pregnancy, and the Child. New York: Raven Press, 1982;53–59.
35. Bherkdal T, Bahna SL. The course and outcome of pregnancy in women with epilepsy. Acta Obstet Gynecol Scand 1973;52:245–248.
36. Wilhelm J, Morris D, Hotham N. Epilepsy and pregnancy—a review of 98 pregnancies. Aust N Z J Obstet Gynaecol 1990;30–34:290–295.
37. Nelson KB, Ellenberg JH. Maternal seizure disorder, outcome of pregnancy, and neurologic abnormalities in the children. Neurology 1982;32:1247–1254.
38. Monson RR, Rosenberg L, Hartz SC. Diphenylhydantoin and selected congenital malformations. N Engl J Med 1973;289:1049–1052.
39. Egenaes J. Outcome of Pregnancy in Women with Epilepsy—Norway 1967–1978: Complications during Pregnancy and Delivery. In D Janz et al. (eds), Epi-

lepsy, Pregnancy, and the Child. New York: Raven Press, 1982;81–85.

40. Janz D, Fuchs V. Are antiepileptic drugs harmful when given during pregnancy? Ger Med Mon 1964;9:20–22.

41. Robertson IG. Breech presentation associated with anticonvulsant drugs. J Obstet Gynecol 1982;4:174–177.

42. Von Mullers-Kuppers M. Embryopathy during pregnancy caused by taking anticonvulsant. Acta Paedopsychiatr 1964;30:401–405.

43. Speidel BD, Meadow SR. Maternal epilepsy and abnormalities of the fetus and newborn. Lancet 1972;2:839–843.

44. Baptisti A. Epilepsy and pregnancy. Am J Obstet Gynecol 1928;35:818–824.

45. Philbert A, Dam M. The epileptic mother and her child. Epilepsia 1982;23:85–99.

46. Shapiro S, Hartz SC, Siskind V, et al. Anticonvulsant and parental epilepsy in the development of birth defects. Lancet 1976;1:272–275.

47. Beck-Mannagetta, Drees B, Janz D. Malformation and Minor Anomalies in the Offspring of Epileptic Parents: a Retrospective Study. In D Janz et al. (eds), Epilepsy, Pregnancy and the Child. New York: Raven Press, 1982;317–323.

48. LinKoch S, et al. Major Malformations in Children of Epileptic Parents—Due to Epilepsy or Its Therapy? In D Janz et al. (eds), Epilepsy, Pregnancy and the Child. New York: Raven Press, 1982;313–315.

49. Strickler SM, Dansky LV, Miller RN, et al. Genetic predisposition of phenytoin induced birth defects. Lancet 1985;1:746–749.

50. Buehler VA, Dalimont D, Van Waes M, Finnell RH. Prenatal prediction of the fetal hydantoin syndrome. N Engl J Med 1990;332:567–572.

51. Lindhout D, Omtzigt JG. Pregnancy and the risk of teratogenicity. Epilepsia 1922;33[Suppl 4]:41–48.

52. Janz D. On Major Malformations and Minor Anomalies in the Offspring of Parents with Epilepsy: Review of the Literature. In D Janz et al. (eds), Epilepsy, Pregnancy, and the Child. New York: Raven Press, 1982;211–223.

53. Hauser WA, Hesdorffer DC. Epilepsy, Frequency, Causes, and Consequences. New York: Demos Publications, 1990.

54. Bustamante SA, Stumpff LC. Fetal hydantoin syndrome in triplets: a unique experiment of nature. Am J Dis Child 1978;132:978–979.

55. Nakane T, Okuma T, Takahashi R, et al. Multi-institutional study on the teratogenicity and fetal toxicity of antiepileptic drugs: a report of a collaborative study group in Japan. Epilepsia 1980;21:663–680.

56. Okuma T, Takahashi R, Wade T, et al. A Collaborative Study of the Teratogenicity and Fetal Toxicity of Antiepileptic Drugs in Japan. In JA Wada and JK Penry (eds), Advances in Epileptology: The Xth Epilepsy International Symposium. New York: Raven Press, 1980;511–517.

57. Annergers JF, Hauser WA, Elveback LR, et al. Congenital malformations and seizure disorders in the offspring of parents with epilepsy. Int J Epidemiol 1978;7:241–247.

58. Hanson JW, Smith DW. The fetal hydantoin syndrome. J Pediatr 1995;87:285–290.

59. Seip M. Growth retardation, dysmorphic facies, and minor malformations following massive exposure to phenobarbital in utero. Acta Paediatr Scand 1976;65:617–621.

60. Jones KL, Lacro RV, Johnson KA, Adams J. Pattern of malformations in the children of women treated with carbamazepine during pregnancy. N Engl J Med 1989;320:1661–1666.

61. DiLiberti JH, Farndon PA, Dennis NR, Curry DJR. The fetal valproate syndrome. Am J Med Genet 1984;19:473–481.

62. Rudd NL, Freedom RM. A possible primidone embryopathy. J Pediatr 1979;94:835–837.

63. Zackai EH, Mellman WJ, Neiderer B, Hanson JW. The fetal trimethadione syndrome. J Pediatr 1975;87:280–284.

64. Delgado-Escueta AV, Janz D. Consensus guidelines: preconceptual counseling, management, and care of pregnant women with epilepsy. Neurology 1992;42:149–160.

65. Guidelines for the Care of Women of Childbearing Age with Epilepsy. Commission on Genetics, Pregnancy, and the Child, International League Against Epilepsy. Epilepsia 1993;34:588–589.

66. Bjerkedal T, Czeizel A, Goujard J, et al. Valproic acid and spina bifida. Lancet 1982;2:1096.

67. Omtzigt JG, Los FJ, Grobbee DE, et al. The risk of spina bifida aperta after first trimester valproate exposure in a prenatal cohort. Neurology 1991;42[Suppl 5]:119–125.

68. Rosa FW. Spina bifida in infants of women treated with carbamazepine during pregnancy. N Engl J Med 1991;324:674–677.

69. Feldman GL, Weaver DD, Lovrien EW. The fetal trimethadione syndrome: report of an additional family and further delineation of this syndrome. Am J Dis Child 1977;131:1389–1392.

70. Finnell RH, Nau H, Yerby MS. Teratogenicity of Antiepileptic Drugs. In RH Levy, RH Mattson, BS Meldrum (eds), Antiepileptic Drugs (4th ed). New York: Raven Press, 1995;209–229.

71. Dansky LV, Andermann E, Sherwin AL, et al. Maternal epilepsy and congenital malformations: a prospective study with monitoring of plasma anticonvulsant levels during pregnancy. Neurology 1980;3:15.

72. Lindhout D, Rene JE, Hoppener A, Meinardi H. Teratogenicity of antiepileptic drug combinations with special emphasis on epoxidation (of carbamazepine). Epilepsia 1984;25:77–83.

73. Kaneko S, Otani K, Fukushima Y, et al. Teratogenicity of antiepileptic drugs: analysis of possible risk factors. Epilepsia 1988;29:459–467.

74. Tanganelli P, Regesta G. Epilepsy, pregnancy, and major birth anomalies: an Italian prospective, controlled study. Neurology 1992;42[Suppl 5]:89–93.

75. Dansky LV. Outcome of Pregnancy in Epileptic Woman: A Prospective Evaluation of Genetic and Environmental Risk Factors [Ph.D. Thesis]. Montreal: McGill University, 1989.

76. Maxwell JD, Hunter J, Stewart DA, et al. Folate deficiency after anticonvulsant drugs: an effect of hepatic enzyme induction. BMJ 1972;1:297–299.

77. Janz D. Antiepileptic drugs and pregnancy: altered utilization patterns and teratogenesis. Epilepsia 1982;23[Suppl 1]:S53–S63.

78. Dansky LV, Rosenblatt DS, Andermann E. Mechanisms of teratogenesis: folic acid and antiepileptic therapy. Neurology 1992;42[Suppl 5]:32–42.

79. Dansky LV, Andermann E, Rosenblatt D, et al. Anticonvulsant, folate levels, and pregnancy outcome: a prospective study. Ann Neurol 1987;21:176–182.

80. Biale Y, Lewenthal H. Effect of folic acid supplementation on congenital malformations due to anticonvulsant drugs. Eur J Obstet Gynecol Reprod Biol 1984;18:211–216.

81. Zhu MX, Zhou SS. Reduction of the teratogenic effects of phenytoin of folic acid and a mixture of folic acid, vitamins, amino acids: a preliminary trial. Epilepsia 1989;30:246–251.

82. Prevention of neural tube defects: results of the Medical Research Council Vitamin Study. MRC Vitamin Study Research Group (Nicolas Wald). Lancet 1991;338:131–137.

83. Recommendations for the use of folic acid to reduce the number of cases of spina bifida and other neural tube defects. MMWR Morb Mortal Wkly Rep 1992;41:1–7.

84. Yerby MS. Pregnancy and Teratogenesis. In MR Trimble (ed), Women and Epilepsy. New York: Wiley, 1991;163–191.

85. Horning MG, Stratton C, Wilson A, et al. Detection of 5-(3-4)-diphenylhydantoin in the newborn human. Anal Lett 1974;4:537–82.

86. Pacifici GM, Colizzi C, Giuliani L, Rane A. Cytosolic epoxide hydrolase in fetal and adult human liver. Arch Toxicol 1983;54:331–341.

87. Wells PG, Zubovits JT, Wong ST, et al. Modulation of phenytoin teratogenicity and embryonic covalent binding by acetylsalicylic acid, caffeic acid and alpha-phenyl-N-E-butylinitrone: implications for bioactivation by prostaglandin synthetase. Toxicol Appl Pharmacol 1983;97:192–202.

88. Nau H, Scott WJ. Weak acids may act as teratogens by accumulating in the basic milieu of the early mammalian embryo. Nature 1986;323:276–278.

89. Lindhout D. Commission reviews teratogenesis and genetics in epilepsy. World Neurol 1989;4:3–7.

90. Goldman AS, Van Dyke DC, Gupta C, Katsumata M. Elevated glucocorticoid receptor levels in lymphocytes in children with the fetal hydantoin syndrome. Am J Med Genet 1987;28:607–618.

91. Andermann E, Dansky L, Kinch RA. Complications of Pregnancy, Labor, and Delivery in Epileptic Women. In D Janz, M Dam, A Richens et al. (eds), Epilepsy, Pregnancy, and the Child. New York: Raven Press, 1982;61–74.

92. Dansky LV, Andermann E, Andermann F, et al. Maternal Epilepsy and Congenital Malformations: Correlation with Maternal Plasma Anticonvulsant Levels during Pregnancy. In D Janz, M Dam, A Richens et al. (eds), Epilepsy, Pregnancy and the Child, New York: Raven Press, 1982;251–258.

93. Fedrick J. Epilepsy and pregnancy: a report from the Oxford record linkage study. BMJ 1973;2:442–448.

94. Mountain KR, Hirsh J, Gallus AS. Neonatal coagulation defect due to anticonvulsant drug treatment in pregnancy. Lancet 1970;1:265–268.

95. Montouris GD, Fenichel GM, Mclain LW. The pregnant epileptic: a review and recommendations. Arch Neurol 1979;36:601–603.

96. Bleyer WA, Skinner AL. Fetal neonatal hemorrhage after maternal anticonvulsant therapy. JAMA 1976;235:626.

97. Bossi L. Neonatal Period Including Drug Disposition in Newborns: Review of the Literature. In D Janz et al. (eds), Epilepsy, Pregnancy, and the Child. New York: Raven Press, 1982;327–341.

98. Deblay MF, Vert P, Andre M, et al. Transplacental vitamin K prevents hemorrhagic disease of infants of epileptic mothers. Lancet 1982;1:1247.

99. Argent AC, Rothberg AD, Pienaar N. Precursor prothrombin status in the mother-infant pairs following gestational anticonvulsant therapy. Pediatr Pharmacol 1983;4:183–187.

100. Davies VA, Argent AC, Staub H. Precursor prothrombin status in patients receiving anticonvulsant drugs. Lancet 1985;1:126–128.

101. Srinivasan G, Seeler RA, Tiruvury A, et al. Maternal anticonvulsant therapy and hemorrhagic disease of the newborn. Obstet Gynecol 1982;59:250–252.

102. Svigos JM. Epilepsy and pregnancy. Aust N Z J Obstet Gynaecol 1984;24:182–185.

103. Krumholz A. Pregnancy. In PJ Goldstein, BJ Stern (eds), Neurological Disorders of Pregnancy (2nd rev ed). Mount Kisco, NY: Futura Publishing, 1992;25–50.

104. Hill RM, Verniaud WM, Horning MG, et al. Infants exposed in utero to antiepileptic drugs: a prospective study. Am J Dis Child 1974;127:645–653.

105. Ramsay RE, Slater JD. Effects of antiepileptic drugs on hormones. Epilepsia 1991;32[Suppl 6]:S60–S67.

106. Morrell MJ. Guidelines for the care of women with epilepsy. Neurology 1998;51[Suppl 4]:21–27.

Section D

Psychiatric and Behavioral Issues

Chapter 19

Nonepileptic Psychogenic Spells: A Neurologist's Perspective

Susan M. Palac and Andres M. Kanner

Pseudoseizures or nonepileptic seizures (NESs) are paroxysmal events that mimic (or are confused with) epileptic seizures but do not result from epileptic activity. NESs can be the expression of organic or psychogenic processes. The type of organic disorders often confused with epileptic seizures include convulsive syncope,[1] various forms of sleep disorders (e.g., the automatic behavior displayed during episodes of excessive daytime somnolence in obstructive sleep apnea), parasomnias (e.g., sleepwalking, rapid eye movement sleep behavior disorder, and night terrors),[2] and cataplectic or sleep paralysis episodes of narcolepsy.[3] Other forms of organic NESs include complicated migraines and certain types of movement disorders.[4] A detailed discussion of organic pseudoseizures can be found in Chapter 1 of this book. NESs resulting from a psychogenic process are the most frequent types of nonepileptic paroxysmal events and are the focus of this chapter.

NESs caused by psychogenic processes have been labeled with various eponyms over the last two centuries; in the nineteenth century, Charcot referred to these attacks as *hysteroepilepsy*.[5] His treatment recommendations included ovarian compressors and were based largely on the theory of the ancient Greeks that such attacks were due to the "wandering of the uterus throughout the body, away from its normal location in the pelvis." More recent terms have included *NESs, psychogenic seizures*, and *hysterical seizures*. We avoid using the term *seizure*, as many patients are unable to discriminate between the concepts of "psychogenic" versus "epileptic" processes and get fixated on the word "seizure." Instead, we use the term *spells*, and we refer to these nonepileptic events as *nonepileptic psychogenic spells* (NEPSs). This term helps to differentiate the nonepileptic nature of these attacks from epileptic seizures and conveys their probable psychogenic cause.

The incidence of NEPSs ranges from 10% to 40% among patients referred to epilepsy centers for the evaluation of poorly controlled seizures.[5-8] Sigurdardottir and Olafsson found the population-based incidence of NEPSs to be 1.4 per 100,000 in Iceland compared to an incidence of 35 per 100,000 for true epilepsy among persons older than 15 years of age.[9] NEPSs are much more common in women than men; 60–75% of patients are women in most series.[5-12] The onset of NEPSs most often occurs in the third and fourth decades of life,[5,11,13,14] although they have been described in children and the elderly.[10,15-18]

Several comprehensive review articles on the diagnosis of NEPS have been published since the advent of video-electroencephalogram (V-EEG).[5-8,19,20] Undoubtedly, such literature has increased awareness of NEPSs among clinicians, resulting in fewer patients with NEPSs that are misdiagnosed as epilepsy. However, studies have demonstrated that clinical phenomena associated with NEPSs can occur in certain types of epileptic seizures. This fact is still under-recognized by many clinicians and may lead to an inverse diagnostic problem (i.e., patients with epilepsy being falsely diagnosed with NEPSs). In this chapter, we focus on this specific problem. We also review two other issues that are relevant to neurologists evaluating patients with NEPSs: (1) predictors of NEPSs outcome and (2) presentation of an NEPS diagnosis.

Diagnostic Limitations of Clinical Phenomena in Nonepileptic Psychogenic Spells

In an early study using V-EEG, King et al.[8] found that referring physicians were able to correctly predict the diagnosis of NEPSs in only 50% of cases. As stated previously, since King's study was published, physicians have become more familiar with NEPSs. Yet there is evidence of an inappropriate overuse of the diagnosis of NEPSs. A number of patients that are given this diagnosis on the sole basis of clinical phenomena are later found to experience either epileptic seizures or organic NESs. For example, Parra et al.[21] studied 100 consecutive patients who were undergoing diagnostic V-EEG. Referring physicians correctly suspected a diagnosis of epileptic seizures in only 9 (43%) of 21 patients, whereas 12 (57%) patients were incorrectly thought to have NEPSs. This misdiagnosis was especially likely in patients with clinical seizures of mesial frontal or parietal lobe origin. To confuse matters further, there are a significant number of patients who experience epileptic seizures and NEPSs. The reported incidence of their coexistence varies from 7% to 37%, with most studies reporting an incidence of approximately 10–20%.[10,12,14,21–25]

A misdiagnosis of NEPSs as epileptic seizures and vice versa exposes patients to ineffective, costly, and potentially dangerous treatments. Various studies have reported that 69–78% of NEPS patients have been treated with antiepileptic drugs (AEDs),[14,26] all of which have the potential for serious side effects. Approximately 10% of patients with NEPSs have been misdiagnosed at some point with status epilepticus and treated accordingly, resulting in the administration of multiple unnecessary parenteral medications, which has caused respiratory arrest in some cases.[10,14,26–28]

In the pursuit of diagnostic accuracy, many investigators have attempted to identify clinical phenomena that may help to differentiate NEPSs from epileptic seizures.[8,10–14,29] The clinical semi-

ology of NEPSs is quite diverse and can vary from spells with intense motor activity, mimicking generalized tonic-clonic seizures, to nonconvulsive episodes consisting of motionless staring and unresponsiveness. The suspicion of a diagnosis of NEPSs is easier in convulsivelike events. The diagnosis of nonconvulsive NEPSs, on the other hand, may be impossible without concurrent electrographic recordings. In the next section, we review the reliability of clinical phenomena in the diagnosis of NEPSs.

Are Nonepileptic Psychogenic Spells Nonstereotypic?

For a long time, we have thought of NEPSs as events with nonstereotypic semiology (within patients), whereas the reverse was used as a clinical sign supportive of a diagnosis of epileptic seizures. Yet the clinical semiology of NEPSs, much like epileptic seizures, can often be stereotypic in individual patients. In four separate studies, 60–90% of patients with NEPSs had spells that varied little from event to event.[10,12,13,29] However, even when clinical features and their sequence are relatively stereotypic, the duration of seizures in patients with NEPSs tends to be more variable than in those with epileptic seizures.

Motor Phenomena in Nonepileptic Psychogenic Spells

In convulsivelike NEPSs, motor manifestations can include cloniclike, myocloniclike, and toniclike movements of the extremities and trunk. Gates et al.[11] reviewed videotapes of patients with NEPSs and noted that cloniclike movements were out of phase and asynchronous in the upper extremities, as opposed to in phase and synchronous during epileptic seizures. However, Leis et al.[14] were not able to make this same distinction in their analysis of the motor phenomena of NEPSs.

Among the more typical motor phenomena of convulsive NEPSs, we think of violent thrashing of the extremities or the entire body, or both, opisthotonic arching of the back, pelvic thrusting motions, and side-to-side head movements. These phenomena have been thought to be frequent and unique to

NEPSs.[11,12] Today, however, we know that all of these signs may be seen in epileptic seizures. Geyer et al.,[30] for example, found pelvic thrusting to be equally common in frontal lobe seizures and NEPSs. Thrashing movements have also been recognized in multiple studies as a frequent expression of seizures of mesial-frontal origin.[31–34] By the same token, these types of symptoms may not be as frequent in NEPSs as previously thought. Thus, Leis et al.[14] reported that pelvic thrusting motions were rare in their NEPS patients.

Vocalizations in Nonepileptic Psychogenic Spells

Vocalizations consisting of shouting, screaming, grunting, and understandable speech have often been associated with a diagnosis of NEPSs.[11,13,14,29] Vocalizations are more likely to occur in the middle of NEPSs, unlike epileptic seizures, in which vocalizations usually occur at the onset of the event. In addition, in NEPSs, vocalizations are usually more complex in nature (groaning, gagging, true speech), whereas in epileptic events, vocalizations are typically more primitive, such as grunting or a simple shout.[11] Yet we have also found an affect-laden ictal cry in seizures of orbitofrontal and mesial-temporal origin (A. Kanner, *unpublished data*). Vocalizations in the presence of shedding of tears supports the diagnosis of NEPSs.[35]

Incontinence and Self Injury in Nonepileptic Psychogenic Spells

Until recently, reports of incontinence and self injury during events were usually considered by clinicians as phenomena likely to exclude a diagnosis of NEPSs. This perception, however, has been proven to be erroneous. Incontinence has been reported to range between 10% and 44% in NEPSs, most commonly urinary incontinence, but fecal incontinence has also been described.[10,19,29,36]

Bruising and minor lacerations from falls, followed by tongue biting (which may be severe enough to cause bleeding)[36] are among the more common injuries reported in patients with NEPSs. Severe injuries, including facial bone fractures, are less common but have also been reported and tend to occur in patients with a psychiatric history of suicide attempts.[36]

Nonconvulsive Nonepileptic Psychogenic Spells

Nonconvulsive NEPSs can mimic absence or partial complex seizures, or both; their actual nature may go unrecognized until patients are referred for V-EEG with a presumed diagnosis of intractable epilepsy. For example, Leis et al.[14] found this type of NEPS to be the most common clinical manifestation in their patients. Patients may be unresponsive, exhibiting a motionless stare. Semipurposeful movements that simulate motor automatisms of complex partial seizures have also been described during NEPSs.[13] Frequently, however, patients who appear to be unresponsive during an NEPS may be actually responsive to external stimulation, and some may even respond verbally to different types of stimulation. More commonly, patients remain nonverbal but display active avoidance to noxious and non-noxious stimuli or resist attempts at eye opening, or both. These findings should alert the physician to the possibility of NEPSs, but they are not specific and do not by themselves rule out that the event may be epileptic.

Distinguishing Nonepileptic Psychogenic Spells from Epileptic Seizures

From the previous discussion, it is apparent that a diagnosis of NEPSs based solely on clinical semiology may lead to a misdiagnosis of epileptic seizures as NEPSs. Epileptic seizures arising from frontal and parietal lobes, especially the mesial structures, are those most commonly misdiagnosed as NEPSs. Indeed, complex partial seizures of mesial frontal origin can present with complex automatisms, often with bizarre features that mimic the typical phenomena of NEPSs. These include kicking or pedaling motions of the lower extremities; thrashing and flailing motions of the extremities or entire body, at times with very violent thrusts; and affect-laden vocalizations, such as screams and loud cries. Other phenomena that may contribute to the diagnostic confusion include a preserved consciousness in seizures originating in supplementary sensory motor area, despite bilateral tonic posturing, and the absence of postictal lethargy or confusion. Kanner et al.[32] compared the clinical phenomena of supplementary sensory motor seizures to those of NEPSs. They found clinical phenomena suggestive of NEPSs in 82% of all seizures recorded in 91% of the frontal lobe epilepsy patients studied.

The atypical clinical phenomena of these seizures are frequently coupled with undetected interictal and ictal epileptiform activity on scalp EEG recordings. The difficulty identifying epileptiform discharges results from the great amount of muscle and movement artifact masking the underlying epileptic activity. The inability of the angle subtended by scalp electrodes to identify the source of the epileptic activity in mesial or orbitofrontal regions is another contributing cause to this problem (see the following discussion). Thus, it is not surprising that these seizures are frequently confused with NEPSs.[19,31–34]

There are certain clinical features that may help the clinician distinguish this type of frontal lobe seizure from NEPSs. First, frontal lobe seizures are significantly shorter in duration (mean duration, 28–51 seconds) than NEPSs (mean duration, 76–176 seconds).[32,34] In addition, there is a clear tendency for frontal lobe seizures to occur predominantly during sleep, whereas NEPSs always occur during wakefulness.[32,34] Clinicians need to be aware that patients may report that NEPSs arise out of sleep. However, V-EEG monitoring should demonstrate an awake EEG pattern preceding the onset of the NEPSs.[37,38] Benbadis et al.[37] coined the term *preictal pseudosleep* to describe the state of wakefulness, although appearing asleep, in these patients with NEPSs.

Simple and complex partial seizures in which epileptic activity originates or propagates to the supplementary sensory motor area display a tonic posturing in abduction of the upper extremities that Kanner et al.[32] found to be specific to frontal lobe seizures. The same study demonstrated a stereotypic quality of the thrashing movements of frontal lobe seizures, whereas that was not the case with NEPSs. Although the clinical features of NEPSs in a patient can be stereotypic, thrashing movements are rarely stereotypic in NEPSs. Also, turning to a prone position during the seizure strongly supports a diagnosis of a frontal lobe, rather than a nonepileptic, seizure.[34]

In summary, when clinicians are evaluating patients with paroxysmal events that have atypical features, they should look for one or more of the outlined clinical phenomena. Their presence should serve as an alert to the likelihood of an epileptic seizure disorder. Furthermore, these observations clearly indicate that a diagnosis of NEPSs should never be established without V-EEG confirmation.

Maximizing the Diagnostic Yield of Auxiliary Tests

Because clinical phenomena are often unreliable in distinguishing NEPSs from epileptic and organic nonepileptic paroxysmal events, we must complement our evaluation with a variety of tests. These include ambulatory monitoring and V-EEG telemetry, measurements of serum concentrations of creatine phosphokinase (CPK) and prolactin, neuropsychologic tests, and psychiatric evaluations.

Video-Electroencephalogram Monitoring

The electrographic diagnosis of NEPSs is based on the recording of one of the patient's typical events in the absence of any electrographic change from their baseline awake activity. Yet, as stated previously, scalp recordings may not readily detect interictal and ictal epileptiform activity, especially when it originates from mesial frontal, mesial parietal, and, occasionally, mesial temporal structures. In addition, scalp recordings fail to reveal any electrographic changes in up to 75% of simple partial seizures.[12] This is because scalp electrodes detect epileptiform activity only if a cortical area of 6 cm^2 or more has been synchronously activated. Thus, reliance solely on EEG recordings to make a diagnosis of NEPSs can clearly be misleading.

Accordingly, in the presence of paroxysmal events that are not associated with any loss of consciousness and normal concurrent EEG recordings, clinicians must consider the possibility of a diagnosis of simple partial seizures before concluding that they are NEPSs. In the presence of events with unresponsiveness, bizarre clinical phenomena, and concurrent unchanged EEG recordings, a diagnosis of mesial frontal or parietal lobe seizures should be considered. A diagnosis of NEPSs is more likely in the absence of the clinical signs typical of the frontal lobe seizures listed previously and if these events can be induced and stopped with the use of suggestive techniques.

In an effort to identify "masked epileptiform patterns," electroencephalographers have relied on the use of the following special electrodes: orbitofrontal, sphenoidal, and the 10-10 (closely spaced) electrodes. Orbitofrontal electrodes and the use of 10-10 electrodes over the parasagittal areas can help to identify ictal activity of mesial and orbitofrontal origin.[39,40] Often, the ictal pattern consists of a subtle, rhythmic theta activity over parasagittal regions[33] that may be masked by overlying muscle artifact. Accordingly, the use of digital systems is of the essence, as recordings need to be reformatted with different settings (sensitivity and filters) than those used for data acquisition. The type of clinical phenomena displayed by the patient can help the clinician decide which electrodes to add: sphenoidal electrodes if the semiology is suggestive of mesial temporal seizures, or orbitofrontal and 10-10 sagittal electrodes if the semiology is suggestive of seizures of mesial-frontal lobe origin.

It should be emphasized that, to definitively diagnose NEPSs, an event recorded during V-EEG monitoring must be the patient's typical event. To that end, it is essential that the recorded spells on videotape be reviewed with family or others who have previously witnessed the events. Recording events with no concurrent EEG changes that differ from the patient's typical spell may occur in any patient that is highly suggestible, and such a recording should never, by itself, lead to a diagnosis of NEPSs.

Role of Interictal Epileptiform Discharges

Interictal EEGs are reported to be abnormal in 23–50% of patients with NEPSs.[29,41–43] Although diffuse or focal slowing is the most common abnormality, interictal epileptiform activity is seen in 35–50% of patients with NEPSs.[42,43] The presence of interictal epileptiform activity in recordings of patients with a documented NEPS raises the possibility of comorbid occurrence of NEPSs and epileptic seizures or of a prior history of epileptic seizures. As stated previously, this comorbidity has been reported in 10–40% of patients with NEPSs. It is therefore essential that clinicians investigate whether other types of events, different than those recorded,

have been witnessed in the past. A careful history often yields the description of classic epileptic seizures that occurred years before the evaluation and that are probably well controlled with AEDs. Devinsky et al.[12] have shown that the semiologies of NEPSs and epileptic seizures differ from each other in patients with comorbid disorders.

Furthermore, the possibility of comorbid occurrence of NEPSs and epileptic seizures must always be considered when planning to discontinue or lower AED doses. Parra et al.[42] found that up to 96% of patients with NEPSs had a typical event within the first 48 hours of V-EEG. Accordingly, we recommend maintaining the patient's usual AED doses during that time. This minimizes the risk of facilitating the occurrence of an epileptic seizure early in the monitoring study of patients with NEPSs and epilepsy. It has been our experience that once an epileptic seizure has been recorded, clinicians prematurely conclude that all the events are epileptic, leading to a false-negative diagnosis of NEPSs.

Induction of Nonepileptic Psychogenic Spells

Several studies have found the use of induction protocols to be helpful in provoking NEPSs.[12,14,29,41,44–47] Ensuring that a typical event is captured early in the course of V-EEG has become a greater concern to epileptologists, especially since the advent of managed care that has limited the duration of hospital stays. Among these patients, 37–91% were reported to respond to induction of their typical NEPSs, with most studies reporting a successful induction in 77–84%.[12,14,41,44–47] Clearly, the sensitivity of induction for NEPSs appears high. Although most studies report the specificity of induction of NEPSs to be 100%,[12,41,45,47] there have been reports of epileptic seizures triggered by induction. Walczak et al.[46] reported that 10% of patients with epilepsy experienced seizures after induction; others have reported similar findings.[21,23] Therefore, a positive induction does not document a diagnosis of NEPSs, and to avoid this type of error, induction protocols should not be carried out in the absence of concurrent electrographic recordings.

In the majority of protocols, induction consists of intravenous infusion of a saline solution after the patient has been told that he or she is being given a medication likely to induce seizures.[12,41,44–46] Lancman et al.[47] described placing an alcohol-soaked patch on the patient's neck after informing the patient that this was likely to provoke a seizure. These latter two protocols carry the risk that patients may realize that they have been deceived. To avert that possibility, we base our induction protocol on the use of hyperventilation or photic stimulation, or both,[14,29] two techniques that are commonly used in EEG studies to facilitate the occurrence of seizures.

Indeed, induction protocols that are based on the use of a placebo raise serious ethical issues and may jeopardize the patient-physician relationship, the patient's trust of all physicians, and the patient's acceptance of the diagnosis of NEPSs. This issue has been discussed in the literature and remains controversial.[48,49] Those who advocate the use of induction protocols argue that such protocols pose no potential physical harm to the patient. They postulate that, by aiding in the accurate diagnosis of NEPSs, induction may help to prevent the patient from receiving inappropriate, potentially harmful AEDs and the incorrect diagnosis of epilepsy, with its potential psychological and social hardships. These advocates thus argue that the use of induction techniques is ethically justifiable.[48] Although we advocate the use of induction protocols, we are against the use of techniques that may lead patients to feel deceived. Furthermore, there is no evidence that the use of a placebo yields a higher sensitivity or specificity than using hyperventilation or photic stimulation.

In light of the issues regarding the specificity and ethics of induction protocols, the recent study by Parra et al.[42] is particularly noteworthy. This study addressed the question of whether induction protocols are necessary during V-EEG monitoring to elicit NEPSs. Of 100 patients admitted for V-EEG monitoring studies, 87 experienced their typical event, and 82 of these did so spontaneously without induction. Among the patients with NEPSs, 96% experienced their typical event without induction in the initial 48 hours. The results of this study are congruent with an earlier study by Slater et al.,[45] in which 75% of patients with NEPSs had spontaneous events without induction. Based on the results of these studies, the physician can expect to be able to make an accurate diagnosis of NEPSs in most patients with V-EEG monitoring in a timely manner, without having to resort to induction protocols.

Neuroimaging Studies

Magnetic Resonance Imaging Studies

Contrary to old beliefs, patients with NEPSs may have abnormal neurologic examinations, EEG studies, and magnetic resonance imaging (MRI) studies. In a recently published study of 45 patients with NEPSs, 43% had an abnormal MRI.[50] Although MRI findings do not confirm or rule out a diagnosis of NEPSs, the presence of a structural lesion in mesial frontal or parietal regions should lead the physician to seriously reconsider the diagnosis of NEPSs.

Single Photon Emission Computed Tomography

Single photon emission computed tomography (SPECT) can be of great assistance in documenting a diagnosis of mesial frontal or parietal epilepsy, provided that the radionuclide marker is injected at the time of the event (ictal SPECT). The epileptogenic zone is represented by an area of hyperperfusion on ictal SPECT. On the other hand, interictal SPECT yields unreliable data in patients with epilepsy and is of no diagnostic value.[51–54]

SPECT studies are not expected to show any changes in NEPSs, but conflicting data have appeared in the literature. For example, Willmore et al.[55] found that 70% of patients with NEPSs had focal abnormalities on interictal SPECT. On the other hand, in patients injected during NEPSs, Price et al.[56] found no abnormalities. Similarly, Spanaki et al.[57] found no quantitative differences in ictal SPECT scans in patients injected during NEPSs. Again, these data support the unreliable nature of interictal SPECT data.

Laboratory Tests

Serum CPK levels were found to be elevated after 15% of generalized tonic-clonic seizures but not after partial seizures or NEPSs in a study by Wyllie et al.[58] The levels of CPK peak between 18 and 24 hours postictally. Thus, a high serum CPK after a convulsive event is suggestive of an epileptic seizure, but normal CPK does not confirm the diagnosis of NEPSs. The gap of 18–24 hours between event and peak serum concentrations makes this a useful test to consider in outpatients.

Serum prolactin levels are commonly elevated after generalized tonic-clonic seizures and complex partial seizures of temporal lobe origin, provided that levels are drawn within 20–30 minutes of seizure onset. Prolactin levels are generally not elevated after simple partial seizures, complex partial seizures of frontal lobe origin, or NEPSs.[59–62] However, a recent study by Alving did report a statistically significant increase in prolactin levels in patients after NEPSs.[63] Another study reported a significant rise in serum prolactin levels after episodes of hypotensive syncope.[64] All this evidence raises concerns regarding the reliability of serum prolactin levels in differentiating epileptic seizures from NEPSs.

Neuropsychological and Psychiatric Assessment

Despite the fact that NEPSs are an expression of presumed psychopathologic processes, neurologists and psychiatrists have yet to develop a clear understanding of these processes. There is a widespread misconception among clinicians that NEPSs are events with the sole aim of attaining a secondary gain. In many patients, however, no gains can be identified. In reality, the psychopathology of NEPSs is complex and is an expression of a variety of psychopathogenic processes. These include conversion, somatization, dissociative, factitious, and malingering disorders[65,66] that may occur in association with psychiatric disorders, such as major depression, anxiety, and personality disorders, among others.[67]

Neuropsychological Profiles

Neuropsychological assessments of patients with NEPSs have been performed in an attempt to develop personality and psychological profiles that can distinguish them from patients with epilepsy. Using the Minnesota Multiphasic Personality Inventory (MMPI), Wilkus et al.[68] described a pattern resulting from high scores on the hysteria and hypochondriasis scales and somewhat lower scores on the depression scale. They called this pattern the

conversion V. They suggested that the presence of this profile could differentiate patients with NEPSs from those with epilepsy. Others[69] were not able to replicate these results, however. Since then, the use of personality profiles in identifying patients with NEPSs has been a matter of controversy that remains unresolved.[7,70–72]

In our opinion, the presence of a conversion V pattern cannot be considered by itself as diagnostic evidence of NEPSs but, when present, can be supportive evidence of the diagnosis. On the other hand, a normal MMPI profile, although not excluding a diagnosis of NEPSs, should serve as an inducement to reconsider this diagnosis. We illustrate this point with the following example of a patient of ours.

A 36-year-old man was referred to our institution with a diagnosis of NEPSs that was reached after two ambulatory EEG studies had captured his events without concurrent EEG changes. On both occasions, his wife witnessed transient loss of awareness of his surroundings associated with "laughter." Although the patient was willing to accept the diagnosis of NEPSs, he denied any stressor, and no psychopathology could be elicited during a psychiatric interview. After a normal neuropsychological evaluation that included a normal MMPI profile, we admitted the patient for V-EEG telemetry. Recurrent episodes were recorded during the initial 24 hours, without any concurrent EEG changes, and no spikes were recorded interictally. Despite these findings, the short duration of his events, their uncanny stereotypic quality, and the affectless grinning led us to suspect that his episodes could be epileptic seizures. An ictal SPECT demonstrated an area of hyperperfusion in the right mesial parietal region, thus suggesting that this patient's spells were epileptic seizures. This was confirmed by the total cessation of events after he was started on phenytoin. This case exemplifies how a completely normal neuropsychological and MMPI profile can serve as a "red flag," alerting the clinician to the possibility of a misdiagnosis of epileptic seizures as NEPSs.

Psychiatric Profiles and Treatment Outcomes

Psychopathology and treatment of NEPSs are two of the areas least explored by neurologists and psychiatrists alike. The following problems may explain the lack of success in the treatment of patients with NEPSs: (1) the heterogeneity of NEPSs with respect to their psychopathogenic mechanisms, which have yet to be understood; (2) the lack of established priorities in the treatment process of NEPSs; and (3) the poor communication between neurologists and psychiatrists—a bizarre phenomenon that, sadly, is endemic in many medical institutions in the United States and other countries.

The heterogeneity of NEPS psychopathology is clearly reflected in the diverse outcomes that are often independent of any therapeutic intervention. For example, in a prospective study of 45 consecutive patients with NEPSs carried out at the Rush Epilepsy Center,[50] 13 stopped having NEPSs once presented with the diagnosis; five of these patients did not receive any type of psychotherapeutic intervention. Ten patients stopped having NEPSs for a period of 3–4 months, whereas the remaining 20 patients continued having NEPSs in an uninterrupted pattern, albeit at a lower frequency than before the diagnostic evaluation. Patients from the three outcome groups differed with respect to their psychiatric profiles. Patients with persistent NEPSs after presentation of the diagnosis had a significantly higher frequency of recurrent major depression, dissociative and personality disorders, and a history of chronic abuse (physical, sexual, emotional, or a combination of these). Patients who stopped having NEPSs for a period of 3–4 months displayed a significantly higher frequency of denial of stressors and psychosocial problems, refusal of treatment recommendations, and development of new somatic symptoms after disclosure of diagnosis. Conversely, a single episode of major depression was the one common diagnosis among patients who stopped having NEPSs, although no psychiatric pathology was identified in some of these patients.

In this study, as noted previously, the patients with persistent NEPSs experienced chronic abuse (many since childhood). In our opinion, a process of dissociation is used as a defense mechanism by these patients, initially to fend off the traumatic experiences they were enduring. Later on, this same defense is used in other situations that are perceived as uncomfortable but not necessarily traumatic experiences. This phenomenon constitutes a process of "learned dissociation." Accordingly, when these patients are told "good news; you do not have epilepsy," the paroxysmal episodes do not cease. In our experience, the events continue until the patient has made the connection between the process of dissociation and the actual NEPSs.

Among patients who stop experiencing NEPSs for a period of time after diagnosis, a conversive process most likely mediates the recurrence of NEPSs. These patients tend to deny the presence of any problem and are more likely to develop other somatic symptoms, in addition to NEPSs.

In some patients in whom NEPSs completely resolve after the diagnosis is presented, no psychopathology is identified. This suggests that our understanding of pathogenesis, as well as our ability to uncover etiologic factors, is limited. However, it also supports the clinical observation that some patients may have excellent outcomes without psychiatric or psychological intervention.

This study serves to highlight the complexity of the psychopathogenic mechanisms that mediate NEPS occurrence. In addition, it shows that having an available psychiatric profile of the patient may help clinicians to predict the outcome of NEPSs after diagnosis and thus plan appropriate treatment strategies. For example, patients with a history of abuse and recurrent depressive episodes are expected to continue having NEPSs. Accordingly, the first goal of therapy is to ensure the patient's acceptance of the diagnosis of NEPSs and his or her understanding that these events do not require AEDs and that visits to the local emergency room may result in unnecessary exposure to potentially harmful therapies.

Other studies seem to support our findings. The factors found in studies to be predictors of poor outcome among patients with NEPSs include full-scale intelligence quotient of less than 80 and a past history of violent behavior,[73] history of abuse,[50] and additional psychiatric disorders.[24,50,74] Some studies have shown long duration of NEPSs before diagnosis to be predictive of poor outcome,[15,24,74,75] whereas others have not.[10,72] Factors predictive of good NEPS outcome include an independent existence,[10] current employment,[36,72] and acceptance of the diagnosis of NEPSs.[72,73,75]

Psychiatric profiles cannot differentiate patients with NEPSs and those with epilepsy. Indeed, psychiatric disturbances are common (50–90%)[24,65] in patients with NEPSs, but so are they in patients with epilepsy. Affective disorders are the most common comorbid psychiatric illnesses in patients with NEPSs and epilepsy. As exemplified by the findings of the study cited in the previous discussion, patients with NEPSs have a higher prevalence of post-traumatic stress disorder, frequently resulting from a history of sexual or physical abuse in childhood, or both,[65,66,76–78] and dissociative disorders,[12,24,25,65,66,79] than do patients with epilepsy. Using structured psychiatric clinical interviews, Bowman and Markand[65] found that most patients with NEPSs presented with features of several different maladaptive personality styles, especially avoidant, borderline, and histrionic personality styles, rather than a single personality disorder, but these are not specific to NEPSs.

Practical Aspects of the Treatment of Nonepileptic Psychogenic Spells

What should be the first priority in the treatment of NEPS patients? As with any medical or psychiatric disorder, the immediate goal of therapy is to remove any threat to the patient's physical well being. In the case of NEPSs, that threat is the potential that physicians may continue to misdiagnose the patient's events as epileptic seizures. It is often the case that NEPSs present as recurrent events that fail to respond to changes in AEDs and therefore are managed as cases of refractory epilepsy. This, in turn, unnecessarily exposes patients to high-dose AEDs that can result in serious, and unnecessary, iatrogenic morbidity. In one study, approximately 53.8% of NEPS patients were receiving AEDs, and 66.7% had taken these drugs in the past.[80] In other series, the percentages are even higher.[13,14,29] The most serious iatrogenic morbidity can result when NEPS patients present to the emergency room with repetitive spells and are mistakenly suspected of having status epilepticus. Pakalnis et al.[81] investigated 20 such patients with repetitive NEPSs. In more than 50% of these patients, events continued, despite aggressive therapy with AEDs, until respiratory arrest and intubation occurred. Thus, the immediate goal of therapy is to ensure that both patient and family have accepted the fact that the spells are not epileptic. This precludes the patient's going (or being taken)

to an emergency room after having NEPSs and thus minimizes the risk of potentially serious iatrogenic problems. It should be recognized, however, that the acceptance that the paroxysmal events are not epileptic *does not necessarily* require the *initial* acceptance by the patient of a psychogenic cause. In our opinion, the acceptance of a psychogenic cause for NEPSs should be the second and not necessarily the first goal of the therapeutic process.

Needless to say, acceptance that the paroxysmal events are not epileptic and acceptance of a psychogenic cause are dependent on the way the diagnosis is presented to the patient. Shen et al.[82] developed a protocol to present a diagnosis of NEPS to patients. This protocol contains seven main points. The first point consists of showing the patient video recordings of the spells without comment regarding the diagnosis. This serves to confirm that the recorded events are indeed the patient's typical spells. The second point involves an explanation, in positive terms, of the nonepileptic nature of the spells. The third one calls for an acknowledgment that the nature of the event is yet to be established, and that its cause may not be found. Further, the ineffectiveness of AEDs for the spells, and hence the possibility of discontinuing AEDs, is discussed. Shen et al. introduce the possibility of a psychogenic cause of the spells in their fourth point by telling the patient that in many cases, such events may be "related to upsetting emotions of which the patient is not aware."[82] An evaluation by a psychiatrist, psychologist, or counselor is then suggested. In Shen's protocol, the fifth point concerns reassuring the patient that he or she is not "crazy."[82] Next, they specifically ask the patient whether they have experienced any sexual abuse, because such abuse is often encountered in patients with these spells. Finally, Shen et al. tell their patients that the spells may spontaneously resolve and that "although one component is subconscious in nature, one can exert a conscious voluntary effort to abort these attacks."[82]

Although Shen's protocol for divulging the diagnosis of NEPS to patients is exemplary in many aspects, we disagree with several points of this approach. In our opinion, patients should never be told that their NEPS are psychogenic without historical and psychological evidence to support such suppositions. In the absence of such evidence, it is better to simply acknowledge that the nature of the events is unclear. In our discussions with patients, we raise the possibility of a psychogenic process in the context of a differential diagnosis of the etiology of the spells. We are careful to emphasize to the patient that such a process is only one of several possible explanations for the events. During this part of the discussion, we introduce the concept that some patients with these types of events have a history of sexual abuse. However, in contrast to the protocol of Shen et al., we do not restrict the association to sexual abuse. We also include any history of physical or emotional trauma. Frequently, we offer the example of war veterans to illustrate such an association. We explain that exposure to very traumatic experiences, like combat, demands that the mind take extreme measures to protect itself from the overwhelming pain associated with such experiences by disconnecting itself from the surrounding traumatic situation. We add, "If our mind could not protect itself in that manner, we would not be human, but superhuman." Such an explanation conveys to patients the sense that they have nothing of which to be ashamed and gives patients the opportunity to freely acknowledge their abuse without shame or guilt. In fact, it has been our experience that after this statement, most patients with such a history volunteer the information spontaneously.

It is only after an extensive discussion and explanation of the diagnosis, as cited previously, that we ask patients if they think that their episodes may be related to a psychogenic process, provided that they have not already volunteered this possibility. From this point on, we guide the discussion according to the answers we get from the patient. If patients accept the possibility of a psychogenic process as a cause of their spells, we encourage them to elaborate on their reasons and cite examples that may illustrate potential conflicts, and we suggest that they undergo complete neuropsychological and psychiatric evaluations. If patients acknowledge a history of abuse or of other traumatic experiences, we ask them to recall how they dealt with such situations when they occurred. It has been our experience and that of others that most patients have no recollection of the actual traumatic event(s). We use that lost memory to illustrate the phenomenon of dissociation by reiterating the fact that when an individual is facing a traumatic experience, his or her mind automatically protects itself by blocking any awareness of

its surroundings. We then add that "this is similar to what may happen when you are having a spell" and go on to explain that after repeated traumatic experiences, one's mind may learn to automatically shut out the outside world, *even in the presence of less traumatic situations*. We repeat the statement that "there is only so much trauma one person can endure before fending off the traumatic experience from one's mind." Usually, patients with a history of abuse can easily relate to these observations. This, in fact, begins the therapeutic process. We emphasize to these patients that their process of dissociation is most likely to continue until they learn with the assistance of a counselor to identify the precipitants, which, by now, need not necessarily be of a traumatic nature.

In the case in which patients *adamantly refute* the possibility of any psychogenic cause to their events, we suggest that they undergo a neuropsychological and neuropsychiatric evaluation to rule out that possibility. We emphasize that the unconscious nature of the involved processes may preclude patients from recognizing an underlying psychological cause of their events. At the same time, we acknowledge the possibility that their spells may not have a psychogenic cause and that we may not be able to find a cause by the completion of the evaluation. We always add, "If we don't look for it, we'll never find it. It's better to thoroughly explore whether there is any possible psychogenic cause."

Although we also tell our patients that their spells may stop occurring just through the knowledge that they are not epileptic in nature, we do not suggest to them that they can consciously stop their events. Our reasons for this omission are threefold: (1) unless the patient is malingering (which accounts for a minority of the cases), we do not believe that the patients have a conscious control over the occurrence of their events, at least at the beginning of treatment; (2) patients (and family members) may interpret such a suggestion as an accusation that they are voluntarily faking the events, which, in turn, raises their resistance to accept the diagnosis further; and (3) we are convinced that exertion of control over the events may eventually occur with the proper treatment.

Patients are told that we would like to continue following them in the outpatient clinic, and we ask them to keep a diary in which they are to write down the circumstances surrounding the occurrence of future events if they continue. We do not push patients to accept a psychogenic cause of their spells when it becomes obvious that they are not ready to do so. In our opinion, the best course to take in these circumstances is to continue to build a relationship with the patient. At the same time, we continue reminding patients that the spells are not epileptic (and that no other organic cause has been identified). In our experience, patients eventually accept our recommendation for psychiatric treatment after a few months. During this time, we are at least able to achieve our primary therapeutic goal—that is, that their spells are not treated as epileptic seizures by other physicians.

Occasionally, patients may be adamant that there is some organic or epileptic process triggering their spells and that we have erred in our evaluation and diagnosis. In such patients, we are likely to suspect a fictitious or malingering disorder. However, we try to keep an open mind when dealing with them. We review the diagnostic process with patients and family and illustrate to them on videotape and EEG tracings the differences between epileptic seizures and NEPSs. If the diagnosis was based on an ambulatory EEG study (Digitrace), we repeat the evaluation in an inpatient V-EEG monitoring unit with the use of special electrodes, as indicated previously. In fact, we have had three patients in whom an erroneous diagnosis of NEPSs was reached with ambulatory EEG studies. Two of the three patients had neuropsychological testing that failed to reveal any propensity for conversive disorder. A correct diagnosis of epilepsy was established during prolonged V-EEG. In short, we must always consider the fact that patients who disagree with the diagnosis of NEPSs may be correct.

Beyond the presentation of the diagnosis to the patient, there is a paucity of information available to guide the physician in formulating an appropriate treatment plan for the patient with NEPSs. Various types of psychiatric treatment have been recommended, including pharmacotherapy, usually with antidepressant medications; individual psychotherapy; family therapy; hypnosis; behavioral modification; and art and music therapy.[73,83,84] However, to date, no controlled study has been conducted to assess the effectiveness of these therapies. The results of studies that have assessed the effects of psychiatric treatment for NEPSs are contradictory and confusing. Several published studies reported better outcome in patients receiving psychotherapy compared to those who did not.[10,23,25,75,84] Other studies showed no difference in the recurrence of NEPSs for patients who received psychotherapy and those who did not.[15,24,36,72,74] Even with no treatment, 34–53% of patients with NEPSs become event free over time.[10,24,36,72] In fact, a significant number of patients with NEPSs become event free shortly after being informed of the diagnosis.[15,84,85]

The final question to address pertains to the issue of how long the neurologist should continue studying these patients. It is common for neurologists to completely transfer the care of NEPS patients to a psychiatrist immediately after disclosure of the diagnosis. We believe, however, that the neurologist's involvement should not stop at the time of diagnosis. Instead, it should continue until the patient has established a therapeutic relationship with a psychotherapist or psychiatrist. The patient should always be included in the decision-making process of when to stop seeing the neurologist.

Conclusion

In this chapter, we have highlighted diagnostic and treatment-related issues in NEPSs that have received relatively little attention but have paramount impact on the evaluation and management of these patients. There is no question that, as neurologists are becoming more familiar with NEPSs, they are able to suspect and recognize this type of event with greater facility. The same cannot be said about the general practitioner, and additional efforts to educate the non-neurologist are required, given the potentially serious morbidity associated with the misdiagnosis of NEPSs as epileptic seizures. By the same token, neurologists need to consider the limitations of clinical phenomena in making a reliable diagnosis of NEPSs and to always consider the possibility of epileptic seizures that mimic NEPSs. To avoid such diagnostic errors, patients need to undergo a V-EEG monitoring study. Although ambulatory studies may also be very useful, the risk of false-positive and false-negative findings is higher with these types of studies.

Undoubtedly, knowledge of the patient's psychiatric profile can assist neurologists in predicting outcome, presenting the diagnosis of NEPSs, and planning treatment strategies together with the psychologist or psychiatrist. In our opinion, the primary goal of the neurologist is to ensure that the patient has accepted the diagnosis of NEPSs and avoids visits to the emergency room when NEPSs occur. Achieving this goal minimizes iatrogenic morbidity for these patients.

References

1. Prensky AL. An Approach to the Child with Paroxysmal Phenomenon with Emphasis on Nonepileptic Disorders. In JM Pellock, WE Dodson, BFD Bourgeois, (eds), Pediatric Epilepsy: Diagnosis and Therapy. New York: Demos Publications, 2001;97–116.
2. Pedley TA. Differential diagnosis of episodic symptoms. Epilepsia 1983;24[Suppl 1]:S31–S44.
3. Thach BT. Sleep apnea in infancy and childhood. Med Clin North Am 1985;69:1289–1315.
4. Marsden CD. Supplementary Sensorimotor Area. In HO Luders (ed), Advances in Neurology (vol 70). Philadelphia: Lippincott–Raven, 1996;467–470.
5. Krumholz A. Nonepileptic seizures: diagnosis and management. Neurology 1999;53[Suppl 2]:S76–S83.
6. Bowman ES. Pseudoseizures. Psychiatr Clin North Am 1998;21:649–657.
7. Chabolla DR, Krahn LE, So EL, Rummans TA. Psychogenic nonepileptic seizures. Mayo Clin Proc 1996;71:493–500.
8. King DW, Gallagher BB, Murvin AJ, et al. Pseudoseizures: diagnostic evaluation. Neurology 1982;32:18–23.
9. Sigurdardottir KR, Olafsson E. Incidence of psychogenic seizures in adults: a population-based study in Iceland. Epilepsia 1998;39:749–752.
10. Meierkord H, Will B, Fish D, et al. The clinical features and prognosis of pseudoseizures diagnosed using video-EEG telemetry. Neurology 1991;41:1643–1646.
11. Gates JR, Ramani V, Whalen S, et al. Ictal characteristics of pseudoseizures. Arch Neurol 1985;42:1183–1187.
12. Devinsky O, Sanchez-Villasenor F, Vazquez B, et al. Clinical profile of patients with epileptic and nonepileptic seizures. Neurology 1996;46:1530–1533.
13. Gulick TA, Spinks IP, King DW. Pseudoseizures: ictal phenomena. Neurology 1982;32:24–30.
14. Leis AA, Ross MA, Summers AK. Psychogenic seizures: ictal characteristics and diagnostic pitfalls. Neurology 1992;42:95–99.
15. Wyllie E, Friedman D, Luders H, et al. Outcome of psychogenic seizures in children and adolescents compared with adults. Neurology 1991;41:742–744.
16. Wyllie E, Glazer JP, Benbadis S, et al. Psychiatric features of children and adolescents with pseudoseizures. Arch Pediatr Adolesc Med 1999;153:244–248.
17. Andriola MR, Ettinger AB. Pseudoseizures and other nonepileptic paroxysmal disorders in children and adolescents. Neurology 1999;53[Suppl 2]:S89–S95.
18. Fakhoury T, Abou-Khalil B, Newman K. Psychogenic seizures in old age: a case report. Epilepsia 1993;34:1049–1051.
19. Lesser RP. Psychogenic seizures. Neurology 1996;46:1499–1507.
20. Kanner AM, Iriarte J. Psychogenic Pseudoseizures: Semiology and Differential Diagnosis. In P Kotagal, HO Luders (eds), The Epilepsies: Etiologies and Prevention. San Diego: Academic, 1999;509–517.
21. Parra J, Iriarte J, Kanner AM. Are we overusing the diagnosis of psychogenic non-epileptic events? Seizure 1999;8:223–227.
22. Holmes MD, Wilkus RJ, Dodrill CB, et al. Coexistence of epilepsy in patients with nonepileptic seizures. Epilepsia 1993;34[Suppl 2]:13.
23. Lesser RP, Lueders H, Dinner DS. Evidence for epilepsy is rare in patients with psychogenic seizures. Neurology 1983;33:502–504.
24. Lempert T, Schmidt D. Natural history and outcome of psychogenic seizures: a clinical study in 50 patients. J Neurol 1990;237:35–38.
25. Krumholz A, Niedermeyer E. Psychogenic seizures: a clinical study with follow-up data. Neurology 1983;33:498–502.
26. Benbadis SR. How many patients with pseudoseizures receive antiepileptic drugs prior to diagnosis? Eur Neurol 1999;41:114–115.
27. Rechlin T, Loew TH, Joraschky P. Pseudoseizure "status." J Psychosom Res 1997;42:495–498.
28. Howell SJ, Owen L, Chadwick DW. Pseudostatus epilepticus. Q J Med 1989;71:507–519.
29. Luther JS, McNamara JO, Carwile S, et al. Pseudoepileptic seizures: methods and video analysis to aid diagnosis. Ann Neurol 1982;12:458–462.
30. Geyer JD, Payne TA, Drury I. The value of pelvic thrusting in the diagnosis of seizures and pseudoseizures. Neurology 2000;54:227–229.
31. Williamson PD, Spencer DD, Spencer SS, et al. Complex partial seizures of frontal lobe origin. Ann Neurol 1985;18:497–504.
32. Kanner AM, Morris HH, Luders H, et al. Supplementary motor seizures mimicking pseudoseizures: some clinical differences. Neurology 1990;40:1404–1407.
33. Morris HH, Dinner DS, Luders H, et al. Supplementary motor seizures: clinical and electrographic findings. Neurology 1988;38:1075–1082.
34. Saygi S, Katz A, Marks DA, et al. Frontal lobe partial seizures and psychogenic seizures: comparison of clini-

cal and ictal characteristics. Neurology 1992;42:1274–1277.

35. Bergen D, Ristanovic R. Weeping as a common element of pseudoseizures. Arch Neurol 1993;50:1059–1060.

36. Peguero E, Abou-Khalil B, Fakhoury T, et al. Self-injury and incontinence in psychogenic seizures. Epilepsia 1995;36:586–591.

37. Benbadis SR, Lancman ME, King LM, et al. Preictal pseudosleep: a new finding in psychogenic seizures. Neurology 1996;47:63–67.

38. Thacker K, Devinsky O, Perrine K, et al. Nonepileptic seizures during apparent sleep. Ann Neurol 1993;33:414–418.

39. Kanner AM. Psychogenic seizures and the supplementary sensorimotor area. Adv Neurol 1996;70:461–466.

40. Bare MA, Burnstine TH, Fisher RS, et al. Electroencephalographic changes during simple partial seizures. Epilepsia 1994;35:715–720.

41. Cohen RJ, Suter C. Hysterical seizures: suggestion as a provocative EEG test. Ann Neurol 1982;11:391–395.

42. Parra J, Kanner AM, Iriarte J, et al. When should induction protocols be used in the diagnostic evaluation of patients with paroxysmal events? Epilepsia 1998;39:863–867.

43. Metrick ME, Ritter FJ, Gates JR, et al. Nonepileptic events in childhood. Epilepsia 1991;32:322–328.

44. Bazil CW, Kothari M, Luciano D, et al. Provocation of nonepileptic seizures by suggestion in a generalized seizure population. Epilepsia 1994;35:768–770.

45. Slater JD, Brown MC, Jacobs W, Ramsay RE. Induction of pseudoseizures with intravenous saline placebo. Epilepsia 1995;36:580–585.

46. Walczak TS, Williams DT, Berten W. Utility and reliability of placebo infusion in the evaluation of patients with seizures. Neurology 1994;44:394–399.

47. Lancman ME, Asconape JJ, Craven WJ, et al. Predictive value of induction of psychogenic seizures by suggestion. Ann Neurol 1994;35:359–361.

48. Devinsky O, Fisher R. Ethical use of placebos and provocative testing in diagnosing noncpileptic seizures. Neurology 1996;47:866–870.

49. Burack JH, Back AL, Pearlman RA. Provoking nonepileptic seizures: the ethics of deceptive diagnostic testing. Hastings Cent Rep 1997;4:24–33.

50. Kanner AM, Parra J, Frey M, et al. Psychiatric and neurologic predictors of psychogenic pseudoseizure outcome. Neurology 1999;53:933–938.

51. Newton MR, Berkovic SF, Austin MC, et al. SPECT in the localisation of extratemporal and temporal seizure foci. J Neurol Neurosurg Psychiatry 1995;59:26–30.

52. Duncan R. The clinical use of SPECT in focal epilepsy. Epilepsia 1997;38[Suppl 10]:39–41.

53. Spencer SS. The relative contributions of MRI, SPECT, and PET imaging in epilepsy. Epilepsia 1994;35[Suppl 6]:S72–S89.

54. Won HJ, Chang KY, Cheon JE, et al. Comparison of MR imaging with PET and ictal SPECT in 118 patients with intractable epilepsy. Am J Neuroradiol 1999;20:593–599.

55. Willmore LJ, Wheless JW, Curtis VL, et al. SPECT abnormalities in patients with nonepileptic seizures. Epilepsia 1992;33[Suppl 3]:53–54.

56. Price HE, Rosenbaum DH, Rowan AJ, et al. Measurement of regional cerebral blood flow by SPECT in nonepileptic seizure disorder patients. Epilepsia 1992;33[Suppl 3]:54.

57. Spanaki MV, Spencer SS, Corsi M, et al. The role of quantitative ictal SPECT analysis in the evaluation of nonepileptic seizures. J Neuroimaging 1999;9:210–216.

58. Wyllie E, Luders H, Pippenger C, et al. Postictal serum creatine kinase in the diagnosis of seizure disorders. Arch Neurol 1985;42:123–126.

59. Meierkord H, Shorvon S, Lightman S, et al. Comparison of the effects of frontal and temporal lobe partial seizures on prolactin levels. Arch Neurol 1992;49:225–230.

60. Dana-Haeri J, Trimble MR, Oxley J. Prolactin and gonadotrophin changes following generalised and partial seizures. J Neurol Neurosurg Psychiatry 1983;46:331–335.

61. Laxer KD, Mullooly JP, Howell B. Prolactin changes after seizures classified by EEG monitoring. Neurology 1985;35:31–35.

62. Collins WC, Lanigan O, Callaghan N. Plasma prolactin concentrations following epileptic and pseudoseizures. J Neurol Neurosurg Psychiatry 1983;46:505–508.

63. Alving J. Serum prolactin levels are elevated also after pseudoepileptic seizures. Seizure 1998;7:85–89.

64. Oribe E, Amini R, Nissenbaum E, et al. Serum prolactin concentrations are elevated after syncope. Neurology 1996;47;60–62.

65. Bowman ES, Markand ON. Psychodynamics and psychiatric diagnoses in pseudoseizure patients. Am J Psychiatry 1996;153:57–63.

66. Bowman ES. Nonepileptic seizures: psychiatric framework, treatment, and outcome. Neurology 1999;53[Suppl 2]:S84–S88.

67. American Psychiatric Association. Diagnostic and Statistical Manual of Mental Disorders (4th ed). Washington: American Psychiatric Association, 1994.

68. Wilkus RJ, Dodrill CB, Thompson PM. Intensive EEG monitoring and psychological studies of patients with pseudoepileptic seizures. Epilepsia 1984;25:100–107.

69. Vanderzant CW, Giordani B, Berent S, et al. Personality of patients with pseudoseizures. Neurology 1986;36:664–668.

70. Wilkus RJ, Dodrill CB. Factors affecting the outcome of MMPI and neuropsychological assessments of psychogenic and epileptic seizure patients. Epilepsia 1989;30:339–347.

71. Kalogjera-Sackellares D, Sackellares JC. Personality profiles of patients with pseudoseizures. Seizure 1997;6:1–7.

72. Storzbach D, Binder LM, Salinsky MC, et al. Improved prediction of nonepileptic seizures with combined MMPI and EEG measures. Epilepsia 2000;41:332–337.

73. McDade G, Brown SW. Non-epileptic seizures: management and predictive factors of outcome. Seizure 1992;1:7–10.

74. Walczak TS, Papacostas S, Williams DT, et al. Outcome after diagnosis of psychogenic nonepileptic seizures. Epilepsia 1995;36:1131–1137.

75. Buchanan N, Snars J. Pseudoseizures (non epileptic attack disorder)—clinical management and outcome in 50 patients. Seizure 1993;2:141–146.

76. Bowman ES, Markand ON. The contribution of life events to pseudoseizure occurrence in adults. Bull Menninger Clin 1999;63:70–88.

77. Alper K, Devinsky O, Perrine K, et al. Nonepileptic seizures and childhood sexual and physical abuse. Neurology 1993;43:1950–1953.

78. Griffith JL, Polles A, Griffith ME. Pseudoseizures, families, and unspeakable dilemmas. Psychosomatics 1998;39:144–153.

79. Alper K, Devinsky O, Perrine K, et al. Dissociation in epilepsy and conversion nonepileptic seizures. Epilepsia 1997;38:991–997.

80. Lancman ME, Brotherton TA, Asconape JJ, et al. Psychogenic seizures in adults: a longitudinal study. Seizure 1993;2:281–286.

81. Pakalnis A, Drake ME, Phillips B. Neuropsychiatric aspects of psychogenic status epilepticus. Neurology 1991;41:1104–1106.

82. Shen W, Bowman ES, Markand ON. Presenting the diagnosis of pseudoseizure. Neurology 1990;40:756–759.

83. Nash JL. Pseudoseizures: etiologic and psychotherapeutic considerations. South Med J 1993;86:1248–1252.

84. Aboukasm A, Mahr G, Gahry BR, et al. Retrospective analysis of the effects of psychotherapeutic interventions on outcomes of psychogenic nonepileptic seizures. Epilepsia 1998;39:470–473.

85. Berkhoff M, Briellmann RS, Radanov BP, et al. Developmental background and outcome in patients with nonepileptic versus epileptic seizures: a controlled study. Epilepsia 1998;39:463–469.

Chapter 20

Psychiatric Comorbidity in Epilepsy

Adarsh K. Gupta, Alan B. Ettinger,
and Deborah M. Weisbrot

The patient's emotional reactions to his seizures, his family, and to his social situations are less important determinants of psychiatric disorder than the site and type of epileptic discharge.[1]

The history of epilepsy is closely associated with the development of psychiatry. Throughout history, epilepsy patients have been considered to be prone to psychopathology.[2] Although there is substantial agreement on the definition of a seizure (i.e., an excessive, synchronous, abnormal firing pattern of neurons associated with alteration in neurologic function), there is much controversy about the wide range of psychological effects that epilepsy may produce. Seizure disorders can have psychosocial consequences, neuropsychological effects, seizure-related behavioral manifestations, and medication-induced behavioral changes. The biopsychosocial model for understanding the vast spectrum of altered behaviors emphasizes the value of a multi-disciplinary approach in the management of epilepsy patients.

Biological factors affecting the behavior in epilepsy patients are diverse and multifactorial. They include effects of antiepileptic drugs (AEDs), effects of epilepsy on behavior (mood, personality, cognition), dysfunction of focal brain areas (particularly limbic system) affecting neuroendocrine and autonomic functions, and alterations in neurochemistry and electrophysiology.

In earlier times, social stigmas associated with epilepsy were regarded as demonic possession, punishment for sins, bewitchment, or even a contagious disease[3] and were linked to insanity.[4] In recent times, we have learned that many psychosocial problems afflict epilepsy patients, including a perceived stigma and problems of self image, fear of having seizures witnessed by others, feelings of helplessness and social exclusion, lack of social support, limitations on important activities of daily living such as driving, limitations on employment, and potential detrimental effects on interpersonal relationships.[5] Marriage rates are lower in people with epilepsy (especially men) than in healthy individuals, and "dependence" is often an obstacle. If seizures are poorly controlled, then the disorder confers many restrictions and social stigmas and adversely affects family dynamics.

Sorting out biological factors from maladaptive reactions to a disorder can be difficult. Although many researchers believe that psychosocial obstacles and disease-related stress predispose an individual to psychological symptoms, others contend that biological variables are more important. Studies that fail to consider all such possible variables may be biased and have limited validity.[4]

In reviewing research in this field, careful attention must be paid to the definitions given for the seizure characteristics and psychiatric diagnoses. For example, numerous studies have associated behavioral features with right- or left-sided temporal seizures, relying on limited interictal electroencephalogram (EEG) recordings. However, the use of invasive electrode techniques during video-EEG (V-EEG) monitoring has demonstrated extratemporal seizure activity in patients thought to have purely temporal interictal epileptiform activity. Moreover, patients who have demonstrated unilateral temporal interictal activity have also demonstrated contralateral or bilateral seizures during prolonged recordings. Thus, the conclusions of such studies may be suspect.

Another pervasive problem is that there are few controlled studies comparing epilepsy patients to patients with other disorders. Given many of the unique characteristics of epilepsy, it may be impossible to adequately control for numerous variables. Confounding variables may produce spurious associations between seizure characteristics and specific behavioral abnormalities. Many studies are performed at tertiary referral centers that evaluate epilepsy patients with more severe seizure disorders and other associated medical and psychosocial complications. Findings among such patients may have little to do with conditions that affect the general epilepsy population.

Prevalence of Psychiatric Comorbidity in Epilepsy

The prevalence of epilepsy is estimated to be 0.7%, suggesting that approximately 2 million people in the United States are affected.[6,7] Furthermore, over the course of one's lifetime, the likelihood of experiencing a single seizure is estimated to be 9% for people living in the Western world.[6–8] However, the frequency of psychiatric disturbance in adult epilepsy is poorly understood, with vastly different estimates among various studies. In an epidemiologic survey of medical practices in England conducted by Pond and Bidwell,[9] 29% of patients had psychological difficulties, and at least half of these patients demonstrated "neurotic symptoms." Smith et al.[10] found a higher rate of behavioral abnormalities among epilepsy patients compared with healthy controls on a self-report measure (profile of mood state), but they did not examine other chronic illnesses. Although these studies suggest a higher rate of psychopathology in epilepsy, others have not found this.[11,12]

Most pediatric epilepsy studies argue forcefully for higher rates of psychopathology in epilepsy. The often-quoted Isle of Wight Study[13] included 12,000 children and was based on interviews and standardized questionnaires completed by parents and teachers. The authors found that psychiatric disorders occurred in 8% of the general population, 16% of children with chronic medical disorders, 29% of children with idiopathic epilepsy, and 58% of epilepsy cases associated with structural lesions above the foramen magnum. The rates of psychiatric disturbance in this study were higher than those found in some other investigations.[14,15] Another study comparing children with newly diagnosed epilepsy to those with newly diagnosed diabetes mellitus and matched healthy controls found the frequency of psychiatric disturbance was higher in epilepsy group.[16] However, only one measure of psychiatric disturbance was administered, and there was no neurologic comparison group.

The issue of whether epilepsy patients are particularly vulnerable to psychiatric disturbance remains unresolved. However, it may be more useful for the clinician to focus on identifying specific risk factors in the individual patient. Factors to consider include (1) central nervous system (CNS) influences, such as seizure disorder duration, localization and etiology, as well as cognitive impairments; (2) medication-induced factors, such as medication-induced cognitive impairments with associated coping difficulties; and (3) psychosocial factors.[17]

Neural Mechanisms of Psychiatric Disturbance in Epilepsy

The neurologic mechanisms that cause psychiatric comorbidity in patients with epilepsy are complex and multifactorial. One area that may lend insight into this relationship is the possible link between epilepsy and schizophrenialike psychosis,[4,18–20] broadly classified as (1) epilepsy and psychosis sharing a *common neuropathology* that may be localized or widespread in the brain or (2) psychosis being due to a *repetitive electrical disturbance*, directly or through the development of neurophysiologic or neurochemical abnormalities. Both mechanisms may be operative, the former being primary and the latter modifying the presentation (contributing to the exacerbation and remissions or may also be the proximate cause).[21] Other possible factors, such as psychological issues, neurotoxicity of AEDs, drug-induced deficiencies (e.g., folic acid), and abnormal experiences, might also contribute.

Neuropathologic and Neurochemical Correlates of Psychosis in Epilepsy

Many studies have shown that temporal lobe epilepsy (TLE) is associated with temporal lobe pathology, including sclerosis and, in some cases, neuronal loss.[22–24] In a large series of subjects with histories of temporal lobectomy, Taylor[25] reported that epilepsy patients with schizophrenialike psychosis were less likely to have *mesial temporal sclerosis* and more likely to have *alien tissue lesions* (small tumors, hamartomas, and focal dysplasias). In a study by Roberts et al.,[26] 40% of patients with schizophrenialike psychosis and epilepsy had mesial temporal sclerosis, 20% had gangliomas, and 20% had no lesions (vs. 49 %, 4%, and 15% of the total epilepsy group, respectively). Histories of birth injuries, head injury, and febrile seizures were not over represented in the group with schizophrenialike psychosis. The frequency of alien tissue tumors and early onset of seizures suggested a developmental lesion in medial temporal structures that had been physiologically active from an early age.

In an extensive magnetic resonance imaging study, Conlon et al.[27] examined the brain morphometry of patients with schizophrenia and TLE. He reported that some of morphologic abnormalities (large ventricles, small hippocampus) were common to both disorders. Bruton et al.[19] examined 661 brains from four groups of patients with epilepsy: (1) those with *Diagnostic and Statistical Manual of Mental Disorders*, *Third Edition–Revised* (*DSM-III-R*) diagnosis of schizophrenia, (2) those satisfying the criteria for an organic psychosis but not schizophrenia, (3) inpatients who did not have psychosis, and (4) outpatients who did not have psychosis. Both groups of psychotic epilepsy patients differed from the nonpsychotic groups with greater *ventricular enlargement, periventricular gliosis,* and *focal brain damage.* The frequency of temporal lobe pathology was similar among the four groups. TLE was not more common in epilepsy with schizophrenia than in other groups. All the schizophrenic patients had generalized seizures, irrespective of whether they had other types of seizures as well. The time between seizure onset and onset of schizophrenic symptoms was 5–38 years. These pathologic findings were similar to those documented in schizophrenic patients without epilepsy.[28,29] The epilepsy patients with schizophrenia were further distinguished from other groups (including the nonschizophrenic psychotic group), by a large number of minute lesions on thick-walled blood vessels throughout the white matter (not attributable to age effects). Bruton et al.[19] concluded that temporal lobe pathology usually associated with TLE is unlikely to account for the development of schizophrenia, and other pathologic changes must be responsible.

Trimble[30] noted that structural brain damage in patients with TLE is largely confined to the temporal lobe, whereas the metabolic changes that have been documented in epilepsy patients with psychosis extend beyond this region. He contends that it is unlikely that epilepsy and psychiatric disturbance have the same organic basis. A positron emission tomography (PET) study using O^{15} H_2O demonstrated lower oxygen extraction ratios in the frontal, temporal, and basal ganglia regions of psychotic patients with epilepsy than in nonpsychotic epileptic patients.[31] TLE has been correlated with hypometabolism in ipsilateral temporal lobe and surrounding regions.[32,33] This hypometabolism has recently been related to impaired cognitive performance in patients with epilepsy.[34]

Psychosis as a Direct Consequence of the Epileptic Disturbance

Seizures may result in ictal, postictal, and interictal psychosis (see Psychosis and Epilepsy). Speculated mechanisms include continuous subictal activity, a homeostatic mechanism that reduces epileptic excitability, and neurochemical and neuroendocrine changes produced by seizures. These may account for acute or subacute psychiatric disturbances but seem inadequate to cause chronic schizophrenialike psychosis.

Kindling and Long-Term Potentiation

Graham and Goddard[35,36] first described the phenomenon of "kindling" as a possible model for the development of seizure foci and partial epilepsy. In animal experiments, repetitive subthreshold electrical stimulation produces a *self-sustaining focus* and then can generate seizure discharges in the absence of external stimulation. Such seizures may spread to lead to *secondary generalization*. Throughout the process of kindling, there is gradual reduction in the threshold of the stimuli needed to induce seizures. Limbic structures are the most vulnerable part of the brain to kindling, possibly explaining why TLE is such a common form of epilepsy.

Long-term potentiation (LTP) is an enhancement of synaptic efficacy that follows high-frequency stimulation of an afferent pathway. Postsynaptic neurons show a larger response to an excitatory stimulus than they did before tetanization.[37,38] The enhancement of the synaptic efficacy is homosynaptic (i.e., specific to the input that has been tetanized), and the postsynaptic response to other afferent inputs is normal. This may be the physiologic mechanism underlying kindling.[36,39] LTP has been implicated in many areas of CNS and is regarded as the robust model of synaptic changes during the formation of memories.[37] Most LTP is mediated by activation of *N*-methyl-D-aspartate (NMDA) receptors; NMDA antagonists prevent the induction but not the maintenance of LTP.[37]

Secondary Epileptogenesis

The phenomenon of mirror and daughter foci may be related to kindling.[40–42] According to theories of *mirror foci*, the epileptogenic focus in the temporal lobe is associated with the development of an independent seizure focus in the contralateral homotopic brain region. In the case of *daughter foci*, nontemporal focal structural lesions produce independent temporolimbic seizures ipsilateral to the structural abnormality. This explains the paradoxical but relatively common finding of TLE in patients with focal structural lesions in the parietal and occipital lobes.[43] Studies of behavioral and pharmacologic kindling in animals and development of mirror foci suggest that the potential exists for repetitive epileptiform discharges to facilitate subsequent propagation along specific pathways that may cause interictal disturbance. In an analogous fashion, electrical and pharmacologic kindling of ventral tegmentum and amygdaloid kindling by ropathology have been theorized to be a basis for

cocaine and apomorphine in a cat[44] have been suggested as model for psychoses.

The critical role of limbic cortices for establishing multimodal associations and their susceptibility to kindling and LTP may help to explain why they are also the most common substrate for the emergence of *reflex epilepsy*. In this condition, sensory stimuli (e.g., certain odors or visual stimuli) or specific cognitive process (e.g., reading, imagining an event, or mental arithmetic) can trigger TLE. Reflex epilepsy may also relate to *psychological kindling*, in which the epilepsy-inducing stimulus is an endogenous pattern of neural activity rather than an exogenously administered electrical or chemical stimuli.

The long duration of epilepsy before the onset of psychosis, frequency of partial seizures, limbic origin of seizures, and phenomenon of forced normalization (see Brief Interictal Psychosis) are consistent with the kindling hypothesis. However, there are limitations to this hypothesis: (1) Kindling has not been definitively proven to occur in humans; (2) the relationship of psychosis to seizures is variable in terms of age of onset, duration, and frequency; (3) LTP, although long term, is not permanent and decays gradually over time; and (4) patients usually have generalized seizures and widespread pathology. Postlobectomy psychosis may be a result of downstream kindling due to persistent ictal activity or decreased seizure frequency.[45]

Development of Plastic Regenerative Changes

Repetitive seizure activity can contribute to the production of aberrant plastic regenerative changes, affecting particularly the medial temporal lobes. Stimulation of hippocampus leads to an anomalous axonal sprouting from dentate granule cells before the development of seizures.[46] The studies of temporal lobectomy specimens have shown expansion of glutamatergic presynaptic mossy fibers and an increase in perforated postsynaptic densities on granule cell densities.[47] These changes are possibly produced by increased expression of messenger RNA for *c-fos* and nerve growth factors by recurrent limbic seizures. The aberrant regeneration and the resultant "miswiring" alone or in combination with underlying neu-schizophrenialike psychosis.

Figure 20-1. Possible pathophysiologic mechanisms for the association between epilepsy and schizophrenialike psychosis. (LTP = long-term potentiation.) (Modified from P Sachdev. Schizophrenia-like psychosis and epilepsy: the status of the association. Am J Psychiatry 1998;155[3]:325–336.)

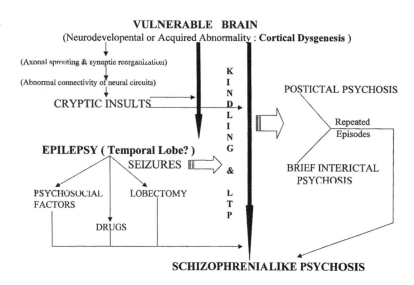

Model for Pathogenesis of Psychosis in Epilepsy

Sachdev[31] proposed a synthesis of various hypotheses contributing to pathogenesis of psychosis in epilepsy. According to this view, epilepsy patients who develop chronic schizophrenialike psychosis have a brain lesion that makes them vulnerable to psychosis (Figure 20-1). This lesion may be neurodevelopmental, leading to cortical dysgenesis or acquired through such events as trauma, hypoxia, and infection. The abnormality may be widespread but is particularly likely to involve limbic structures, leading to abnormalities of connectivity of these structures to their afferent and efferent projection regions. The abnormality is likely to cause electrical storms in the limbic cortex, with seizures occurring at an early age. Seizures or subclinical electrographic discharges may exacerbate the abnormality via kindling mechanisms or the regenerative changes involving axonal sprouting and synaptic reorganization. Over time, these may progressively disrupt functional systems and lead to schizophrenialike psychosis. Seizures, by the presence of continuous subictal activity or by their modulation of pre- and postsynaptic glutamatergic and gabaminergic activity, modulate the expression of the psychosis or act as brakes, sometimes leading to impression of antagonism (see Brief Interictal Psychosis). The picture is further complicated by long-term AED therapy with its potential for neurotoxicity and psychosocial factors related to epilepsy.

Temporal Lobe Personality Traits

Personality traits are influenced by developmental and social environments, gender, intelligence, medication, genetic factors, and other biological and environmental factors. TLE is associated with alteration in neurotransmitters, neuropeptides, neuroendocrine function, metabolism, synaptic connectivity, and neuronal populations, among other pathophysiologic changes associated with epilepsy.

Epilepsy-related behavioral changes may be positive, as exemplified by many famous individuals with epilepsy in politics, religion, and arts and sciences. Dostoyevsky is classically cited for having one notorious feature of a temporal lobe personality trait (i.e., hypergraphia). He described the relationship between his writing and epilepsy in a letter to his brother (Aug. 27, 1849): "Whenever formerly I had such nervous disturbances, I made use of them for writing; in such a state I could write much more and much better than usual."[48] Hypergraphia occurs in 7–10% of TLE patients.[49,50] It is the driven nature of the writing, the preoccupation with personal detail, its exces-

Table 20-1. Opposite Behaviors after Bilateral Temporal Lobectomy (Klüver-Bucy Syndrome) and Temporal Lobe Epilepsy

Klüver-Bucy Syndrome (Sensory-Limbic Disconnection)	Temporal Lobe Epilepsy (Sensory-Limbic Hyperconnection)
Hypersexuality	Hyposexuality
Hypermetamorphosis of attention	Viscosity of thinking
Placidity	Emotional intensity

sive quantity, and the repetitive moralistic and philosophic content that tend to be characteristic of TLE.

The recognition of aberrant personality traits is interesting in light of enhanced understanding of the role of the limbic system (including mesial temporal regions) in emotion and behavior, along with the recognition that the temporal lobe is the most common site of onset of partial seizures.[51] More recently, Geschwind and co-workers[52–54] renewed the interest and controversy concerning personality alterations among patients with epilepsy. In 1975, Waxman and Geschwind[53] noted interictal behavioral syndrome consisting of "hyposexuality, hyperreligiosity, hypergraphia, and viscosity in thinking." This represented a reverse of a "Klüver-Bucy syndrome (hypersexuality, hypermetamorphosis of attention, and placidity)," (i.e., a syndrome of sensory-limbic hyperconnection).[55] Geschwind proposed that kindling may affect the amygdala, producing a limbic spike focus and that such an

abnormality of the limbic system could alter perception of and response to stimuli, resulting in behavioral or personality changes[54] (Table 20-1).

In an attempt to lend more validity to the concept of a TLE syndrome, Bear and Fedio[56] designed a self-report instrument, the Bear-Fedio Index (BFI), which focused on behaviors believed to be related to TLE. This was administered to the patients with "left and right temporal foci," to patients with neuromuscular disorders, and to healthy controls. The authors contended that BFI differentiated epilepsy patients from neuromuscular patients and controls. They argued that there were lateralizing traits as well (Table 20-2), and that the measure provided strong evidence of a specific TLE personality syndrome.

The Bear and Fedio study has been criticized for selection bias with inappropriate control groups and use of a nonvalidated questionnaire response format. Some believe that the BFI simply identifies nonspecific psychopathology. Subsequent studies failed to replicate the results of Bear and Fedio.[51,57,58] Rodin and Schmlts[59] attempted to replicate the findings of Bear and Fedio using temporal and generalized epilepsy groups as well as "control" groups (pain clinic patients, psychiatric patients, and healthy individuals). They could not demonstrate a specific syndrome for patients with temporal lobe seizure foci or replicate laterality findings. The issue of selective temporal lobe seizure foci and specific behaviors is the crux of the controversy. However, the BFI was not developed to separate the epilepsy and psychiatric patients or those with temporal versus frontal foci.[60] Devinsky[61] argues that the BFI consistently demonstrates that TLE patients have behavioral traits different from those of control subjects without epilepsy or behavioral disorders. Despite the continuing controversy, the BFI has helped to expand the focus on behavioral issues in epilepsy research.

Many studies since the 1950s have reported an association of specific personality traits with temporolimbic epilepsy.[62–66] These have included deepened emotionality, humorlessness, hyposexuality, anger, religiosity,[67] enhanced philosophic preoccupation, moralism, obsessional thinking, paranoia, circumstantiality, viscosity (enhanced social cohesiveness), and hypergraphia (extensive writing and drawing).[68] Clinical experience and many studies suggested that behavioral changes occur that defy traditional syndrome categorization. However, the

Table 20-2. Lateralization of Temporal Lobe Personality Features According to Bear and Fedio

Right-Sided TLE	Left-Sided TLE
Elation or sadness	Anger
Obsessiveness	Paranoia
Viscous personality (cohesive interpersonal style promoting prolonged verbal contact)	Dependence
	Negative self-image
	Concerns with personality destiny

TLE = temporal lobe epilepsy.

increased awareness of the range of behavioral changes and their risk factors and increased understanding of their mechanisms involved may lead to identification of patients at risk and preventive strategies, as well as earlier detection and treatment.

Psychosis and Epilepsy

This section reviews the phenomenology of psychosis in epilepsy (mechanisms are discussed earlier). The prevalence of psychosis in epilepsy is not well established; overall estimates, including interictal and peri-ictal cases, range from 5% to 9%.[69] Psychotic syndromes have traditionally been classified according to their temporal relationship to seizure events as ictal, postictal (or preictal), and interictal.

Ictal Psychosis and Delirium

Complex partial seizure (CPS)–associated symptoms may resemble psychosis but are more accurately described as a *delirium*. The symptoms are usually brief but, rarely, in cases of status epilepticus, can last from hours to days. They may present with a wide range of perceptual, behavioral, cognitive, and affective symptoms, often in association with automatisms involving oral activity, picking at clothes, and paucity of speech or mutism.[70,71] *Psychosis* is not synonymous with delirium. In psychosis, alertness and attention are relatively preserved, and delusions and hallucinations are more organized. Prolonged nonconvulsive seizures (absence or partial complex) may be more difficult to recognize, are usually associated with varying degrees of altered awareness, and can last from hours to days, especially if untreated.

Simple partial status may also produce affective, autonomic, and psychiatric symptoms that may include hallucinations and delusions but with clear consciousness. Insight about the unreality of symptoms is usually preserved.[69] Petit-mal status alters consciousness and may cause motor symptoms, such as eyelid fluttering and myoclonic jerks, and may superficially resemble psychosis, but delusions and hallucinations are lacking.

Ictal psychosis is defined as psychotic symptoms that occur during a seizure. Proving the presence of seizure can be challenging, because EEG changes may not be detectable in some cases of simple partial status. Most of these seizures originate in the temporal lobe, but the focus is extratemporal in 30% of patients, usually in dorsolateral, prefrontal, or cingulate cortex. Seizures emanating from extratemporal areas notoriously lack obvious scalp EEG changes.[72]

Kindrick and Gibbs[73] used implanted electrodes to study the electrophysiologic disturbance in schizophrenia and in the psychosis of TLE; spike discharges in medial temporal and frontal regions were demonstrated in both patient groups. Sem-Jacobsen[74] and Heath[75] reported similar abnormal electrical discharges that did not spread beyond amygdala, hippocampus, and septal regions in schizophrenic as well as "epileptic psychosis" patients. Attempts to confirm or refute these findings have not been made, perhaps owing to ethical constraints against the use of depth electrodes for research purposes. The question of whether chronic psychosis in clear consciousness can be a direct consequence of continuous seizure activity restricted to deep brain structures has generated much controversy. Most epileptologists consider this extremely unlikely,[69] but this long-held idea remains current.[22]

Postictal Psychosis

In *postictal psychosis* (PIP), brief psychotic symptoms follow the termination of a seizure. It is much less common than chronic interictal psychosis, and there is only a handful of case series. PIP usually follows seizure clusters[76] or a recent exacerbation in seizure frequency that may be related to withdrawal of anticonvulsants, often as a part of a V-EEG–monitoring procedure.[77,78] The incidence of PIP in various epilepsy-monitoring facilities has been reported from 6% to 10%.[78,79] The psychosis may be referred to as peri-ictal, rather than postictal, if it develops gradually and in parallel with increasing seizure frequency. However, there is no reason to believe that this distinction is meaningful clinically or for its pathophysiology.

Clinical Features

Kanner[80] and others noted some common features among PIP patients:

1. PIP usually occurs after a 12- to 72-hour lucid interval[81] between seizure termination and

the onset of psychotic symptoms. PIP should be distinguished from the commonly encountered confusional state that immediately follows seizures and that usually resolves within minutes.

2. PIP typically lasts more than 24 hours to several days[76,78] and, rarely, weeks.[77]

3. The mental status change may include some clouding of consciousness during the lucid interval, which may extend to the initial period of psychosis. Psychotic symptoms are pleomorphic (persecutory, referential, grandiose, somatic and religious delusions, hallucinations, and catatonia).

4. Affective symptoms are also common.[76,82]

5. The majority of patients have partial complex seizures that are secondarily generalized before PIP.

6. Epilepsy is often present for more than 10 years before the onset of psychosis.[76,78,79]

7. There is typically prompt response to low-dose neuroleptic medication or benzodiazepines, or both.

Implications of Postictal Psychosis in Patients Undergoing Vigilance-Controlled Electroencephalogram Monitoring

Kanner et al. reported that presence of PIP was associated with bilateral ictal foci in 89% of cases.[83] Umbrich et al.[84] found similar results and also noted that patients with PIP and interictal psychosis had a lower intelligence quotient and the absence of mesial temporal sclerosis. Devinsky et al.[85] found a higher frequency of bilateral-independent interictal foci in 20 patients with PIP compared to 150 controls.

Kanner[80] suggested that, in patients undergoing a V-EEG study, the clinician should be aware of (1) occurrence of *de novo* clusters of secondary generalized tonic-clonic seizures (or complex partial seizures), (2) bilateral independent ictal foci, (3) past psychiatric history of depression or psychosis, and (4) insomnia or mild thought disorder between 12 and 72 hours after the last seizure.

The occurrence of PIP has important diagnostic and therapeutic implications for the neurologists. If the previously mentioned symptoms are identified, then a neuroleptic such as low-dose risperidone (1–2 mg) can be administered. If PIP predictably occurs after most or all seizure clusters, then neuroleptic medication can be given at the time of the cluster to prevent PIP. In patients manifesting PIP, bilateral-independent ictal foci should be suspected, with important implications for epilepsy surgery patients. PIP patients may therefore require longer V-EEG monitoring studies to record greater numbers of seizures or use of intracranial electrodes to confirm the seizure foci. If recording with depth or subdural electrodes is considered, then prophylactic treatment with low-dose risperidone or haloperidol can avert the occurrence of PIP during the invasive V-EEG monitoring studies.

The pathogenetic mechanisms for PIP are poorly understood. Changes in postsynaptic dopamine receptor sensitivity may be relevant.[86,87] PIP has also been conceptualized as a phenomenon akin to Todd's paralysis, indicating a postictal inactivation of cortical regions involved in the ictal event, which usually include bilateral medial temporal structures.[69]

Brief Interictal Psychosis

Brief psychotic episodes can also occur when seizures are infrequent or fully controlled. Psychosis exacerbations may last from a few days to weeks but are usually self-limited. They may be difficult to distinguish from PIP in the face of frequent seizures; clinical presentations of psychosis may be similar. The psychotic manifestations of alternative psychosis (defined later) were identified after a *long duration of seizure disorder.* Wolf[89] noted a 15.2-year history of epilepsy in 23 patients with this type of psychosis. Tellenbach[88] reported the presence of premonitory symptoms, such as insomnia, anxiety, feelings of oppression, and withdrawal, as heralding the psychosis. Wolf[89] suggested that treatment with anxiolytics at this stage may prevent the development of psychosis.

Some have contended that brief psychoses typically alternate with seizures in an antagonistic fashion.[22] This *alternating psychosis* promptly resolves once the seizures recur.[90] Landolt[91] coined the term *forced normalization* and defined it as "the phenomenon characterized by the fact that, with the occurrence of psychotic states, the EEG becomes more normal or entirely normal as compared with previous or subsequent EEG findings." As Wolf and Trimble[92] pointed out, the term is misleading because of difficulty in translating Landolt's intent from the original German. Wolf[89] called this phenomenon *paradoxic normalization*, and

Tellenbach[88] suggested the term *alternative psychosis*. This aspect of antagonism prompted Cerletti and Bini to treat psychiatric disorders, especially schizophrenia, with electrically induced seizures.[93] Numerous theories about the mechanism of paradoxic normalization have been suggested.[94] One theory focuses on dopamine, whose antagonists may provoke seizures, whereas agonists increase or precipitate psychosis but have anticonvulsant properties. Such a relationship between epileptiform activity and psychotic symptoms would have important clinical implications, because treating one disorder could result in worsening the other. Reid and Mothersill[95] concluded that alternative psychosis should be treated by reducing or discontinuing AEDs until overt seizure recurrence causes a remission of psychotic symptoms. After that, AEDs should be reintroduced slowly. The existence of alternative psychosis remains controversial, or, if it does exist, then it is probably very rare in clinical practice.[90] In general, clinicians should not be inhibited from treating psychosis in the face of a seizure disorder.

Chronic Interictal Psychosis

Prevalence

The unique etiologic relationship between epilepsy and chronic interictal psychosis or schizophrenialike psychosis has been alluded to under Neural Mechanisms of Psychiatric Disturbance in Epilepsy.[22] An influential study by Slater and Beard[21] reported 69 patients with epilepsy and interictal schizophrenic disorder and noted that these disorders occurred together more frequently than expected by chance. Most subsequent studies indicate that 7–12% of patients with epilepsy develop a psychotic disorder, usually a chronic, interictal schizophrenic illness.[96] In a study involving 1,611 outpatients with epilepsy, Mendez et al.[97] found that interictal schizophrenic disorders were 9–10 times more common among patients with epilepsy than among control subjects with other neurologic disorders. The schizophrenic disorder may be especially associated with CPSs. One study found psychosis in 12% of 1,675 patients with CPSs of temporal lobe origin, especially on the left, compared with fewer than 1% of 6,671 patients with

generalized epilepsy.[98] In conclusion, patients with epilepsy have a severalfold greater risk for a psychotic schizophreniclike illness compared to the general population, and the risk is particularly high for patients with CPSs.

Location of Seizures in Chronic Interictal Psychosis

Many studies indicate that psychosis in epilepsy is *preferentially associated with TLE*,[21,98–100] especially of *mesial temporal origin*. Epigastric[101] and other autonomic auras[97] are very common. Sachdev[22] argued that the structural abnormality in epileptic psychosis is not lateralized[20,27] and is possibly bilateral, but the functional abnormality is predominantly left sided, as indicated by most EEG and imaging studies.[32,100,102–104]

Risk Factors for Development of Chronic Interictal Psychosis

In a review of 14 studies, Trimble[96] found the mean interval between the onset of epilepsy and the development of psychotic symptoms to be 15 years (range, 11–21 years). Patients with an earlier age of epilepsy onset (enduring through puberty) were at higher risk for psychosis.[20,26,105] Others noted risk factors, including severe epilepsy with episodes of status epilepticus,[21] multiple seizure types,[12] and resistance to the treatment.[106] Unlike ictally related psychotic episodes, chronic interictal psychosis has no direct relationship to individual seizures.[96,97] Schizophrenialike psychosis has been reported in 3–28% of the patients undergoing temporal lobectomy for treatment of intractable seizures,[22] usually developing months or years after the surgery.

Clinical Presentation of Chronic Interictal Psychosis

Slater et al.[21,107] argued that the psychiatric features of interictal psychosis are different from those seen in schizophrenia. The features commonly associated with schizophrenia, such as a family history of schizophrenia, abnormal premorbid personality traits, catatonic phenomenon, and loss of warm affective responses and interpersonal relationships, are less common in patients with interictal psychosis. The schizophrenic disorder resembles an episodic schizoaffective psychosis with prominent paranoia, positive symptoms, relatively preserved affect, and normal premorbid personality.[96,100] Perez and Trimble[100] found that only 50% of patients with epilepsy and psychosis could be diagnosed as schizophrenic, and 92% of those had *nuclear schizophrenia* according to Schneiderian first-rank symptoms (i.e., audible thoughts; voices arguing or discussing, or both; voices commenting; somatic passivity experiences; thought withdrawal; thought broadcasting; delusional perceptions; and all other experiences involving volition, made affects, and made impulses).

Many investigators have found a relative lack of negative symptoms and a more benign course for interictal psychosis,[21,108] but supportive, controlled studies are lacking. Indeed, in a study by Mendez et al.,[97] the epilepsy with psychosis group did not differ from the nonepileptic-schizophrenic comparison subjects on any psychosis item except increased suicidal behavior in the former.

Treatment of Psychosis in Epilepsy

The management of psychosis in epilepsy patients is similar to that in patients with or without epilepsy, with a few caveats. Nonpharmacologic interventions should also be considered where applicable. The use of neuroleptics in patients with epilepsy should be guided primarily by the etiology of psychosis and whether the psychosis is ictal, postictal, or interictal. Ictal psychosis is best treated by addressing seizure control. Postictal psychosis is more common than ictal psychosis and usually does not require long-term use of antipsychotic drugs. The short-term use of neuroleptics or benzodiazepines may be warranted for postictal psychosis.

Unlike peri-ictal psychosis, the treatment of interictal psychosis does warrant consideration of long-term use of neuroleptic drugs. Data concerning the appropriate neuroleptic drugs for patients with epilepsy are largely anecdotal, and there is a paucity of well-designed studies with sufficient numbers to estimate the epileptogenic risk of individual agents. When selecting a specific antipsychotic medication, one must consider the risk of lowering seizure threshold and potential drug inter-

actions (these topics are discussed in more detail under Effects of Psychotropic Agents on Seizure Threshold). Although it is essential that the risk of seizure occurrence always be considered when starting neuroleptic medications, it should never be a reason not to treat a patient in need of antipsychotic medication. Most neuroleptic drugs can cause EEG changes consisting of slowing of background activity when used at high doses. In addition, some of these drugs, particularly clozapine, can cause paroxysmal electrographic changes in the form of interictal sharp waves and spikes.[109] This type of epileptiform activity, however, is not predictive of seizure occurrence. Data from studies by Tiihonen et al.[110] suggest that severe disorganization of EEG recordings is a more likely predictor of seizure occurrence.

McConnell[111] summarized the available data on use of neuroleptics in epilepsy patients with the following recommendations:

1. Clozapine, chlorpromazine, and loxapine should be avoided, if possible, in epilepsy patients because of their clearly increased epileptic potential. If clozapine is needed, then coadministration of AEDs such as valproic acid (VPA) may lower the risk of seizures.

2. Among the traditional neuroleptics, haloperidol may be the drug of choice in epilepsy patients. However, given the risk of extrapyramidal side effects, atypical neuroleptics may be considered. If long-term treatment is necessary, then risperidone and sulpiride may have less lowering of the seizure threshold and fewer extrapyramidal effects. Only limited data are available on other atypical neuroleptics, such as olanzapine, quetiapine, and ziprasidone, but their epileptogenic risk is probably low.

3. Trifluoperazine, fluphenazine, molindone, and thioridazine are other reasonable alternatives, in that they probably have less effect on seizure threshold than others.

4. Regardless of the neuroleptic selected, doses should be *initiated low* and *titrated slowly* with monitoring of seizure frequency and severity.

5. Neuroleptic (when possible) and AED levels should be monitored in those receiving both.

6. The use of neuroleptics should be primarily guided by the etiology of the psychosis and whether psychosis is ictal, postictal or interictal. Psychosis related to AED use should be treated

with switching to an alternative antiepileptic rather than neuroleptic therapy.

Depressive Disorders in Epilepsy

Prevalence

Depression is a frequent neuropsychiatric disturbance in patients with epilepsy, occurring in 11–60% of cases.[112–114] There are at least four controlled studies that indicate that depression is significantly more common in epilepsy versus other chronic disorders.[56,115–117] Depression is particularly prevalent among those with CPSs.[118–121] Most investigators report a twofold greater frequency of interictal depression among patients with seizures than among comparable disabled individuals.[12,59,112,113] Depression is also the most common reason for psychiatric hospitalization of epilepsy patients. There is consensus that the risk of suicide related to depression is at least four to five times greater in epileptic patients than in the general population,[122–124] and those with TLE have a 25 times greater risk than that expected in the general population.[122]

The relationship between epilepsy and depression has been recognized since the time of Hippocrates, who observed a relatively high frequency of "melancholia" among epileptics, as well as the fact that "melancholics were more prone to develop epilepsy."[125] Interestingly, recent research indicates that depression may actually be a risk factor for epilepsy.[7] This is not to say that depression causes epilepsy, but rather that an underlying disturbance may give rise to both conditions, with depression symptoms occurring first. In one study,[126] newly diagnosed epilepsy patients had a seven times higher risk of depression than a control group.

Most of our knowledge of depression among epilepsy patients is based on uncontrolled studies conducted at tertiary referral centers comprised of patients with more severe forms of epilepsy. The true prevalence of different types of depressive disorders in the general population of epileptic patients has yet to be established. Moreover, the clinical picture of depression seen in the epilepsy patients may not meet the DSM IV criteria for the affective disorders, and it has been considered to be an "atypical depression" (as discussed under Clinical Presentation of Depression in Epilepsy).

Etiologic Factors for Pathogenesis of Depression

Possible risk factors for depression in epilepsy can be organized into three broad categories: neurobiological, psychosocial, and iatrogenic. These dimensions can be viewed as potentially interacting rather than exclusive and independent. Recognizing these risk factors may lend insight into nature and treatment of chronic interictal depression.

Neurobiological Risk Factors

According to several salient studies, risk factors for depression in epilepsy include

1. Late onset of seizures: Mignone et al.[127] noted that patients with late onset seizures had higher depression scores on the Minnesota Multiphasic Personality Inventory than did those with earlier onset.

2. Partial seizures: Interictal depression is not frequent among patients with partial seizures that involve the limbic circuitry (i.e., TLE).[112,117,128,129] Dikmen et al.[130] found Minnesota Multiphasic Personality Inventory depression scale scores to be higher in patients *who had CPSs with secondary generalization* than in those with primary generalized seizures.

3. Presence of auras: Patients with *auras consisting of psychiatric symptoms* may have a higher rate of depression than those with partial seizures without auras or those with auras consisting of motor, sensory, or autonomic symptoms.[131]

4. Laterality: The issue of laterality and risk for development of depression in TLE has been a topic of considerable recent interest. Some authors believe that left temporal focus may be a predisposing factor in depression.[112,116,120,128,132] Victoroff et al.[121] recently reported a significant correlation between interictal left-sided temporal lobe hypometabolism and depression. Imaging studies support an increased *risk of depression in patients with left temporal lobe seizure origin* with concomitant PET, single-photon emission com-

puted tomography, or neuropsychological evidence of frontal lobe dysregulation.[133–135]

5. Recent use of PET and single-photon emission computed tomography in the preoperative assessment of intractable seizures has helped to clarify some of the complexities involved.[136] These studies show that the zone of hypometabolism or decreased blood flow can extend into extratemporal regions, especially frontal and subcortical regions.[136,137] This is consistent with neuropsychological findings of impaired frontal lobe functions in some of the patients with documented TLE.[138] The *combination of left temporal lobe origin and concomitant frontal lobe dysregulation* may form a potential neurobiological substrate for depression in seizures of left TLE.[139]

6. Genetic predisposition: Some investigators suggest that epilepsy patients with a family history of an affective disorder have a higher risk of developing depression than do patients lacking a genetic predisposition. Robertson and Trimble[140] concluded, "Depression is not directly interlinked with epileptic variable *per se*, but it is probably the outcome of multiple factors in the genetically predisposed individual." Alterations of various *biochemical systems* involving norepinephrine, dopamine, serotonin, and GABA as well as dysfunction of the hypothalamic-pituitary axis may contribute to the etiology of both epilepsy and mood disorders.[141] Animal studies show that chronic seizures are associated with sleep disturbances with decreased rapid eye movement sleep.[69] AEDs such as barbiturates and benzodiazepines suppress rapid eye movement sleep.[142] This chronic sleep deprivation may cause various abnormal behaviors, personality changes, and mood disorders.

Psychosocial Risk Factors

Multiple psychological factors can contribute to the occurrence of depression in epilepsy. A large body of literature has addressed the relationship between the depression and so-called "external locus of control" in relation to epilepsy.[143] The repeated exposure to essentially random, adverse events (seizures) over which the patient has minimal volitional control leads to fears and vulnerability. An external locus of control is more prevalent among children with epilepsy compared to children with other chronic disorders.[144] Another elaboration of this relationship termed *learned helplessness* has been found to apply to the epilepsy-depression relationship.[145] Other commonly encountered stresses include the patient's lack of acceptance and poor adjustment to epilepsy,[146] the stigma associated with a diagnosis of epilepsy, and the experience of discrimination. Living with epilepsy promotes dependence on the spouse or social support to make a significant adjustment in lifestyle, such as relinquishing driving or changing jobs to ensure that seizure precautions can be closely observed.[147–149] Other difficulties faced by individuals with epilepsy include maintaining employment or insurance coverage; disinclination to participate in sports, neighborhood activities, or social relationships; and a high divorce rate.

Iatrogenic Risk Factors

The relationship between AEDs and mood and cognitive abnormalities has been reported with many of the older as well as the new compounds. Barbiturates (phenobarbital and primidone) have been implicated in AED-associated depression in a number of investigations. Major depression was noted in 40% of patients receiving phenobarbital versus 4% in those receiving carbamazepine in one classic study.[150,151] Some of the earlier papers reported that *barbiturates* and *phenytoin* (PHT) can cause reduction of *folic acid* levels, which may have some relationship with depression.[152–154] Suicidal ideation is higher in patients using phenobarbital. TGB, topiramate, vigabatrin (VGB),[155–157] and felbamate are newer AEDs reported to occasionally cause symptoms of depression. AEDs with mood-stabilizing properties, such as carbamazepine and VPA, occasionally cause depression but with a significantly lower frequency than other AEDs.[158]

Clinical Presentation of Depression in Epilepsy

The recognition of depression in patients with epilepsy is often ignored for a variety of reasons, including the patient's tendency to minimize psychiatric symptoms for fear of being further stigmatized, atypical presentation of depression in epilepsy, and because clinicians fail to ask about the psychiatric symptoms or minimize their importance. Depressive disorders can be conveniently classified as ictal, peri-ictal, or interictal, depending on their temporal relationship between psychiatric symptoms and seizure occurrence.

Interictal Depression

Interictal depressive disorder is the most frequently recognized psychiatric disorder in patients with epilepsy.[116] However, most interictal depressive disorders do not meet formal DSM-IV criteria for major depression. In a study by Mendez,[159] 50% of epilepsy patients were classified to have atypical depression according to DSM III-R criteria. Atypical features included more paranoia and psychotic symptoms that were peri-ictal and resolved with antiepileptic treatment. These patients were also reported to have increased *irritability* and *emotionality*. The psychotic features may have been part of a major depressive disorder (MDD), representing a more severe form of disorder (MDD with psychotic features) or part of a schizoaffective disorder coexisting with an affective component.

Blumer emphasized the pleomorphic pattern of the affective disorder in epilepsy (consistent with Kraepelin's observations in 1923) and coined the term *interictal dysphoric disorder*.[160] The symptoms have an intermittent course and are categorized into *depressive-somatoform*, consisting of depressed mood, anergia, vague pains, insomnia, and the like, and *affective*, characterized by irritability, euphoric mood, fear, and anxiety. All of these have been considered to be depressive equivalents.[118,161–164] Because of its relative milder severity, interictal dysphoric disorder's diagnosis and treatment is often neglected.

Many studies suggest that interictal depression in epilepsy mimics a dysthymic disorder, with endogenous features and an intermittent course[112,128,133,159,164,165] with a symptom-free period of days to weeks. In a severe form, the pattern may be similar to double depression, which is a chronic dysthymic disorder with a superimposed MDD.[160]

Ictal and Peri-Ictal Affective Symptoms

Ictal Depression and Mania. Mood change can accompany partial seizures in which symptoms of depression or mania consist of its sole presentation. Williams[166] examined 2,000 epilepsy patients considered to be living normal lives. Out of these, 100 experienced ictal emotions, 65 were noted as having *ictal fear,* and another 21 as experiencing a depression of varying severity.[166] In eight patients, ictal depression persisted in the postictal period, lasting up to 3 days, and five patients developed suicidal ideation with one suicide completion. *Ictal laughter* and *crying* have been documented, mostly presenting as CPSs with the former more frequent than the latter.[167] However, in these events, the patient's experience of the true emotion is variable.

If mood change is the only symptom of partial seizures, then diagnosis may be difficult. Ictal affective symptoms are usually brief and stereotyped, occurring out of context and often associated with other ictal phenomenon. Common symptoms are fear and sadness; other symptoms include guilt, anhedonia, and suicidal ideation. As the seizure evolves from simple to complex partial, depression symptoms are followed by alteration in consciousness.[168–170]

Peri-Ictal Depression and Mania. *Peri-ictal mania* is unusual, and few case reports exist. Williams found nine patients who experienced "pleasure" peri-ictally, with three noting "elation."[166] Manic symptoms usually follow an increased seizure frequency during a "normal period" after the ictal events.[21,171,172] *Peri-ictal depression* presents as a dysphoric mood before or after the seizure event.[166,169,173] In children, dysphoria manifests as irritability, poor frustration tolerance, or aggressive behavior.[174] A recent study[175] reported postictal depression in 56 of 100 patients with poorly controlled partial seizure patients, with a mean duration of 37 hours. Postictal depression is more common in patients with *unilateral frontal* or *temporal seizure focus* without lateral predominance.[83]

Suicide in Epilepsy

Among all patients with epilepsy, the estimated risk of death by suicide is 3–22% or four to five times higher than those for general population.[123] Among those with CPSs of temporal lobe origin, the risk of suicide is as much as 25 times greater.[122] Furthermore, as many as one-third of all patients with epilepsy have attempted suicide at some point in time.[112] Successful suicide attempts have occurred more frequently with interictal depression. Brief peri-ictal psychotic or depressive episodes can also lead to sudden acts of suicide.[176–178] Risk factors for suicide in epilepsy include TLE, a history of psychiatric hospitalization[179,180] (indicator of severe psychiatric pathology), and epilepsy severe enough to warrant treatment in a tertiary epilepsy center. Patients are most likely to complete suicide when they have psychosis with paranoid hallucinations, agitated compunction to kill themselves, and occasional ictal command hallucinations to commit suicide.[181]

Treatment of Depression in Epilepsy

Comorbid depression in epilepsy is under-recognized and undertreated.[139] There are only a few double-blind, placebo-controlled studies of therapy of depression in epilepsy patients.[182] As an initial approach, it is imperative to determine whether the patient's depressive symptoms are peri-ictal or interictal. Peri-ictal depression is best treated with optimization of AED therapy rather than the use of psychotropics, which may further lower the seizure threshold. Interictal symptoms are much more common than are peri-ictal symptoms, and their etiology may be multifactorial. The management of interictal depression involves addressing the patient's psychological and psychosocial issues. Involvement of a *multidisciplinary team* consisting of a neurologist, psychiatrist, social worker, and epilepsy nurse may be helpful. Treatment issues for depression in epilepsy can be categorized under the following categories.

Reevaluate the Anticonvulsant Regimen

Potential contribution of AED's adverse psychotropic effects should be examined:

1. Depressive symptoms may reflect side effects or toxic reaction to barbiturates and PHT,[150,151] as well as the newer AEDs.[155–157]
2. Discontinuation of AEDs with mood-stabilizing effects, such as carbamazepine or VPA, can provoke depressive, hypomanic, or manic symptoms. Clinicians should determine the timing of the onset of depressive symptoms relative to initiation or change of AED.
3. Polypharmacy: Many AEDs can adversely affect the mental state of epilepsy patients, some of whom show overt psychiatric illness.[183] If possible, treat seizures with one AED rather than with several. A reduction in the number of AEDs can improve mood, demeanor, and cognitive function.[184–186]
4. Consider the use of psychoactive AEDs.[187] The psychotropic properties of AEDs are particularly important in the management of depression.[188] These medications may relieve some behavioral symptoms through direct psychotropic properties or through their effects on seizure control.[189] Carbamazepine, VPA, lamotrigine (LTG), and gabapentin (GPN) can be considered for their mood-stabilizing effects.

Use of Antidepressants to Treat Depression in Epilepsy

Antidepressant's Effect on Lowering Seizure Threshold. Many psychotropic agents (antidepressants and antipsychotics) have the theoretical capacity to lower the seizure threshold.[190–192] Most antidepressants block the reuptake of norepinephrine or serotonin, or both, at the synaptic cleft. These neurotransmitters can have a anticonvulsant effect in animals and humans.[193] However, it appears that a reuptake blockade of *neurotransmitters* (the proposed antidepressant action) is not the cause of proconvulsant action, as observed in many of these drugs.[188,194,195] Studies in epilepsy-prone rats found that depletion of brain monoamines with reserpine did not change the incidence of seizures caused by large doses of the antidepressant desipramine.[193]

Clinicians can be reassured that the use of antidepressants in epilepsy patients does not usually pose a significant problem, and the risk can be significantly minimized by appropriate measures. Tricyclic antidepressants (TCAs) are more likely to increase seizure frequency than are selective monoamine oxidase-A inhibitors (MAOIs) and selective serotonin reuptake inhibitors (SSRIs).[160,182,196–198] The incidence of seizures with different antidepressant and antipsychotic medications is displayed in Tables 20-3 and 20-4. The following strategy may be helpful in the use of antidepressants:

1. Commence therapy at a low dose and then increase it slowly. Psychotropic drugs are most convulsive when introduced rapidly or given in high doses.

2. Monitor the plasma levels of AEDs and antidepressant drugs (specifically TCAs). There are no reports in the literature of TCA-induced seizures at therapeutic plasma concentrations. Patients who present with seizures on therapeutic dosage of TCAs have been found to be slow metabolizers of these drugs.[182,199–202]

3. Depression in epilepsy patients may respond to less than the recommended dosages (approximately equivalent to half) for nonepileptic patients.[163,203–205] Therefore, treat with the lowest effective dosage and review regularly.

Choice of Antidepressants. SSRIs should be considered as a *first-line treatment* in depressed patients with epilepsy.[206] SSRIs, generally well tolerated in overdose, have a favorable adverse effects profile (vs. TCAs), and their propensity for causing seizures is low.[204,207] The major concern with their use is drug interactions with AEDs because of their effects on hepatic P-450 cytochrome metabolic enzyme systems (see under Drug Interactions). Currently used SSRIs include fluoxetine, sertraline, paroxetine, fluvoxamine, citalopram, roboxetine, and venlafaxine. Fluoxetine may have a higher seizure induction frequency in comparison with others (0.2% vs. 0.1% for paroxetine).[200] Nefazodone, trazodone, and mirtazapine are also considered to pose a minimal risk in the event of overdose. Monoamine oxidase inhibitors, types A and B, including maclobemide (not released in the United States), appear to be safe drugs for use in epilepsy[158] but are used less frequently because of other potentially serious side effects.

TCAs are effective but have the risk of cardiotoxicity and severe complications with overdoses. Among the TCAs, doxepine may be less epileptogenic, and clomipramine may be more epileptogenic than others. Maprotiline and amoxapine should be avoided because of high seizure potential with overdose.[200,208,209]

Bupropion should also be avoided because of its low therapeutic index.[158,200,210,211]

Lithium carbonate (the first antimanic drug used to treat bipolar patients) is often used to augment the antidepressant action of SSRIs and TCAs and is

Table 20-3. Relative Seizure Risk during Therapeutic Use of Psychotropics

High Risk	Intermediate Risk	Low Risk
Antidepressants		
Bupropion (HD)	(MD to LD)	
Clomipramine (HD)	(MD to LD)	
Maprotiline (HD)	(MD to LD)	
	Fluoxamine	
	TCA	(LD)
	(HD to MD)	
	Venlafaxine	Fluoxetine
		MAO inhibitors
		Mirtazapine
		Nefazodone
		Paroxetine
		Sertraline
		Trazodone
Antipsychotics		
Chlorpromazine (HD)	(MD to LD)	
Clozapine (HD to MD)	(LD)	Fluphenazine
	Olanzapine	
	Quetiapine	Haloperidol
	Thioridazine	Molindone
		Pimozide
		Risperdone
		Trifluoperazine

HD = high dose; LD = low dose; MAO = monoamine oxidase; MD = moderate dose.

considered to have problems for its use in epilepsy patients. Its use includes changes in EEG recordings and lowering of seizure threshold at therapeutic dosages in epileptic and nonepileptic patients.[158]

Drug Interactions between Antiepileptic Drugs and Antidepressant Medications. Before making a decision for use of an antidepressant in epilepsy patients, carefully consider the potential drug interactions between AEDs and antidepressants. A detailed listing of such drug interactions is covered later in this chapter (also see Chapter 26).

When the metabolic route for two drugs (e.g., an SSRI and an AED) involves the same cytochrome P-450 isoenzyme in liver, significant drug interactions can occur owing to induction or inhibition of metabolism. AEDs with *enzyme-inducing properties*

Table 20-4. Psychotropic and Anticonvulsant Drug Interactions

Antiepileptic Drugs	Psychotropic Drug Class			
	Antidepressants	Neuroleptics	Antimanics	Anxiolytics
Barbituates	Barbituate may ↓ TCA level ↑ Sedative effects of TCAs and MAOIs SSRIs may ↑ the phenobarbital levels	↑ Sedation with clozapine and CBZ ↓ Neuroleptic levels	VPA may ↑ barbiturate levels ↓ CBZ levels	Phenobarbital may ↓ benzodiazepine levels Additive sedative effects
Carbamazepine	CBZ ↓ TCA levels ↑ Levels of CBZ with fluoxetine and fluvoxamine	↓ Neuroleptic levels: Haldol, Olanzapine, and risperidone CBZ and Clozaril, both may induce leukopenia	↑ Lithium levels Neurotoxicity reported in absence of lithium ↑ Lithium + CBZ can have additive antithyroid effects	CBZ may ↓ benzodiazepine levels
Valproate	One report of ↓ VPA Half-life with amitriptyline SSRIs may ↑ VPA levels	Chlorpromazine may ↑ VPA levels VPA may ↑ neuroleptic levels ↓ Total clozapine level, unbound, unchanged	↓ VPA levels with CBZ	VPA ↑ diazepam effects by displacing it from protein binding
Phenytoin	TCAs may ↑ PHT levels PHT may ↓ TCA level Fluoxetine may cause PHT toxicity	Phenothiazines may ↑ or ↓ PHT levels PHT may ↓ clozapine levels	Possible risk of ↑ lithium toxicity	PHT may ↓ benzodiazepine levels, additive sedation Benzodiazepines may ↑ or ↓ PHT levels
Lamotrigine	—	—	VPA may ↓ LTG metabolism (by 25%), LTG ↑ by twofold CBZ ↓ lamotrigine concentration by 40%	—
Topiramate	—	—	CBZ results in ↓ topiramate levels VPA: slight ↓ in level of both drugs	—

↑ = increase; ↓ = decrease; CBZ = carbamazepine; LTG = lamotrigine; MAOIs = monoamine oxidase inhibitors; PHT = phenytoin; SSRIs = selective serotonin reuptake inhibitors; TCA = tricyclic antidepressants; VPA = valproic acid.

(PHT, carbamazepine, phenobarbital, and primidone) can increase the metabolism of antidepressants, thus requiring an adjustment in their dosages. This pharmacokinetic effect is not caused by newer AEDs such as GPN, LTG, and topiramate. On the other hand, some SSRIs can alter AEDs metabolism by inhibiting several isoenzymes of the cytochrome P-450 system. These include fluvoxamine, fluoxetine, and paroxetine. Sertraline and citalopram are less likely to have interactions with AEDs.[212–215]

Electroconvulsive Therapy

Electroconvulsive therapy is an effective treatment for patients with severe major depression, especially when it is accompanied with psychotic features. It is usually considered when MDD is refractory to medications.[216] Electroconvulsive therapy is not contraindicated in depressed patients with epilepsy[217] and can actually raise the seizure threshold considerably during the course of several procedures.[158] Lithium should be discontinued 5 days before electroconvulsive therapy because of increased risk for prolonged seizures and memory loss.

Psychotherapy

The patient's psychological factors and psychosocial maladjustment are important issues contributing to affective disorders in epilepsy patients. Psychotherapy is largely neglected in the care of epilepsy patients. The selection of a psychiatric intervention (cognitive-behavioral, supportive, group and family therapy, biofeedback, or relaxation techniques) depends on different aspects of the patient, including intelligence, personality characteristics, family support, coping skills, and social environment. Issues of "self-esteem, dependency, fear of loss of control, helplessness, stigmatization, marital and job difficulties"[143–149] are crucial and need to be addressed in the frame of psychotherapeutic interventions. An initial effort toward the education of patient and family members about relevant topics (e.g., understanding of epilepsy, comorbidity of psychiatric disorders, medications, and availability of the possible resources) may also help the overall therapeutic endeavor.

Fear and Anxiety Disorders in Epilepsy

There are fewer studies of epilepsy and anxiety disorders than of depression or psychosis, perhaps because of difficulty in separating the normal or situational anxiety accompanying a chronic disease from a "pathologic or endogenous" anxiety. There is a close association between anxiety and depression, with many of the same factors precipitating both affective states. The DSM IV describes 11 anxiety disorders; however, the more relevant disorders in the context of epilepsy are panic disorder (with or without agoraphobia), generalized anxiety disorder (GAD), and obsessive-compulsive disorder (OCD).

Prevalence of Anxiety Disorders in Epilepsy

Anxiety disorders are the leading psychiatric comorbidity in epilepsy. Williams[166] found that 65 of 2,000 patients (3%) experienced ictal fear. In a large epidemiologic study in the United States, epilepsy patients were reported to have a six times higher incidence of panic disorder than controls.[218] Currie et al.[118] found that 19% of their 666 TLE patients had anxiety disorders. However, the prevalence of anxiety disorders was found to be even higher (31.67%) among the patients with intractable seizures admitted to V-EEG monitoring units for presurgical evaluation.[219] At our tertiary epilepsy center,[220] 57% of the adult epilepsy patients met criteria for high anxiety as measured by the Spielberger State-Trait Anxiety Inventory[221]; there was a strong relationship between a number of psychological difficulties and anxiety.

Etiologic Risk Factors for Anxiety Disorders in Epilepsy

As in depression, these factors are multidimensional and mutually interacting rather than exclusive and independent. They are broadly considered under the descriptors neurobiological, psychosocial, and iatrogenic.

Neurobiological Factors

Seizure localization, type, and severity may play an important role in the presentation of anxiety symptoms. Fear and anxiety are common ictal symptoms in TLE[166] and have been localized to *anteromedial temporal lobe*[222] or other limbic regions.[223] Recent brain-imaging studies using PET[224] and magnetic resonance imaging[225] suggest that the *disturbance in nonepileptic panic disorder may be localized to the temporal lobes as well*. This and other case reports[226–228] describe panic attack as a symptom with clear-cut pathologic CNS disorders. Perini and Mendius[229] reported that anxiety disorders were higher among patients with epileptic foci *lateralized to the left hemisphere*, compared to those on right. Penfield and Jasper used electrical stimulation to evoke fear responses in patients undergoing a presurgical evaluation for intractable seizure,[222] whereas Gloor et al.[223] were able to elicit anxiety symptoms with stimulation of the *amygdala*. Theoretically, *kindling mechanisms* may be responsible for development of interictal anxiety states by repeated seizures of the amygdala, resulting in its neuronal hyperexcitability.[230]

Iatrogenic Factors

Anxiety is a significant AED side effect, as noted in patients treated with topiramate,[231] VGB,[232] and felbamate.[233] Depression and anxiety symptoms are frequently reported symptoms induced by *withdrawal of AEDs* among patients undergoing V-EEG monitoring for evaluation of intractable seizures or in preparation for clinical drug trials.[234–236] Bladin[237] reported a high incidence of anxiety disorders (54% of his 107 patients) as a *postsurgical outcome* of anterotemporal lobectomy for intractable seizures.

Psychosocial Factors

Patient anxieties related to their epileptic condition may be very severe and are often under-recognized by clinicians. *Fear of death, brain damage*, and *mental deterioration* were particularly prominent anxieties reported in a survey of epilepsy patients at one center.[238] In parents of children with epilepsy, there may be another set of anxieties that can lead them to be *overprotective* or *overindulgent*, leading to a transmission of fearfulness to their children. The psychological and psychosocial factors, discussed in the etiology of depression and epilepsy, may also contribute. Anxiety and depression may be related to *learned helplessness*, a reaction to the unpredictable, uncontrollable aversive event of a seizure. In this situation, a patient with epilepsy may adopt a passive, victimized stance, which may lead to anxiety and depression.[239–241] Another factor is the stigma commonly associated with having seizures.

Clinical Presentation of Anxiety Disorders in Epilepsy

Anxiety disorders can present during the peri-ictal, ictal, or interictal period. The peri-ictal anxiety disorder has been reported,[242] but ictal fear (which needs to be differentiated from panic disorder) is more frequent.[166] Interictal anxiety disorder is seen most commonly in clinical practice. The latter may be comorbid with depressive disorders.

Ictal Fear

Jackson[243] was the first to describe how fear could be a part of an ictus itself rather than an anticipatory reaction to an oncoming seizure. Fear can be an isolated symptom of a simple partial seizure without other ictal phenomenon, or it can be the "aura" of a seizure that evolves. Autonomic symptoms (e.g., palpitations, tachycardia, shortness of breath, shaking, flushing or pallor, nausea and a rising epigastric sensation) can accompany ictal fear in simple partial seizures, whereas typical automatism-related movements may be seen with CPSs. Some authors claim that patients with ictal fear exhibit more psychopathology than do other patients with CPSs,[244,245] but this association has been refuted.[246] Although fear is not a frequent enough symptom during seizures to be a primary cause of anxiety in most epilepsy patients, ictal fear may be associated with higher rates of anxiety interictally.[244]

Panic Disorder

Health professionals dealing with epilepsy should strongly consider *panic disorder* in the differential diagnosis of paroxysmal neurologic events. Panic disorder is characterized by spontaneously occurring episodes of intense fear or discomfort reaching a peak within 10 minutes and is associated with numerous physical symptoms.[247] According to DSM IV, the diagnosis of panic disorder[248] requires at least 4 of the following 13 symptoms: palpitations, sweating, trembling, shortness of breath, sensation of choking, chest pain, abdominal discomfort, dizziness, derealization, fear of loss of control or death, paraesthesias, or chills. Panic disorder may be associated with anticipatory anxiety or phobic avoidant behavior, or both (in that case called *panic disorder with agoraphobia*). Symptoms of panic disorder may overlap with partial seizures. In panic disorder, consciousness is preserved during the event and symptoms may last several minutes to hours (vs. several seconds to minutes in ictal fear),[249] and it is usually not associated with postepisode confusion. A careful history, along with routine EEG or V-EEG monitoring, when indicated, is helpful in distinguishing these two disorders. However, the scalp EEG does not always detect very localized discharges.[250] Furthermore, patients may have epilepsy and panic disorder.[251]

Obsessive-Compulsive Disorder

In DSM IV,[248] OCD is characterized by recurrent obsessions or compulsions that are excessive and unreasonable. Obsessionality has been attributed to patients with TLE,[55] as are compulsions, particularly writing.[252] Tourette's syndrome, postencephalitic Parkinson's disease, and Sydenham's chorea may overlap with OCD, suggesting that organic factors may contribute to its pathophysiology. As with OCD in nonepileptic populations, OCD patients tend to be reluctant to reveal their symptoms; thus comorbid OCD may be unrecognized. Pathophysiologic factors, such as limbic system abnormalities in these two disorders, particularly involving the amygdala, may overlap.[253] Stimulation of the amygdala may produce both anxiety and "forced thinking," which, symptomatically, closely resembles obsessions. Although cases of linking epilepsy and OCD have been reported, a clear-cut relationship between the two conditions has yet to be demonstrated.[254]

Generalized Anxiety Disorder

Generalized anxiety disorder is more frequently found among patients with partial seizures related to limbic foci, but a higher prevalence has also been reported in patients with generalized epilepsy. The etiopathogenesis of interictal anxiety disorder (GAD) is complex, and a clear neurobiological link between GAD and epilepsy has not been established. Psychological mechanisms to explain interictal anxiety (GAD) are multiple and complex and include fear of seizure recurrence, issues surrounding locus of control, learned helplessness, and various psychosocial factors.

Treatment of Anxiety Disorders in Epilepsy

As in depression, a multidisciplinary approach to the management of anxiety disorders is most effective. This includes pharmacologic management of anxiety, cognitive behavioral therapy, individual and group psychotherapy, and stress reduction techniques.

Antidepressant drugs also have anxiolytic properties, but selecting the agent and titrating the dose requires patience and extra attention to multiple factors discussed earlier (e.g., potential for lowering seizure threshold, side effect profile, CP-450 drug interaction of SSRIs with AEDs).

Benzodiazepines are commonly prescribed to treat anxiety, although abrupt withdrawal of benzodiazepines should be avoided, as this may precipitate withdrawal seizures. *Clonazepam* is effective in the treatment of panic disorder,[255] and, because of its usefulness as an adjunctive treatment of seizure disorders, it is frequently used in this population. Its long half-life renders it better tolerated and less addicting.

Aggressive Behavior in Epilepsy

Although aggressive behavior in epilepsy has provoked public interest and is occasionally used as a legal defense, study of this phenomenon is limited. The literature is based mainly on anecdotal reports. Misconceptions linking epilepsy with violence have disproportionately emphasized the nature of this relationship[256] and aggravate the psychosocial stigma already associated with epilepsy. Most directed aggression in epilepsy correlates less with seizures than with indirect factors such as psychosis, "episodic dyscontrol" (intermittent explosive disorder with ictal-like feature), subnormal intelligence, lower socioeconomic status, prior head injuries, and possible orbitofrontal damage.[257–259]

Ictal aggression is rare. Primary ictal aggression results from ictal discharges involving the areas of the brain responsible for aggression. Secondary ictal aggression results from a disinhibition of social behavior by an ictal EEG discharge. Aggressive behavior exhibited during a seizure is usually nondirected and clumsy, leading to little risk of injury from a patient. Dangerous acts of violence are exceptional.[260,261] In a study of 5,400 epilepsy patients, only 19 had possible ictal aggressive behavior. Most patients with a higher degree of aggression were mentally impaired and had a history of psychiatric disorders and interictal aggressive behaviors. Ictal aggressive behavior is seen mainly in association with CPSs of frontal or temporal lobe origin.

In the postictal confusional period, usually after more severe convulsive episodes, adverse verbal or physical behaviors may occur.[262] Because the postictal state is self limited, there is usually no need for specific physical or pharmacologic intervention. Patients in postictal states should receive verbal stimulation that helps to reorient them; such patients should not be physically restrained, as this may elicit aggressive behavior. Behavioral abnormalities in nonepileptic patients may be sometimes confused with seizures (see Chapter 19). V-EEG monitoring can distinguish episodic dyscontrol from epileptic activity.

Sexuality and Epilepsy

Both men and women with epilepsy experience disturbance of sexual arousal and a lowered sexual drive.[263,264] Women with TLE have 14–20% amenorrhea rates, and more than 50% have some form of menstrual dysfunction.[265,266] One-third of the cycles are anovulatory, compared to 8% among healthy controls.[267] Fertility is reduced to 69–80% of the expected number of offsprings.[268] Men with TLE have 49–71% rates of diminished potency or sexual interest.[269,270] Besides hyposexuality, there are case reports of sexual deviation, mostly fetishism and transvestism, but a statistical relationship between sexual perversions and epilepsy has not been convincingly demonstrated.

Although controversial, some data suggest that sexual interest and function may be more impaired among patients with epilepsy of temporal lobe origin than with generalized or focal motor seizures. An earlier age of onset is associated with more severe hyposexuality, whereas seizure onset after puberty correlates with better sexual health. Although there is no direct correlation of seizure frequency to severity of hyposexuality, *seizure cessation* with medication or surgery may increase sexual interest.[271] Sexual dysfunction in patients with epilepsy[272,273] may partly be due to AED-induced hepatic metabolism of sex hormones. Many studies on hormonal and endocrine effects report an *increase in plasma sex hormone–binding globulin*, at least partly caused by AED hepatic induction; an increase in luteinizing hormone and follicle stimulating hormone; and a decrease in free testosterone and free testosterone fraction.[271]

Sexual dysfunction may also be due to central mechanisms, particularly *limbic dysfunction* from a seizure focus, causing hyposexuality and hormonal abnormalities.[274] Limbic regions have direct and reciprocal connections with hypothalamic nuclei. Stimulation and ablation of specific amygdaloid nuclei can alter the release of luteinizing hormone, follicle-stimulating hormone, thyroid-stimulating hormone, and prolactin.[275] Furthermore, estrogen and progesterone receptors on limbic neurons can directly influence the threshold for seizure activity.[276] Estrogen has convulsant properties, and progesterone has anticonvulsant effects. Catamenial epilepsy (i.e., the perimenstrual increase of seizures in women with epilepsy) may reflect the epileptogenic effect of high estrogen concentrations relative to those of progesterone.[277,278]

Cognitive Impairment in Epilepsy

Most patients with epilepsy lead normal lives with minimal or no cognitive impairments; however, some patients develop significant cognitive deficits in the domain of attention, psychomotor abilities, and memory. Cognitive and psychiatric disruptions can interact with one another to further exacerbate neurobehavioral functioning and thereby dramatically reduce quality of life.[279]

Cognitive Dysfunction (Major Types of Dysfunction Seen)

Cognitive functioning is the product of complex interaction of neuronal circuits that govern motivation, attention, language, memory, executive functions, intelligence, and other mental abilities (see Table 20-5, which summarizes cognitive domains and how they can be affected in epilepsy). Neuropsychological tests results for different cognitive domains and for different epilepsy syndromes are reviewed elsewhere.[138,279–281]

Risk Factors for Cognitive Dysfunction

Patients with *symptomatic epilepsy* are more likely to have impaired intellect than are those with idiopathic epilepsy.[282] *Pre-existing brain damage* is an important variable but may not entirely explain neuropsychological deficits. Factors related to epi-

Table 20-5. Domains of Cognitive Functioning Affected by Epilepsy

Domain	Affected Function	Functions not Affected
Language	Anomia	Comprehension
	Fluency/word generation	Repetition
	Oral reading	Writing
Attention	Simple attention (digit span)	Complex attention
	Simple reaction time	Divided/choice reaction time
	Sustained concentration	
	Vigilance	
Memory	Consolidation and delayed recall	Remote memory
	Verbal memory (e.g., paragraph)	Factual information
	Verbal learning (e.g., word lists/pairs)	
	Nonverbal memory (e.g., designs, faces)	
Executive systems	Concept formation	Impulse control
	Perseveration	Self-monitoring
	Cognitive flexibility	
	Alteration of cognitive set	
Visuospatial	Most areas not affected	Constructional ability
		Perception and integration
		Neglect and hemi-inattention
Sensory/integrative	Most areas not affected	Tactile perception
		Praxis
		Cross-modal integration
Motor	Fine motor dexterity	Gross motor strength
	Motor sequencing	Tone, reflexes, coordination
	Psychomotor speed	
Intelligence	Varies	Varies

Source: Reproduced wth permission from K Perrine. Cognitive deficits in epilepsy and contribution to psychopathology. Neurology 1999;55(Suppl 2):S39–S45.

lepsy may contribute to cognitive disturbances.[283] Among seizure-related variables, age of onset, duration of epilepsy, seizure type, and seizure frequency have been examined. Early age of onset is a poor prognostic factor for intelligence. Dodrill[284] examined the long-term effects of seizures on psychological tasks and noted that a lifelong history of more than 100 convulsions is associated with decreased functioning in a variety of areas. Seidenberg et al.[285] reported improved intellectual functioning with decreased seizure frequency after a test-retest interval.

Seizure Type and Pattern of Cognitive Dysfunction

Patients with TLE are particularly vulnerable to disturbances of language and memory.[286,287] Left TLE patients may have *fixed long-term deficits* on tests of verbal list learning, cued verbal recall,

and semantic encoding, whereas patients with right TLE may perform poorly on tests of nonverbal memory.[288,289] *Accelerated forgetting* occurs in some TLE patients, characterized by normal retention of new information over hours to days but amnesia for information from longer time periods.[290,291] This accelerated forgetting may reflect the disruptive effects of seizures on the long-term consolidation of new information.[275]

Patients with *generalized seizures* have more deficits of *attention* and *concentration* compared to patients with focal seizures. Patients with generalized *absence seizures* show minimal interictal cognitive dysfunction. If absences are frequent, then impaired performance in the classroom setting may lead to educational underachievement. Even "subclinical focal discharges" may cause transient cognitive impairment on selective tasks during brief interictal EEG focal discharges.[292]

A dementia of epilepsy[106] is characterized by cognitive deterioration but is different from progressive parenchymatous degenerative dementias. Retrospective studies[293] indicate that such a dementia may be associated with multiple factors, such as generalized tonic-clonic seizures with recurrent head injury and the prescription of certain AEDs—notably, PHT and primidone.

Etiology of Cognitive Deficits in Epilepsy

Cognitive deficits in epilepsy can arise from multiple interacting factors. The most common causes are ongoing cortical disruption caused by the seizures and interictal discharges, AEDs, underlying neuropathology, and head trauma. TLE may be associated with *atypical patterns of hemispheric specialization*, probably because of the cerebral reorganization that induces it. For example, left-handed and right cerebral dominance for language are more common in TLE than in the general population.[275]

Head trauma is a frequent cause of epilepsy and is usually associated with some degree of cognitive impairment, particularly from contusions, shearing of white matter, or regions of encephalomalacia. Among patients with *symptomatic epilepsy, neoplasms* or *vascular malformations* should be considered. Vascular malformations, such as angiomas, cavernomas, or arteriovenous malformations, do not usually cause cognitive deficits directly, unless they are large or cause major hemorrhages. Small, slow-growing tumors are not usually associated with discrete cognitive deficits, but more rapid-growing neoplasms, such as high-grade astrocytomas, may be more obviously complicated by cognitive decline. *Infectious processes* leading to epilepsy can have profound effects on cognition. Encephalitis can cause severe memory impairments. PHT-associated encephalopathy has been discussed since the early descriptions of dilantin dementia by Rosen.[294] However, it affects only a minority of patients, and other metabolic factors, such as folate deficiency, may be involved.

Cognitive Effects of Antiepileptic Drugs

Extensive reviews on cognitive effects of AEDs[282,295] are briefly summarized here. Generally, the data favor the newer AEDs, carbamazepine, sodium valproate, and VGB, and emphasize more cognitive impairments with *PHT* and *phenobarbital.*[296–299] Phenobarbital and primidone can affect psychomotor speed and vigilance,[300] cognitive speed,[301] motor functions,[302] memory and concentration, and intelligence quotient.[303,304]

Limited data suggest that *newer AEDs have fewer side effects* than standard AEDs. Studies targeting the effects of TGB,[305] GPN,[306] LTG,[307] and VGB[308] demonstrated few to no effects on neuropsychological functioning, although high doses of these medications can cause sedation, altered mood, or even psychosis.[309] However, topiramate has gained recent notoriety for occasionally inducing psychomotor slowing, language impairments, difficulty with concentration, confusion, and psychiatric disturbances (see under Psychiatric or Behavioral Effects of Antiepileptic Drugs).

Cognitive impairment with specific AEDs is usually related to dosages that produce high therapeutic or *toxic AED blood levels.*[310] Irrespective of the specific agents used, polytherapy substantially raises the risk of cognitive impairments. Therefore, in patients on *polytherapy*, reducing the number of administered AEDs improves cognitive function over a wide range of cognitive abilities.[311] Considerable *individual variations* in drug tolerance for different AEDs should also be considered. The impairment associated with AEDs tends to affect concentration, attention, and psychomotor abilities more than memory functions. Memory deficits can result from recurrent seizures, temporal lobe lesions, or temporal lobectomy. Conversely, memory functions have been known to improve after *effective control of seizures* with AEDs or surgery (especially in the nondominant temporal lobe).

Mental Status Examination or Neuropsychological Testing and Localization of Seizures

Many epilepsy patients who complain of cognitive difficulties perform fairly well on the commonly used Mini-Mental State Examination administered by clinicians. Such bedside exams may identify gross cognitive deficits that occur in dementia or stroke but are not sensitive for mild to moderate cognitive impairments common to epilepsy patients.

Formal neuropsychological testing is often required.

Patients with generalized epilepsy have mild, generalized, cognitive deficits. Patients with partial seizures may show lateralized patterns of cognitive deficits, reflecting the unilateral seizure focus. For example, a left temporal lobe seizure focus may be associated with anomia and verbal memory deficits (list generation tasks deficits).[312] Although impairments in recall of geometric figures or faces would be expected with right temporal seizures, recent studies have not confirmed this.[280] Seizures with frontal lobe onset can result in executive function deficits, including problems in complex motor speed, sequencing, concept formation, set shifting, and inhibition of competing responses. Patients with a parietal lobe focus may show deficits in more complex or cross-modal functions, such as praxis, reading, writing (if the focus is in the left parietal lobe), and constructional ability (if the focus is in right parietal lobe).

Optimizing cognitive functioning in epilepsy patients depends on understanding the factors underlying the cognitive deficits. Decreasing the frequency of seizures with rational use of AEDs can improve cognitive function. Psychiatric disorders can coexist and exacerbate the cognitive deficits.

Quality of Life Assessment

Health-related quality of life includes aspects of physical, psychological, and social well being for people with epilepsy. A recent study by Herman et al.[313] reported that comorbid interictal psychiatric symptoms are elevated among patients with TLE compared to healthy controls and appear to be modestly associated with increasing chronicity (duration) of epilepsy. The study also concludes that comorbid emotional-behavioral distress is specifically associated with a significantly poorer health-related quality of life and suggests that quality of life research should devote greater attention to the potential impact of comorbid psychiatric distress.

Recently developed quality of life in epilepsy (QOLIE) questionnaires can be used to assess the effects of seizures and medications on cognitive function, memory, mood, and physical health as perceived by the patient. The information derived from QOLIE is often inadequately elicited in the typical clinical interview,[314] because clinicians tend to focus on seizure type and frequency rather than the way in which a seizure affects a patient's quality of life. The QOLIE self-report[315] measure helps direct the clinician's attention to important domains, including seizure worry, overall quality of life, emotional well being, cognitive effects, medication effects, social function, and overall health. The more detailed 89-item QOLIE survey may be most useful for the research purposes. A more simplified 31-item version has also been developed.

Many physicians may find the abbreviated 10-item QOLIE measure to be most efficient for use in the clinical setting. The QOLIE-10 assesses worries related to seizures, emotional well being, energy and fatigue, cognitive function, medication effects, social function, and overall quality of life. The QOLIE-10 can be obtained free of charge by contacting the publisher[316] (Figure 20-2).

Psychiatric or Behavioral Effects of Antiepileptic Drugs

AEDs can influence the mental state. Behavior and cognition in patients with epilepsy are affected by other factors in addition to AEDs. These factors include the age at seizure onset, the seizure type, the seizure etiology, laterality, CNS lesions, hereditary factors, premorbid psychiatric status, and numerous psychosocial factors. Most reports are anecdotal, and these factors must be controlled in AED studies.[317–322] Dodrill[323,324] reviewed more than 90 studies and concluded that "contamination of drug effects with factor of subject selection" and "lack of standardized method for behavioral assessment" were prevalent.

The *behavior toxicity profile* of most drugs is complex, because a particular drug may influence one aspect of behavior positively and another negatively. The behavioral effects of AEDs may be dose related, or there may be subacute and chronic changes. Other factors that can predispose to behavioral effects of AEDs include the duration of AED therapy, use of polytherapy, exposure of developing neuronal structures to maternal AEDs, and CNS injury, malnutrition, and intercurrent illness.[325,326] The physician needs to be aware of behavior-related effects of AEDs. Suppressing sei-

Version 1.0

Patient Inventory

Patient's Name: _____ Today's Date: _____

Gender: ☐ Male ☐ Female   Birthdate: ___ / ___ / ___

Have you completed this questionnaire prior to today's visit?   ☐ Yes   ☐ No

MD Name: _____

Instructions: Please **circle** one number for each question. If you are unsure about how to answer a question, please give the best answer you can and write a comment or explanation in the margin. Please feel free to ask someone to assist you if you need help reading or marking this form.

HOW MUCH OF THE TIME DURING THE PAST 4 WEEKS . . .

	All of the time	**Most** of the time	**Some** of the time	**A Little** of the time	**None** of the time
1. Have you had a lot of energy?	1	2	3	4	5

	None of the time	**A Little** of the time	**Some** of the time	**Most** of the time	**All** of the the time
2. Have you felt downhearted and blue?	1	2	3	4	5

	Not at all	A **Little**	**Somewhat**	A **Lot**	A **Great Deal**
3. Has your epilepsy or anti-epileptic medication caused trouble with driving?	1	2	3	4	5

DURING THE PAST 4 WEEKS, HOW MUCH HAVE YOU BEEN BOTHERED BY . . .

	Not At All Bothered	A **Little**	**Somewhat**	A **Lot**	**Extremely** Bothered
4. Memory difficulties?	1	2	3	4	5
5. Work limitations?	1	2	3	4	5
6. Social limitations?	1	2	3	4	5

Figure 20-2. The Quality of Life in Epilepsy Inventory: QOLIE-10. (Reprinted with permission from Post Graduate Service.)

zures at the expense of deterioration in the patient's behavior is not ideal. It can impair quality of life and adversely affect the family.

Mechanism of Behavioral Toxicity

AEDs have behavioral effects via a number of direct and indirect mechzanisms. The *direct effects* of AEDs, *dose-related* and *non–dose related*, occur with prenatal exposure in human and animal studies and have been studied in vitro using cultured mammalian neurons.[327] The mechanism of direct effects is not clear, although in vitro study findings include reductions in neuronal density, changes in neuronal morphology, and changes affecting various neurotransmitters (e.g., decrease in high-affinity uptake of GABA, choline acetyltransferase activity, benzodiazepine binding, or calcium uptake or effects on tropic substrates).[327] Psychiatric effects occur with acute or subacute elevation of serum AEDs.[328] *Chronic effects are typically unrelated to serum levels.*[329]

Indirect effects of AEDs can produce behavioral disturbances. These effects include folate deficiency, hepatotoxicity, hyperammonemia; electro-

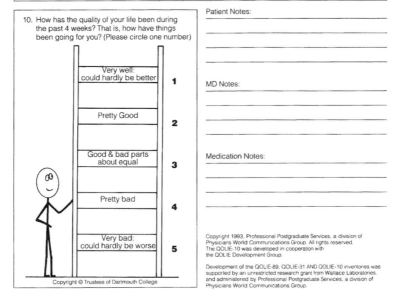

Figure 20-2. *continued*

lyte imbalances (e.g. hyponatremia), anemia, forced normalization, and effects on monoamine, neuropeptides, and endocrine function. The behavioral manifestations of AEDs could also be related to polypharmacy, AEDs' withdrawal effects, and drug interactions with psychotropics.

Biochemical and Endocrine Changes

Hyponatremia is a common side effect of carbamazepine and oxcarbazepine that can lead to behavioral changes.[330] Hepatotoxicity and *hyperammonemia*-related behavioral changes occur commonly with use

of valproate. *Folate deficiency* (with use of phenobarbital, primidone, and PHT), leading to depression, psychosis, delirium, or dementialike picture, was postulated by Reynolds[153] in the 1970s; however, there is not much data to support this. AEDs can also result in *hormonal changes* (e.g., decline in free androgen levels and compensatory increase in luteinizing hormone[331]) by induction of hepatic enzymes and increased synthesis of sex hormone–binding globulin. AEDs may also have a direct effect on the hypothalamic-pituitary-adrenal axis.[332] *Somatostatin*, a neuropeptide with epileptogenic effect, is linked with mood changes; carbamazepine may diminish somatostatin activity. AEDs' effects on behavior can be linked to other factors, including variable suppression of different groups of cortical neurons with "unregulated release of limbic mechanisms," and altered neurotransmitter levels (relevant to both epilepsy and behavior), such as norepinephrine and GABA.[326]

Behavioral Effects of Specific Antiepileptic Drugs

The reader is referred to a number of excellent reviews on this topic, including Devinsky[295] and Gates[333] (Table 20-6).

Older Antiepileptic Drugs

Phenobarbital. "Paradoxic" side effects of phenobarbital include hyperactivity, irritability, and belligerence occurring in up to 40% of children,[326] and an agitated confusional state occurs in organically impaired, demented, or elderly patients. These effects may or may not be dose related but are likely to be exacerbated by increasing doses.[334] Domizo et al.[335] reported that 76% of the children treated with phenobarbital showed one or more of the behavioral symptoms, as compared to only 31% of those treated with other AEDs. The most frequently observed behavioral disturbance was *hyperactivity*. Barbiturates can cause *sedation, mood shifts*, and increased *aggression* and *depression*[336] with *suicidal* ideation, intent, and acts. In children with epilepsy, depression and suicidal ideation were 10 times higher in patients treated with phenobarbital versus carbamazepine.[337]

Phenytoin. Unlike an ideal AED that has linear kinetics (i.e., change in serum concentration is proportional to the change in dose at any point on the curve), PHT poses a unique challenge because of its *nonlinear kinetics*. PHT changes from first-order to saturation kinetics at the lower end of therapeutic range; thus, beyond that point, a small increase in dose can result in a dramatic increase in serum concentration.[338] The dose and concentration side effects of PHT are well established and include cognitive impairment, ataxia, poor concentration, and dyskinesia. These side effects seen with toxic PHT levels (acute phenytoin encephalopathy) are reversible.[339]

Although a dose-related sedation may occur, a paradoxic *excited delirium* may be seen with therapeutic or toxic PHT levels.[339] A "toxicity"[340] characterized by lethargy, confusion, ataxia, and impaired intellectual functioning with personality changes (and slowing of the alpha rhythm, as well as the appearance of delta waves in the EEG) has been reported even with PHT blood levels between 10 and 20 μg/ml. An older literature describes a "chronic cumulative encephalopathy,"[326] which is unassociated with neurologic toxic signs[183] but includes intellectual impairment and memory disturbances.

Carbamazepine. The principal dose-related effects of carbamazepine include diplopia, cognitive viscosity, lethargy, and movement disorders. There are few reports of negative psychiatric or behavioral effects of carbamazepine. It has been used in prophylaxis of bipolar disorder, acute mania, and in personality disorders with symptoms of impulsivity and behavioral dyscontrol. Some of the reported adverse effects from carbamazepine include irritability, mania, and personality changes. Its adverse effects may be related to polypharmacy, the active 10-, 11-epoxide metabolite, or to the development of hyponatremia.[341,342]

Valproic Acid. VPA has antimanic and mood-stabilizing properties.[343] Dose-related side effects of VPA include gastrointestinal upsets, tremor, increased blood ammonia levels, somnolence, cognitive viscosity, and thrombocytopenia. Trimble[344] and Smith[345] noted sodium valproate to have fewer overall cognitive effects than PHT and barbiturates. However, at higher levels, impairment in recall and concentration has been noted. Idiosyncratic reactions to VPA include hepatic failure, a confusional syndrome that can progress to coma or stupor, and pancreatitis. This may occur in absence of elevated ammonia or other liver dysfunction and is supported by the presence of high-voltage frontally predominant delta activity on the EEG.[346]

Mental retardation and use of multiple AEDs may increase the risk of valproate-induced hyperammonemia, which may manifest as lethargy and confusional-irritable state.[347] The hyperammonemia may occur without apparent liver dysfunction. However, Murphy and Marquard observed hyperammonemia without apparent consequence in a large group of cognitively impaired patients.[348] Cognitive impairment is mostly associated with

Table 20-6. Behavioral Effects of Antiepileptic Drugs

Drug Class	GABAergic Potency	Antiglutametergic Potency	Negative Effects	Positive Effects
Barbiturates	++	–	Sedation, depression, cognitive impairment, aggression, learning deficits, sexual dysfunction, hyperactivity and irritability in children	Anxiolytic/hypnotic
Benzodiazepines	++	–	Confusion, depression, aggression, irritability, cognitive impairment, disinhibition	Anxiolytic/hypnotic, antimanic (clonazepam)
Phenytoin	–	–	Sedation, ataxia, confusion, may cause depression, progressive encephalopathy	Partially sedating, possibly antiaggressive
Carbamazepine	+	+	Depression, irritability, sexual dysfunction, mania	Mild antidepressant, antimanic treatment of aggression
Valproate	++	+	Progressive encephalopathy, depression, extrapyramidal effects	Antimanic, a mild antidepressant
Felbamate	+	++	Depression, apathy, psychosis irritability, agitation	Activation, weight loss
Gabapentin	++	++	Sedation, ataxia, aggression/hyperactivity	Mood stabilizer, treatment of bipolar disorder, panic and anxiety disorder
Lamotrigine	–	+	Dizziness, ataxia, additive toxicity with carbamazepine	Partially activating, mood stabilizer, treatment of mania and depression
Topiramate	+	++	Sedation, confusion, cognitive deficits	Probable mood stabilizer, weight loss
Tiagabine	++	–	Sedation, psychosis (few cases), depression	Anxiolytic, treatment of tardive dyskinesia?
Vigabatrin	++	–	Sedation, depression, psychosis, hyperactivity, dyskinesia	Less effect on cognition

– = none; + = mild; ++ = moderate.

higher blood ammonia levels (>100 μg/ml in polypharmacy and >150 μg/ml in monotherapy), and carnitine supplementation may help to ameliorate this in many patients.

Ethosuximide. Ethosuximide is used primarily to treat absence seizures. It may occasionally cause confusion, sleep disturbance, and a wide assortment of behavioral changes, such as aggressive activity, depression, hostility and psychosis.[336]

Newer Antiepileptic Drugs

Felbamate. *Felbamate* is a meprobamate analog that appears to act by NMDA antagonism with potentiation of GABA activity.[349] It has been observed to cazuse secondary mania and irritability,[350] probably owing to its stimulantlike properties. Dose-related side effects include insomnia, loss of appetite, nausea, and weight loss. For many patients, these side effects result in a regression to their ideal body weight and the need for less sleep.

However, an irreversible idiosyncratic side effect—*aplastic anemia* (with an incidence of 1 in 5,000) and *hepatic failure* severely limit its use. McConnell et al.[233] noted the occurrence of apathy states as well as depression and psychosis related to its use.

Vigabatrin. Vigabatrin (γ-vinyl-GABA; VGB), an enzyme-activated irreversible inhibitor of GABA-aminotransferase, is used for treatment of patients with partial seizures. The British literature contains numerous reports of VGB causing depression and psychosis.[155,351–353] Risk factors include severe epileptic disorders, a sudden reduction in seizure frequency, and a history of psychosis. In children with static encephalopathies or hyperactive behavior, VGB (especially in high doses) may exacerbate hyperkinesia.[354,355] Caution is therefore advised when using VGB in patients with established psychopathology or static encephalopathies.

Gabapentin. The mechanism of action of GPN is not firmly established. It is not an agonist of the GABA receptor. GPN may facilitate release of GABA at times of excessive rates of neuronal firing. A number of reports suggest that GPN may promote an improved sense of well being independent of seizure reduction.[356–359] Based on open-label case reports, GPN may have anxiolytic and antimanic effects,[356,360,361] although rigorous controlled trials are needed. There are several reports of severe behavioral disturbance, including hyperactivity and aggression in children (especially developmentally disabled) receiving GPN.[362–364] The most common side effects of GPN are drowsiness, somnolence, and generalized fatigue.

Lamotrigine. Lamotrigine's mechanism of action involves stabilizing neuronal membranes by inhibiting sodium channels and glutamate-mediated excitation. It is a promising new agent with few adverse cognitive and psychiatric effects. Double-blind, placebo-controlled studies found LTG to be effective in bipolar depression[365] and in treatment-refractory rapid-cycling bipolar disorder.[366] Common side effects are skin rash, somnolence, headache, tremor, and nausea. In mentally retarded epilepsy patients, LTG was associated with positive and negative behavioral effects. Beran and Gibson[367] noted the development of aggressive or violent behavior, or both, in 14 of 19 patients who received LTG, whereas one patient demonstrated improvement in behavior. Ettinger et al.[368] reported 3 of 20 MR epilepsy patients receiving LTG who developed new or worsened hyperactivity, irritability, and stereotypy. Another four patients, however, exhibited positive psychotropic effects, including reduction in irritability and hyperactivity, decreased lethargy, and better social engagement. The reasons for these disparate effects were unclear, and serum LTG levels did not predict who developed positive versus negative symptoms.

Topiramate. Topiramate is a weak carbonic anhydrase inhibitor that blocks voltage-dependent Na$^+$ and Ca$^+$ channels. There is a significant amount of anecdotal data that reports potential adverse effects on cognitive dysfunction[369,370] (considered by the manufacturer to be a reflection of excessively rapid titration in its early use). More recently, a placebo-controlled trial by Faught[371] found that topiramate was associated with dose-related CNS side effects, including *headache, somnolence, mental slowing*, and *dull thinking*. In a 2-year follow-up study, Guberman[372] reported 36% of patients with memory impairments and 22% with cognitive slowing, suggesting that such side effects may persist beyond the initial phase. However, more studies are required to determine the incidence of these side effects with more recently recommended slower titration. Betts et al.[373] reported 12 patients with severe psychiatric disturbance (including psychosis and depression), representing 15% of their patients treated with topiramate. In long-term safety data involving controlled and open trials with topiramate, psychosis was reported in 3% (30 of 1,001) of patients.

Tiagabine. TGB is a new AED that acts as a potent inhibitor of GABA uptake into neurons and glia. It is a generally well-tolerated AED with a CNS side effect spectrum similar to most AEDs, including dizziness, headache, ataxia, and nervousness.[374] Data concerning the psychotropic profile of TGB are limited and equivocal. One study in intractable epilepsy patients demonstrated improvements in mood among patients converted to TGB monotherapy. Mood elevation was not correlated with seizure reduction, suggesting that positive psychotropic benefits may be independent of antiepileptic effects.[305] Limited case series also note potential benefit in bipolar disorder.[375] Trimble et al.[376] reported 5 cases of psychosis among their 65 patients; Sackellares et al.[377] found a rate of 0.8%, compared to 0.4% in control subjects.

Rational Use of Antiepileptic Drugs to Minimize Adverse Behavioral Effects

General Model for Optimizing Psychiatric Outcome with Use of Antiepileptic Drugs

Ketter[378] proposed a general approach on how to optimize psychiatric outcome when AEDs are administered to epilepsy patients. This approach integrates neurochemical mechanisms, activity in animal models of psychiatric disturbance, and clinical observations of psychotropic effects in psychiatric disorders in epilepsy. Accordingly, two categories of AEDs are identified on the basis of their psychotropic profiles (see Table 20-6). One group has "sedating" effects in association with fatigue, cognitive slowing, and weight gain, as well as possible anxiolytic and antimanic effects. These actions may be related to potentiation of *GABA-inhibitory neurotransmission* induced by drugs such as barbiturates, benzodiazepines, valproate, GPN, TGB, and VGB. The other group is associated with predominant *attenuation of glutamate excitatory neurotransmission* and has "activating" effects with activation, weight loss, and possibly anxiogenic and antidepressant effects. This group includes felbamate and LTG. Topiramate, with GABAergic and antiglutamatergic actions, may have "mixed" profiles. Ketter[378] suggests a testable hypotheses that better psychiatric outcomes in seizure disorder patients are achieved by treating patients with baseline *activated* profiles (insomnia, agitation, anxiety, racing thoughts, weight loss) with *sedating* predominantly GABAergic drugs and, conversely, those with baseline *sedated* or anergic profiles (hypersomnia, fatigue, apathy, depression, sluggish cognition, weight gain) with *activating* predominantly antiglutamatergic agents. Although this model provides a general framework for use of AEDs in relation to behavioral issues, a systematic clinical investigation is needed to assess the use of this general proposition and define exceptions to these broad principles.

Genetic, Developmental, and Age Factors in Choosing an Antiepileptic Drug

Genetic variations may cause individual differences in enzyme production, protein binding, and end-organ sensitivity. Idiosyncratic behavioral reactions to AEDs may be related to these individual variations in the metabolism of the drugs.[326,379,380] Many of the reported behavioral side effects from AEDs have occurred in developmentally disabled patients.[363] LTG is reported to have mixed results in this population[367,368,381] Another study[382] found VGB to be associated with more behavioral problems than LTG or GPN.

Susceptibility to behavioral changes from AEDs varies among *different age groups*. Children and the elderly are particularly vulnerable to effects of phenobarbital, which may cause hyperactivity, irritability, or confusion. Most behavioral effects of GPN have been reported in children. Long-term treatment with AEDs, particularly PHT and phenobarbital, can affect development, behavior, and cognitive function in children.[383,384] AED effects on the CNS may interfere with appropriate development of psychosocial patterns of behavior, cognitive structures, and language development at crucial developmental stages in the child's life.[385] The relative advantage of controlling seizures must be balanced against this possibility. Drug pharmacokinetic and pharmacodynamic properties are significantly different in elderly patients, and various factors influence the drug action, including hepatic or renal dysfunction, increased plasma-free levels of the drug (due to decreased albumin and protein binding), and decreased body fats. For this reason, AED concentrations should be checked regularly.

Polypharmacy and Drug Interactions

Studies of polypharmacy show that polypharmacy increases the risk of behavioral toxicity and therefore should be avoided whenever monotherapy is feasible. The older AEDs have well-known effects on each other's metabolism that affect their total and free-serum levels.[386] There is growing evidence that reduction in polypharmacy leads to improvement in mood, personality, behavior, and cognitive functioning, thus enhancing quality of life.[296,299,387,388] The reader is referred to Chapter

26 for a detailed review of various pharmacokinetic interactions between AEDs and between AEDs and psychotropic agents.

Examples

Phenobarbital may increase the metabolism of PHT, but the two compete for microsomal enzymes, thus potentially increasing the half-life of the other. Carbamazepine may decrease the levels of PHT by increasing its metabolism. Among the newer AEDs, felbamate causes increases in PHT and valproate levels and decreases carbamazepine levels. Carbamazepine and PHT may both decrease LTG levels, whereas valproate increases LTG levels. Behavioral changes can also be expected when AEDs are used along with psychotropics. Carbamazepine can increase the metabolism of haloperidol and result in decreases of its plasma levels to greater than or equal to one-half.[389] This may result in exacerbation of psychotic symptoms.

Antiepileptic Drugs and Withdrawal Syndromes

Excessively rapid reduction of barbiturates and benzodiazepines can result in withdrawal effects, including anxiety, irritability, psychosis, and delirium.[248,390–394] However, up to 40% of epilepsy patients withdrawing from PHT, carbamazepine, and valproate develop moderate to severe psychiatric symptoms, including anxiety, panic, depression, psychosis, mania, and mixed mood states.[395] Withdrawal-emergent psychopathology can begin in the final week of AED tapering and tends to resolve within 2 weeks of restarting original AEDs.

Effects of Psychotropic Agents on Seizure Threshold (Choosing a Psychotropic Agent)

Because of the high frequency of psychopathology in epilepsy, psychotropic agents are commonly prescribed in this patient population. A growing area of concern has been the potential risk of eliciting seizures through their effects on the seizure threshold. Our understanding of these risks is limited by a number of problems well summarized by Edwards (e.g., use of concomitant medications that

may also adversely affect the seizure threshold, withdrawal from drugs or alcohol inducing seizures, inclusion of subjects with predisposition factors for seizures, seizures being poorly defined in some reports, and bias inherent to retrospective data).[200,396–398] Animal models do not necessarily predict drug effects in humans.[399]

Risk Factors Contributing to Drug-Induced Seizures

Overall, the risk of eliciting seizures with psychotropic drugs is low and should not preclude the addition of most types of agents. Seizure risk is higher in the presence of *clinical factors*, including personal or family history of seizures, mental retardation, brain injury, CNS neoplasms, head trauma, secondary dementia, an abnormal EEG pattern (especially epileptiform abnormalities), and CNS vascular disease. *Drug-related factors* that can potentially increase the seizure risk include use of high doses of psychotropics, rapid escalation in dose, concomitant therapy with other drugs that lower the seizure threshold, overdose, history of substance abuse, and withdrawal from alcohol or anxiolytics.[200,400–402]

Risk of Seizures after Psychotropic Drug Overdose

Seizures induced by psychotropics usually occur in the context of high doses. Most reports of seizure-related morbidity after overdose concern the cyclic antidepressants; the incidence varies from 4% to 20%.[403,404] A meta-analysis of 26 studies (2,536 patients) with seizures induced by TCA overdoses found an overall seizure incidence of 8.4%.[405] Seizures usually occur within 3–6 hours after TCA ingestion and are uncommon after 24 hours.[406,407] There are mixed reports about the value of TCA levels (one study demonstrated levels above 1,000 ng/ml[404] and QRS duration of less than 0.1 seconds[407] in predicting the occurrence of seizures.[408] Among the cyclic antidepressants, there was a statistically significant increase in the risk of seizures after amoxapine and maprotiline overdose (24.5% and 12.2%, respectively) compared to TCA and trazadone overdose (3% and 0%, respectively).[409]

SSRIs, a new class of antidepressants (Table 20-7), are safer than cyclic antidepressants after overdose. However, the relative seizure risk with overdose of newer antidepressants is not well defined, as seizures have been reported with fluoxetine, sertraline, fluvoxamine, and venlafaxine in overdose situations.[410–413] In the overdose, cyclic antidepressants carry a higher risk of causing seizures than do most antipsychotic agents. An Australian report of 299 consecutive antipsychotic drug overdose cases indicated a seizure incidence of only 1% among patients who had taken a single drug.[414] However, seizures occurred in 6 of 10 cases of loxapine overdose.[415] Because of the small number of reported cases, the relative risk of seizures among antipsychotics is not clear.

Risk of Seizures during Therapeutic Use of Psychotropic Drugs

Antidepressants

The reported risk of seizures associated with routine doses of antidepressants ranges from 0.1% to 4.0%,[200] although most series show a risk of less than 1%. Some authors suggested that certain TCAs (e.g., imipramine, amitriptyline, and especially maprotiline and clomipramine)[401,416] carry a higher risk of lowering the seizure threshold than trazodone, SSRIs, or MAOIs. A multicenter trial of clomipramine in the treatment of patients with OCD reported seizures in 2.1% of patients receiving more than 300 mg per day and in 0.48% of patients receiving less than 250 mg per day.[417] Overall, seizures associated with TCAs use are estimated to occur in less than 0.6% of cases.[200,396] The mechanism responsible for lowering the seizure threshold is not understood but appears to be independent of the antidepressant effect. Seizures often occur within days of introduction of the drug, whereas the antidepressant effect may take weeks to occur.[398] If a TCA is to be used, then one retrospective series suggests that doxepin may have the lowest risk of eliciting seizures.[418]

Other antidepressants, amoxapine and bupropion, are thought to have an especially high risk of seizure,[315] although the evidence is not conclusive. The high rates of seizures associated with bupropion administration, however, may have had more to do with the excessively high doses (450–900 mg per day, with a seizure incidence of 1%) tested in premarketing trials than with the true risk associated with more moderated therapeutic doses.[419]

Table 20-4 summarizes relative seizure risk associated with psychotropic agents. Some evidence suggests that SSRIs and MAOIs may occasionally demonstrate anticonvulsant properties.[399,420,421] Because of the overall low incidence of seizures and the relatively small number of patients exposed, differences in seizure risk among these agents cannot be discerned with confidence.

Antipsychotic Agents

Overall, antipsychotic agents carry an approximate 1% risk for seizures, with specific agents having notably higher rates.[422] Some authors suggest that butyrophenones (e.g., haloperidol) have a lower risk of seizures than the phenothiazines (e.g., chlorpromazine).[5] Phenothiazines have been reported to produce seizures even among patients with no history of epilepsy.[423] The aliphatic class of phenothiazines (e.g., chlorpromazine) is thought to be associated with particularly high risk, although the literature does not provide adequate comparative data to other classes of agents. Seizures often occurred shortly after initiation of phenothiazines or after increasing the maintenance dosage and were more often observed in patients with identified CNS disease.[424]

The minimal neuronal excitability demonstrated in animal hippocampal slice studies with the administration of molindone (a dihydroindolone),[425] as well as anecdotal clinical evidence,[18] suggests that this drug may be an optimal choice for epilepsy patients who require an antipsychotic drug. Theoretically, *fluphenazine* and *haloperidol* are potential alternatives; despite increasing neuronal excitability, they have high potency and, therefore, low dose requirements.[398]

The more recently marketed atypical antipsychotic agents offer the advantage of few or none of the extrapyramidal effects commonly associated with previously described agents. However, clozapine has attracted much attention for its dose-related significant risk of seizures, estimated at 3.5% overall. Frank epileptiform activity (general-

Table 20-7. Seizures: Risk Related to Use of Newer Antidepressants and Antipsychotic Agents

New Antidepressants	Therapeutic Use in Premarketing Trials	Overdose	Comments
Fluoxetine (Prozac)	0.1% risk in placebo-controlled trials; 0.2% incidence in all trials	Reported	0.2% incidence of seizures with placebo in comparative trials.
Fluoxamine (Luvox)	0.2% incidence	Reported	—
Mirtazapine (Remeron)	One seizure in 2,796 treated patients (0.04%)	No seizures in eight reported cases	—
Nefazodone (Serzone)	One patient	One patient (multidrug overdose)	Recurrence of *petit mal* seizures in a patient with prior history of this seizure.
Paroxetine (Paxil)	0.1% incidence	No seizures in single-dose overdose	—
Sertraline (Zoloft)	None in depression trials; 0.2% incidence in OCD trials	Not reported	Three of four patients with seizures. OCD trials had a personal or family history of seizures.
Venlafaxine (Effexor)	0.26% incidence (eight patients)	Reported	Five of eight patients with seizures in therapeutic use received <150 mg/day.
New antipsychotic agents			
Clozapine (Clozaril)	3.5% incidence; cumulative incidence of 5% at a year	Reported	
Olanzapine (Zyprexa)	0.9% incidence	Not reported	
Quetiapine (Seroquel)	0.9%	Not reported	
Risperidone (Risperdal)	0.3% incidence	Reported	

OCD = obsessive-compulsive disorder.
Source: Adapted from Physicians' Desk Reference. Montvale, NJ: Medical Economics Company, 2000.

ized spike and wave) may be induced by this drug. However, generalized spikes are not equivalent to frank seizures, and their presence should not necessarily lead to discontinuation of the drug.[426] Drug-induced seizures may be generalized tonic-clonic or myoclonic. It has been argued that, in the absence of other medication alternatives, even the occurrence of seizures should not necessarily lead to discontinuation of clozapine, because other measures, such as reduction of a dose or addition of an antiepileptic drug such as valproate, may be taken. The risk of seizures associated with other recently introduced antipsychotic agents, such as risperidone, seems to be substantially less than that associated with clozapine. In the premarketing tri-als, the risk of seizures with risperidone was 0.3%[427] (see Table 20-7).

Agents Used in Bipolar Disorder

Lithium may reduce the seizure threshold, but most cases have been reported with lithium intoxication, especially when levels exceed 3 mEq/liter.[419,423] EEG may demonstrate epileptiform abnormalities during routine lithium dosing. Because other antiepileptic drugs, such as carbamazepine, valproate, GPN, LTG, and topiramate, have been used to treat seizures and bipolar disorders, these medications may be more optimal than lithium.

Anxiolytics

Benzodiazepines, which are commonly used to treat anxiety, also have antiepileptic effects. Seizures associated with use of benzodiazepines usually occur in the context of benzodiazepine withdrawal. Despite the level of concern about seizure-inducing properties of psychotropic agents, available evidence suggests that these drugs can usually be used safely in epilepsy patients. Current data do not provide a very accurate assessment of relative risk, except for the strongest (e.g., clozapine) or weakest (e.g., MAOIs) culprits. Clinicians are still faced with making a drug choice for their patients in the absence of evidence-based guidelines. Table 20-3 suggests relative seizure risk associated with selected psychotropic agents on the basis of available clinical literature and case reports.[428]

Drug Interactions between Psychotropic and Antiepileptic Drugs

Because of high frequency of psychiatric and epileptic comorbidity, psychotropic agents and AEDs are often prescribed concomitantly. Careful attention must be given to potential drug interactions that could lead to toxicity and reduced efficacy of one or both classes of drugs.

Drug interactions could be classified as pharmacodynamic or pharmacokinetic. Pharmacodynamic interactions occur at the receptor site or other sites of action. Pharmacokinetic interactions occur as a result of interference with a drug's absorption, distribution, metabolism, or excretion. They may be additive, synergistic, or antagonistic. The cytochrome P-450 system is the main hepatic enzyme system for the metabolism of drugs. Because the psychotropics and AEDs may use the same isoenzyme systems, knowledge of the P-450 system with respect to psychotropic and AED metabolism is clinically important. The details of these interactions are discussed in Chapter 26.

Table 20-5 displays examples of potential drug interactions among AEDs and psychotropic agents, although one may extrapolate these effects to the general class of medications in many cases. As mentioned before, antiepileptic drugs, including PHT, carbamazepine, and especially barbiturates (phenobarbital and primidone), induce hepatic metabolism and may result in reduction in the levels of concomitantly administered medications. Carbamazepine may increase the metabolism of haloperidol—for example, resulting in a decrease in plasma haloperidol levels of as much as 50% or greater.[389] There is potential negative interaction between clozapine and carbamazepine,[158] both of which are associated with leukopenia, and, if combined, then there is potential synergistic effect on the white blood cell count. VPA inhibits hepatic metabolism and can result in elevated levels of concomitant drugs. GPN has minimal drug interactions with nonpsychotropic agents and is expected to have similar minimal interactions with psychotropic agents as well. LTG tends to have minimal effects on concomitant medications but is vulnerable to effects of enzyme inhibition or induction resulting from a concomitant medication.

Recently introduced antidepressant agents deserve special mention. SSRIs inhibit different isoenzymes of hepatic P-450 cytochrome systems.[429] This leads to potential risk of reduced metabolism (and elevated serum levels) of those concomitantly administered AEDs that are typically metabolized in the liver. Among the AEDs, GPN would therefore be expected to be minimally affected by such drug interactions. Clinically based case reports of such interactions are only beginning to appear in the literature. Variations in the specific isoenzymes inhibited by the various SSRIs may help to explain why, for example, fluoxetine and fluvoxamine may result in elevated levels of carbamazepine[430] and PHT,[431] whereas these AEDs drug levels seem to be unaffected by sertraline, paroxetine, and citalopram.

Fluoxetine, sertraline, and paroxetine are all highly protein bound, which could result in competition for protein-binding sites and a higher unbound fraction of anticonvulsant. Further experience is needed to assess the actual clinical risk.

The combination of MAOIs and TCA can result in hypertensive crisis. Because of chemical similarity of carbamazepine and tricyclic agents, the combination of MAOIs and carbamazepine should be avoided.[399] Perhaps for similar reasons, the combination of carbamazepine and SSRIs may cause a hyperserotonergic state called *serotonin syndrome*, which is characterized by mood changes, tremor, myoclonus, shivering, delirium, and, less commonly, seizures. This syndrome usually remits spontaneously with withdrawal of the responsible agents, although supportive measures, including the addition of other AEDs, may be indicated.[432]

Conclusion

The study of epilepsy and its psychiatric comorbidity gives us a unique opportunity to expand our understanding of brain-behavior relations. The symptom complex of TLE provides excellent opportunity for increasing our understanding of limbic physiology. We now know that there is no single epileptic personality that defines all patients with epilepsy. Our understanding of mood and thought disorder in epilepsy remains poorly defined and is an area of active investigation. Modern care of persons with epilepsy goes beyond attempts to control seizures and requires consideration of broader issues related to cognitive, psychiatric, and social functioning. Optimizing the quality of life in patients with epilepsy needs careful assessment of these issues. The rational use of antiepileptic and psychotropic drugs requires knowledge of psychiatric and cognitive effects of AEDs, the risk of seizures posed by use of psychotropics, and drug-drug interactions.

References

1. Warrington EK, James M. Visual apperceptive agnosia: a clinico-anatomical study of three cases. Cortex 1988;24:1–32.
2. Kraepelin E. Psychiatrie (8th ed). Leipzig, Germany: Johann Ambosius Barltz, 1923.
3. Jilek W. The epileptic's outcast role and its background: a contribution to the social psychiatry of seizure disorders. J Oper Psychiatry 1979;10:127–133.
4. Trimble M.R. Treatment of Epileptic Psychoses. In The Psychoses of Epilepsy. New York: Raven Press, 1991;150–163.
5. Ettinger AB, Jandorf L, Berdia A, et al. Felbamate-induced headache. Epilepsia 1996;37(5):503–505.
6. Hauser WA, Pedley TA. Epidemiology, Pathology, and Genetics of Epilepsy. In J Engel Jr, TA Pedley (eds), Epilepsy: A Comprehensive Textbook. Philadelphia: Lippincott–Raven, 1998;9–230.
7. Robb P. Focal Epilepsy: The Problem, Prevalence, and Contributing Factors. In D Purpura, JK Penry, RD Walter (eds), Neurosurgical Management of the Epilepsies. New York: Raven Press, 1975;11–22.
8. Manford M, Hart YM, Sander JW, et al. National General Practice Study of Epilepsy (NGPSE): partial seizures patterns in a general population. Neurology 1992;42:1911–1917.
9. Pond DA, Bidwell BH. A survey of epilepsy in 14 general practices: II. Social and psychological aspects. Epilepsia 1959;60:285–299.
10. Smith DB, Craft BR, Collins J, et al. Behavioral characteristics of epilepsy patients compared with normal controls. Epilepsia 1986;27:760–768.
11. Standage KF, Fenton GW. Psychiatric symptom profiles of patients with epilepsy: a controlled study. Psychol Med 1975;5:152–160.
12. Whitman S, Hermann BP, Gordon AC. Psychopathology in epilepsy: How great is the risk? Biol Psychiatry 1984;19:213–236.
13. Rutter M, Graham P, Yule WA. A Neuropsychiatric Study in Childhood. Philadelphia: J.B. Lippincott, 1970.
14. Cavazzuti GB. Epidemiology of different types of epilepsy in school age children of Modena, Italy. Epilepsia 1980;21:57–62.
15. Holdsworth L, Whitmore K. A study of children with epilepsy attending ordinary schools. I. Their seizure patterns, progress, and behavior in school. Dev Med Child Neurol 1974;16:746–755.
16. Hoare P. The development of psychiatric disorder among schoolchildren with epilepsy. Dev Med Child Neurol 1984;26:3–13.
17. Perrine K and Congett S. Neurobehavioral Problems in Epilepsy. In O Devinsky (ed), Neurologic Clinics. Philadelphia: W.B. Saunders, 1994;129–152.
18. Mendez MF, Grau R, Doss RC, Taylor JL. Schizophrenia in epilepsy. Neurology 1993;43:1073–1077.
19. Bruton CJ, Stevens JR, Frith CD. Epilepsy, psychosis, and schizophrenia: clinical and neuropathological correlations. Neurology 1994;44(1):34–42.
20. Slater E, Beard AW, and Glithero E. The schizophrenia-like psychosis of epilepsy. Br J Psychiatry 1963;109:95–105.
21. Sachdev P. Schizophrenia-like psychosis and epilepsy: the status of the association. Am J Psychiatry 1998;155:(3):325–336.
22. Adam C, Baulac M, Saint-Hilaire JM, et al. Value of magnetic resonance imaging-based measurements of hippocampal formations in patients with partial epilepsy. Arch Neurol 1994;51(12):130–138.
23. Hugg JW, Laxer KD, Matson GB, et al. Neuron loss localizes human temporal lobe epilepsy by in vivo proton magnetic resonancy spectroscopic imaging. Ann Neurol 1993;34:788–794.
24. Jackson GD, Kuzniecky RI, and Cascino GD. Hippocampal sclerosis without detectable hippocampal atrophy. Neurology 1994;44(1):42–46.
25. Taylor D. Factors influencing the occurrence of schizophrenia-like psychosis in patients with psychosis. Psychol Med 1975;5:249–254.
26. Roberts GW, Done DJ, Bruton C, Crow TJ. A "mock up" of schizophrenia: temporal lobe epilepsy and schizophrenia-like psychosis. Biol Psychiatry 1990;28:127–143.

27. Conlon P, Trimble MR, Rogers D. A study of epileptic psychosis: using magnetic resonance imaging. Br J Psychiatry 1990;156:231–235.

28. Bruton CJ, Crow TJ, Frith CD, et al. Schizophrenia and brain: a perspective clinico-neuropathological study. Psychol Med 1990;20(2):285–304.

29. Roberts G. The cellular biology of functional psychosis. Trends Neurosci 1990;13:207–211.

30. Trimble M. Kindling, Epilepsy and Behavior. In TG Bolwig, MR Trimble (eds), The Clinical Relevance of Kindling. Chichester, England: Wiley, 1989;177–190.

31. Gallhofer B, Trimble MR, Frackowiak R, et al. A study of cerebral blood flow and metabolism in epileptic psychosis using positron emission tomography and oxygen-15. J Neurol Neurosurg Psychiatry 1985;48:201–206.

32. Henry TR, Mazziotta JC, Engel J., Interictal metabolic anatomy of mesial temporal lobe epilepsy. Arch Neurol 1993;50:582–589.

33. Radtke RA, Hanson MW, Hoffman JM, et al. Temporal lobe hypometabolism on PET: predictor of seizure control after temporal lobectomy. Neurology 1993;43:1088–1092.

34. Rausch R, Henry TR, Ary CM, et al. Asymmetric inzterictal glucose hypometabolism and cognitive performance in epileptic patients. Arch Neurol 1994;51:139–144.

35. Goddard G. Development of epileptic seizures through brain stimulation at low intensity. Nature 1967;214:1020–1021.

36. Goddard G. The kindling model of epilepsy. Trends Neurosci 1983:275–279.

37. Bliss TV, Collingridge GL. A synaptic model of memory: long-term potentiation in hippocampus. Nature 1993;361(5091):31–39.

38. Bliss TV, Lomo T. Long-lasting potentiation of synaptic transmission in the dentate area of the anesthetized rabbits following stimulation of the perforant path. J Physiol (Lond) 1973;232:331–356.

39. Wada JA, Tsuchimochi H. Cingulate kindling in Senegalese baboons, Papio papio. Epilepsia 1995;36:1142–1151.

40. Morrell F. Secondary epileptogenesis in man. Arch Neurol 1985;42:318–335.

41. Morrell F, Tsuru N, Hoeppner TJ, et al., Secondary epileptogenesis in the frog forebrain: effects of inhibition of protein synthesis. Can J Neurol Sci 1975;2:407–418.

42. Morrell F. Physiology and Histochemistry of the Mirror Focus. In HH Jasper, AA Ward, A Pope (eds), Basic Mechanisms of Epilepsy. Boston: Little, Brown, 1969;357–374.

43. Stamm JS, Rosen SC. Learning on somesthetic discrimination and reversal tasks by monkey with epileptogenic implants in anteromedial temporal cortex. Neuropsychologia 1971;9:185–191.

44. Sato M. Long-lasting hypersensitivity to methamphetamine following amygdaloid kindling in cats: the relationship between limbic epilepsy and the psychotic state. Biol Psychiatry 1983;18:525–536.

45. Stevens J. Psychiatric consequences of temporal lobectomy for intractable seizures: a 20–30 year follow-up of 14 cases. Psychol Med 1990;20:529–545.

46. Sutula T, He XX, Cavazos J, Scott G. Synaptic reorganization in the hippocampus induced by abnormal functional activity. Science 1988;239:1147–1150.

47. Babb TL, KW, Pretorius JK. Synaptic reorganization of mossy fibers into molecular layer in human epileptic fascia dentata. Abstracts of the Society for Neuroscience 1988;88:351.

48. Geschwind N. Dostoievsky's epilepsy. In Blumer D (ed), Psychiatric aspects of epilepsy. Washington, DC: American Psychiatric Press, 1984;325–334.

49. Hermann BP, Whitman S, Arnston P. Hypergraphia in epilepsy: Is there a specificity to temporal lobe epilepsy? J Neurol Neurosurg Psychiatry 1983;46:848–853.

50. Hermann BP, Whitman S, Wyler AR, et al. The neurological, psychosocial and demographic correlates of hypergraphia in patients with epilepsy. J Neurol Neurosurg Psychiatry 1988;51:203–208.

51. Mungas D. Interictal behavior abnormality in temporal lobe epilepsy: a specific syndrome or nonspecific psychopathology? Arch Gen Psychiatry 1982;39:108–111.

52. Geschwind N. The clinical setting of aggression in temporal lobe epilepsy. Neural basis of violence and aggression. St. Louis: Warren H Green, 1975;273–281.

53. Waxman S, Geschwind N. The interictal behavior syndrome in temporal lobe epilepsy. Arch Gen Psychiatry 1975;32:1580–1586.

54. Geschwind N. Behavioral changes in temporal lobe epilepsy. Psychol Med 1979;9:217–219.

55. Bear DM. Temporal lobe epilepsy—a syndrome of sensory-limbic hyperconnection. Cortex 1979;15:357–384.

56. Bear DM, Fedio P. Quantitative analysis of interictal behavior in temporal lobe epilepsy. Arch Neurol 1977;34:454–467.

57. Naugle RI, Rodgers DA. Personality inventory responses of males with medically intractable seizures. J Pers Assess 1992;59(3):500–14.

58. Hermann B, Reil P. Interictal personality and behavioral traits in temporal lobe and generalized epilepsy. Cortex 1981;17:125–128

59. Rodin E, Schmaltz S. The Bear-Fedio personality inventory and temporal lobe epilepsy. Neurology 1984;34:591–596.

60. Bear D. Interictal behavioral syndrome in temporal lobe epilepsy. J Neuropsychiatry 1989;1:308–311.

61. Devinsky O, Najjar S. Evidence against the existence of a temporal lobe epilepsy personality syndrome. Neurology 1999;53(5 Suppl 2):S 13 –25.

62. Falconer M. Reversibility by temporal-lobe resection of the behavioral abnormalities of temporal lobe epilepsy. N Engl J Med 1973;289:451–455.

63. Hill D. Psychiatric disorders of epilepsy. Med Press 1953;229:473–475.

64. Pond D. Psychiatric aspects of epilepsy. J Med Prof 1957;3:1441–1451.
65. Taylor D. Mental state and temporal lobe epilepsy; a correlative account of 100 patients treated surgically. Epilepsia 1972;13:727–765.
66. Trimble M. Personality disorders in epilepsy. Neurology 1983;33:1332–1334.
67. Dewhurst K, Beard AW. Sudden religious conversions in temporal lobe epilepsy. Br J Psychiatry 1970;117:497–507.
68. Bear D, Fedio P. Quantitative analysis of interictal behavior in temporal lobe epilepsy. Arch Neurol 1997;34:454–467.
69. Engel J, et al. Neurobiological Evidence for Epilepsy-Induced Interictal Disturbances. In DB Smith, DM Treiman, and MR Trimble (eds), Neurobehavioral Problems in Epilepsy. New York: Raven Press, 1991;97–111.
70. Lee SI. Nonconvulsive status epilepticus. Arch Neurol 1985;42:778–781.
71. Scholtes FB, Renier WO, Meinardi H. Non-convulsive status epilepticus: causes, treatment, and outcome in 65 patients. J Neurol Neurosurg Psychiatry 1996;61:93–95.
72. Williamson PD, Spencer SS. Clinical and EEG features of complex partial seizures of extratemporal origin. Epilepsia 1986;27(Suppl 2):S46–S63.
73. Kendrick JF, Gibbs FA. Origin, spread and neurosurgical treatment of psychomotor type of seizure discharge. Neurosurg 1957;14:270–284.
74. Sem-Jacobson CW. Depth electrographic observations on psychotic patients: a system related to emotional behavior. Acta Psychiatr Scand 1959;34:412–416.
75. Heath RG. Common clinical characteristics of epilepsy and schizophrenia: clinical observation and depth electrode studies. Am J Psychiatry 1962;118:1013–1026.
76. Logsdail SJ, Toone BK. Postictal psychoses: a clinical and phenomenological description. Br J Psychiatry 1988;152:246–252.
77. Savard G, Andermann F, Olivier A, Remillard GM. Postictal psychosis after partial complex seizures: a multiple case study. Epilepsia 1991;32:225–231.
78. Kanner AM, Stagno S, Kotagal P, Morris HH. Postictal psychiatric events during prolonged video-electroencephalographic monitoring studies. Arch Neurol 1996;53:258–263.
79. Kanemoto K, Takeuchi J, Kawasaki J, Kawai I. Characteristics of temporal lobe epilepsy with mesial temporal sclerosis, with special reference to psychotic episodes. Neurology 1996;47:1199–1203.
80. Kanner A. Psychosis of epilepsy: a neurologist's perspective. Epilepsy and Behavior 2000;1:219–227.
81. Kanner AM, Stagno S, Kotagal P, Morris HH. Postictal psychosis events during prolonged video-EEG monitoring studies. Arch Neurology 1996;53:258–263.
82. Kanemoto K, Kawasaki J, Kawai I. Postictal psychosis: a comparison with acute interictal and chronic psychoses. Epilepsia 1996;37:551–556.

83. Kanner A, Soto A. Ictal recordings in postictal psychosis and postictal depression (abstract). Neurology 1998;50:A397.
84. Umbricht D, Degreef G, Barr WB, et al. Postictal and chronic psychoses in patients with temporal lobe epilepsy. Am J Psychiatry1995;152:224–231.
85. Devinsky O, Abramson H, Alper K, et al. Postictal psychosis: a case control study of 20 patients and 150 controls. Epilepsy Res 1995;20:247–253.
86. So NK, Savard G, Andermann F, et al. Acute postictal psychosis: a stereo EEG study. Epilepsia 1990;31:188–193.
87. Ring, HA, Trimble MR, Costa DC, et al. Striatal dopamine receptor binding in epileptic psychosis. Biol Psychiatry 1994;35:375–380.
88. Tellenbach H. Epilepsie als anfallsleiden und psychose: ueber alternative psychosen paranoider praegung bei 'forcierter normalisierung' (Landolt) des elektroenzephalogramms epileptischer. Nervenarzt 1965;36:190–202.
89. Wolf P. The clinical syndromes of forced normalization. Jpn J Psychiatry Neurol 1984;38:187–192.
90. Pakalnis A, Drake ME Jr, John K, Kellum JB. Forced normalization. Acute psychosis after seizure control in seven patients. Arch Neurol 1987;44:289–292.
91. Landolt H. Serial Electroencephalographic Investigations during Psychotic Episodes in Epileptic Patients and During Schizophrenic Attacks. In L deHass (ed), Lectures on Epilepsy. London: Elsevier Sciences, 1958;91–133.
92. Wolf P, Trimble MR. Biological antagonism and epileptic psychosis. Br J Psychiatry 1985;146:272–276.
93. Weiner RD. EEG Related to Electroconvulsive Therapy. In JR Hughes, WP Wilson (eds), EEG and Evoked Potentials in Psychiatry and Behavioral Neurology. Boston: Butterworth, 1983;101–126.
94. Wolf P. Acute Behavioral Symptomatology at Disappearance of Epileptiform EEG Abnormality. Paradoxical or 'Forced Normalization.' In DB Smith, DM Treiman, MR Trimble (eds), Advances in Neurology. New York: Raven Press, 1991;127–142.
95. Ried S, Mothersill I. Forced Normalization: The Clinical Neurologist's Review. In M Trimble, B Schmitz (eds), Forced Normalization and Alternative Psychoses of Epilepsy. Bristol, PA: Wrightson Biomedical, 1998;77–84.
96. Trimble MR. The Psychoses of Epilepsy. New York: Raven Press, 1991.
97. Mendez MF, Grau R, Doss RC, Taylor JL. Schizophrenia and epilepsy: seizure and psychosis variables. Neurology 1993;43:1073–1077.
98. Gibbs FA. Ictal and non-ictal psychiatric disorders in temporal lobe epilepsy. J Nerv Ment Dis 1951;113:522–528.
99. Bruens JH. Psychosis in epilepsy. Psychitr Neurol Neurochir 1971; 74:174–192.

100. Perez MM, Trimble MR. Epileptic psychosis-diagnostic comparison with process schizophrenia. Br J Psychiatry 1980;137:245–249.

101. Kristensen O, Sindrup HH. Psychomotor epilepsy and psychosis. Acta Neurol Scand 1987;57:361–379.

102. Marshall JE, Syed GM, Fenwick PB, Lishman WA. A pilot study of schizophrenia-like psychosis in epilepsy using single photon emission computerised tomography. Br J Psychiatry, 1993. 163:32–36.

103. Fujimoto T, et al. Proton magnetic resonance spectroscopy of temporal lobe in epileptic psychosis and schizophrenia (abstract). Epilepsia 1995;36(Suppl 3):S 174.

104. Sherwin I. Psychosis associated with epilepsy: significance of the laterality of the epileptogenic lesion. J Neurol Neurosurg Psychiatry 1981;44:83–85.

105. Lindsay J, Ounsted C, Richards P. Longterm outcome in children with temporal lobe seizures I: Social outcome and childhood factors. Dev Med Child Neurol 1979;21(285–298):630–636.

106. Trimble MR, Ring HA, Schmitz B. Neuropsychiatric Aspects of Epilepsy. In B Fogel, R Schiffer, S Rao (eds), Neuropsychiatry. Baltimore: Williams & Williams, 1996;771–803.

107. Slater E, Beard AW, Glithero E. Schizophrenia-like psychoses of epilepsy: relation between ages of onset. Br J Psychiatry 1963;115:599–603.

108. Perez MM, Trimble MR, Murray NM, Reider I. Epileptic psychosis: an evaluation of PSE profiles. Br J Psychiatry 1985;146:155–163.

109. Toth P, Frankenberg F. Clozapine and seizures: a review. Can J Psychiatry 1994;39:236–239.

110. Tiihonen J, Nousiainen U, Hakola P, et al. EEG abnormalities associated with clozapine treatment (letter). Am J Psychiatry 1991;148:1406.

111. McConnell H, Duncan D. Treatment of Psychiatric Comorbidity in Epilepsy. In HW McConnell, PJ Snyder (eds), Psychiatric Comorbidity in Epilepsy. Washington, DC: American Psychiatric Press, 1998;300–301.

112. Mendez MF, Cummings JL, Benson DF. Depression in epilepsy. Significance and phenomenology. Arch Neurol 1986;43:766–770.

113. Kogeorgos J, Fonagy P, Scott D. Psychiatric symptom patterns of chronic epileptics attending a neurological clinic: a controlled investigation. Br J Psychiatry 1982;140:236–243.

114. Rutter M, Tizard J, Yule W. Isle of Wight Studies, 1964–1974. Psychol Med 1976;6:313–332.

115. Ring HA, Trimble MR. Depression in Epilepsy. In SE Starkstein, RG Robertson (eds), Depression in Neurologic Diseases. Baltimore: John Hopkins University Press, 1993.

116. Altshuler L. Depression in Epilepsy. In O Devinsky, WH Theodore (eds), Epilepsy and Behavior. New York: Wiley-Liss, 1991.

117. Dodrill CB, Batzel LW. Interictal behavioral features of patients with epilepsy. Epilepsia 1986;27(Suppl 2):64–76.

118. Currie S, Heathfield KW, Henson RA, Scott DF. Clinical causes and prognosis of temporal lobe epilepsy: a survey of 66 patients. Brain 1971;94:173–190.

119. Dongier S. Statistical study of clinical and electroencephalographic manifestations of 536 psychotic episodes occurring in 516 epileptics between clinical seizures. Epilepsia 1959;1:117–142.

120. Roy A. Some determinants of affective symptoms in epileptics. Can J Psychiatry, 1979;24:554–556.

121. Victoroff JI, Benson F, Grafton ST, et al. Depression in complex partial seizures: electroencephalography and cerebral metabolic correlates. Arch Neurol 1994;51:155–163.

122. Barraclough B. Suicide and Epilepsy. In EH Reynolds, MR Trimble (eds), Epilepsy and Psychiatry. Edinburgh: Churchill Livingstone, 1981;72–76.

123. Matthews W, Barabas G. Suicide and epilepsy: a review of the literature. Psychosomatics 1981;22:515–524.

124. Wannamaker BB. Unexplained mortality in epilepsy: a perspective on death of persons with epilepsy. Paper presented at the 15th Epilepsy International Symposium, Washington, DC, 1983.

125. Lewis A. Melancholia: a historical review. J Ment Sci 1934;80:1–42.

126. Forsgren L, Nystrom L. An incident case referent study of epileptic seizures in adults. Epilepsy Res 1990;6:66–81.

127. Mignone RJ, Donnelly EF, Sadowsky D. Psychological and neurological comparisons of psychomotor and non-psychomotor epileptic patients. Epilepsia 1970;11:345–359.

128. Indaco A, Carrieri P, Nappi C. Interictal depression in epilepsy. Epilepsy Res 1992;12:45–50.

129. Septien L, Giroud M, Didi-Roy R. Depression and partial epilepsy: relevance of laterality of the epileptic focus. Neurol Res 1993;15:136–138.

130. Dikman S, et al. Validity of the Minnesota Multiphasic Personality Inventory (MMPI) to psychopathology in patients with epilepsy. J Nerv Ment Dis 1983;171:114–122.

131. Bromfield EB, Altshuler L, Leiderman DB. Cerebral metabolism and depression in patients with complex partial seizures. Epilepsia 1990;31:625.

132. Robertson M. Ictal and Interictal Depression in Patients with Epilepsy. In M Trimble (ed), Aspects of Epilepsy and Psychiatry. New York: Wiley, 1986;213–233.

133. Hermann BP, et al. Mood state in unilateral temporal lobe epilepsy. Biol Psychiatry 1991;30:1205–1218.

134. Broomfield E, et al. Cerebral metabolism and depression in patients with complex partial seizures. Arch Neurol 1992;49:617–623.

135. Schmitz EB, et al. Psychiatric profiles and patterns of cerebral blood flow in focal epilepsy: interactions between depression, obsessionality, and perfusion related to the laterality of the epilepsy. J Neurol Neurosurg Psychiatry 1997;62:458–463.

136. Henry TR. Functional neuroimaging with positron emission tomography. Epilepsia 1996;37:1141–1154.

137. Jokeit H, et al. Prefrontal asymmetric interictal glucose hypometabolism and cognitive impairment in patients with temporal lobe epilepsy. Brain 1997;120:2283–2294.

138. Hermann BP, Wyler AR, Richey, ET. Wisconsin Card Sorting Test performance in patients with complex partial seizures of temporal lobe origin. J Clin Exp Neuropsychol 1988;10:467–476.

139. Wiegatz P, et al. Co-morbid psychiatric disorder in chronic epilepsy: recognition and etiology of depression. American Academy of Neurology 1999;53(Suppl):S3–S8.

140. Robertson MM, Trimble MR. Depressive illness in patients with epilepsy: a review. Epilepsia 1983;24(Suppl 2):S109–116.

141. Robertson MM. Depression in patients with epilepsy: an overview and clinical study. In MR Trimble (ed), The Psychopharmacology of Epilepsy. Chichester, England: Wiley, 1985.

142. Johnson LC. Effects of anticonvulsant medication in sleep patterns. In MB Sterman, MN Shouse, P Passouant (eds), Sleep and Epilepsy. New York: Academic Press, 1982;381–394.

143. Lefcourt HM. Locus of control: current trends in theory and research. Hillsdale, New Jersey: Erlbaum, 1976.

144. Matthews WS, G Barabas, Ferrari M. Emotional concomitants of childhood epilepsy. Epilepsia 1982;23(6):671–681.

145. Hermann BP, Wyler AR. Depression, locus of control, and the effects of epilepsy surgery. Epilepsia 1989;30:332–338.

146. Chaplin J, Yepez R, Shorvon S. A quantitative approach to measuring the social effects of epilepsy. Neuroepidemiology 1990; 9:151–158.

147. Hermann BP, Whitman S. Psychosocial predictors of interictal depression. J Epilepsy 1989;2:231–237.

148. Dell J. Social dimensions of epilepsy: stigma and response. In S Whitman, B Hermann (eds), Psychopathology in Epilepsy. New York: Oxford University Press, 1986;185–210.

149. Dodrill C. Neuropsychology. In J Laidlaw, A Richens, D Chadwick (eds), A Textbook of Epilepsy (4th edition). London: Churchill Livingstone, 1993.

150. Robertson MM, Trimble MR, Townsend HRA. Phenomenonology of depression in epilepsy. Epilepsia 1987;28:364–372.

151. Rodin EA. Differences between patients with temporal lobe seizures and those with other forms of epileptic attacks. Epilepsia 1976;17:313.

152. Reynolds EH. Antiepileptic drugs and Psychopathology. In MR Trimble (ed), The Psychopharmacology of Epilepsy. Chichester, England: Wiley, 1985.

153. Reynolds EH, et al. Folate deficiency in depressive illness. Br J Psychiatry 1970; 117:287–292.

154. Trimble MR, Corbett JA, Donaldson D. Folic acid and mental symptoms in children with epilepsy. J Neurol Neurosurg Psychiatry 1980;43:1030–1040.

155. Ring H, Reynold E. Vigabatrin and behavioral disturbance. Lancet 1990; 335:970.

156. Ring H, Heller A, Farr I. Vigabatrin: rational treatment for chronic epilepsy. J Neurol Neurosurg Psychiatry 1990; 53:1051–1055.

157. Ring H, Reynolds E. Vigabatrin. In T Pedley (ed), Recent Advances In Epilepsy, Vol. 5. Edinburgh, UK: Churchill Livingstone, 1992;177.

158. McConnell H, Duncan D. Treatment of Psychiatric Comorbidity in Epilepsy. In H McConnell, P Snyder (eds), Psychiatric Comorbidity in Epilepsy. Washington: American Psychiatric Press, 1998;245–361.

159. Mendez MF, et al. Interictal depression in epilepsy: relationship to seizure variables. J Nerv Ment Dis 1993;181:444–447.

160. Blumer D. Antidepressant and double antidepressant treatment for the affective disorder of epilepsy. J Clin Psychiatry 1997;58:3–11.

161. Robertson M. Epilepsy and Mood. In M Trimble (ed), Epilepsy, Behavior and Cognitive Function. New York: Wiley, 1988;145–147.

162. Robertson M. Depression in patients with epilepsy reconsidered. In T Pedley (ed), Recent advances in epilepsy, Vol. 4. Edinburgh, UK: Churchill Livingstone, 1988;205.

163. Robertson M. Depression in patients with epilepsy: an overview. Semin Neurol 1991;11:182–189.

164. Blumer D. Epilepsy and Disorders of Mood. In D Smith, D Treiman, M Trimble (eds), Neurobehavioral Problems in Epilepsy. New York: Raven Press, 1991;185–195.

165. Blumer D, Montouris G, Herman B. Psychiatric morbidity in seizure patients on a neurodiagnostic monitoring unit. J Neuropsychol Clin Neurosci 1995;7:445–456.

166. Williams D. The structure of emotions reflected in epileptic experiences. Brain 1956; 79:29.

167. Robertson MM. Affect and mood in epilepsy: an overview with a focus on depression. Acta Neurol Scan 1992;86:127–132.

168. Betts T. Depression, Anxiety and Epilepsy. In E Reynolds, M Trimble (eds), Epilepsy and Psychiary. New York: Churchill and Livingstone, 1981;60–71.

169. Weil A. Depressive reactions associated with temporal lobe uncinate seizures. J Nerv Ment Dis 1955;121(121):505–510.

170. Daly D. Ictal affect. Am J Psychiatry 1958;115:97–108.

171. O'Shea. Hypomania and epilepsy. Br J Psychiatry 1988;15:571.

172. Humphries SR, Dickinson PS. Hypomania following complex partial seizures. Br J Psychiatry 1988;15:571–572.

173. Mulder D, Daly D. Psychiatric symptoms associated with lesions of temporal lobe. JAMA 1952;150:173–176.

174. Perrine K, Congett S. Neurobehavioral problems in epilepsy. Neurol Clin North Am 1994;12:129–152.

175. Soto A, Kanner A, Hershkovitz L. Postictal psychiatric symptoms in patients with poorly controlled seizures: a prevalence study (abstract). Epilepsia 1997;38(Suppl 8):155.

176. Tucker G, Price T, Johnson V. Phenomenology of temporal lobe dysfunction: a link to atypical psychosis—a series of cases. J Nerv Ment Dis 1986;174:348–356.

177. Lindsay J, Ounsted C, Richards P. Longterm outcome in children with temporal lobe seizures: III: Psychiatric aspects in childhood and adult life. Dev Med Child Neurol 1979;21:630–636.

178. Prudhomme C. Epilepsy and suicide. J Nerv Ment Dis 1941;94:722–731.

179. Khron W. Causes of death among epileptics. Epilepsia 1963;4:315–321.

180. Silanpaa M. Medico-social prognosis of children with epilepsy: epidemiological study and analysis of 245 patients. Acta Paediat Scand 1973;62(Suppl 237):3–104.

181. Mendez MF, Doss RC. Ictal and psychiatric aspects of suicide in epileptic patients. Int J Psychiatry Med 1992;22:231–237.

182. Kalichman M. Neurochemical correlates of the kindling model of epilepsy. Neurosci Biobehav Rev 1982;6:165–181.

183. Trimble MR, Reynolds EH. Anticonvulsant drugs and mental symptoms. Psychol Med 1976;6:169–178.

184. Albright P, Bruni J. Overview of recent research in depression. Arch Gen Psychiatry 1985;42:797–799.

185. Giordani B, et al. Improvement in neuropsychological performance in patients with refractory seizures after intensive diagnostic and therapeutic intervention. Neurology 1983;33:489–493.

186. Trimble T, Perez M. Quantification of psychopathology in adult patients with epilepsy. In BM Kulig, H Menardi, Stoses GL, (eds), Conference Proceedings of WOPSASSEPY I 1990. 1982;118–126.

187. Pollack MH, Scott EL. Gabapentin and lamotrigine: novel treatments for mood and anxiety disorders. CNS Spectrums 1997;2:56–61.

188. Robertson MM, Trimble MR. The treatments of depression in patients with epilepsy: a double blind trial. J Affect Disord 1985;9:127–136.

189. Post RM, Uhde TW, Joffe RT. Anticonvulsant Drugs in Psychiatric Illness: New Treatment Alteratives and Theoretical Implications. In MR Trimble (ed), The Psychopharmacology of Epilepsy. New York: Wiley, 1985;141–171.

190. Itil TM, Soldatos C. Epileptogenic side effects of psychotropic drugs: practical recommendations. JAMA 1980;244:1460–1463.

191. Luchins D, Oliver AP, Wyatt RJ. Seizures with antidepressants; an in vitro technique to assess relative risk. Epilepsia 1984;25:25–32.

192. Oliver AP, Luchins DH, Wyatt RJ. Neuroleptic induced seizures. Arch Gen Psychiatry 1982;39:206–209.

193. Matthews C. The neuropsychology of epilepsy: an overview. J Clin Exp Neuropsychol 1992;14:133–143.

194. Dailey J, Naritoku D. Antidepressants and seizures: clinical anecdotes overshadow neuroscience. Biochem Pharmacol 1996; 52:1323–1329.

195. Jobe P, Laired H. Neurotransmitter abnormalities as determinants of seizure susceptibility and intensity in the genetic models of epilepsy. Biochem Pharmacol 1981;30:3137–3144.

196. Blumer D, Heilbronn M, Himmelhoch J. Indications for carbamazepine in mental illness: Atypical psychiatric disorder or temporal lobe syndrome? Compr Psychiatry 1988;29:108–122.

197. Power B, Hackett L, Dusci L. Antidepressant toxicity and the need for identification and concentration monitoring in overdose. Clin Pharmacokinet 1995;29:154–171.

198. Swinkels J, Jonghe J. Safety of antidepressants. Int Clin Psychopharmacol 1995;9(Suppl 4):19–25.

199. Snead O. On the sacred disease: the neurochemistry of epilepsy. Int Rev Neurobiol 1983;24:93–180.

200. Rosenstein DL, Nelson JC, Jacobs SC. Seizures associated with antidepressants: a review. J Clin Psychiatry 1993;54(8):289–99.

201. Preskorn SH, Fast GA. Tricyclic antidepressant-induced seizures and plasma drug concentration. J Clin Psychiatry 1992;53(5):160–162.

202. Benet L, Schawartz J, Oie S. Design and Optimization of Dosage Regimens: Pharmacokinetics Data. In J Hardman, et al. (eds), The Pharmacological Basis of Therapeutics. New York: McGraw-Hill, 1996;1707.

203. Blumer D, Zielinski J. Pharmacological treatment of psychiatric disorders associated with epilepsy. J Epilepsy 1988;1:135–150.

204. Fromm G, Amores C, Thies W. Imipramine in epilepsy. Arch Neurol 1972;27:198–204.

205. Legg N, Amores C, Thies W. Clinical note: seizures and EEG activation after trimipramine. Epilepsia 1974;15:131–135.

206. Rasmussen J, Johnson A. Incidence of seizures during treatment with antidepressants, including the new selective serotonin re-uptake inhibitor paroxetine. Proc 5th World Congr Biol Psychiatry 1991:40–41.

207. Peck A, Stern W, Watkinson C. Incidence of seizures during treatment with tricyclic antidepressant drugs and buprorion. J Clin Psychiatry 1983;44:197–201.

208. Litovitz TL, Troutman WG. Amoxepine overdose: seizures and fatalities. JAMA 1983;250:1069–1071.

209. Merigan KS, Browning RG, Leeper KV. Successful treatment of amoxepine-induced refractory status epilepticus with propofol. Acad Emerg Med 1995;2(2):128–133.

210. Horne RL, et al. Treatment of Bulimia with bupropion a multicenter controlled trial. J Clin Psychiatry 1998;49(7):262–266.

211. Johnston JA, et al. A 102-center prospective study in association with bupropion. J Clin Psychiatry 1991;52:450–477.

212. Grimsley S, Jann M, Carter J. Increased carbamazepine plasma concentration after fluoxetine co-administration. Clin Pharmacol Ther 1991;50:10–15.

213. Pearson H. Interaction of fluoxetine with carbamazepine. J Clin Psychiatry 1990;51:126.

214. Fritze J, Unsorg B, Lanczik M. Interaction between carbamazepine and fluvoxamine. Acta Psychiatr Scand 1991;84:583–584.

215. Delucchi G, Calabrese J. Anticonvulsants for the treatment of manic depression. Cleve Clin J Med 1989;56:756–761.

216. Figiel GS, et al. Electroconvulsive Therapy. In AF Schatzberg, CB Nemeroff (eds), Textbook of Psychopharmacology (2nd ed). Washington: American Psychiatric Press, Inc., 1998.

217. Post R, Putnam F, Uhde T. Electroconvulsive Therapy as an Anticonvulsant: Implications for Its Mechanism of Action in Affective Illness. In S Malitz, H Sackeim (eds), Electroconvulsive Therapy: Clinical and Basic Research Issues. New York: NY Academy of Sciences, 1986.

218. Neugebauer R, et al. Comorbidity of panic disorder and seizures: Affinity or artifact? J Anx Dis 1993;7:21–35.

219. Victoroff J, *DSM-III-R* Psychiatric diagnosis in candidates for epilepsy surgery: lifetime prevalence. Neuropsychiatry Neuropsychol Behav Neurol 1994;7:87–97.

220. Francis S, et al. Anxiety in epilepsy (abstract). Epilepsia 1996;37(Suppl 5):3.

221. Spielberger CD, Gorusch RL, Lushene RE. STAI Manual for the State-Trait Anxiety Inventory. Palo Alto, CA: Consulting Psychologists Press, 1970.

222. Penfield W, Jasper H. Epilepsy and the functional anatomy of the human brain. Boston: Little, Brown, 1954.

223. Gloor P, et al. The role of limbic system in experiential phenomenon of temporal lobe epilepsy. Ann Neurol 1982;12:129–144.

224. Reiman EM, et al. The application of positron emission tomography to the study of panic disorder. Am J Psychiatry 1986;143:469–477.

225. Flor-Henry P. Schizophrenic-like reactions and affective psychoses associated with temporal lobe epilepsy: etiological factors. Am J Psychiatry 1969;126:400–404.

226. Drubach DA, Kelly MP. Panic disorder associated with a right paralimbic lesion. Neuropsychitr Neuropsychol Behav Neurol 1989;2:282–289.

227. Ghadirian AM, Gauthier S, Bertrand S. Anxiety attacks in a patient with right temporal lobe meningioma. J Clin Psychiatry 1986;47:270–271.

228. Wall M, Tuchman M, Mielke D. Panic attacks and temporal lobe seizures associated with a right temporal lobe arteriovenous malformation: case report. J Clin Psychiatry 1985;46:143–145.

229. Perini G, Mendius R. Depression and anxiety in complex partial seizures. J Nerv Ment Dis 1984;172:287–290.

230. DePaulis A, et al. Anxiogenic-like consequences in animal models of complex partial seizures. Neurosci Biobehav Rev 1997;6:767–774.

231. Doose DR, et al. Single-dose pharmacokinetics and effects of food on the bioavailability of topiramate, a novel antiepileptic drug. J Clin Pharmacol 1996;36:884–891.

232. Ring HA, et al. Vigabatrin and depression. J Neurol Neurosurg Psychiatry 1993;56:925–928.

233. McConnell H, et al. Neuropsychiatric side effects related to treatment with felbamate. J Neuropsychiatry Clin Neurosci 1996;8:341–346.

234. Trimble MR. Neuropsychiatric Consequences of Pharmacotherapy. In J Engel, TA Pedley (eds), Epilepsy: a Comprehensive Textbook. Philadelphia: Lippincott–Raven, 1997;2161–2170.

235. Theodore WH. Abrupt Withdrawal of Antiepileptic Drugs for Intensive Video-EEG Monitoring. In E Wyllie (ed), The Treatment of Epilepsy: Principles and Practice. Philadelphia: Lea & Febiger, 1993;1009–1013.

236. Malow BA, et al. Carbamazepine withdrawal: effects of taper rate on seizure frequency. Neurology 1993;43:2280–2284.

237. Bladin PF. Psychosocial difficulties and outcome after temporal lobectomy. Epilepsia 1992;33:898–907.

238. Mittan RJ, Locke GE. Fear of seizures: epilepsy's forgotten problem. Urban Health 1982;40(January/February):38–39.

239. Seligman MEP. Helplessness. San Francisco: Freeman, 1975.

240. Hermann BP. Psychopathology in epilepsy and learned helplessness. Med Hypotheses 1979;5:723–729.

241. Devillis RF, Devillis BM. Epilepsy and learned helplessness. Basic and Applied Social Psychology 1980;1(3):241–253.

242. Betts TA. Neuropsychiatry. In J Laidlaw (ed), A Textbook of Epilepsy. Churchill Livingstone, 1993:397–457.

243. Jackson JH. Lectures on the Diagnosis of Epilepsy. In J Taylor (ed), Selected Writings Of John Hughlings Jackson, Vol. 1. London: Holder and Stoughton, 1931;276.

244. Hermann BP, et al. Interictal psychopathology in patients with ictal fear: a quantitative investigation. Neurology 1982;32:7–11.

245. Devinsky O, et al. Ictal fear in temporal lobe epilepsy: association with interictal behavioral changes. J Epilepsy 1992;4.

246. Stagno SJ, et al. Self-report inventory responses of patients with childhood onset epilepsy with ictal fear. Paper presented at American Epilepsy Society Annual Meeting, 1989, Boston, MA.

247. Spitz MC. Panic disorder in seizure patients: a diagnostic pitfall. Epilepsia 1991;32(Suppl 1):33–38.

248. DSM-IV, *Diagnostic and Statistical Manual of Mental Disorders. DSM-IV.* DSM-IV, ed. A.P. Association. Washington: American Psychiatric Association Press, 1994.

249. Sheehan DV. Current concepts in psychiatry: panic attacks and phobias. N Engl J Med 1982;307:156–158.

250. Devinsky O, Sato S, et al. Fear episodes due to limbic seizures with normal scalp EEG. A subdural electro-

graphic study. J Clin Psychiatry 1989;50:28–30.
251. Dantendorfer K, Amering M, et al. Is there a pathophysiological and therapeutic link between panic disorder and epilepsy? Acta Psychiatr Scand 1995;91:430–432.
252. Waxman SG, Geschwind N. Hypergraphia in temporal lobe epilepsy. Neurology 1974;24:629–638.
253. Kanner AM, et al. Remission of obsessive-compulsive disorder following right temporal lobectomy. Neuropsychtry Neuropsychol Behav Neurol 1993;6:126–129.
254. Kettle PA, Marks IM. Neurological factors in obsessive compulsive disorders: two case reports and a review of the literature. Br J Psychiatry 1986;149:315–319.
255. Pollack MH, et al. Clonazepam in the treatment of panic disorder and agoraphobia: a one year follow-up. J Clin Psychopharmacol 1986;6:302–304.
256. Fenwick P. The nature and management of aggression in epilepsy. J Neuropsychiatry Clin Neurosci 1989;1:418–425.
257. Herzberg JL Fenwick PB. The aetiology of aggression in temporal lobe epilepsy. Br J Psychiatry 1988;153:50–55.
258. Mendez MF, Doss RC, Taylor JL. Interictal violence in epilepsy: relationship to behavior and seizure variables. J Nerv Ment Dis 1993;181:566–569.
259. Stevens JR, Hermann B. Temporal lobe epilepsy, psychopathology and violence: the state of the evidence. Neurology 1981;31:1127–1132.
260. Niedermeyer E. Psychological-Psychiatric Aspects. In E Niedermeyer (ed), The Epilepsies: Diagnosis and Management. Baltimore: Williams & Wilkins, 1990;213–218.
261. Delgado-Escueta AV, et al. The nature of aggression during epileptic seizures. N Engl J Med 1981;305:711.
262. Devinsky O, Vazquez B. Behavioral changes associated with epilepsy. In O Devinsky (ed), Neurologic Clinics 1993;127–149.
263. Morrell MJ, Guldner GT. Self-reported sexual function and sexual arousability in women with epilepsy. Epilepsia 1996;37:1204–1210.
264. Murialdo G, et al. Sex hormones and pituitary function in male epileptic patients with altered or normal sexuality. Epilepsia 1995;36:360–365.
265. Herzog A, et al. Reproductive endocrine disorders in women with partial seizures of temporal lobe origin. Arch Neurol 1986b;43:341–346.
266. Cogen P, Antunes J, Correl J. Reproductive function in temporal lobe epilepsy: the effect of temporal lobectomy. Surg Neurol 1979;12:243–246.
267. Cummings L, Morrell M, Giudice L. Ovulatory function in epilepsy. Epilepsia 1995;36:353–357.
268. Dansky L, Andermann E, Andermann F. Marriage and fertility in epileptic patients. Epilepsia 1980;1:261–271.
269. Blumer D. Changes of sexual behavior related to temporal lobe disorders in man. J Sex Res 1970;6:173–180.
270. Herzog AG, et al. Reproductive endocrine disorders in men with partial seizures of temporal lobe origin. Arch Neurol 1986;43:347–350.
271. Toone BK. Sexual Disorders in Epilepsy. In TA Pedley, BS Meldrum (eds), Recent Advances in Epilepsy. New York: Churchill Livingstone, 1987;233–259.
272. Hoffman H, Kahlert T. The effects of prolonged anticonvulsant treatment on the sexual hormone of male epileptic patients. Nervenarzt 1981;52:715–717.
273. Toone BK, Wheeler M, Fenwick PBC. Sex hormone changes in male epileptics. Clin Endocrinol (Oxf) 1980;12:391–395.
274. Spark RF, Wills CA, Royal H. Hypogonadism, hyperprolactinemia, and temporal lobe epilepsy in hyposexual men. Lancet 1984;1(8374):413–416.
275. Schomer DL, O'Connor M, Paul S, et al.. Temporolimbic Epilepsy and Behavior. In MM Mesulam (ed), Principles of Behavioral and Cognitive Neurology. New York: Oxford University Press, 2000;373–397.
276. Gloor P. The Temporal Lobe and the Limbic System (2nd ed). New York: Oxford University Press, 1997.
277. Herzog AG, et al. Temporal lobe epilepsy: an extrahypothalamic pathogenesis for polycystic ovarian syndrome? Neurology 1984;34:1389–1393.
278. Herzog AG, et al. Neuroendocrine dysfunction in temporal lobe epilepsy. Arch Neurol 1982;39:133–135.
279. Perrine K. Cognitive deficits in epilepsy and contribution to psychopathology. Neurology 1999;55(Suppl 2):S39–S45.
280. Barr W, Consortium B. The right temporal lobe and memory: a critical reexamination. J Int Neuropsychol Soc 1995;1:139–149.
281. Herman W, Consortium B. Memory functions and verbal learning ability in patients with complex partial seizures of temporal lobe origin. Epilepsia 1987;28:547–554.
282. Trimble MR, Thompson PJ. Neuropsychological Aspects of Epilepsy. In I Grant, KM Adam (eds), Neuropsychological Assessment of Neuropsychiatric Disorders. New York: Oxford University Press, 1986;321–346.
283. Klove H, Matthews CG. Psychometric and adaptive abilities in epilepsy with different aetiology. Epilepsia 1966;7:330–338.
284. Dodrill C. Correlates of generalized tonic-clonic seizures with intellectual, neuropsychological, emotional and social functions in patients with epilepsy. Epilepsia 1986;27:191–197.
285. Seidenberg M, et al. Changes in seizure frequency and test-retest scores on the WAIS. Epilepsia 1981;22:75–83.
286. Bergin PS, et al. The effects of seizures on memory for recently learned material. Neurology 1995;45:236–240.
287. Corsi PM. Human Memory and the Medial Temporal Region of the Brain [dissertation]. Montreal, Quebec, Canada: McGill University; 1972.
288. Barr WB. Examining the right temporal lobe's role in nonverbal memory. Brain Cogn 1997;35:26–41.
289. Davis M. Neurobiology of fear responses: the role of the amygdala. J Neuropsychiatry Clin Neurosci 1997;9:382–402.

290. Kapur N, et al. Very long-term amnesia in association with temporal lobe epilepsy: evidence for a multistage consolidation process. Brain Cogn 1997;35:58–70.

291. O'Connor M, et al. Accelerated forgetting in association with temporal lobe epilepsy and paraneoplastic syndrome. Brain Cogn 1997;35:71–84.

292. Binnie C. Monitoring Seizures. In M Trimble, EH Reynolds (eds), What Is Epilepsy? Vol. 7. Edinburgh, UK: Churchill Livingstone, 1986;330–338.

293. Trimble M. Cognitive Hazards of Seizure Disorders. In M Trimble (ed), Chronic Epilepsy, Its Prognosis and Management. New York: Wiley, 1989,

294. Rosen J. Dilantin Dementia. Trans Am Neurol Assoc 1966;93:273.

295. Devinsky O. Cognitive and behavioral effects of AEDs. In Annual Course of the American Epilepsy Society: New Developments in Antiepileptic Drug Therapy. New Orleans, 1994.

296. Thompson P, Huppert F, Trimble M. Phenytoin and cognitive functions; effects on normal volunteers and implications for epilepsy. Br J Clin Psychol 1981;20:155–162.

297. Thompson P, Trimble M. Comparative effects of anticonvulsant drugs on cognitive functioning. Br J Clin Prac 1982;18 S(Suppl):154–156.

298. Smith D. Cognitive Effects of Anticonvulsant Drugs. In D Smith, D Treiman, M Trimble (eds), Advances in Neurology. New York: Raven Press, 1991;197–224.

299. Duncan JS, Shorvon SD, Trimble MR. Effects of removal of phenytoin, carbamazepine, and valproate on cognitive function. Epilepsia 1990;31(5):584–591.

300. Nolte R, et al. Effects of Phenytoin and Primidone-Monotherapy on Mental Performance in Children. In S Johannessen, et al. (eds), Antiepileptic Therapy: Advances in Drug Monitoring. New York: Raven Press, 1980.

301. MacLeod C, Decaban A, Hunt E. Memory impairment in epilepsy patients: selective effects of phenobarbital concentrations. Science 1978;202:1102–1104.

302. Ozdirim E, Renda Y, Epir S. Effects of phenobarbital and phenytoin on the behavior of epileptic children. Adv Epileptol 1978;13:120–123.

303. Camfield C, et al. Side effects of phenobarbital in toddlers: behavioral and cognitive aspects. J Pediatr 1979;95:361–365.

304. Farwell J, et al. Phenobarbital for febrile seizures—effects on intelligence and seizure recurrence. N Engl J Med 1990;322:364–369.

305. Dodrill CB, et al. Effects of tiagabine monotherapy on abilities, adjustment, and mood. Epilepsia 1998;39(1):33–42.

306. Leach JP, et al. Gabapentin and cognition: a double blind, dose ranging, placebo controlled study in refractory epilepsy. J Neurol Neurosurg Psychiatry 1997;62:372–376.

307. Marciani MG, et al. Lamotrigine add-on therapy in focal epilepsy: electroencephalographic and neuropsychological evaluation. Clin Neuropharmacol 1998;21:41–47.

308. Monaco F, et al. Lack of association between vigabatrin and impaired cognition. J Int Med Res 1997;25:296–301.

309. Thomas L, et al. Vigabatrin and behaviour disorders. Epilepsy Res 1996;25:21–26.

310. Meador K, Loring D. Cognitive Effects of Antiepileptic Drugs. In O Devinsky, W Theodore (eds), Epilepsy and Behavior. New York: Wiely-Liss, 1991;151–170.

311. Thompson P, Trimble M. Anticonvulsant drugs and cognitive functions. Epilepsia 1982;23:531–594.

312. Jones-Gotman M. Commentary: Psychological Evaluation-Testing Hippocampal Function. In J Engel (ed), Surgical Treatment of Epilepsies. New York: Raven Press, 1987;203–211.

313. Hermann B, et al. Comorbid psychiatric symptoms in temporal lobe epilepsy: association with chronicity of epilepsy and impact on quality of life. Epilepsy and Behavior 2000;1:184–190.

314. Cramer JA, et al. A brief questionnaire to screen for quality of life in epilepsy: the QOLIE-10. Epilepsia 1996;37(6):577–582.

315. Ettinger AB, Perrine K. Psychiatric/Psychosocial Issues in Epilepsy. In J French, et al. (eds), Epilepsy Update. Norwalk, CT: GEM Communications, 1996;13–24.

316. QOLIE, Quality of Life in Epilepsy. Postgraduate Services, Attention: QOLIE Study Services, 400 Plaza Drive, Secaucus, NJ 07094.

317. Adachi N, et al. Effects of the laterality of interictal discharge an antiepileptic drugs on cognitive function in temporal lobe epilepsy: a preliminary study. Jpn J Psychiatry Neurol 1993;47:366–367.

318. Bennett T. Cognitive Effects of Epilepsy and Anticonvulsant Medications. T Bennett (ed), The Neuropsychology of Epilepsy. New York: Plenum, 1992;73–95.

319. Brown S, McGown M, Reynolds E. The influence of seizure types and medications on psychiatric symptoms in epileptic patients. Br J Psychiatry 1986;148:300–304.

320. Iivanainen M. Effects of Antiepileptic Drugs on Maturation of the Human Body. In P Morselli, C Pippenger (eds), Drug Therapy in Pediatrics. New York: Raven Press, 1983;65–73.

321. Meador KJ, et al. Comparative cognitive effects of phenobarbital, phenytoin, and valproate in healthy adults. Neurology 1995;45(8):1494–1499.

322. Trimble M. Neuropsychiatric complications of epilepsy and its drug treatment. Eur J Neurol 1996;3(Suppl 3):21–28.

323. Dodrill C. Behavioral Effects of Antiepileptic Drugs. In D Smith, D Treimann, M Trimble (eds), Advances in Neurology. New York: Raven Press, 1991;213–224.

324. Dodrill C. Effects of Antiepileptic Drugs on Behavior. In O Devinsky (ed), Epilepsy and Behavior. New York: Wiley-Liss,1991;37–46.

325. Reynolds E. Mental effects of antiepileptic medications: a review. Epilepsia 1983;24(Suppl 2):S85–S95.

326. Rivinus TM. Psychiatric effects of the anticonvulsant regimens. J Clin Psychopharmacol 1982;2:165–192.

327. Ransom B, Elmorek J. Effects of Antiepileptic Drugs on the Developing Central Nervous System. In D Smith, D Treiman, M Trimble (eds), Advances in Neurology. New York: Raven Press, 1991;225–237.

328. Kato H. Antiepileptic drugs and psychiatric disorders: mechanisms involved in manifestation of psychic symptoms of high blood levels of antiepileptics. Folia Psychiatrica et Neurologica Japonica 1983;37:283–290.

329. Kugoh T, Hosokawa K. Pharmacodynamic factors in the occurrence of psychiatric symptoms patients with epilepsy. Folia Psychiactrica et Neurologica Japonica 1983;37:277–282.

330. Yassa R, et al. Carbamazepine and hyponatremia in patients with affective disorder. Am J Psychiatry 1988;145(3):339–342.

331. Toone B. Epilepsy and Sexual Life. In A Hopkins, S Shorvon (eds), Epilepsy. London: Chapman and Hall, 1995;557–564.

332. Snyder P, Badura L. Chronic administration of sodium valproate slows pubertal maturation in inbred DBA/2J mice: skeleton, histological and endocrinological evidence. Epilepsy Res 1995;20(3):203–211.

333. Gates J. Side Effects Profile and Behavioral Consequences of Antiepileptic medications. Epilepsy and Behavior 2000;1(3):153–159.

334. Cramer J, Mattson R. Toxicity. In R Levy, et al. (eds), Antiepileptic Drugs (4th ed). New York: Raven Press, 1995;817–822.

335. Domizo S, et al. Antiepileptic therapy and behavioral disturbances in children. Childs Nerv Syst 1993;9:272–274.

336. Stagno SJ. The Epidemiology of Epilepsy. In E Wyllie (ed), The Treatment of Epilepsy: Principles and Practice. Philadelphia: Lea & Febiger, 1993;1149–1162.

337. Brent DA, et al. Phenobarbital treatment and major depressive disorder in children with epilepsy. Pediatrics 1987;80:909–917.

338. Browne T, LeDuc B. Chemistry and Biotransformation. In Levy RH, et al. (eds), Antiepileptic Drugs (4th ed). New York: Raven Press, 1995;283–300.

339. Dam M. Phenytoin: toxicity, ed. DM Woodbury, JK Penry, CE Pippenger. New York: Raven Press, 1982;247–256.

340. Perlo VP. Unrecognized Dilantin Intoxication. In S Locke (ed), Modern Neurology. Boston: Little, Brown,1969;589–597.

341. Gillham R, et al. Concentration-effects relationships with carbamazepine and its epoxide on psychomotor and cognitive function in epileptic patients. J Neurol Neurosurg Psychiatry 1988;51:929–933.

342. Kastner T, Friedman D, Pond W. Carbamazepine-induced hyponatremia in patients with mental retardation. Am J Ment Retard 1992;96(5):536–540.

343. Calabrese JR, Delucchi GA. Spectrum of efficacy of valproate in 55 patients with rapid-cycling bipolar disorder. Am J Psychiatry 1990;147:431–434.

344. Trimble M, Thompson P. Sodium valproate and cognitive function. Epilepsia 1984; 25(S):S60–S64.

345. Smith DB, et al. Results of a nationwide Veterans Administration cooperative study comparing the efficacy and toxicity of carbamazepine, phenobarbital, phenytoin, and primidone. Epilepsia 1987;28(Suppl 3):S50–S58.

346. Sackellares J, Lee S, Dreifuss F. Stupor following administration of valproic acid to patients receiving other antiepileptic drugs. Epilepsia 1979;20:697–703.

347. Williams C, Tiefenbach S, McRaynolds J. Valproic acid-induced hyperammonemia in mentally retarded adults. Neurology 1984;34:550–553.

348. Murphy J, Marquard K. Asymptomatic hyperammonemia in patients receiving valproic acid. Arch Neurol 1982;39:591–592.

349. Rho J, Donevan S, Rogawski M. Mechanism of action of anticonvulsant felbamate: Opposing effects of N-methyl-D-aspartate and γ-aminobutyric acid A receptors. Ann Neurol 1994;35:229–234.

350. Hill R, Stagno S, Tesar G. Secondary mania associated with the use of felbamate. Psychosomatics 1995;36:404–406.

351. Brodie MJ, McKee PJW. Vigabatrin and psychosis. Lancet 1990;335:1279.

352. Robinson M, Richens A, Oxley R. Vigabatrin and behavior disturbances (letter). Lancet 1990;335:504.

353. Sander JWAS, et al. Vigabatrin and psychosis. J Neurol Neurosurg Psychiatry 1991;54(5):435–439.

354. Dulac O, et al. Vigabatrin in childhood epilepsy. J Child Neurol 1991;6(Suppl):2S30–2S37.

355. Appelton R. The role of vigabatrin in the management of infantile epileptic syndromes. Neurology 1993;43(Suppl 5):S21–S23.

356. Ojemann L, et al. Long-term treatment with gabapentin for partial epilepsy. Epilepsy Res 1992;13:159–165.

357. Dimond K, et al. Effect of gabapentin (Neurontin) on mood and well being in patients with epilepsy. Prog Neuropsychopharmacol Biol Psychiatry 1996;20:407–417.

358. Harden C, Pick L. Alterations in mood and anxiety in epilepsy patients treated with gabapentin (abstract). Epilepsia 1996;37(Suppl 5):137.

359. Brodie MJ, Richens A, Yuen A. Double-blind comparison of lamotrigine and carbamazepine in newly diagnosed epilepsy. Lancet 1995;345:468–476.

360. McElroy SL, et al. A pilot trial of adjunctive gabapentin in the treatment of bipolar disease. Ann Clin Psychiatry 1997;6(2):99–103.

361. Ryback RS, Brodsky L, Manasifi F. Gabapentin in bipolar disorder (letter to the editor). J Neuropsychiatry Clin Neurosci 1997;9:301.

362. Lee DO, et al. Behavioral side effects of gabapentin in children. Epilepsia 1996;37:87–90.

363. Tallian KB, et al. Gabapentin associated with aggressive behavior in pediatric patients with seizures. Epilepsia 1996;37(5):501–502.

364. Wolf SM, et al. Gabapentin toxicity in children manifesting as behavioral changes. Epilepsia 1995;36(2):1203–1205.

365. Calabrese J, et al. A double-blind placebo controlled study of lamotrigine monotherapy in outpatients with bipolar I depression. J Clin Psychiatry 1999;60:79–80.

366. Frye M, et al. Gabapentin and lamotrigine monotherapy in mood disorder: an update (abstract). Proc Annu Meet Am Psychiatric Assoc 1998:150.

367. Beran RG, Gibson RJ. Aggressive behaviour in intellectually challenged patients with epilepsy treated with lamotrigine. Epilepsia 1998;39(3):280–282.

368. Ettinger AB, et al. Positive and negative psychotropic effects of lamotrigine in epilepsy patients with mental retardation. Epilepsia 1998;39:874–877.

369. Rosenfeld W, et al. Topiramate: effective dosing enhances potential for success. Epilepsia 1992;33(Suppl):118.

370. Rak I, Isacoff J. Topiramate add-on therapy in medically intractable epilepsy: clinical features of cognitive effects. Epilepsia 1993;34(Suppl):44.

371. Faught E, et al. Topiramate placebo controlled dose-ranging trial in refractory partial epilepsy using 200, 400 and 600 mg doses. Neurology 1996;46:1684–1690.

372. Guberman J, et al. Canadian long-term experience with topiramate. Epilepsia 1996;37(Suppl):67.

373. Betts T, Smith K, Khan G. Severe psychiatric reactions to topiramate (abstract). Epilepsia 1997;38(Suppl 3):64.

374. Rowan AJ, et al. Safety and efficacy of three dose levels of tiagabine HCl versus placebo as adjunctive treatment for complex partial seizures. Epilepsia 1994;35(Suppl 8):54.

375. Kaufman KR. Adjunctive tiagabine treatment of psychiatric disorders: three cases. Ann Clin Psychiatry 1998;10(4):181–184.

376. Trimble M, et al. Psychosis with tiagabine (abstract). Epilepsia 1997;38(Suppl):40–41.

377. Sackellares J, Deaton R, Sommerville K. Incidence of psychosis in controlled tiagabine trials (abstract). Epilepsia 1997;38(Suppl 3):67.

378. Ketter TA, Post RM, Theodore WH. Positive and negative psychotropic effects of antiepileptic drugs in patients with seizure disorders. Neurology 1999;53(5 Suppl 2):S52–S66.

379. Kutt H. Interactions with Antiepileptic Drugs Involving Multiple Mechanisms. In P Morselli, S Garrantini, S Cohen (eds), Drug Interactions. New York: Raven Press, 1974.

380. Weber W. Relationship of Genetic Factors to Drug Reactions. In L Meyer, H Peck (eds), Drug Induced Disease. Experta Medica Foundation, 1972;33–59.

381. Serra L, Gallicchio B, Serra F. Lamotrigine monotherapy for treatment of learning and behavioral disorders in epileptic children (abstract). Epilepsia 1997;38(Suppl 3):130.

382. Bhaumik S, et al. A naturalistic study of the use of vigabatrin, lamotrigine and gabapentin in adults with learning disabilities. Seizure 1997;6:127–133.

383. Calandre E, et al. Cognitive effects of long-term treatment with phenobarbital and valproate in school children. Acta Neurol Scand 1990;81:504–506.

384. Corbet JA, Trimble MR, Nicol TC. Behavioral and cognitive impairment in children with epilepsy: the longterm effects of anticonvulsant toxicity. J Am Acad Child Psychiatry 1985;24(17):17–23.

385. Trimble M. Anticonvulsant Drugs and Psychosocial Development: Phenobarbitone, Sodium Valproate, and Benzodiazepines. In P Morselli, C Peppenger, J Penry (eds), Therapy in Paediatrics. New York: Raven Press, 1983;201–217.

386. Tollefson G. Psychiatric implications of anticonvulsant drugs. J Clin Psychiatry 1982;41(9):295–302.

387. Milano CG.o.S.o.E., Long-Term Intensive Monitoring in the Difficult Patient. In Gardner-Thorpe (ed), Antiepileptic Drug Monitoring. Turnbridge Wells, England: Pittman, 1977.

388. Schain R, Ward J, Guthrie D. Carbamazepine as an anticonvulsant in children. Neurology 1977;27:476–480.

389. Ketter T, Post R, Wothington K. Principles of clinically important drug interactions with carbamazepine, II. J Clin Psychopharmacol 1991;11(5):306–312.

390. Demers-Desrosiers L, Nestoros J, Vaillancourt P. Acute psychosis precipitated by withdrawal of anticonvulsant medications. Am J Psychiatry 1978;135:981–982.

391. De Bard M., Diazepam withdrawal syndrome of anticonvulsant medication: a case with psychosis, seizure, and coma. Am J Psychiatry 1979;136:104–105.

392. Sironi V, et al. Interictal acute psychosis in temporal lobe epilepsy during withdrawal of anticonvulsant therapy. J Neurol Neursurg Psychiatry 1979;42:724–730.

393. Zaret BS, Cohen RA. Reversible valproic acid-induced dementia: a case report. Epilepsia 1986;27:234–240.

394. Hauser P, et al., Benzodiazepine withdrawal delirium with catatonic features. Arch Neurol 1989;46:696–699.

395. Ketter T, et al. Anticonvulsant withdrawal—emergent psychopathology. Neurology 1994;44:55–61.

396. Edwards, Antidepressants and Seizures: Epidemiological and Clinical Aspects. In MR Trimble (ed), The Psychopharmacology of Epilepsy. Chichester, England: Wiley, 1985;119–139.

397. Garcia PA, et al. Phosphorus magnetic resonance spectroscopic imaging in patients with frontal lobe epilepsy. Ann Neurol 1994;35:217–221.

398. Markowitz JC, Brown RP. Seizures with neuroleptics and antidepressants. Gen Hosp Psychiatry 1987;9:135–141.

399. Stoudemire A, Fogel BS. Psychiatric Care of the Medical Patient. New York: Oxford University Press, 1993;475–476.

400. Davidson J. Seizures and bupropion: a review. J Clin Psychiatry 1989;50:256–261.

401. Skowron D, Stimmel G. Antidepressants and risk of seizures. Pharmacotherapy 1992;12:18–22.

402. Toone BK, Fenton GW. Epileptic seizures induced by psychotropic drugs. Psychol Med 1977;7:265–270.

403. Starkey I, Lawson A. Poisoning with tricyclic and related antidepressant—a ten year review. QJM 1980;193:33–49.
404. Biggs J, et al. Tricyclic antidepressants overdose: incidence of symptoms. JAMA 1977;238:135–138.
405. Frommer D, et al. Tricyclic antidepressant overdose: a review. JAMA 1987;257:521–526.
406. Ellison D, Pentel P. Clinical features and consequences of seizures due to cyclic antidepressants overdose. Am J Emerg Med 1989;7:5–10.
407. Boehnert M, Lovejoy F. Value of QRS duration versus the serum drug level in predicting seizures and ventricular arrhythmias after an acute overdose of tricyclic antidepressants. N Engl J Med 1985;313:474–479.
408. Foulke G, Albertson T. QRS interval in tricyclic antidepressant overdose: inaccuracy as a toxicity indicator in emergency settings. Ann Emerg Med 1985;16:160–163.
409. Wedin G, et al. Relative toxicity of cyclic antidepressants. Ann Emerg Med 1986;15:797–804.
410. Garnier R, et al. Acute fluvoxamine poisioning. J Int Med Res 1993;21:197–208.
411. Catalano G, et al. Paediatric sertraline overdose. Clin Neuropharmacol 1998;21:59–61.
412. Riddle M, Brown N, Dzubinski P. Fluoxetine overdose in adolescents. J Am Acad Child Adolesc Psychiatry 1989;28:587–588.
413. Zhalkovsky B, Walker D, Bourgeois J. Seizure activity and enzyme elevations after venlafaxine overdose. J Clin Psychopharmacol 1997;17:490–491.
414. Buckley N, et al. Cardiotoxicity more common in thioridazine overdose than with other neuroleptics. J Toxicol Clin Toxicol 1995;33:199–204.
415. Peterson C. Seizures induced by acute loxapine overdose. Am J Psychiatry 1981;138:1089–1091.
416. Jabbari B, et al. Incidence of seizures with tricyclic and tetracyclic antidepressants. Arch Neurol 1985;42:480–481.
417. DeVeaugh-Geis J, Landau P, Katz R. Preliminary results from a multicenter trial of clomipramine in obsessive-compulsive disorder. Psychopharmocol Bull 1989;25:36–40.
418. Ojemann LM, Baugh-Bookman C, Dudley D. Effect of psychotropic medications on seizure control in patients with epilepsy. Neurology 1987;37:1525–1527.
419. Alldredge BK, Simon RP. Drugs That Can Precipitate Seizures. In SR Resor, H Kutt (eds), The Medical Treatment of Epilepsy. New York: Marcel Dekker, 1992;497–523.
420. Favale E, et al. Anticonvulsant effect of fluoxetine in humans. Neurology 1995;45(10):1926–1927.
421. Prediville S, Gale K. Anticonvulsant effect of fluoxetine on focally evoked limbic motor seizures in rats. Epilepsia 1993;34(2):381–384.
422. American Hospital Formulary Service. In GK McEvoy, K Litvac, OH Welsh, et al. (eds), Drug Information. Bethesda, MD:American Society of Hospital Pharmacists, 1994.
423. Garcia PA, Alldredge. Drug-induced seizures. Neurol Clin 1994;12(1):85–99.
424. Logothetis J. Spontaneous epileptic seizures and electroencephalographic changes in the course of phenothiazine therapy. Neurology 1967;17:869–877.
425. Remick PA, Fine SH. Antipsychotic drugs and seizures. J Clin Psychiatry 1979;40:78–80.
426. Devinsky O, Pacia SV. Seizures during clozapine therapy. J Clin Psychiatry 1994:55(Suppl B):153–156.
427. Jansen P. Risperdal (package insert). Titusville, NJ, 1996.
428. Alldredge, BK. Seizure risk associated with psychotropic drugs: clinical and pharmacokinetic considerations. Neurology 1999;53(Suppl):S68–S75.
429. Nemeroff CB, DeVane CL, Pollock BG. Newer antidepressants and the cytochrome P450 system. Am J Psychiatry 1996;153(3):311–320.
430. Applied Therapeutics. Drug interactions newsletter and updates. Vancouver: Applied Therapeutics, Inc, 1995.
431. Rapeport WG, et al. Absence of a sertraline-mediated effect on the pharmacokinetics and pharmacodynamics of carbamazepine. J Clin Psychiatry 1996;57(Suppl 1):20–23.
432. Dursun SM. Toxic Serotonin Syndrome. In SP Kutcher (ed), Child and Adolescent Psychopharmacology News, 1996;4–5.

Chapter 21

Recognition and Management of Psychiatric Disorders in Childhood Epilepsy

Gerald Novak

All physicians caring for children with epilepsy have encountered patients whose behavioral problems were more severe and disabling than their seizures. Although the existence of this phenomenon is well recognized, a review of the literature summarized in the following discussion reveals that the spectrum of psychopathology in children with epilepsy is broad. Problems outside of the disruptive behavioral disorders remain relatively underdiagnosed and undermanaged. The challenge of the treating physician is to recognize these complications of epilepsy and to maintain control of the seizures while modifying therapy. This may include the withdrawal of offending antiepileptic drugs (AEDs) or the introduction of effective psychotropic drugs. In formulating the strategy to manage these problems, the physician must address the following questions: What is the prevalence of psychiatric disorders in epileptic children? What is the best way to screen for them? What kinds of behavioral problems predominate? What factors are associated with increased risk? What is the long-term outcome? What measures should be taken to treat these problems?

Prevalence of Behavioral Disorders in Children with Epilepsy

Nearly all investigators have reported a high prevalence of behavioral problems in children with epi-

lepsy.[1–19] This finding holds for a variety of outcome measures: higher ratings for problem behaviors on standardized questionnaires (Tables 21-1 and 21-2); a higher proportion with a history of psychiatric consultation or treatment with psychotropic medication[20,21]; and a higher proportion with a diagnosis of a psychiatric disorder, based on either structured interview or unblinded clinical assessment (Table 21-3). Several studies are based on population surveys,[8,13,15,16,18] although most have recruited cases from hospital-based epilepsy clinics.[1–7,9–12,14,17,19] With few exceptions,[1,22–25] children with epilepsy consistently display more behavioral problems than comparison groups, including controls drawn randomly from the same geographic region,[8,13] matched nonepileptic classroom peers,[1,2] siblings of children with epilepsy,[2–4] and children with chronic medical disorders, including diabetes mellitus,[2,3,5] asthma,[6,7] juvenile rheumatoid arthritis,[26] congenital heart disease,[8] and cerebral lesions without epilepsy.[13]

Identification of a Behavioral Disorder

Given the high prevalence of behavioral problems in this population, all children should be screened for them on their initial evaluation in the epilepsy clinic, even if symptoms are not reported. The targets of inquiry are patterns of behavior falling outside of the range expected for gender and age and causing

Table 21-1. Children with Epilepsy and Comparison Groups Meeting Criteria for Behavioral Problems on Screening Questionnaires

Study	Source of Patients	Scale	Criterion	Epilepsy Patients Meeting Criterion	Nonepileptic Comparison Group
Hackney and Taylor (1976)	Hospitalized epileptic and epilepsy clinic	Rutter Teacher's Questionnaire	>13	Hospitalized: 17/30 (57%) Epilepsy clinic: 5/30 (17%)	Inpatient psychiatric: 18/30 (60%) Normal peers: 3/30 (10%)
Hoare (1984a, 1984b)	Epilepsy clinic	Rutter Questionnaire		Newly diagnosed	Siblings of newly diagnosed epileptic children
		Parent	>13	13/29 (45%)	2/23 (8.7%)
		Teacher	>9	13/29 (45%)	4/23 (17%)
				Chronic	Siblings of chronic epileptic children
		Parent	>13	14/29 (48%)	7/23 (30%)
		Teacher	>9	12/29 (41%)	7/23 (30%)
					Newly diagnosed diabetic
		Parent			5/29 (17%)
		Teacher			5/29 (17%)
					Chronic diabetic
		Parent			6/36 (17%)
		Teacher			5/36 (14%)
					Healthy controls
		Parent			10/113 (8.8%)
		Teacher			10/113 (8.8%)
Hoare and Kerley (1991)	Epilepsy clinic	Rutter Questionnaire			Siblings of epileptic children
		Parent	>13	54%	12%
		Teacher	>9	48%	25%
Austin et al. (1992, 1994)	Epilepsy clinic	Child Behavior Checklist	> Ninety-eighth percentile, total behavior	34/127 (27%)	Chronic asthma: not stated, but lower internalizing and externalizing scores than epileptic patients
Hoare and Mann (1994)	Epilepsy clinic	Child Behavior Checklist	> Ninety-third percentile, total behavior	16/62 (25%)	Diabetes: 10/91 (11%)
McDermott et al. (1995)	Population based	Behavior Problem Index	> Ninetieth percentile, any of six behaviors	38/121 (31%)	Heart disease: 60/225 (21%) Well children: 334/3616 (8.5%)
Wirrell et al. (1997)	Population based	Structured interview that assessed psychosocial function	Patient admitted to "psychiatric or emotional problems in past"	30/56 (54%)	Juvenile rheumatoid arthritis: 19/61 (31%)

Table 21-2. Prevalence of Children with Epilepsy Meeting Criteria for a Behavioral Problem on Screening Questionnaires

Study	Source of Patients	Scale	Criterion	Epilepsy Patients Meeting Criterion
Dorenbaum et al. (1985)	Epilepsy clinic	Child Behavior Checklist	> Ninety-eighth percentile; either internalizing, externalizing, or total behavioral or social competence	9/38 (24%)
Corbett et al. (1985)	Epilepsy clinic	Rutter Parent and Teacher Questionnaire	>13 Parent, >9 teacher	Parent: 174/312 (56%) Teacher: 134/312 (43%)
Dunn et al. (1997)	Epilepsy clinic	Child Behavior Checklist	> Eighty-fifth percentile, total behavior	10/42 (24%)
Ettinger et al. (1998)	Epilepsy clinic	Child Depression Inventory Child Manifest Anxiety Scale	>13 > Eighty-fifth percentile	12/42 (29%) 7/42 (16%)
Dunn et al. (1999)	Epilepsy clinic	Child Depression Inventory–Child Behavior Checklist–Youth Self Report	>12 > Eighty-fifth percentile, Anxiety/Depression Subscale	26/115 (22.6%) 24/115 (21%)

impairment in one or more areas of function. Standardized questionnaires are widely used by physicians to screen for behavioral problems. The use of these scales implies that deviant behaviors fall along a continuum of severity and that higher ratings have significance as an indication of the amount of functional impairment. If the aim is to recognize patients with behavioral disorders, the criteria for the validity of a questionnaire are its sensitivity (the likelihood that a child with a behavioral disorder may have a deviant score) and its specificity (the likelihood that a deviant score actually indicates a behavioral disorder). Some questionnaires in use, such as the Child Behavior Checklist (CBCL),[27] have been referenced to a clinical "golden standard" and accurately differentiate children referred to behavioral clinics from their unaffected peers. However, this validation may not have been established for populations of children with chronic illnesses, such as epilepsy, and it may be unclear which point on the rating scale corresponds to a high likelihood of a clinical diagnosis. Of nine reported cohorts of epileptic children rated on the CBCL,[5,6,9,19,23,28–31] only one was also evaluated by structured psychiatric interview.[19] In this study, 7 of 39 children were diagnosed with major depressive disorders using the Kiddie-Schedule for Affective Disorders and Schizophrenia; their mean total behavioral score on the CBCL was approximately the ninetieth percentile, but ratings for the Anxiety or Depression subscale of the CBCL were not presented.

There is excellent data on the validity of the Rutter Scales in children with epilepsy. In the Isle of Wight study,[13] ratings above the cutoff on the Parent and Teacher Scales identified 54.5% and 53%, respectively, of 10- to 11-year-old children in the general sample who were eventually diagnosed with a psychiatric disorder, and 80% of such children were diagnosed with epilepsy or other chronic physical handicaps. This scale was subsequently used in at least eight other studies, mainly in Britain.[1,2,4,10,18,24,32,33]

Ratings for a deviant behavior may be inflated by ambiguous items on a questionnaire that may actually reflect epileptic behavior (e.g., incontinence, inattention, twitching or other unusual movements; see Perrin et al.[34]). Deletion of potentially ambiguous items on the CBCL did not affect the ratings of diabetic children and their controls,[35] but the effect of this correction has not been measured in epileptic children.

Some scales have been carefully validated in the diagnosis of a specific psychiatric disorder, such as

Table 21-3. Children with Epilepsy Meeting Criteria for the Diagnosis of a Psychiatric Disorder

Study	Source of Patients	Scale	Criterion	Epilepsy Patients Meeting Criterion	Nonepileptic Comparison Group
Rutter et al. (1970)	Population based	Interview	Clinical diagnosis	Uncomplicated epilepsy: 18/63 (29%)	Age-matched controls: 144/2,189 (6.6%)
				Epilepsy with structural lesion: 7/12 (58%)	Other chronic disorders: 16/138 (12%)
					Cerebral lesions without epilepsy: 9/24 (38%)
Sillanpaa (1973)	Population based	Interview	Clinical diagnosis (psychoneurotic)	72/197 (37%)	—
Ounsted et al. (1966)	Clinic; all temporal lobe epilepsy	Unblinded clinical assessment	Hyperactive	26/100 (26%)	—
			Catastrophic rage	36/100 (36%)	—
			Either	47/100 (47%)	—
Steffenburg et al. (1996)	Population based; mentally retarded epileptic	Interview	Autistic spectrum problems	40/90 (44%)	—
			Attention deficit hyperactivity disorder	6/90 (7%)	—
			Other	7/90 (8%)	—
			Uncategorizable/demented	32/90 (36%)	—
			No psychiatric diagnosis	5/90 (6%)	—
Caplan et al. (1997)	Epilepsy clinic: complex partial seizures	Diagnostic interview for children and adolescents	DSM-III	20/30, including schizophrenia-like psychosis: 6; disruptive behaviors: 9; affective/anxiety: 3	—
	Primarily generalized epilepsy	Kiddie-Schedule for Affective Disorders and Schizophrenia (K-SADS)	DSM-IV	13/24, including disruptive behaviors: 8; affective/anxiety: 5	—
Hackett et al. (1998)	Population based	Interview	International Statistical Classification of Diseases, 10th Revision, any diagnosis	6/17 (35%)	—
Brent et al. (1987)	Epilepsy clinic	K-SADS	DSM-III, affective disorder	11/39 (28%)	—

DSM-III = Diagnostic and Statistical Manual of Mental Disorders, Third Edition; DSM-IV = DSM, Fourth Edition.

depression (the Children's Depression Inventory[36]) or attention deficit hyperactivity disorder (ADHD; the ADHD Questionnaire[37]). For screening, a broader diagnostic spectrum is more desirable, complemented with subscales that target specific symptom clusters or diagnoses. Thus, the CBCL includes a total behavioral score, as well as eight "narrow band" scales of specific problem behaviors and two "broad-band" scales—internalizing symptoms (e.g., schizoid, depressed, uncommunicative, obsessive-compulsive, and somatic complaints) and externalizing symptoms (e.g., hyperactive, aggressive, and delinquent). Subscales are usually derived empirically from factor analysis of responses to all of the items on the questionnaire,[27] not by the theoretical fit of each item to an actual clinical diagnostic category. Some tests, however, are based directly on the fourth edition of the *Diagnostic and Statistical Manual of Mental Disorders* (*DSM-IV*), such as the Child Symptom Inventory.[38]

Structured interviews are often used to attain a high degree of diagnostic specificity in clinical research; this is necessary to ensure that patients selected for therapeutic trials are diagnostically "pure." They may be used as a means to validate the specificity of questionnaires and unblinded clinical assessment. However, some children with psychosocial impairment fall short of criteria for any single diagnosis on these interviews.[39] Ultimately, the most important part in the evaluation of a possible psychiatric disorder in a child with epilepsy is the estimation of the degree of impairment in everyday life; questionnaires and rating scales may sensitize the clinician and direct his or her focus, but there is no substitute for open-ended questions and common sense in the interpretation of the child's responses.

Types of Behavioral Disorders Seen in Epileptic Children

A review of many published studies does not reveal a consistent pattern of behavioral disorders in children with epilepsy. This reflects differences in the clinical makeup of the populations studied, as well as differences in nosology and methods of assessment. Most studies fail to support the notion of a distinctive pattern of deviant behavior, when

epileptic children of normal intelligence are compared to nonepileptic children with behavioral disorders. In the Isle of Wight study,[13] the proportion of children classified by a standardized interview as neurotic or antisocial or having mixed psychiatric disorder symptoms did not differ between epileptic children with and without structural brain lesions and the general population. Similarly, Hackney et al.[1] found no differences in the relative proportions of children that met the criteria on the Rutter Parent and Teacher Questionnaires for neurotic, antisocial, and mixed symptoms when comparing four groups: hospitalized epileptic patients, psychiatric inpatients, epileptic schoolchildren, and their peers, matched for age and gender.

A different picture emerges when more severely impaired children are included. Using the Rutter Questionnaires, Corbett et al.[10] found a relatively high proportion of antisocial symptoms (42%) in a residential school for epileptic children, of whom 60% were mentally retarded. There is clearly an over-representation of autistic spectrum disorders in the epileptic population; Sillanpaa[16] noted psychosis ("chiefly of the autism . . . type") in 26 out of 242 children (11%), and Steffenburg et al.[15] noted autistic spectrum disorders (including autistic disorder, Asperger syndrome, autisticlike conditions, and autistic traits) in 40 of 90 (44%) children with active epilepsy and mental retardation (MR).

An interictal psychosis, described as schizophrenialike, appears to be more common in adults with partial epilepsy than in the general population.[40] Of Ounsted's original series of 100 children with temporal lobe epilepsy, 9 of 87 who reached adulthood without moderate to severe MR developed a schizophreniform psychosis.[40] A left-sided focus (seven of nine), frequent childhood seizures (eight of nine), male gender (eight of nine), and continuation of seizures into adulthood (nine of nine) were associated factors. Caplan et al.[17] diagnosed a schizophrenialike psychosis in 6 of 30 children with complex partial seizures (CPSs), but none in 24 children with primarily generalized epilepsy (PGE). The Kiddie Formal Thought Disorders Rating Scale[41] was used to rate a videotaped interview from each child. With verbal intelligence quotient (IQ) as a covariate, ratings for illogical thinking were higher for the CPS group than for the PGE group, which, in turn, did not differ from a group of healthy controls. The ratings were highest for psychotic children. Among children with disruptive behavior disorders but no psychosis, ratings for illogical thinking were higher in the CPS group than in the PGE group. There were no group differences for children with affective or anxiety disorders or for those with no psychiatric diagnosis. In the CPS group, multiple regression of the illogical thinking scores showed the significant effect of the diagnosis of psychosis and of three factor scores derived from the revised Wechsler Intelligence Scale for Children[42]: verbal comprehension, freedom from distractibility, and perceptual organization. There was no effect of seizure control, age of onset, electroencephalogram (EEG) focus laterality, or number of AEDs. Thus, thought disorder, with or without psychosis, may be more common in children with complex partial seizures. These children may be at greater risk for the development of psychosis in adulthood.

Another cluster of problems that appears to be more common in children with epilepsy is the disruptive behavioral disorder group: ADHD, oppositional defiant disorder, and conduct disorder. The symptoms that define the *DSM-IV* diagnostic criteria for the disruptive behavioral disorders fall into several categories: impulsivity or hyperactivity; inattention or distractibility; opposition and defiance; and rule-breaking behaviors that include physical aggression, destruction of property, deceit and theft, and truancy.[43] The existence of these categories and their subtypes as distinct clinical entities, their regions of overlap, and the precise criteria that define their diagnostic thresholds are sure to change with the accrual of new data and shifts in expert consensus. Because of this, it is impossible to compare the prevalence of these disorders across studies that have occurred at different times and used different screening instruments.

Studies that rely on unblinded global clinical assessment generally report a higher frequency of hyperactivity in epileptic children than in the general population. Sillanpaa[16] observed hyperactivity in 80 of 210 patients (38%) in a population study, whereas Ounsted[44] found it in 70 of 830 patients (8%) in a hospital clinic. Ounsted[14] reported an even higher prevalence in a study of 100 children with temporal lobe epilepsy, many of whom were medically intractable: 26 were hyperactive, 36 displayed episodes of "catastrophic rage," and 47 had at least one of these problems. Similarly, high estimates of

hyperactivity have appeared when global impressions were sought from teachers (Sturniolo and Galetti[45]: 24 of 41 children with idiopathic epilepsy) or from parents (Harvey et al[46]: 14 of 63 children with new-onset temporal lobe epilepsy).

Hyperactivity and oppositional behaviors are highly associated. If these symptoms are co-reported, the prevalence of hyperactivity may be underestimated if other disruptive behaviors are assigned diagnostic precedence. Thus, in the Isle of Wight study,[13] Rutter classified 9 of 34 children with psychiatric disorders as antisocial but only four as hyperactive. These diagnostic categories were mutually exclusive.

Questionnaires appear to be more sensitive to hyperactivity when completed by parents than when completed by teachers: Aman et al. (New Zealand),[22] Berg et al. (Britain),[24] and Epir et al. (Turkey)[47] found that ratings for hyperactivity on the Conners Teacher Rating Scale[48] did not differ between epileptic patients and matched controls, whereas Stores et al.[49] found higher ratings for hyperactivity only on the Conners Parent Rating Scale[48] in children with absence and partial epilepsy compared to healthy controls. McDermott et al.[8] found a higher proportion of epileptic children with elevated scores for the hyperactivity factor on the parent-reported Behavior Problem Index[50,51] than in healthy controls and children with congenital heart disease. The proportion remained higher when the comparison was limited to children who met the criteria for any of the six deviant behaviors on this questionnaire.

Few studies have applied *DSM-IV* criteria for the diagnosis of ADHD to children with epilepsy. Five studies differing widely in composition found that 14–37% of children met these criteria (Table 21-4).[17,52–55] Dunn et al.[52] used *DSM-IV* criteria in a study of 158 children, allowing for differentiation of predominantly inattentive, hyperactive, and combined subtypes. Children were more commonly inattentive (22%) than combined (12%) or hyperactive (2.5%), a reversal of the predominance of the combined subtype seen in the nonepileptic population.

Risk Factors for Behavioral Problems in Childhood Epilepsy

The prevalence of behavioral disorders varies widely across the sample of studies seen in Tables

Table 21-4. Children with Epilepsy Meeting Criteria for Diagnosis of Attention Deficit Hyperactivity Disorder

Study	Source of Patients	Criteria	Method	Patients Meeting Criteria
Dunn et al. (1999)	Epilepsy clinic	*DSM-IV*	Parent questionnaires (Child or Adolescent Symptom Inventory-4)	58/158 (36.7%)
Semrud-Clikeman and Wical (1999)	Epilepsy clinic	*DSM-III-R*	Semistructured parent interview (modified Kiddie-Schedule for Affective Disorders and Schizophrenia [K-SADS])	12/33 (36%)
Williams et al. (1998)	Epilepsy clinic	*DSM-III-R*	Not stated	11/79 (14%)
Caplan et al. (1997)	Epilepsy clinic, complex partial seizures	*DSM-III*	Diagnostic Interview for Children and Adolescents	9/30 (30%)
	Epilepsy clinic, primarily generalized epilepsy	*DSM-IV*	K-SADS	6/24 (25%)
Hempel et al. (1995)	Epilepsy clinic	*DSM-III-R*	Not stated	40/109 (37%)

DSM-III-R = Diagnostic and Statistical Manual of Mental Disorders, Revised Third Edition; DSM-IV = DSM, Fourth Edition.

21-1 and 21-3, even when the same outcome measure is used. Behavioral disorders in children with epilepsy must result from the interaction of the many factors that differ among these studies. Hermann et al.[30] proposed a multietiologic model for psychopathology in childhood epilepsy. Etiologic factors fell into four domains: demographic, biological, pharmacologic, and psychosocial. This model provides a useful framework for this review.

Demographic Factors

Age

Austin et al.[6] and Hermann et al.[30] found that age was inversely correlated with behavioral ratings on the CBCL, but this effect disappeared on multivariate analysis. Most other investigators found a similar prevalence of behavioral problems in children of all ages with epilepsy.[8,13,22]

Gender

Males predominate among children with psychiatric diagnoses, especially in those with disruptive behavioral disorders. This is confirmed in several studies[22,30,32,50] of children with epilepsy. Ounsted[14] found that, among children with temporal lobe epilepsy, boys were two times more likely than girls to exhibit hyperactivity, and 1.5 times more likely to have rage episodes. However, the observed relative risks are lower than the approximately fourfold male preponderance for ADHD, as diagnosed in North America.[56]

Other studies found no significant gender differences in the rates of behavioral problems.[4,13] McDermott et al.[8] found a male preponderance for antisocial and hyperactive behaviors in the general population as well as in children with congenital heart disease, whereas rates for nearly all behavioral problems were similar for boys and girls with epilepsy, except for anxiety (which was more common in girls). These studies suggest that epilepsy tends to elevate the rate of behavioral problems independent of gender.

Other investigators found an interaction of gender with other factors. Aman et al.[22] found that boys with partial seizures had a higher rating for socialized aggression on the Revised Behavior Problem Checklist.[57] Austin et al.[58] found that girls with a high initial seizure severity were rated by their mothers as having more severe thought, attention, and social problems. On follow-up, those girls whose seizures remained severe after 4 years were the only children with epilepsy whose ratings for internalizing and externalizing behaviors on the CBCL actually worsened.[59]

Socioeconomic Status

Surprisingly, socioeconomic status has a small and inconsistent effect on the prevalence of behavioral disorders in children with epilepsy. Rutter et al.[13] noted a higher prevalence of psychiatric disorders in children whose fathers were manual laborers. McDermott et al.[8] found higher ratings for hyperactivity and peer conflict in children with epilepsy whose family income fell below the 1988 federal poverty index; the magnitude of this effect was greater for these children than it was for healthy controls and children with cardiac disease. Hermann et al.[30] found that income was directly proportional to ratings for social competence, but not for problem behaviors. Several other investigators found no effect,[6,11] perhaps because a more homogenous sample was studied.

Biological Factors

The biological factors that may account for behavioral disorders include those related to the epilepsy itself, as well as those resulting from the other brain disorders that may be associated with epilepsy.

Types of Epilepsy Associated with Behavioral Disorders

Of all of the abnormalities of function in the epileptic brain, which ones ought to take theoretical precedence as a cause for disturbed behavior? Our hypotheses are generated from clinical observation and are limited by the ways in which we classify seizures, epileptic syndromes, and etiologies and by the way in which we quantify their severity. Therefore, it is not surprising that no single type of epilepsy has been consistently linked to an increased overall risk of psychopathology.

There are additional problems on the level of description that hamper this effort. According to

the criteria of the International League Against Epilepsy (ILAE), patients with epilepsy may be classified by seizure type,[60] syndrome,[61] and etiology.[62] Older studies generally classified patients only by seizure type, and their terminology and diagnostic boundaries do not always correspond with the current ILAE criteria. Because similar seizure types may be seen in different epilepsy syndromes, patients grouped by seizure type may confound different prognoses, treatments, and neurologic comorbidities. Some types of seizures are easily confounded, including generalized absence and complex partial seizures, primarily generalized tonic-clonic and partial with secondary generalization seizures, and the variety of seizure types seen in the infant. There is probably a systematic underestimation of partial seizures and of the presence of structural lesions, especially in the older literature, in younger patients and early in the course of epilepsy. The use of ancillary tests, such as neuroimaging or EEG, in lateralizing and localizing the origin of the seizure is inconsistent between and within studies. The use of specific EEG findings (e.g., midtemporal spikes) as the main explanatory variable is likely to confound different seizure types and syndromes that may share one or more electrophysiologic features. Finally, few studies examine interobserver consistency of the classification of epilepsy at the level of syndrome and etiology,[63] which must be presumed to be low when considering studies originating in different institutions and in different decades.

Other possible biological risk factors may differ systematically between different types of epilepsy, including the age of onset, age of the patient at the time of study, presence of an associated encephalopathy besides epilepsy, seizure frequency and severity, and choice of AED. Therefore, these factors must be accounted for whenever different types of epilepsy are compared.

In the Isle of Wight study, Rutter et al.[13] observed the highest prevalence of psychiatric disorder in children with epilepsy and known structural cerebral lesions (7 of 12; 58%). In a cohort of children with temporal lobe epilepsy, Ounsted[14] observed that children with a history of "gross cerebral insult" or status epilepticus were more likely to exhibit hyperactivity or "catastrophic rage." Therefore, it might be expected that the highest risk of psychiatric disorder exists in children with symptomatic partial epilepsy. However, the majority of studies analyzing type of epilepsy as a risk factor for behavioral problems have based their analyses on seizure type alone, not on epilepsy syndrome or etiology.

Several studies have failed to observe a difference in behavioral disorders for different types of epilepsy.[6,11,16,19,64] When an effect of seizure type is found, it is nearly always by univariate analysis, favoring partial rather than generalized seizures, with other factors often significant as well. Considering a group of children with low seizure frequency on monotherapy, Aman et al.[22] found higher ratings for conduct disorder on the Conners Teacher Rating Scale and for socialized aggression on the Revised Behavior Problem Checklist in boys with partial seizures. No pair-wise comparison of ratings by AED was significant. The highest ratings for socialized aggression were seen for children on valproate, a drug that is more commonly used in generalized epilepsies. Pooling new-onset and chronic epileptic children, Hoare[2] observed a higher risk of behavioral disorders for complex partial seizures, as well as for focal EEG abnormalities, polypharmacy or treatment with phenytoin, and high seizure frequency. Hoare and Kerley[4] found a higher risk with focal EEG abnormalities, young age of onset, high seizure frequency, and polypharmacy, whereas seizure type alone was not significant. Hoare and Mann[5] found that duration of treatment and male gender made a greater contribution to more deviant scores on the CBCL than did ILAE seizure type or severity. Looking only at patients with uncomplicated epilepsy (i.e., idiopathic and cryptogenic etiology), Rutter et al.[13] found that a significantly higher fraction of children with psychomotor seizures had a psychiatric disorder (six of eight) than those with other seizure types (12 of 55) and that age of onset and frequency were not significant factors.

A more favorable prognosis may exist for some patients with idiopathic partial epilepsies. Loiseau et al.[65] found a more favorable psychosocial outcome in young adults with a prior history of benign rolandic epilepsy than for childhood absence epilepsy. Camfield et al.[21] noted a more favorable outcome for children with simple partial seizures. Hermann et al.[66] found that children with "focal nontemporal epilepsies" had a lower score for aggression on the CBCL than did children with

temporal lobe epilepsy (although comparison with generalized seizures was not significant).

Hermann et al.[30] emphasize the need to use multivariate techniques in disentangling the confounding effects of multiple biological factors. Univariate tests showed that mixed seizure types were associated with higher ratings of internalizing symptoms and lower ratings of social competence on the CBCL and that symptomatic etiology was associated with higher ratings of externalizing symptoms, but these were not significant predictors on multivariate analysis. Seizure type (partial versus generalized) was not significant even on univariate analysis.

Severity and Frequency

The independent contribution of high seizure frequency to behavioral disorders is supported by studies that included this factor in multivariate analysis.[6,30] Studies that have shown no effect of seizure frequency have generally comprised populations with infrequent seizures[11,13,64] or a more severely affected population with a high baseline prevalence of behavioral disorder.[1] It is unclear whether the positive relationship between seizure frequency and rate of behavioral disturbance is linear, exponential, or a threshold effect, and whether it is modified by the duration of epilepsy. Thus, the effect may be accounted for by a relatively small group of patients with frequent seizures (approximately 20–30% of children with epilepsy in clinical practice) or by a larger group of patients with infrequent, but continuing, seizures. Indeed, the identification of a threshold effect of seizure frequency on behavioral disorder would have strong implications in deciding whether the criterion for success in the management of epilepsy should be anything less than a seizure-free state.

Age of Onset and Duration

Younger age of onset is associated with a greater risk of psychiatric disorder in many studies.[4,5,14] This may be confounded with seizure type, etiology, AED, and duration of epilepsy. Controlling for these factors on multivariate analysis, Hermann et al.[30] found a positive correlation of age of onset with externalizing behaviors on the CBCL. However, this has not been a consistent finding; in the

Isle of Wight study,[13] age of onset of epilepsy did not differ in children with and without psychiatric disorder, and Austin et al.[6] found no uni- or multivariate correlation with any behavior on the CBCL.

The effect of duration of epilepsy must be interpreted with care. Given that it represents the difference between current age and the age of onset, it may be influenced by either or both factors. The smaller the age range of the study population, the more duration simply mirrors the inverse effect of age of onset. Only one multivariate study analyzed this variable; Hermann et al.[30] found duration to be inversely correlated with social competence.

Laterality

Determination of seizure laterality in these studies has been based principally on the EEG, not on seizure semiology or neuroimaging. Comparing 27 children with either pure left or right temporal spike foci (23 had complex partial seizures), Camfield[20] found no difference for behavioral ratings on the Personality Inventory for Children.[67] Hoare[2] found children with right-sided slowing on EEG were more likely to exceed cutoff scores on the Rutter Parent Scale, whereas Corbett et al.[10] found that several items on the Rutter Parent and Teacher Scales were more commonly endorsed in children with left temporal spikes (including destruction of property, worrying, irritability, fussiness, and resentfulness or aggression). There were major differences in the makeup of all three studies: Camfield's patients were drawn from a population sample, all had normal intelligence, and two-thirds had infrequent seizures (less than two per year); half of Hoare's sample had new-onset seizures, and all were attending ordinary school; Corbett's population was comprised exclusively of children with "complicated epilepsy" attending a hospital school specialized for childhood epilepsy. Thus, effects of laterality have not been separated effectively from other important clinical factors.

Mild Cognitive Impairment and Mental Retardation

Mild degrees of cognitive impairment may be associated with behavioral disorder. In a group of children administered an adaptation of the Luria-Nebraska neuropsychological test battery, those falling below the median score had higher ratings for aggression and total behavioral problems and lower ratings for social competence on the CBCL than those who were above the median.[29]

Given a higher rate of psychiatric disorders among children with MR, this might be expected to be a significant risk factor in the epilepsy population. Some psychiatric diagnoses are highly associated with both epilepsy and cognitive subnormality (e.g., autistic spectrum disorders[15,68]). This relationship may reflect independent contributions from MR. Hoare and Kerley[4] found no difference in the Rutter Scale scores between children with normal intelligence and those with mild to moderate MR. Rutter et al.[13] found a higher proportion of psychiatric disorder in children with severe MR (50%) and those with an IQ less than 85 (28%) than in those with a higher IQ (12%). Ounsted et al.[14] reported that 24 of 26 hyperactive children and all 15 children with hyperactivity and rage attacks fell below the sample median IQ of 90. However, additional factors (e.g., gross cerebral insult or prior status epilepticus) were present in 23 of 24 and all 15, respectively. The effect of MR may be entirely independent of epilepsy; Lewis et al.,[25] controlling for severity of cognitive impairment, found no difference in intellectually disabled children with and without epilepsy for any of the six scales on the Developmental Behaviour Checklist.[69] Unless children without epilepsy are included, a true interaction of MR and epilepsy cannot be deduced.

Pharmacologic Factors

A clinician's first priority is to monitor for immediate and obvious adverse behavioral effects of AEDs, particularly when a new drug is started or when its dose is increased. These effects may be predictable and dose related, such as sedation with benzodiazepines and barbiturates, or idiosyncratic and unrelated to dose, such as psychosis after initiation of vigabatrin. Nearly all AEDs have been implicated in some way.

An equally serious concern is the existence of subtle, chronic adverse behavioral effects that may be subthreshold diagnostically but are enough to impair function. Several studies have examined this by comparing patients on different AED regimens.[2,4,6,30] The risk may be increased in patients receiving more than one AED. Dose-related side effects may be magnified through pharmacokinetic increases in AED serum levels, and superadditive effects may emerge through pharmacodynamic interactions, even when AED levels are unchanged. Hoare[2] and Hoare and Kerley[4] found higher Rutter Scale scores in children on polypharmacy. However, polypharmacy may be associated with other risk factors, such as duration of epilepsy and medical intractability. Thus, in Hermann's study,[30] polypharmacy was positively correlated on univariate tests with externalizing behavior and inversely correlated with social competence on the CBCL, but it was not a significant independent factor on multivariate tests. Similarly, polypharmacy was not associated with CBCL ratings on uni- or multivariate tests in Austin et al.'s study.[6]

The most consistent adverse effects of monotherapy are reported for barbiturates. Thirty-six percent to 61% of children present with sedation, inattention, or hyperactivity.[70–74] This may be anticipated and easily detected. Significant mood symptoms may emerge on barbiturates. Ferrari[75] noted lower self-esteem and more anxiety in children on phenobarbital compared to those on carbamazepine and ethosuximide, and Brent[19] diagnosed major depressive disorder in 6 of 15 children on phenobarbital and in only 1 of 24 on carbamazepine. All three patients taken off phenobarbital improved; remarkably, three patients remained depressed on phenobarbital at the time of follow-up 13–30 months later.[76]

Several studies found no differences among non-barbiturate monotherapies.[24,50] Conflicting evidence for behavioral effects has been reported for carbamazepine and valproate. On multivariate testing, Hermann et al.[30] found a positive correlation for carbamazepine and externalizing problem scores on the CBCL, whereas Bailet[64] found lower scores on this scale for carbamazepine than valproate. Aman[22] noted a higher rating for socialized aggression on the Revised Behavioral Problem Checklist for valproate than for carbamazepine and phenytoin. Given the inconsistency of these results and their relatively small magnitude, it is not possible to conclude that a real difference between these AEDs exists.

Psychosocial Factors

Hermann[30] conceives of psychosocial forces as a fourth domain of factors that determine psychopathology in children with epilepsy: "those factors thought to be related to the stress and tension associ-ated with living with the disorder, the widely discussed stigma and discrimination, as well as other factors, such as loss of social support." The following putative psychosocial factors have been measured in the families of children with epilepsy: parental marital status[6,13] and marital satisfaction,[4] stressful events experienced by members of the family,[4,6] family adaptive resources,[6] parental knowledge of and attitude toward epilepsy,[4,33] and psychopathology in parents and siblings.[3,4,19,24] Several related characteristics of the child may also be included: self perception and self-esteem,[4–7] dependency,[4,77] estimation of disease severity,[4,12] and perception of the locus of control.[12]

The risk of psychiatric problems in children from single-parent households has not been consistently shown to be greater (no effect: Austin,[6] Rutter,[13] McDermott[8]; positive association: Hoare and Kerley,[4] Hermann[30]). The marital satisfaction of parents of children with epilepsy was similar to that of the general population in one study,[4] but these families experience a greater amount of external stress, which correlates with higher ratings for behavioral problems in the children.[4,6] When measured, relative familial strengths have equally strong inverse correlations with these problems.[6]

Measures of parental attitudes toward epilepsy are strongly correlated with the parent's ratings of problem behaviors in their child. Thus, parents who assigned a high probability that a variety of daily life problems would occur in children with epilepsy also produced high ratings for their child's behavior problems on the Rutter Scale (and higher than the teacher's ratings for the same children).[4] When scored on a semistructured interview, maternal statements about children with epilepsy were more emotionally charged than were statements about their nonepileptic siblings, and maternal criticism and hostility were associated with higher ratings for antisocial and hyperactive behavior in the child.[33]

Parents of children with epilepsy may[24] or may not[3,4] have more psychopathology than the general population. However, parental psychopathology is more frequent when the child has a psychiatric disorder, whether in new-onset or chronic epilepsy patients.[3] This may be especially true for affective disorders: Brent[19] diagnosed major depressive disorders in five of six phenobarbital-treated children with a positive family history in a first-degree relative, but only in one of nine without. There appears to be a greater incidence of psychiatric disturbance in siblings of children with chronic epilepsy than in siblings of new-onset cases or in the general population.[3]

In general, children's self ratings on the Piers-Harris Self-Concept Scale[4,7,58] and the Harter Self-Esteem Questionnaire[5] as well as their ratings for dependency[4,77] were strongly related to parental ratings on the CBCL and the Rutter scales. In addition, these measures may be important clues to the existence of depression. Dunn et al.[52] found three psychosocial measures in the child that independently predicted of depression on the Children's Depression Inventory: youth's attitude toward epilepsy, youth satisfaction with family relationships, and unknown locus of control or external locus of control for socially powerful others. These measures were more predictive than gender, current age, age of onset, or a composite measure of seizure severity.

Thus, although psychiatric symptoms may be associated with ratings on these measures of psychosocial function, the direction of the association is not always clear. Is it possible to identify a set of psychosocial attributes that independently determine the child's vulnerability to the development of a psychiatric disorder, given a challenge such as epilepsy? Or are these psychosocial attributes part of the same continuum of behavioral symptoms expanded to include the child's family? Is psychosocial maladjustment simply another manifestation of an underlying psychiatric disorder?

Prognosis, Short and Long Term

A few studies have repeated behavioral measures in children with epilepsy over relatively short time periods, finding either a stable but persistent elevation in scores[64] or a tendency to improve.[28,63] In a 4-year follow-up study, children with asthma and epilepsy improved in ratings for internalizing and externalizing behaviors on the CBCL, with one exception: girls whose seizures remained relatively severe worsened in both of these measures.[59]

Several studies followed patients to young adulthood. Following Ounsted's original cohort of 100 children with temporal lobe epilepsy into early adulthood, Lindsay et al.[78,79] diagnosed a psychiatric disorder in 26 of 87. Nine had a schizophreniform psychosis, 12 had an antisocial personality disorder, and five were neurotic (e.g., anxious or depressed). A history of childhood rage episodes was predictive of psychiatric diagnoses in general, and male gender and severe or frequent seizures were predictive of psychosis or antisocial personality. A history of childhood hyperactivity or a disordered home was not predictive of psychiatric disorder. Thirty of 95 survivors were unable to live independently. Factors predictive of this outcome on univariate analysis included an IQ less than 90, age of onset of less than 2 years 4 months, severe seizures, frequent seizures (more than one per day), and childhood hyperactivity or rage episodes. Outcome has been less severe in population-based studies. In a prospectively studied cohort of childhood absence epilepsy followed to at least 18 years of age, Wirrell[26] found that 8 of 19 patients still having seizures reported ongoing psychiatric or emotional difficulties, but only 1 of 37 patients was seizure free. Jalava et al.[80] reported follow-up in a cohort at a mean of 35 years, none of whom had MR or other neurologic deficits. Psychiatric disorders, most commonly neuroses, were seen in 23% of patients but only 7% of controls, and the group differences were significant even for the two-thirds who were seizure free and off medication. The group as a whole had less education, more unemployment, and less marriage, and individuals often endorsed the statement that they had little or no control over their life.[81] A somewhat different picture emerges from the studies of Kokkonen et al.[82] Patients with childhood-onset epilepsy had a rate of psychiatric disorder similar to nonepileptic controls but more frequent psychosocial problems, including less education and greater dependency. This outcome was related more to coexisting cognitive impairment than to the severity or activity of the epilepsy. A greater rate of psychiatric disturbance, especially depression, was seen in a group of nonretarded, nonepileptic patients with spina bifida or cerebral palsy compared to nonretarded epileptic patients without motor deficits.[83]

Management Strategies

Is a Change in Antiepileptic Therapy Indicated?

A first step in managing behavioral problems is to ascertain the recency of the onset of symptoms and, in acute situations, to identify and remove the possible triggers. A variety of symptoms, especially hyperactivity, irritability, and aggression, may appear in the immediate postictal period, usually resolving over days. These sometimes may be difficult to differentiate from treatment-emergent symptoms elicited by new AEDs started after an increase in seizures; an iatrogenic cause must be suspected when the symptoms endure. Barbiturates produce hyperactivity, irritability, or aggressive behavior in 36–61% of patients.[70–74] Given the association of depression with barbiturates,[19,75] a medication change should be strongly considered in any child who exhibits mood symptoms at any time after initiating this medication, especially in the presence of a positive family history of a mood disorder. Vigabatrin produced an acute psychosis in 3.4% of adults who participated in controlled randomized trials, compared to 0.6% on placebo,[84] and moderate to severe hyperactivity was observed in 25% of children in open-label studies.[85] Behavioral effects are less likely to appear with other AEDs, but most commonly these consist of restlessness and irritability in the context of sedation.[72] In children with coexisting ADHD, these sedative-hypnotic effects are likely to worsen all symptoms, especially when the agent is phenobarbital or a benzodiazepine.[56]

Withdrawal of AEDs may elicit behavioral symptoms independent of the exacerbation of seizures. In addition to abstinence syndromes produced by discontinuation of barbiturates and benzodiazepines, withdrawal-emergent psychopathology was seen in 12 of 32 adults acutely withdrawn from phenytoin, valproate, and carbamazepine.[86] Most commonly, these included anxiety and depression, but panic, mania, and psychosis were also seen. The symptoms emerged in the final week of medication taper before an actual increase in seizures, and the severity of symptoms was not related to that experienced before withdrawal.

Is a Psychosocial Intervention Indicated?

Given the association of behavioral problems with family stress, lack of family resources, negative parental attitudes toward epilepsy, and the child's lack of self-esteem, an assessment of the psychosocial state of the child and his or her family is imperative. The psychosocial distress of the child and his

family should not be tolerated as the inevitable consequence of the stress of active epilepsy. The following recommendations are based on standards of good clinical practice. It is remarkable that there is no study that allows us to compare the results of psychosocial interventions in epileptic and nonepileptic children with behavioral disorders.

As a matter of good clinical practice, psychosocial intervention should begin with the first contact with the patient. The most important part of the diagnostic process is its communication to the patient. It is necessary to convey an accurate prognosis, as well as a realistic estimate of the risks and the necessity of health-related limitations of activity. Happily, this often involves presenting a more favorable prognosis than the family expects, and many inappropriate concerns and limitations may be debunked. Communication can bolster the child's self-esteem and guide the family in setting appropriate limitations on the child's unruly behavior. The physician must also inquire about sources of parental stress, including marital discord, financial embarrassment, and loss of employment.

Chronic academic failure is an additional source of stress and discouragement. The physician, more than any other professional, is best qualified to disentangle the contributions of chronic encephalopathy, continued seizures, and AEDs to academic achievement and to interpret the results of psychoeducational testing.

It is often necessary for follow-up treatment to include behavioral modification and supportive family therapy. Given the limitation of clinic time and lack of formal training in the psychotherapeutic technique shared by most physicians treating the child's epilepsy, this requires referral to a psychiatrist, clinical psychologist, or clinical social worker. Unfortunately, financial considerations may limit the choice of therapist and duration of intervention. These needs remain unmet in many children with epilepsy in North America.

Is Pharmacotherapy Indicated?

It should always be a high priority, once a major depressive disorder is suspected, to assess the risk of suicide. This is a clear risk in adults with comorbid epilepsy and depression, and Brent et al.[19] observed suicidal ideation in 7 of 15 children treated with phenobarbital. However, reports of suicide in children with epilepsy and adolescents are scarce.

In the treating of an affective disorder, the physician may consider exploiting the positive psychotropic effects of some AEDs. There has been a growing body of evidence from controlled randomized trials that support the efficacy of these agents in adults with affective disorders. As reviewed by Post et al.,[87] carbamazepine can effectively treat acute mania and rapid-cycling bipolar disorder, but it is not effective in treating monopolar or bipolar depression. It may also be efficacious in treating agitated or disruptive behaviors in other disorders, including schizophrenia and schizoaffective disorder.[88] Valproate has efficacy in the treatment of classic, mixed, and rapid cycling bipolar disorder[89] and acute mania.[90] Lamotrigine is effective in the treatment of bipolar depression and the maintenance of rapid-cycling bipolar disorder.[91,92] In patients with epilepsy, a meta-analysis of three controlled-randomized trials showed fewer adverse events corresponding to depression on lamotrigine than on placebo or other comparator AEDs.[93] In addition, one double-blind study of adult epilepsy patients showed a superiority of lamotrigine over valproate in a variety of patient-rated mood assessments.[94] There is less evidence for the effectiveness of other new AEDs; topiramate[95] and gabapentin[96] have failed in controlled randomized trials as adjunctive agents in bipolar disorder. However, gabapentin has shown efficacy in the treatment of social anxiety.[97] Thus, the evidence of a beneficial psychotropic effect for an AED chiefly rests on the AED's efficacy as a mood stabilizer, with effect profiles varying from one drug to another. Bipolar disorder is a challenging diagnosis in children, and its prevalence in childhood epilepsy is undefined. Therefore, the true efficacy of AEDs in treating mood disorders in children with epilepsy is unknown.

The psychiatric diagnosis most readily made by North American pediatricians and child neurologists in children with epilepsy is ADHD. Given the clear superiority of stimulant medications over other forms of therapy for ADHD, the only issue that remains is the supposed risk of methylphenidate in lowering the seizure threshold. Although the risk is inferred from animal studies, it is reiterated in the *Physicians' Desk Reference*[98] as a warning to patients. Two open-label studies, totaling 40 children, that used the standard 0.3 mg/kg dose of methylphenidate for the treatment of children with epilepsy and ADHD showed no statistically significant effect on seizure frequency.[99,100] Both studies, in addition to that of Semrud-Clikeman and Wical[54] (which did not present data on seizures), showed efficacy in the treatment of the ADHD symptoms. However, Gara and Roberts[101] recently reported dyskinesias and bruxism in two children with epilepsy when methylphenidate was added to valproate. Finally, one report[102] noted an increase in serum levels of phenobarbital and phenytoin with the addition of methylphenidate. Given these precautions, we may conclude that the current standard practice of treating ADHD in children with epilepsy with stimulants, including methylphenidate, is safe.

In treating an epilepsy patient with a psychotropic medication, one must consider the risk of exacerbating seizures with the psychotropic drug and the risk of pharmacokinetic interactions with the AED. The estimate of the risk of seizure exacerbation is based mainly on the reported incidence of seizures in the nonepileptic patients treated with these agents. For most of the tricyclic antidepressants, risk is proportional to dose. Thus, in a 1983 meta-analysis of 98 studies of imipramine that included 5,476 adults,[103] the overall occurrence of seizures was 0.1% for patients prescribed less than 200 mg per day and 0.63% for those prescribed more than 200 mg per day. Similar effects have been noted for amitryptiline and clomipramine.[104] It is likely that the dose effect is ultimately related to serum level. Because the metabolic capacity of the cytochrome P-450 system is affected by age, genetic polymorphisms that vary widely among ethnic groups, and induction or inhibition by other drugs (including many AEDs), the true risk for an individual patient is difficult to estimate. Careful monitoring of serum levels of tricyclics is mandatory for all children, especially those with epilepsy.

The incidence of seizures in patients treated with bupropion was initially high enough to cause its withdrawal from the American market. However, it was reintroduced with the recommendation not to exceed an adult dose of 450 mg per day after it was shown that the occurrence of seizures was 0.44% below this dose and 2.2% above, in doses ranging as high as 900 mg per day.[105] There is much less experience with newer agents, including the selective serotonin reuptake inhibitors and venlafaxine, and the experience that does exist is limited mainly to data from premarketing controlled trials. However, risk generally has been below 0.3% and, in some cases, was below the occurrence in placebo.[104]

Seizures have been reported in patients treated with all antipsychotics. In a large observational study of psychiatric inpatients, Logothetis[106] reported seizures in 10 of 859 patients treated with phenothiazines and in none of 669 who were not treated with these agents. A higher risk was reported in patients with other known nonepileptic neurologic disorders and patients who received larger doses. There has been no large comparison study allowing determination of relative risk among phenothiazines or butyrophenones. The seizure risk may be higher for clozapine (2.9% in premarketing studies[107]), but the use of this agent has been significantly limited owing to the high incidence of agranulocytosis. The seizure risk is lower with other atypical antipsychotics, including olanzepine, risperidone, and quetiapine.[104]

The most significant pharmacokinetic effect of psychotropic agents on AEDs is the inhibition of some cytochrome P-450 enzymes by selective serotonin reuptake inhibitors and, to a lesser extent, the tricyclics. The anticipated effect of this inhibition would be a rise in serum levels of AEDs metabolized by these pathways, including phenobarbital, phenytoin, and carbamazepine.[104] The relative magnitude of the effects among the different psychotropics has not been determined; indeed, as reviewed by Lambert and Robertson,[108] there have been conflicting reports on the interactions of phenytoin with sertraline and carbamazepine with sertraline, fluoxetine, or fluvoxamine. Thus, serum levels of these AEDs should be monitored carefully, when antidepressants are introduced. Because phenytoin, phenobarbital, and carbamazepine are cytochrome P-450 enzyme inducing, the potential effect of these AEDs in lowering serum levels of antidepressants must also be taken into consideration.

Conclusion

Psychiatric disorders are common enough in childhood epilepsy to warrant screening in all cases, either by clinical interview or by standardized questionnaire. The range of symptoms is broad and does not differ from that which is seen in children without epilepsy. Several clinical factors may be associated with an increased risk of psychiatric disorder, but any child with epilepsy may be affected. Psychiatric morbidity may persist into young adulthood, especially in more severe cases of epilepsy. Psychiatric disorders should be managed, not ignored; this may require modification of antiepileptic therapy, psychosocial intervention, or the use of psychotropic medication.

References

1. Hackney A, Taylor DC. A teacher's questionnaire description of children with epilepsy. Epilepsia 1976;17:275–281.
2. Hoare P. The development of psychiatric disorder among schoolchildren with epilepsy. Dev Med Child Neurol 1984;26:3–13.
3. Hoare P. Psychiatric disturbance in the families of children with epilepsy. Dev Med Child Neurol 1984;26:14-19.
4. Hoare P, Kerley S. Psychosocial adjustment of children with chronic epilepsy and their families. Dev Med Child Neurol 1991;33:201–205.
5. Hoare P, Mann H. Self-esteem and behavioural adjustment in children with epilepsy and children with diabetes. J Psychosom Res 1994;38:859–869.
6. Austin JK, Risinger MW, Beckett LA. Correlates of behavioral problems in children with epilepsy. Epilepsia 1992;33:1115–1122.
7. Austin JK, Smith S, Risinger MW, McNelis AM. Childhood epilepsy and asthma: comparison of quality of life. Epilepsia 1994;35:608–615.
8. McDermott S, Mani S, Krishnaswami S. A population-based analysis of specific behavior problems associated with childhood seizures. J Epilepsy 1995;8:110–118.
9. Dorenbaum D, Cappelli M, Hons BA, et al. Use of a child behavior checklist in the psychosocial assessment of children with epilepsy. Clin Pediatr 1985;24:634–637.
10. Corbett JA, Trimble M, Nochol T. Behavioral and cognitive impairments in children with epilepsy: the long-term effects of anticonvulsant therapy. J Am Acad Child Psychiatry 1985;24:17–23.
11. Ettinger A, Weisbrot D, Nolan E, et al. Symptoms of depression and anxiety in pediatric epilepsy patients. Epilepsia 1998;39:595–599.
12. Dunn DW, Austin JK, Huster GA. Symptoms of depression in adolescents with epilepsy. J Am Acad Child Adolesc Psychiatry 1999;38:1132–1138.
13. Rutter M, Graham P, Yule W. A Neuropsychiatric Study in Childhood. Philadelphia: JB Lippincott Co, 1970.

14. Ounsted C, Lidsay J, Norman RM. Biological Factors in Temporal Lobe Epilepsy. Clinics in Developmental Medicine (no. 22). Philadelphia: JB Lippincott Co, 1966.

15. Steffenburg S, Gilberg C, Steffenburg U. Psychiatric disorders in children and adolescents with mental retardation and active epilepsy. Arch Neurol 1996;53:904–912.

16. Sillanpaa M. Medical-social prognosis of children with epilepsy. Epidemiological study and analysis of 245 patients. Acta Pediatr Scand 1973;63[Suppl 237]:1–104.

17. Caplan R, Arbelle S, Guthrie D, et al. Formal thought disorder and psychopathology in pediatric primarily generalized and complex partial epilepsy. J Am Acad Child Adolesc Psychiatry 1997;36:1286–1294.

18. Hackett R, Hackett L, Bhakta P. Psychiatric disorder and cognitive function in children with epilepsy in Kerala, South India. Seizure 1998;7:321–324.

19. Brent D, Crumrine P, Varma R, et al. Phenobarbital treatment and major depressive disorder in children with epilepsy. Pediatrics 1987;80:909–917.

20. Camfield P, Gates R, Ronen G, et al. Comparison of cognitive ability, personality profile, and school success in epileptic children with pure right versus left temporal lobe EEG foci. Ann Neurol 1984;15:122–126.

21. Camfield CS, Camfield P, Smith B, et al. Biologic factors as predictors of social outcome of epilepsy in intellectually normal children: a population-based study. J Pediatr 1993;122:869–873.

22. Aman MG, Werry J, Turbott S. Behavior of children with seizures. J Nerv Ment Dis 1992;180:124–129.

23. Apter A, Aviv A, Kaminer Y, et al. Behavioral profile and social competence in temporal lobe epilepsy of adolescence. J Am Acad Child Adolesc Psychiatry 1991;30:887–892.

24. Berg I, Butler A, Ellis M, Foster J. Psychiatric aspects of epilepsy in childhood treated with carbamazepine, phenytoin, or sodium valproate: a random trial. Dev Med Child Neurol 1993;35:149–157.

25. Lewis JN, Tonge BJ, Mowat DR, et al. Epilepsy and associated psychopathology in young people with intellectual disability. J Paediatr Child Health 2000;36:172–175.

26. Wirrell EC, Camfield C, Camfield P, et al. Long-term psychosocial outcome in typical absence epilepsy. Arch Pediatr Adolesc Med 1997;151:152–158.

27. Achenbach T. Manual for the Child Behavior Checklist/4-18 and 1991 Profile. Burlington, VT: University of Vermont, Department of Psychiatry, 1991.

28. Dunn DW, Austin JK, Huster GA. Behaviour problems in children with new-onset epilepsy. Seizure 1997;6:283–287.

29. Hermann BP. Neuropsychological functioning and psychopathology in children with epilepsy. Epilepsia 1982;23:545–554.

30. Hermann BP, Whitman S, Hughes JR, et al. Multietiological determinants of psychopathology and social competence in children with epilepsy. Epilepsy Res 1988;2:51–60.

31. Mitchell WG, Scheier L, Baker SA. Psychosocial, behavioral, and medical outcomes in children with epilepsy: a developmental risk factor model using longitudinal data. Pediatrics 1994;94:471–477.

32. Kurokawa T, Matsuo M, Yoshida K, et al. Behavioral disorders in Japanese epileptic children. Folia Psychiatr Neurol Jpn 1983;37: 259–266.

33. Hodes M, Garralda ME, Rose G, Schwartz R. Maternal expressed emotion and adjustment in children with epilepsy. J Child Psychol Psychiatry 1999;40:1083–1093.

34. Perrin E, Stein R, Drotar D. Cautions in using the child behavior checklist: observations based on research about children with a chronic illness. J Pediatr Psychology 1991;16:411–421.

35. Holmes CS, Respess D, Greer T, Frentz J. Behavioral problems in children with diabetes: disentangling possible scoring confounds on the child behavior checklist. J Pediatr Psychology 1998;23:179–185.

36. Kovacs M. The Children's Depression Inventory (CDI). Psychopharmacol Bull 1985;21:995–998.

37. DuPaul GJ, Power TJ, Anastopoulos AD, Reid R. ADHD Rating Scale-IV: Checklists, Norms, and Clinical Interpretation. New York: The Guilford Press, 1998.

38. Gadow KD, Sparfkin J. Child Symptom Inventory 4 Norms Manual. Stony Brook, New York: Checkmate Plus Ltd, 1997.

39. Angold A, Costello J, Farmer E, et al. Impaired but undiagnosed. J Am Acad Child Adolesc Psychiatry 1999;38:129–137.

40. Lancman M. Psychosis and peri-ictal confusional states. Neurology 1999;53[Suppl 2]:33–38.

41. Caplan R, Arbelle S, Guthrie D, et al. The Kiddie Formal Thought Disorders Rating Scale (K-FTDS): clinical assessment, reliability, and validity. J Am Acad Child Adolesc Psychiatry 1989;28:208–216.

42. Wechsler D. The Wechsler Intelligence Scale for Children—Revised. New York: Psychological Corporation, 1974.

43. American Psychiatric Association. Diagnostic and Statistical Manual of Mental Disorders (4th ed). Washington: American Psychiatric Association, 1994.

44. Ounsted C. The hyperkinetic syndrome in epileptic children. Lancet 1955;2:303–311.

45. Sturniolo MG, Galetti F. Idiopathic epilepsy and school achievement. Arch Dis Child 1994;70:424–428.

46. Harvey AS, Berkovic SF, Wrennall JA, Hopkins IJ. Temporal lobe epilepsy in childhood: clinical, EEG, and neuroimaging findings and syndrome classification in a cohort with new onset seizures. Neurology 1997;49:960–968.

47. Epir S, Renda Y, Baser N. Cognitive and behavioural characteristics of children with idiopathic epilepsy in a low-income area of Ankara, Turkey. Dev Med Child Neurol 1984;26:200–207.

48. Goyette CH, Conners CK, Ulrich RF. Normative data on revised Conners Parent and Teacher Rating Scales. J Abnorm Child Psychol 1978;6:221–236.

49. Stores G, Williams PL, Styles E, Zaiwalla Z. Psychological effects of sodium valproate and carbamazepine in epilepsy. Arch Dis Child 1992;67:1330–1337.

50. National Center for Health Statistics. Data from the National Health Survey. Parent ratings of behavioral patterns of children, United States. Vital and health statistics. Washington: U.S. Government Printing Office, 1971.

51. Zill N. Behavioral Problem Index Based upon Parent Report. In National Health Interview Survey, Child Health Supplement, 1990. Washington: National Center for Health Statistics, 1990.

52. Dunn DW, Austin JK, Hareziak J, Ambrosius W. Attention deficit hyperactivity disorder and chronic epilepsy in childhood. Epilepsia 2000;41[Suppl 7]:239(abst).

53. Williams J, Griebel M, Dykman RA. Neuropsychological patterns in pediatric epilepsy. Seizure 1998;7:223–228.

54. Semrud-Clikeman M, Wical B. Components of attention in children with complex partial seizures with and without ADHD. Epilepsia 1999;40:211–215.

55. Hempel AM, Frost MD, Ritter F, Farnham S. Factors influencing the incidence of ADHD in pediatric epilepsy patients. Epilepsia 1995;36[Suppl 4]:122.

56. Barkley R. Attention Deficit Hyperactivity Disorder (2nd ed). New York: The Guilford Press, 1998.

57. Quay HC, Peterson DR. Interim manual for the Revised Behavioral Problem Checklist. HC Quay, Box 240074, University of Miami, Coral Gables, Florida 33124.

58. Austin JK, Huster GA, Dunn DW, Risinger MW. Adolescents with active or inactive epilepsy or asthma: a comparison of quality of life. Epilepsia 1996;37:1228–1238.

59. Austin JK, Dunn DW, Huster GA. Childhood epilepsy and asthma: changes in behavioral problems related to gender and change in condition severity. Epilepsia 2000;41:615–623.

60. Proposal for revised clinical and electroencephalographic classification of epileptic seizures. From the Commission on Classification and Terminology of the International League Against Epilepsy. Epilepsia 1981;22:489–501.

61. Proposal for revised classification of the epilepsies and epileptic syndromes. Commission on Classification and Terminology of the International League Against Epilepsy. Epilepsia 1989;30:389–399.

62. Guidelines for epidemiologic studies on epilepsy. Commission on Epidemiology and Prognosis, International League Against Epilepsy. Epilepsia 1993;34:592–596.

63. Berg AT, Levy SR, Testa F, Shinnar S. Classification of childhood epilepsy syndromes in newly diagnosed epilepsy: interrater agreement and reasons for disagreement. Epilepsia 1999;40:439–444.

64. Bailet LL, Turk WR. The impact of childhood epilepsy on neurocognitive and behavioral performance: a prospective longitudinal study. Epilepsia 2000;41:426–431.

65. Loiseau P, Pestre M, Dartigues JF, et al. Long-term prognosis in two forms of childhood epilepsy: typical absence seizures and epilepsy with rolandic (centrotemporal) EEG foci. Ann Neurol 1983;13:642–648.

66. Hermann BP, Black R, Chabria S. Behavioral problems and social competence in children with epilepsy. Epilepsia 1981;22:703–710.

67. Wirt RD, Lachar D, Klincdinst JK, Seat PD. Multidimensional Description of Child Personality. Los Angeles: Western Psychological Services, 1977.

68. Tuchman RF, Rapin I. Regression in pervasive developmental disorders: seizures and epileptiform electroencephalogram correlates. Pediatrics 1997;99:560–566.

69. Einfeld SL, Tonge BJ. Manual for the Developmental Behaviour Checklist. Melbourne, Australia: Monash University Center for Developmental Psychiatry, 1992.

70. Committee on Drugs, American Academy of Pediatrics. Behavioral and cognitive effects of anticonvulsant therapy. Pediatrics 1985;76:644–647.

71. Wolf SM, Carr A, Davis DC, et al. The value of phenobarbital in the child who has had a single febrile seizure: a controlled prospective study. Pediatrics 1977;59:378–385.

72. Herranz JL, Armijo J, Arteaga R. Clinical side effects of phenobarbital, primidone, phenytoin, carbamazepine, and valproate during monotherapy in children. Epilepsia 1988;29:794–804.

73. Vining EP, Mellits ED, Dorsen MM, et al. Psychological and behavioral effects of antiepileptic drugs in children: a double-blind comparison between phenobarbital and valproic acid. Pediatrics 1987;80:165–174.

74. Camfield CS, Chaplin S, Doyle AB, et al. Side effects of phenobarbital in toddlers: behavioral and cognitive aspects. J Pediatr 1979;95:361–365.

75. Ferrari M, Barabas G, Matthews WS. Psychologic and behavioral disturbance among epileptic children treated with barbiturate anticonvulsants. Am J Psychiatry 1983;140:112–113.

76. Brent D, Crumrine P, Varma R, et al. Phenobarbital treatment and major depressive disorder in children with epilepsy: a naturalistic followup. Pediatrics 1990;85:1086–1091.

77. Hoare P. Does illness foster dependency? A study of epileptic and diabetic children. Dev Med Child Neurol 1984;26:20–24.

78. Lindsay J, Ounsted C, Richards P. Long-term outcome in children with temporal lobe seizures. III: Psychiatric aspects in childhood and adult life. Dev Med Child Neurol 1979;21:630–636.

79. Lindsay J, Ounsted C, Richards P. Long-term outcome in children with temporal lobe seizures. I: Social out-

come and childhood factors. Dev Med Child Neurol 1979;21:285–298.

80. Jalava M, Sillanpaa M. Concurrent illnesses in adults with childhood-onset epilepsy: a population-based 35-year follow-up study. Epilepsia 1996;37:1155–1163.

81. Jalava M, Sillanpaa, Camfield C, Camfield P. Social adjustment and competence 35 years after onset of childhood epilepsy: a prospective controlled study. Epilepsia 1997;38:708–715.

82. Kokkonen J, Kokkonen ER, Saukkonen AL, Pennanen P. Psychosocial outcome of young adults with epilepsy in childhood. J Neurol Neurosurg Psychiatry 1997;62:265–268.

83. Kokkonen ER, Kokkonen J, Saukkonen AL. Do neurological disorders in childhood pose a risk for mental health in young adulthood? Dev Med Child Neurol 1998;40:364–368.

84. Ferrie CD, Robinson RO, Panayiotopoulos CP. Psychotic and severe behavioral reactions with vigabatrin: a review. Acta Neurol Scand 1996;93:1–8.

85. Dulac O, Chiron D, Cusami R, et al. Vigabatrin in childhood epilepsy. J Child Neurol 1991;6[Suppl 2]:30–37.

86. Ketter TA, Malow BA, Flamini R, et al. Anticonvulsant-withdrawal-emergent psychopathology. Neurology 1994;44:55–61.

87. Post RM, Ketter TA, Denicoff K, et al. The place of anticonvulsant therapy in bipolar illness. Psychopharmacology 1996;128:115–129.

88. Okuma T, Yamashita I, Takahashi R, et al. A double-blind study of adjunctive carbamazepine vs. placebo on excited states of schizophrenic and schizoaffective disorders. Acta Psychiatr Scand 1989;80:250–259.

89. Bowden CL, Calabreses JR, McElroy SL, Hirschfeld RM. A randomized, placebo-controlled 12-month trial of divalproex and lithium in treatment of outpatients with bipolar I disorder. Divalproex Maintenance Study Group. Arch Gen Psychiatry 2000;57:481–489.

90. Bowden CL, Brugger AM, Swann AC, et al. Efficacy of divalproex and placebo in the treatment of mania. The Depakote Mania Study Group. JAMA 1994;271:918–924.

91. Calabrese JR, Bowden CL, Sachs GS, et al. A double blind placebo-controlled study of lamotrigine monotherapy in outpatients with bipolar I depression. The Lamictal 602 Study Group. J Clin Psychiatry 1999;60:79–88.

92. Calabrese JR, Suppes T, Bowden CL, et al. A double-blind, placebo-controlled prophylaxis study of lamotrigine in rapid cycling bipolar disorder. The Lamictal 604 Study Group. J Clin Psychiatry 2000;61:841–850.

93. Edwards KR, Sackelleres JC, Calabrese JR, et al. The Lamictal Development Team. Presented as a scientific exhibit sponsored by Glaxo-Wellcome Inc, Research Triangle Park, NC 27709 USA; Annual Meeting of the American Epilepsy Society; December 1–6, 2000; Los Angeles, CA.

94. Edwards KR, Kalogjera-Sackelleres D, Sackelleres JC, et al. Lamotrigine monotherapy improves mood in epilepsy: a randomized, double-blind comparison with valproate. Epilepsia 2000;41[Suppl 7]:104 (abst).

95. Calabrese JR. The use of antiepileptic drugs in psychiatry. Presented at the Annual Meeting of the American Epilepsy Society; December 2, 2000; Los Angeles, CA.

96. Frye MA, Ketter TA, Kimbrell TA, et al. A placebo-controlled study of lamotrigine and gabapentin monotherapy in refractory mood disorders. J Clin Psychopharmacol 2000;20:607–614.

97. Pande AC, Davidson JT, Jefferson JW, et al. Treatment of social phobia with gabapentin: a placebo-controlled study. J Clin Psychopharmacol 1999;19:341–348.

98. Arky A. Physician's Desk Reference. Montvale, NJ: Medical Economics Data Production Company, 1994.

99. Gross-Tsur V, Manor O, van der Meere J, et al. Epilepsy and attention deficit disorder: is methylphenidate safe and effective? J Pediatr 1997;130:670–674.

100. Feldman H, Crumrine P, Handen BL, et al. Methylphenidate in children with seizures and attention-deficit disorder. Arch Dis Child 1989;143:1081–1086.

101. Gara L, Roberts W. Adverse response to methylphenidate in combination with valproic acid. J Child Adolesc Psychopharmacol 2000;10:39–43.

102. McConnell HW, Duncan D. Treatment of Psychiatric Comorbidity in Epilepsy. In HW McConnell, PJ Snyder (eds), Psychiatric Comorbidity in Epilepsy. Washington, DC: American Psychiatric Press Inc, 1998;245–361.

103. Peck AW, Stern WC, Watkinson C. Incidence of seizures during treatment with tricyclic antidepressant drugs and bupropion. J Clin Psychiatry 1983;44:197–201.

104. Alldredge BK. Seizure risk associated with psychotropic drugs: clinical and pharmacokinetic considerations. Neurology 1999;53[Suppl 2]:68–75.

105. Davidson J. Seizures and bupropion: a review. J Clin Psychiatry 1989;50:256–261.

106. Logothetis J. Spontaneous epileptic seizures and electroencephalographic changes in the course of phenothiazine therapy. Neurology 1967;17:869–877.

107. Devinsky O, Honigfield G, Patin J. Clozapine-related seizures. Neurology 1991;41:369–371.

108. Lambert MV, Robertson MM. Depression in epilepsy: etiology, phenomenology, and treatment. Epilepsia 1999;40[Suppl 10]:21–48.

Section E

Special Populations

Chapter 22

Pediatric Disorders

Daniel K. Miles

Most pediatric disorders associated with seizures also affect adults. These disorders are discussed in chapters devoted to the various organ systems that they involve. Developmental disabilities in adults and children are covered in Chapter 23. This chapter addresses disorders that affect children, which are not covered in other areas of the text, and focuses on nutritional deficiencies, congenital heart disease (CHD) and other cardiac disorders, infectious diseases, and pediatric renal and rheumatologic disorders. This discussion is intended to assist the practitioner who cares for children with these specific disease conditions. Table 22-1 provides a list of the pediatric disorders discussed in this chapter, as well as other disorders associated with epilepsy in children.

Nutritional Disorders

Biotin

Biotin (vitamin H) is a cofactor for four carboxylation enzymes involved in gluconeogenesis, fatty acid synthesis, propionate metabolism, and leucine catabolism, respectively. Biotin deficiency is manifested by a rash resembling that of seborrheic dermatitis, alopecia, anorexia, metabolic acidosis, developmental delay, ataxia, hearing loss, and seizures.

True biotin deficiency is rare but occurs in association with parenteral hyperalimentation without biotin supplementation[1] and chronic hemodialysis.[2] Ingestion of large quantities of raw egg white can also result in a symptomatic biotin deficiency. Avidin, a component of egg white, so thoroughly binds the biotin that it cannot be absorbed from the intestines.[3] Deficiency of biotinidase, an enzyme that cleaves biotin from polypeptides and permits the biotin to be recycled into other reactions, results in a secondary or relative state of biotin deficiency. Clinical manifestations of biotinidase deficiency are similar to those of biotin deficiency and include seizures.[4]

Recognition of these disorders and initiation of treatment with supplemental biotin, typically a dose of 10 mg per day, can result in dramatic improvement, although neurologic symptoms may persist.[5]

Folate

The vitamin folate is needed for the synthesis of nucleic acids as well as cell growth and division. Although there is no causal relationship between folate deficiency and seizures, it is recognized that antiepileptic medications, including phenytoin, phenobarbital, carbamazepine, and primidone, can cause folate deficiency.[6–9] Complications of such a deficiency include megaloblastic anemia, diarrhea, irritability, affective disorders, dementia, polyneuropathy, and subacute combined degeneration. Neural tube defects, such as spina bifida, are associated with low serum folate levels that may or may not be due to a genetic predisposition.[10] Epilepsy itself is a risk for neural tube defects in offspring. It is

Table 22-1. Selected Pediatric Disorders Associated with Epilepsy

Developmental disorders	Metabolic disorders
Asperger's syndrome	Biotinidase
Attention deficit	Glycine encephalopathy
hyperactivity disorder	Phenylketonuria
Autism	Urea cycle disorders
Cerebral palsy	Maple syrup urine disease
Disintegrative disorder	Menkes disease
Landau-Kleffner	Mitochondrial disorders
syndrome	**Neurocutaneous disorders**
Rett syndrome	Neurofibromatosis
Infectious disorders	Sturge-Weber syndrome
Cat-scratch disease	Tuberous sclerosis
Cerebral abscess	**Nutritional disorders**
Encephalitis	Biotin deficiency
Intrauterine infections	Folate deficiency
Meningitis	Pyridoxine-dependent
Shigellosis	epilepsy
Genetic disorders	**Other systemic disorders**
Angelman's syndrome	Congenital heart disease
Down syndrome	Renal failure
Fragile X syndrome	Hepatic failure
Lowe syndrome	Hemolytic uremic syndrome
Prader-Willi syndrome	Henoch-Schönlein purpura
Williams syndrome	

recommended that women of child-bearing age, particularly those with epilepsy and especially those receiving antiepileptic medications, should be given 0.4 mg or more of folic acid a day.[11]

Pyridoxine

Pyridoxine (vitamin B_6) deficiency is a rare disorder that may be associated with the use of isoniazid, birth control pills, and penicillamine. Disease states, including cancer, celiac disease, and renal failure, have also been linked to the deficient state. Although a pyridoxine-deficient state may be characterized by peripheral neuropathy in adults, it is more commonly associated with refractory seizures (especially infantile spasms) in the neonatal and infantile period.

Pyridoxine-dependent epilepsy is an autosomal recessive disorder recently mapped to chromosome 5q31.[12] Pyridoxine-dependent epilepsy is characterized by severe seizures associated with a markedly abnormal electroencephalogram (EEG) and is

unresponsive to standard antiepileptic therapy. An abnormality of pyridoxine binding to the enzyme glutamic acid decarboxylase may diminish γ-aminobutyric acid and thereby cause seizure activity.[13] Intravenous administration of 50–100 mg of pyridoxine results in seizure control and normalization of the EEG within minutes of treatment. Maintenance therapy is then initiated at 5–300 mg/kg per day.[14] Infantile spasms may respond to pyridoxine therapy as well.

Cardiac Diseases

Congenital Heart Disease

CHD occurs in at least 10 per 1,000 live-born children.[15] The central nervous system is one of the most common sites of complications associated with the cardiac lesions of CHD, and cardiac abnormalities are associated with an increased risk of congenital cerebral defect. The most frequent cause of neurologic dysfunction is hypoxic-ischemic injury, but infective endocarditis (IE), brain abscesses, and cerebral dysgenesis associated with CHD are also etiologies of central nervous system injury. Seizures may be associated with any of these brain abnormalities.

Hypoxic-ischemic central nervous system injury may be due to chronic or acute injury. Chronic hypoxia results from various right-to-left shunting cardiac malformations, and acute hypoxia may occur with cardiac arrest or surgical correction. Central nervous system insults may be global in nature, secondary to hypoperfusion related to cardiac arrest, or focal, owing to occlusive processes associated with thromboembolic phenomena. In the case of children born prematurely with CHD, poor autoregulatory control of cerebral blood flow may further complicate their course and add to the risk of central nervous system pathology. Seizures are one of the more frequent manifestations of the cerebral injury associated with CHD, particularly in the period after surgery to repair a congenital defect.[16]

Before cardiopulmonary bypass, the primary pathophysiologic process underlying cerebral injury associated with CHD was right-to-left shunting. The ability to perform open-heart surgery was a major advance in the treatment of CHD, permitting cardiothoracic surgeons to undertake life-saving procedures on neonates and young infants. Extracorporeal cardiopulmonary support did not, however, overcome all the technical aspects of cardiac surgery in the young child. Although palliative procedures could be performed, surgery that definitively corrected the life-threatening cardiac malformations could only rarely be undertaken owing to the small size of the heart and surgical field and blood that obscured complicated congenital defects. The inability to correct the congenital heart lesions in a single procedure resulted in a series of palliative procedures that was performed over a period of months, if not years, until the infant grew sufficiently to allow the ultimate correction. During this process, infants with CHD continued to experience cerebral injury related to right-to-left shunting and hypoxia, as well as the complications of the many palliative procedures.[17]

The advent of low-flow cardiopulmonary bypass used in conjunction with deep hypothermic circulatory arrest has resulted in definitive repairs undertaken at a much earlier age than in the past. This advance in cardiothoracic surgical procedures has reduced the need for multiple palliative procedures and thus lessened the risk of central nervous system injury by decreasing the time to achieve normalized cardiac function. The progress in this area had resulted in decreased mortality but not diminished morbidity.[18] Morbidity related to factors such as chronic hypoxia and multiple palliative surgical procedures has been reduced. However, severe hemodynamic shock and marked acidosis associated with previously lethal heart malformations, which are now surgically corrected at an early age, continue to elevate morbidity statistics. In addition, newly recognized forms of neurologic morbidity have been related to low-flow cardiopulmonary bypass and deep hypothermic circulatory arrest. Thus, children with CHD survive with little or no cardiac morbidity but prominent neurologic dysfunction.

CHD is a risk factor for IE and brain abscess. The pathogenesis of IE involves high-velocity flow created by an abnormal valve or communication between systemic and pulmonary circulations, resulting in eddying and turbulence that damages endothelium. Platelets and fibrin adhere to the damaged endothelium and form small sterile thrombi. Circulating bacteria adhere to and grow in these thrombi. IE is most often seen in children with CHD. The bacteria most commonly found in IE are those that produce substances like dextran or glycoproteins, which promote platelet aggregation or aid in bacterial adhesion to surfaces. *Streptococci* often cause endocarditis. Vegetations are formed as microorganisms grow in and on the endocardium. The vegetations consist of platelets, fibrin, bacteria, leukocytes, and red cells. Systemic embolization occurs in up to 50% of patients with IE.[19] Neurologic injury occurs in 20–40%[20] of patients. Central nervous system manifestations of IE include cerebrovascular injury, meningitis, brain abscess, and seizures. Lesions of the cerebral vasculature that result from infective emboli are at particular risk of bleeding, and thus anticoagulation is contraindicated in children with IE who develop neurologic symptoms.

Brain abscesses are uncommon in the pediatric population[21]; however, among children with an abscess, nearly 50% have CHD.[22] The peak incidence of brain abscess is between the ages of 4 and 7 years. Cyanotic heart disease represents the greatest risk; polycythemia and right-to-left shunts are associated risk factors. Owing to disturbances of perfusion of the brain's microvasculature, polycythemia results in areas of ischemia in which microbial organisms, which have bypassed the phagocytic-filtering action of the pulmonary capillary bed through a right-to-left shunt, may gain access to necrotic cerebral tissue. Within these localized areas of cerebritis, an abscess may develop.

In approximately 75% of cases, the abscesses are supratentorial and multifocal 20% of the time. The presentation of an abscess is typically insidious, with headache and vomiting being the most common symptoms at the time of diagnosis. Initial symptoms of brain abscess are more likely owing to its intracranial mass effect than to the infectious condition of illness. Partial or generalized seizures may be the first indication of cerebral involvement. Although initially subtle in onset, the cerebral abscess can be rapidly progressive. The patient is often not febrile, and a peripheral white blood cell count may be elevated only mildly. Diagnosis is made by demonstrating enhancement on brain computed tomography (CT). Unless contraindicated by imaging evidence of problematic mass effect, a lumbar puncture should be performed to obtain cerebrospinal fluid for diagnostic studies.

Aggressive management of a cerebral abscess includes surgical resection or aspiration of the lesion in conjunction with antimicrobial treatment. The more typically chosen conservative therapy consists of 6 weeks of antibiotic therapy. A third-generation cephalosporin and an antistaphylococcal agent are commonly used, pending definitive microbial cultures. In the past, brain abscesses were usually attributed to streptococci or *Staphylococcus aureus*. More recently, anaerobic bacteria, in particular *Bacteroides fragilis*, have been diagnosed.

Before the availability of CT scanning, mortality for cerebral abscess was as high as 40%. Two major factors, late diagnosis and the presence of multiple lesions, contributed to the high mortality rate. A dramatic reduction in mortality has resulted from the use of CT scanning and advances in antimicrobial therapy. Epilepsy occurs in approximately 30% of patients with cerebral abscesses, but it may be years before it develops.[22]

Cerebral dysgenesis, often associated with CHD, has been reported in many series. Cerebral dysgenesis has been found in up to 29% of autopsy studies of children with CHD and should be considered in any child with evidence of central nervous system dysfunction.[23] Children with the hypoplastic left-heart syndrome are at particularly high risk of abnormal cerebral development; malformations include microdysgenesis and holoprosencephaly. Epilepsy and other disorders, including motor delays, can be seen in the neonatal period or later in infancy. Diagnosis is made by magnetic resonance imaging (MRI) scan.

Williams Syndrome

Williams syndrome (WS) is characterized by distinctive facial features, mental retardation, cardiovascular disease, and hypercalcemia.[24] WS is a contiguous gene disorder with a critical region deletion at chromosome locus 7q11 that is found in more than 99% of patients with the clinical diagnosis. The disorder is transmitted in an autosomal-dominant manner, but most instances represent de novo deletions. It has a prevalence of 1 in 20,000.

Children with WS have "elfin faces." Features include broad brow, bitemporal narrowing, malar hypoplasia, long philtrum, large lips, wide mouth, small jaw, and large ear lobes. Features change with age, and adults have long faces and necks that give them a gaunt appearance.

Most individuals with WS have some degree of mental retardation. Cognitive delays range from mild to severe. Some have average intelligence.

Cardiovascular abnormalities are due to an elastin arteriopathy in which arteries may be narrowed. Supravalvar aortic stenosis is the most common abnormality and occurs in 75% of patients. Other structural cardiac lesions are peripheral pulmonary stenosis, atrial septal defect, and ventricular septal defect. The cardiac abnormalities are associated with a microdeletion or mutation of the ELN gene at 7q11.23,[25] an area within the much larger WS critical region deletion. The ELN gene is responsible for production of elastin, a structural protein that is a component of elastic fibers in many tissues. The gene defect results in a multifocal intracranial arteriopathy characterized by medial fibroelastic dysplasia, hypertrophied smooth muscle, and disorganized elastin fibers.

The clinical course of WS is notable for a delay in achieving motor milestones that is likely associated with hypotonia and hyperextensible joints. The cognitive features of WS consist of strengths in auditory rote memory and language but weaknesses in visuospatial constructive areas. Sensory defensiveness, perseveration, and attention deficits are also noted. Idiopathic hypercalcemia occurs in 15% of patients; the etiology is unclear. Failure to thrive is seen in 70% of cases. Sudden deaths in patients with WS may result from coronary artery stenosis.[26] Stroke has also been reported in WS patients.[27,28] Seizures, including infantile spasms, have been reported in patients with WS. Seizures may be the presenting manifestation of cerebral infarcts, secondary to cerebral artery stenosis.[29] Six of 16 patients in a series of patients with WS had abnormal EEGs or seizures, and two of those six had infantile spasms.[30]

A multidisciplinary approach to the management of patients with WS is required. Cardiac and kidney function must be monitored along with calcium levels. The significant risk of neurologic disease warrants ongoing evaluations by a neurologist.

Renal Disorders

Congenital Uremia

In children younger than 1 year of age, severe chronic renal failure (function less than 10% of normal) is often associated with a severe subacute progressive encephalopathy.[31] This group of children has a markedly different outcome than children who develop end-stage renal disease after the first year of life. Although 90% of the children in the latter group achieve developmental milestones appropriately,[32] two out of three children with early onset failure or congenital uremia experience seizures and developmental arrest followed by regression and microcephaly.[33]

The encephalopathy associated with congenital uremia is commonly complicated by bulbar dysfunction that often results in death in the first years of life. Neuroimaging typically reveals evidence of enlarged ventricular size and prominent sulci and gyri. These findings may result from true atrophy or "pseudoatrophy" related to the use of corticosteroids.[34]

The cause of congenital uremic encephalopathy is uncertain. Aluminum toxicity is one commonly proposed mechanism for neurologic dysfunction. Hyperphosphatemia resulting from hyperparathyroidism is treated with phosphate binders that contain aluminum. Epidemiologic studies have identified aluminum exposure as a risk factor for encephalopathy. Aluminum may alter cellular repair mechanisms or have adverse effects on neurotransmitter or energy metabolism. Other etiologies have been suggested, including the chronic uremic state itself, malnutrition, hypertension, and lack of psychosocial interaction.

The mechanism underlying seizure activity is unclear; hypertension and aluminum toxicity are the two most commonly suspected factors. Partial and generalized seizures have been reported. Control of hypertension and reduction of the risk of aluminum toxicity should be undertaken in conjunction with the use of an appropriate antiepileptic medication based on seizure classification.

Dialysis

Seizure activity has been reported in 7–10% of children with chronic renal disease undergoing dialysis. Seizures tend to occur during or shortly after dialysis and are most often generalized tonic-clonic. Seizure activity is most likely caused by chemical or osmotic imbalances. Seizures tend to occur during the initial stages of a course of dialysis, when solute changes are most significant. The increased risk of seizure activity associated with hemodialysis, as compared to that of peritoneal dialysis, may also be related to the more rapid rate at which solutes are cleared. Children with a history of seizures are at particular risk of dialysis-associated seizures.[35] The use of an antiepileptic medication depends on the degree to which it is dialyzable.

Hemolytic Uremic Syndrome

Classically seen in infants younger than 2 years of age, hemolytic uremic syndrome (HUS) is characterized by microangiopathic hemolytic anemia, renal cortical necrosis with acute renal insufficiency, and thrombocytopenia resulting from increased platelet utilization. Although most cases are sporadic, a genetic predisposition is suggested by reports of individuals, and at times siblings, who have experienced multiple episodes of HUS. It is thought that the genetic basis for the disease is probably a deficiency of prostacyclin. Small epidemics of HUS have led to the hypothesis of an infectious etiology; it has been associated with viral, *Shigella*, and *Escherichia coli* infections.

Endothelial injury of the vascular bed secondary to viruses, toxins, and immune complexes results in exposure of the subendothelium of the vessel wall and accumulation of platelets. Fibrin deposition follows, causing injury to red blood cell membranes and hemolytic anemia. The microangiopathy involving the capillary bed brings about necrotizing arterial thrombosis. Ischemic lesions are found in the kidney, intestine, myocardium, and the central nervous system.

The clinical course of HUS is often characterized by a prodromal respiratory syndrome that lasts approximately 1 week. Patients then develop abdominal pain, vomiting, and diarrhea. Gross blood is found in the stool of 20% of patients. Renal insufficiency occurs, and microscopic and gross hematuria have been reported. Neurologic dysfunction seen in HUS includes mild confusion, somnolence, coma, and seizures. Evidence of central nervous system involvement is seen in 30–50% of patients.[36,37] Examination of the peripheral blood smear reveals burr cells, helmet cells, and schistocytes, consistent with the presence of microangiopathic hemolysis. Hemoglobin concentration and platelet counts may be greatly diminished, as low as 2 g/dl and 20,000 platelets/mm³, respectively. Urinalysis demonstrates the presence of red blood cells and protein in association with rising blood urea nitrogen and creatinine values. On brain MRI, discrete infarcts with edema and at times hemorrhage may be revealed, most commonly in the internal capsule and subcortical nuclei.[38]

Treatment is centered on transfusion, dialysis, and management of fluid, electrolytes, and hypertension. Other interventions may include anticoagulation, antiplatelet agents, thrombolysis, plasmapheresis, and infusion of gamma globulins, but none of these measures has been studied sufficiently to demonstrate efficacy in a pediatric population.

Lowe Syndrome

The oculocerebrorenal syndrome of Lowe is an X-linked disorder that maps to Xq25-q26 of the long arm of the X chromosome.[39] It is uncertain how the underlying enzyme deficiency, an abnormality of inositol polyphosphate 5-phosphatase,[40] correlates with the clinical presentation of bilateral, congenital cataracts, neurologic dysfunction, and a renal Fanconi's syndrome.

The clinical course is characterized by frontal bossing and deep-set eyes, apparent early in life. Even if cataracts are surgically treated early, vision remains poor. Glaucoma often complicates the picture and is difficult to control. Marked, diffuse hypotonia is present early and contributes to motor delays. Loss of tendon reflexes takes place by the age of 1 year. Cognitive impairment is a prominent feature, and as the child grows older, behavior can be a major problem. Seizures occur in approximately 50% of patients. Partial and generalized seizures, as well as infantile spasms, may occur. No particular seizure pattern is noted; standard use of

antiepileptic medications is recommended. MRI and CT imaging of the brain commonly demonstrate periventricular white matter cystic lesions.[41,42]

Hyperaminoaciduria and proteinuria are due to the Fanconi's syndrome renal dysfunction. Slowly progressive renal dysfunction occurs, but the degree of impairment varies. Renal stones and nephrocalcinosis due to wasting of calcium and phosphate can be present.[43]

Early diagnosis and intervention should avoid dehydration and other complications of the disorder. Vitamin D and alkali should be used to correct acidosis and prevent rickets. Some patients live into the fourth decade. Cardiac and renal failure can be fatal in these patients.

Infectious Disorders

Cat-Scratch Disease

Cat-scratch disease (CSD) is a disorder of childhood characterized by a primary skin lesion and regional lymphadenopathy associated with interaction with and scratches from a cat. The infection is attributed to the organism *Bartonella (Rochalimaea) henselae*. The natural course of the disease is for the enlarged node or nodes to resolve spontaneously over a period of several months.

As many as 22,000 cases of CSD are diagnosed annually in the United States; 80% are in patients under the age of 21 years. CSD occurs worldwide in all races, with a slight predominance in men. A seasonal variability is noted in the incidence of CSD, more commonly occurring in fall and winter. In more than 95% of cases, the history reveals the illness after a scratch or lick from a kitten or cat. The cat probably acts as a vector for the *B. henselae* rather than being infected by it, because skin testing with cat-scratch antigen provokes no response in the animals.[44]

During the course of the disease, the patient does not appear to be ill, even though lymphadenopathy may be quite prominent. Initially, flulike symptoms may be reported, but the primary lesion (a papule or pustule at the site of the scratch) becomes apparent only after 3–10 days. The primary lesion persists for approximately 1–3 weeks, rarely longer, and tender adenopathy is seen approximately 2 weeks after the contact with the cat. The nodes may remain enlarged for months; suppuration is noted in approximately 25% of patients referred to hospitals, but less often in those evaluated in office practices.

Central nervous system involvement is noted in 2–4% of children with CSD. They may develop encephalopathy, meningitis, radiculitis, or polyneuritis. The onset of neurologic symptoms is usually abrupt, taking place within the first month to a month and a half after adenopathy occurs. Seizures, including status epilepticus, occur in 50% of encephalopathic patients.[45,46] Seizures should be treated symptomatically; long-term therapy is not required.

Diagnosis is made clinically if three of the five following criteria exist: a history of animal (usually cat) contact or presence of a scratch or a primary dermal or eye lesion; aspiration of sterile pus from the node (a presumptive diagnostic test for CSD) or negative cultures and serology tests that exclude other etiologic possibilities; a *B. henselae*-based immunofluorescent assay test; a positive skin test to CSD antigen; and node biopsy showing histopathology consistent with CSD, especially if pleomorphic rod-shaped bacilli are demonstrated with the Warthin-Starry silver stain.[47]

CSD is typically a benign, self-limited disease and thus rarely requires active therapy. Management includes reassurance, analgesics, and aspiration of suppurative nodes. In more severely ill individuals, antibiotics can be used. Those reported to have been effective are erythromycin, doxycycline, rifampin, ciprofloxacin, trimethoprim-sulfamethoxazole, and gentamicin. Prognosis is excellent; adenopathy resolves in 2–4 months, and a single occurrence appears to provide immunity for life.

Shigella

Shigellosis is a bacterial enteritis caused by the four groups of *Shigella*. Fever and intestinal and extraintestinal symptoms are characteristics of the infection. Neurologic symptoms, including seizures, are common.

Shigella is divided into four groups and 40 serotypes. It is easily cultured from stool early in the course of diarrhea. *Shigella* infection is usually acquired through ingestion of contaminated food or water. Person-to-person transmission by contaminated hands is common. Humans are hosts for *Shigella*, but animals are not. In developing countries, food and water are important vectors of transmission. Crowding, poor personal hygiene, and the lack of sanitary facilities increase the risk of intrafamily spread of the infection. The rate of infection is greatest in the first 4 years of life. July through October is the peak period for infection in the United States.

Adherence of *Shigella* to intestinal epithelial cell–surface receptor sites alters the brush border of the intestines, resulting in vesicular formation on the cell membrane. Organisms then enter the cell cytoplasm after penetration of the vesicle and spread from one epithelial cell to another.

Clinical manifestations of shigellosis vary from watery stools for several days to high fevers, cramplike abdominal pain, and malaise. With colonic invasion, dysentery occurs. Tenesmus, fecal urgency, and bloody diarrhea are frequent. Symptoms resolve quickly. Fever typically lasts 24 hours, and other symptoms abate within 5–7 days.

Seizures occur in 12–45% of hospitalized patients with culture-proven shigellosis. The seizures are most often seen in children between the ages of 6 months and 4 years.[48,49] The seizure frequency is out of proportion to that expected owing to fever alone. There is debate as to whether the *Shigella* toxin plays a role in the genesis of seizure activity or other neurologic symptoms.[50] Lethargy, confusion, headache, and, rarely, encephalopathy have also been reported. Follow-up studies of patients with seizures in association with *Shigella* infection 6–9 years earlier revealed that 3% had febrile seizures and none had afebrile seizures.[51] Although acute therapy may be indicated in certain cases, no long-term therapy is warranted. Neurologic outcome is good.

Rheumatologic Disorders

Henoch-Schönlein Purpura

Most common in children 4–15 years of age, Henoch-Schönlein purpura (HSP), or anaphylactoid purpura, is a generalized vascular disorder that results from acute aseptic vasculitis involving arterioles and capillaries. Inflammatory changes within and around vessel walls are thought to be associated with hypersensitivity, but only rarely is an allergen detected. Eosinophilia may be detected, and 50% of patients have elevated immunoglobulin A levels.

HSP typically presents with palpable purpura, abdominal pain, and joint pain. The most commonly involved areas are the skin, joints, gastrointestinal tract, and kidneys. The classic distribution of the red maculopapular "palpable purpura" involves the buttocks, posterior thighs, and extensor surfaces of the arms and legs. The lesions spare the face, trunk, palms, and soles. Painful edema of the scalp, joints, and scrotum as well as large-joint arthritis occur. Abdominal pain is colicky and may be associated with emesis and melena. Abdominal complications include perforation and intussusception. Lab studies may reveal anemia due to blood loss, as well as hematuria and proteinuria.

Central nervous system manifestations have been documented in 1–8% of patients. Seizures, headache, and altered states of consciousness may occur.[52-54]

HSP is a self-limited disease that resolves in 6–12 weeks. Recurrences have been reported. The most serious chronic complication is renal failure; 5–10% of patients develop chronic nephritis. Plasmapheresis, steroids, and azathioprine have been used in the treatment of HSP. Early treatment with prednisone and azathioprine prevent the progression of chronic changes and improve outcome.[55]

References

1. Mock DM, deLorimer AA, Liebman WM, et al. Biotin deficiency: an unusual complication of parenteral alimentation. N Engl J Med 1981;304:820–823.
2. Yatzidis H, Koutsicos S, Agroyannis B, et al. Biotin in the management of uremic neurologic disorders. Nephron 1984;36:183–186.
3. Sweetman L, Surh IL, Baker H, et al. Clinical and metabolic abnormalities in a boy with dietary deficiency of biotin. Pediatrics 1981;68:553–558.
4. Wolf B, Grier RE, Allen RJ, et al. Phenotypic variations in biotinidase deficiency. J Pediatr 1983;103:233–237.
5. Ginat-Israeli T, Hurvitz H, Klar A, et al. Deteriorating neurological and neuroradiological course in treated biotinidase deficiency. Neuropediatrics 1993;24:103–106.
6. Reynolds EH. Effects of folic acid on the mental state and fit-frequency of drug-treated epileptic patients. Lancet 1967;1:1086–1088.
7. Davis RE, Woodliff HJ. Folic acid deficiency in patients receiving anticonvulsant drugs. Med J Aust 1971;2:1070–1072.
8. Reizenstein P, Lund L. Effect of anticonvulsant drugs on folate absorption and the cerebrospinal folate pump. Scand J Haematol 1973;11:158–165.
9. Reynolds EH. Folate and Epilepsy. In HF Bradford, CD Mardson (eds), Biochemistry and Neurology. London: Academic, 1976;247–252.
10. Molloy AM, Mills JL, Kirk PN, et al. Folate status and neural tube defects. Biofactors 1999;10:291–294.
11. Fishman MA. Birth defects and supplemental vitamins. Curr Treat Options Neurol 2000;2:117–122.
12. Cormier-Daire V, Dagoneau N, Nabbout R, et al. A gene for pyridoxine-dependent epilepsy maps to chromosome 5q31. Am J Hum Genet 2000;67:991–993.
13. Lott IT, Coulombe T, DiPaolo RV, et al. Vitamin B_6-dependent seizures: pathology and chemical findings in brain. Neurology 1978;28:47–54.
14. Haengeli CA, Girardin E, Paunier L. Pyridoxine-dependent seizures, clinical and therapeutic aspects. Eur J Pediatr 1991;150:452–455.
15. Hoffman JIE. Congenital Heart Disease. In AM Rudolph, JIE Hoffmann, CD Rudolph (eds), Rudolph's Pediatrics (20th ed). Stamford, CT: Appleton & Lange, 1996:1457–1517.
16. du Plessis AJ. Neurologic Disorders Associated with Cardiac Disease. In KF Swaiman, S Ashwal (eds), Pediatric Neurology, Principles and Practice (3rd ed). St. Louis: Mosby, 1999:1385–1402.
17. Newburger JW, Silbert AR, Buckley LP, et al. Cognitive function and age at repair of transposition of the great arteries in children. N Engl J Med 1984;310:1495–1499.
18. Majnemer A, Limperopoulos C. Developmental progress of children with congenital heart defects requiring open heart surgery. Semin Pediatr Neurol 1999;6:12–19.
19. Lutas E, Roberts R, Devereux R, et al. Relation between the presence of echocardiographic vegetations and the complication rate in infective endocarditis. Am Heart J 1986;112:107–113.
20. Saiman L, Prince A, Gersony W. Pediatric infective endocarditis in the modern era. J Pediatr 1993;122:847.
21. Ghosh S, Chandy M, Abraham J. Brain abscess and congenital heart disease. J Indian Med Assoc 1988;88:312.
22. Aebi C, Kauffmann F, Schaad U. Brain abscess in childhood: long-term experiences. Eur J Pediatr 1991;150:282.
23. Miller G, Vogel H. Structural evidence of injury or malformation in the brains of children with congenital heart disease. Semin Pediatr Neurol 1999;6:20–26.

24. Morris DA, Demsey SA, Leonard CO, et al. Natural history of Williams syndrome: physical characteristics. J Pediatr 1988;113:318.

25. Ewart AK, Morris DA, Atkinson K, et al. Hemizygosity at the elastin locus in a developmental disorder, Williams syndrome. Nat Genet 1993;5:11.

26. Bird LM, Billman GF, Lacro RV, et al. Sudden death in Williams syndrome: report of ten cases. J Pediatr 1996;129:926–931.

27. Ardinger RH Jr, Goertz KK, Mattioli LF. Cerebrovascular stenosis with cerebral infarction in child with Williams syndrome. Am J Med Genet 1994;51:200.

28. Soper R, Chaloupka JC, Fayad PB, et al. Ischemic stroke and intracranial multifocal cerebral arteriopathy in Williams syndrome. J Pediatr 1995:126:945.

29. Kaplan P, Levinson M, Kaplan BS. Cerebral artery stenoses in Williams syndrome cause strokes in childhood. J Pediatr 1995;126:943.

30. Mizugishi K, Yamanaka K, Kuwajima K, Kondo I. Interstitial deletion of chromosome 7q in a patient with Williams syndrome and infantile spasms. J Hum Genet 1998;43:178.

31. Foley CM, Polinsky MS, Gruskin AB, et al. Encephalopathy in infants and children with chronic renal disease. Arch Neurol 1981;38:656.

32. Rasbury WC, Fennell FS III, Moris MK. Cognitive functioning of children with end stage renal disease before and after successful transplantation. J Pediatr 1983;1:1327.

33. Polinsky MS, Kaiser BA, Stover JR, et al. Neurologic development of children with severe chronic renal failure from infancy. Pediatr Nephrol 1987;1:157.

34. Baluarte HJ, Gruskin AB, Hiner LB, et al. Encephalopathy in children with chronic renal failure. Proc Clin Dial Transpl Forum 1977; 7:95.

35. Glenn CB, Astley SJ, Watkins SL. Dialysis-associate seizures in children and adolescents. Pediatr Nephrol 1992;6:182.

36. Martin DW, MacDonald KL, White KE, et al. The epidemiology and clinical aspects of the hemolytic uremic syndrome in Minnesota. N Engl J Med 1990;17:1161.

37. Sheth KJ, Swick HM, Haworth N. Neurologic involvement in hemolytic-uremic syndrome. Ann Neurol 1986;19:90–93.

38. Jeong YK, Kim IO, Kim WS, et al. Hemolytic uremic syndrome: MR findings of CNS complications. Pediatr Radiol 1994;24:585.

39. Hoffman GF, Bohles HJ, Burlina A, et al. Physical mapping and genomic structure of the Lowe syndrome gene OCRL1. Hum Genet 1997;99:145.

40. Attree O, Olivos IM, Okabe I, et al. The Lowe's oculocerebrorenal syndrome gene encodes a protein highly homologous to inositol polyphosphate-5-phosphatase. Nature 1992;358:239.

41. Demmer LA, Wippold FJ II, Dowton SB. Periventricular white matter cystic lesions in Lowe (oculocerebrorenal) syndrome. A new MR finding. Pediatr Radiol 1992;22:76.

42. O'Tuama LA, Laster DW. Oculocerebrorenal syndrome: case report with CT and MR correlates. AJNR Am J Neuroradiol 1987;8:555–557.

43. Charnas LR, Bernardini I, Rader D, et al. Clinical and laboratory findings in the oculocerebrorenal syndrome of Lowe, with special reference to growth and renal function. N Engl J Med 1991;324:1318.

44. Margileth AM, Hayden GF. Cat scratch disease: from feline affection to human infection. N Engl J Med 1993;329:53.

45. Hadley S, Albrecht MA, Tarsey C. Cat-scratch encephalopathy: a cause of status epilepticus and coma in healthy young adult. Neurology 1995;45:196.

46. Hahn J, Sum J, Lee K. Unusual MRI findings after status epilepticus due to cat-scratch disease. Pediatr Neurol 1994;10:255.

47. Slater LN, Welch DF. Bartonella Infections Including Cat-Scratch Disease. In WM Scheld, RF Whitley, DH Durack (eds), Infections of the Central Nervous System (2nd ed). Philadelphia: Lippincott–Raven, 1997.

48. Ashkenazi S, Dinari G, Weitz B, et al. Convulsions in shigellosis. Evaluation of possible risk factors. Am J Dis Child 1983;137:1985.

49. Daoud AS, Zaki M, al-Mutairi G, et al. Childhood shigellosis: clinical and bacteriological study. J Trop Med Hyg 1990;93:275.

50. Ashkenazi S, Cleary KR, Pickering LK, et al. The association of shiga toxin and other cytotoxins with the neurologic manifestations of shigellosis. J Infect Dis 1990;161:961.

51. Lahat E, Katz Y, Bistritzer T, et al. Recurrent seizures in children with *Shigella*-associated convulsions. Ann Neurol 1990;28:393.

52. Belman AL, Leicher CR, Moshe SL, et al. Neurologic manifestations of Schönlein-Henoch purpura: report of three cases and review of the literature. Pediatrics 1985;75:687.

53. Ostergaard JR, Storm K. Neurologic manifestations of Schönlein-Henoch purpura. Acta Paediatr Scand 1991;80:339.

54. Ritter FJ, Seay AR, Lahey ME. Peripheral mononeuropathy complicating anaphylactoid purpura. J Pediatr 1983;103:77.

55. Foster BJ, Bernard C, Drummond KN, Sharma AK. Effective therapy for severe Henoch-Schönlein purpura nephritis with prednisone and azathioprine: a clinical and histopathologic study. J Pediatr 2000;136:370.

Chapter 23

Developmental Disabilities and Epilepsy

Ross B. FineSmith

Medical Services for Developmentally Disabled Persons

The term *developmentally disabled* describes a group of individuals with cognitive and physical impairments of heterogenous cerebral etiology that limit independence and function. *Epilepsy* is also of cerebral etiology and refers to those who have experienced two or more unprovoked seizures. The neuropathology associated with a developmental disability (DD) can also be a nidus for seizures.

A DD requires some clarification, because it can manifest in a diverse group of individuals and conditions. Most individuals with a DD are mentally retarded based on formal cognitive testing and assessment of adaptive behaviors. The American Association on Mental Retardation established the following definition: "Mental retardation refers to substantial limitations in present functioning. It is characterized by significantly subaverage intellectual functioning, existing concurrently with related limitations in two or more of the following applicable adaptive skill areas: communication, self-care, home living, social skills, community use, self-direction, health and safety, functional academics, leisure, and work. Mental retardation is manifest before age 18."[1]

There is a similarity in the descriptions of persons with a DD and those with mental retardation, which has resulted in the terms' being used interchangeably in literature and in our culture. The two conditions frequently occur together, but there are distinct differences that make the two groups separate. As previously defined, a person with a DD has a limited ability to live and function independently. This can be a result of a physical or cognitive disability; however, either disability can also occur incidentally. An example of this includes a subgroup of persons with a motor-based DD, such as cerebral palsy (CP) or spina bifida. These individuals can have normal intellectual abilities but still have a severe physical DD. The converse also applies. An individual can meet the requirements to be classified as mentally retarded but is able to live independently and maintain employment. Those with DDs have greater medical need and, until recently, were cared for by large residential institutions. In addition, those with disabling psychiatric disorders, without intrinsic cognitive or physical limitations, may be unable to function independently in our communities solely as a result of their abnormal perceptions and behaviors.

Shift from Residential Institutions to Community Settings

The current trend of deinstitutionalization of individuals with moderate to profound DDs has resulted in a relocation of this population to a variety of community settings, including group homes, sponsored living, supported living arrangements, and supervised apartment living. The medical and neurologic care of these individuals is now the responsibility of those physicians practicing in these locations. Unlike staff physicians employed by developmental centers, most physicians in the community have limited experience with or exposure to persons with significant DDs. This is a result, not of discrimination, but of demographics. These patients were institutionalized and typically did not require treatment from "outside" physicians. The relocation process is a national trend and has resulted in a marked increase in medical consumers with DDs who require medical care in our communities.

There are few facilities that specialize in outpatient medical care for the DD. These centers can be more efficient and effective in caring for this population, because the medical staff is more familiar with the medical, neurologic, and psychiatric conditions and complications that are frequently seen in the developmentally disabled. This may include hypothyroidism and early-onset Alzheimer's disease in people with Down syndrome or severe behavioral outbursts in individuals with autism as a reaction to pain, such as trigeminal neuralgia or migraine. Experienced staff can reduce the need for costly diagnostic studies and the risk of adverse events. The relative cost of caring for individuals with a DD can be higher than that of the nonhandicapped patient, because they are at greater risk for medical and psychiatric complications. For example, patients with a DD are at greater risk for developing epilepsy and have a higher incidence of medically refractory epilepsy; therefore, they require more frequent office visits, laboratory studies, emergency room visits, and neurodiagnostic tests.[2]

Medical care in those with DDs is frequently complicated by their cognitive deficits and maladaptive behaviors, because there can be an inability to describe symptoms and cooperate with diagnostic studies. For more sensitive studies, like magnetic resonance imaging (MRI), conscious sedation by an anesthesiologist may be required and thereby increases the risk of adverse effects from the anesthetic medication. These are also additional costs that place a financial burden on the centers providing medical care to the developmentally disabled, which is complicated by the current healthcare insurance environment.

Epidemiology

The relocation of the developmentally disabled from the institution to the community setting has been especially challenging to those physicians treating epilepsy in the community. The incidence of epilepsy in persons with DDs is 30–50%; as many as 45% of these have medically refractory epilepsy, and most begin having seizures before the age of 5 years.[2–5]

Cause and Effect Relationship of Epilepsy and Encephalopathy—More Than a Comorbidity

The etiology of the seizures is presumed to be due to the same cerebral dysfunction that is responsible for the developmental condition. This seems plausible in conditions that have recognizable neuropathologic correlates on neuroimaging, such as neuronal migration disorders, hypoxic or ischemic disease, and neuronal injury due to infection and traumatic brain injury. However, in those without neuroanatomic evidence or history of brain injury, the association is not as clear. There is a growing body of research that describes the genetics associated with the cellular and molecular mechanisms of some forms of epilepsy and developmental disabilities.[6,7] In addition, the increasingly sensitive MRI and functional imaging are identifying previously undetectable small lesions and heterotopic foci.

The alternative hypothesis implicates epilepsy as a causative factor that results in impaired learning ability and, ultimately, a DD. The electrical dysfunction of a seizure impairs a person's regulated neuronal activity and prevents its ability to function normally. Cognitive processing speed and ability are only temporarily disrupted during a seizure, but a prolonged seizure or frequent seizures can cause permanent disruptive changes. It is therefore plausible that seizures can cause mental retardation in children who would not have been mentally retarded without the occurrence of epilepsy.

The negative impact of seizures on cognitive ability is supported by evidence that early-onset and prolonged seizures in animals can cause selective neuronal cell death[8] and long-term learning deficits. In the surviving neurons, the excessive and abnormal cellular activity that occurs during a seizure can alter the cell's gene expression of ion channels and enzymes. Ion channels and enzymes regulate neuronal signal transduction, and these alterations can cause excessive excitability and hypersynchrony.[9–12]

The hippocampus is sensitive to the hypoxic conditions that accompany early-onset and repetitive seizures. Progressive neuronal injury can result in cumulative cognitive impairment, especially for memory. Abnormal neuronal regrowth and synaptic reorganization have been observed in the resected brain specimens of the epileptogenic hippocampus in humans who have undergone temporal lobe epilepsy surgery.[13–15] This reorganization may result in new "circuits" that are more likely to result in recurrent seizures and impaired learning.

A second proposed mechanism for patients with extratemporal seizures involves a more temporary, but generalized, disruption of processing in the association and integration areas of the brain. Multiple daily seizures may interrupt normal cerebral functioning during the seizure, and learning can continue to be markedly impaired during the postictal phase. After a seizure, the electrochemical abnormalities in the neurons require time to return to their resting membrane potential and resume baseline functioning. The postictal deficits can follow motor seizures as well as more subtle seizures, such as absence and complex partial seizures. If a patient has four to five complex partial seizures per day with a 30-minute postictal interruption in learning and other cognitive functions, 2.5 hours may be affected each day. Cumulatively, this can significantly impact the rate of language acquisition and many other areas of cognition in children, and it can affect adults as well. Under these conditions, epilepsy may be viewed as a progressive disorder that can contribute to or even cause mental retardation.

Multiple variables can confound our ability to dissociate the consequences of epilepsy from a predetermined underlying DD. A better understanding of the cause and effect relationship between repetitive seizures and subsequent cognitive impairment may allow us to target and more effectively treat children at risk for progressive impairments.

The treatment of epilepsy may also contribute to developmental delays in children. Farwell[16] demonstrated that children treated with phenobarbital to prevent recurrent febrile seizures had a significantly lower intelligence quotient than a control group that was not treated. This effect has not been demonstrated with other antiepileptic drugs (AEDs), in part because it would be unethical to follow a randomized untreated control group of children with epilepsy. There have been studies that demonstrated

mild reductions in response times in patients on phenytoin and carbamazepine[17] and improvement when patients were taken off phenytoin, carbamazepine, or valproate.[18]

Last, it is possible that a combination of neuronal injury, a predisposition for learning difficulties, the effects of seizures, and medication result in an impaired learning process in some individuals with epilepsy.

Common Diagnostic Challenges for the Neurologist

Attempting to determine whether a paroxysmal event in a person with a DD is related to seizure activity is complicated by maladaptive behavior, accompanying mental retardation, and, occasionally, a comorbid psychiatric condition. Children and adults with DDs frequently require sedation for studies because of their inability to remain stationary in specific conditions. This is often necessary for both electroencephalogram (EEG) lead placement and neuroimaging. The medications used for sedation frequently cause generalized slowing and excessive beta activity in the EEG pattern. This can be avoided if the individual is admitted to the hospital for a 24-hour EEG study, which allows for recovery from the sedation and return of the EEG pattern to baseline. Simultaneous closed-circuit television capability is available in many larger hospitals and most university centers and allows for excellent electrographic correlation.

If the behaviors or suspected seizures are problematic and studies are unable to be obtained, a medication trial often helps to differentiate the cause. For example, risperidone (Risperdal) or a selective serotonin reuptake inhibitor helps in the treatment of an intermittent explosive disorder but has no effect on complex partial seizures. A selective serotonin reuptake inhibitor escalates manic episodes and, again, does not change the frequency of the events if they are a manifestation of a complex partial seizure. Carbamazepine, valproate, lamotrigine, and gabapentin have been used as "mood stabilizers" and may reduce events related to affective disorders as well as seizures. The AEDs may be the best choice of treatment when etiology cannot be determined and is suspected to be a cyclic affective disorder or seizure related.

Developmental Conditions

The etiology and manifestation of several conditions associated with DDs are reviewed and the role of epilepsy discussed in the following sections. Only the most frequently encountered developmental disorders are addressed.

Cerebral Palsy

The physical disability in CP results in additional burden on caretakers, and the addition of epilepsy results in significant complications to the care and management.

Incidence of Cerebral Palsy

CP occurs in approximately 2.5 per 1,000.0 live births.[19] The prevalence has not been significantly reduced despite widespread improvements in prenatal care, the availability of appropriate pediatric care, and neonatal intensive care units. This may be owing to the fact that those infants now surviving are more ill and recover with a higher rate of morbidity.

A diagnosis of CP is comprised of a combination of findings that include motor delay, positive neurologic signs, persistent primitive reflex activity, and abnormal postural reactions. The diagnosis of CP implies that no active disease is present, and the motor impairment is a result of upper motor neuron dysfunction. It is a diagnosis of exclusion and should not be made after one examination.

Improved and more appropriate medical care has resulted in a 90% survival rate of infants with CP into adulthood. However, children with CP associated with severe mental retardation, nonambulatory status, and required tube feeding have a much shorter survival rate.

Etiology of Cerebral Palsy

A specific cause for most cases of CP is unknown, and when a cause can be identified, it is usually of prenatal origin. The etiology was previously thought to be intrapartum asphyxia, but only 10% of CP is associated with such an event. Prenatal etiologies include cerebral dysgenesis, genetic disorders, in utero infections, and in utero strokes.

Postnatal acquired causes account for approximately 10–18% of CP and include central nervous system infections, trauma, childhood strokes, and severe hypoxic events.

Incidence of Epilepsy in Cerebral Palsy

The incidence of epilepsy in those with CP is 36–42%. This increases to approximately 50% in those with spastic quadriplegia or hemiplegia; however, the incidence was lower in patients with spastic diplegia. Partial seizures were the most frequently reported seizure type, and primary generalized seizures were less common. Primary generalized seizures infrequently occur in the spastic hemiplegic type.[20,21]

Children with spastic quadriplegia more commonly have their initial seizure in the first year of life, and those children with spastic hemiplegia more commonly had their initial seizure after the second year of life. Children with CP had a higher incidence of neonatal seizures and status epilepticus and required more than one AED to control their seizures.[20]

Phenomenology of Cerebral Palsy

The cerebral palsies are characterized by their motor dysfunction, but they are frequently accompanied by additional deficits. The deficits are experienced in the areas of cognition, vision, hearing, language, and behavior. Epilepsy is frequently associated, and approximately 65% of the total CP population has mental retardation.[18,21] There is a correlation with the severity of motor handicap, but individual variation occurs and is considerable.

The clinician must carefully differentiate between primary generalized epilepsy and partial-onset epilepsy that secondarily generalizes. The lateral cerebral spread of epileptiform electrochemical activity can be remarkably rapid, and therefore the clinical description of the event may not provide the information to classify seizure type. When mental retardation is also present, the impaired expressive ability limits the personal history, and the presence of pseudobulbar palsy with dysarthria can completely prevent communicative ability.

Extrapyramidal syndromes may initially be diagnosed as CP, because there are several common elements. These include persistence of primitive neonatal reflexes, hypotonia in infancy, delayed motor development, dysarthria speech, and tone abnormalities in subsequent years. Some extrapyramidal syndromes, such as congenital choreoathetosis, paroxysmal kinesogenic dyskinesia, and nonkinesogenic dyskinesia, manifest with frequent involuntary movements that may be interpreted as seizures.

Antispasticity Medications and Cerebral Palsy

Baclofen is one of the most widely used antispasmodic drugs. It is a structural analog of the inhibitory neurotransmitter γ-aminobutyric acid B (GABA$_B$) subtypes and exerts its effect on the GABA$_A$ receptor subtypes. In 1996, the intrathecal baclofen pump (Medtronic Inc., Minneapolis, MN) was approved by the U.S. Food and Drug Administration. This device provides continuous intrathecal infusion for those patients with severe spasticity who are unable to tolerate higher oral doses of baclofen. Intrathecal baclofen results in a greater effect on spasticity than oral dosing, because higher concentrations of baclofen are delivered directly in the cerebrospinal fluid at approximately 1% of the daily oral dose. First-time seizures or exacerbations of epilepsy with the initiation of baclofen have been reported. In those reports, comorbid conditions, including static encephalopathy, increase the risk for baclofen-related seizures.

In this author's experience, individuals with CP and mental retardation have benefited significantly from the continuous infusion and have tolerated it well. No change in seizure frequency or new-onset seizures has occurred in 20 patients.

Treatment and Outcome of Cerebral Palsy

Good seizure control can be achieved in up to 65% in persons with CP. In prospective studies, 13–20% of patients with CP and epilepsy are able to be successfully withdrawn from AEDs after at least a 1-year seizure-free period. In a retrospective study, a group with epilepsy and CP had a seizure relapse rate of 37% compared to a nonhandicapped control seizure-free rate of 90%.[21] Factors associated with a seizure-free period of 1 year or more in epileptic children with CP were normal intelligence, single seizure type, monotherapy, and spastic diplegia.

Clinicians should be cautious, however, to taper AEDs slowly rather than withdrawing AEDs abruptly, to avoid acute withdrawal seizures. The degree of mental retardation and impairment of ambulatory status in children with CP was more likely to be severe when associated with epilepsy.

Pervasive Developmental Disorders

The broad category of pervasive developmental disorders (PDDs) includes autism, PDDs not otherwise specified, childhood disintegrative disorder, Asperger's syndrome, and Rett syndrome. This group of disorders is heterogeneous and ranges from relatively minor speech and socialization deficits to severe neurodegenerative conditions. The common feature in all PDDs is the child's relatively healthy development until 12–18 months of age. After this period, the child undergoes a regression or loss of previously acquired abilities.

Children with autism or a PDD not otherwise specified experience a regression in (1) communication abilities, (2) reciprocal social interaction, and (3) appropriate play. They become less interested in interacting with others, lose most if not all language that developed until that time, have less eye contact, and begin to display abnormal self-stimulatory mannerisms. This is the most common and therefore the most studied group of children within the PDDs. The majority of this section focuses on this disorder referred to as *autistic spectrum disorder* (ASD).

Rett syndrome, childhood disintegrative disorder, and Asperger's syndrome occur less frequently and are discussed in this chapter only briefly. Rett syndrome is similar to other PDDs with healthy early development until 6–18 months of age. This condition occurs in only girls at a rate of 0.7–1.0 per 10,000. There is deterioration in language, behavior, and cognition and a loss of purposeful hand movements with associated hand wringing, truncal ataxia, and seizures. Seizures most frequently occur between 2 and 10 years of age and can be partial onset or generalized, and treatment depends on seizure type. Girls who develop Rett syndrome frequently exhibit movement disorders, which are frequently difficult to differentiate from focal motor seizures. Childhood disintegrative disorder is far less common, with little information related to epilepsy available. There is a relentless loss of motor abilities and cognitive function in the affected children. There is no significant association between Asperger's syndrome and seizures.

Incidence of Pervasive Developmental Disorder and Epilepsy

The incidence of autism is 4 to 5 patients per 10,000.[22,23] The frequency increases to 10 to 15 per 10,000, when all children with ASD are included.

Approximately 50% of children with ASD have abnormal EEGs, and approximately 30% of these have overt seizures. Tuchman[24] found the most frequent abnormalities were focal or centroparietal spikes (31%), generalized spikes (19%), bilateral or multifocal spikes (19%), generalized slowing (17%), and focal slowing (13%). In addition, those with mental retardation are likely to have generalized slowing.

Seizures can occur in up to 42% of children with autism spectrum disorders at one point in their lives.[24–26] There is a bimodal distribution of seizures, with the first occurring between 2 and 5 years of age and the second in adolescence.[26] The major risk factors for epilepsy in a child with ASD are low cognitive status, motor deficit, and a type of language dysfunction. Children with comorbid severe mental retardation have a 25% chance of developing epilepsy. ASD children who have verbal auditory agnosia, a language disorder characterized by a severe deficit in auditory and phonologic processing, have a 41% chance of developing epilepsy.[27,28] Girls with ASD are at increased risk for seizures. There is a 4 to 1 ratio, with more boys being diagnosed with ASD; however, girls are more likely to experience severe cognitive deficits and seizures.[24]

Phenomenology of Pervasive Developmental Disorder

Clinical seizure identification can be difficult in children with ASD, owing to their unusual behavioral mannerisms and their impaired language ability. Common behaviors in children with ASD can include periods of irritability, hyperactivity, apparent change in awareness, self-injurious behaviors, emotional outbursts, and lack of responsiveness.[29] Simple partial or complex partial seizures may manifest in similar behaviors in children with ASD. The communication deficit limits the ability of the children to describe the sensation or event, which is typically an important component in the diagnosis of a seizure. This lack of expressive language and, presumably, internal language may prevent them from understanding the experience themselves, because language at the interpersonal level plays a role in concept formation.[30,31]

The hypothesis that autistic regression is causally related to subclinical temporal lobe electrical epileptiform activity is controversial. Increasing research supports the Autistic Regression Syndrome phenomenon that may possibly include all children in the ASD classification with an epileptiform EEG.[24] The association of localized EEG findings with language and behavioral dysfunction is more clearly defined in the two epilepsy syndromes Landau-Kleffner syndrome and the syndrome of epilepsy with continuous spike and wave during slow wave sleep (CSWS).[33]

Landau-Kleffner syndrome is an acquired aphasia that manifests between 3 and 8 years of age after an initially healthy development. The onset of aphasia is often insidious, and the most common feature is verbal auditory agnosia[28]; however, different types of aphasia may occur.[32] Spontaneous recovery does occur, but as many as two-thirds are left with permanent language impairment. Autistic features are more likely to occur when the aphasia appears at a younger age. Seizures are present in 70–80% of the children and may appear before or after onset of aphasia.[32] The epileptic foci have been mapped to the left midtemporal cortex on EEG and more specifically to the intrasylvian cortex on magnetoencephalogram studies.[34] The epileptiform discharges are believed to interrupt language function in the superior temporal lobe, and when treatment is effective, there is a resolution of the spike-wave discharges and recovery of speech. The most common types of seizures are atypical absences, atonic seizures, and partial motor seizures with secondary generalization. Prednisone has been the most effective treatment; however, other AEDs have been used with success. More recently, subpial transection of the affected region has been reported with mixed success.[34]

CSWS is also an acquired epileptic condition that can result in deterioration in several neuropsychological functions. Patry first described this condition in 1971, and Tassinari further defended the clinical characteristics observed in the children. Language ability is predominantly affected with accompanying short-term memory deficits, impaired temporospatial orientation, short attention span, hyperkinesias, and, occasionally, aggressive behavior.[35,36]

CSWS is characterized by a sleep-induced EEG pattern consisting of spike-wave discharges occurring for at least 85% of non–rapid eye movement sleep. The average age of onset is 5 years, and the duration of CSWS is between 6 months and 5 years. Children with CSWS often manifest cognitive and behavioral abnormalities similar to those present in ASD.[37] These include language disorders, sensory aphasia, oral-motor apraxia, and a variety of behavioral disorders. A sleep EEG is therefore critical to differentiate the two disorders.

The clinical presentation of CSWS can also be similar to the Landau-Kleffner syndrome. However, CSWS has a more widespread deterioration, and the characteristic awake inter-racial EEG in CSWS has a predominately frontal focus compared to the temporal focus seen in Landau-Kleffner syndrome.[34,35]

Treatment of Pervasive Developmental Disorders

Determining the most appropriate time to consider discontinuation of AEDs after a seizure-free interval depends on a review of traditional risk factors associated with seizure relapse and those factors more specifically identified for individuals with ASD. These factors were discussed in the beginning of this section and include degree of cognitive impairment, type of language disorder, and gender.

Down Syndrome

Down syndrome is frequently diagnosed at birth with the identification of well-defined physical characteristics. These include hypotonia, midface hypoplasia, single palmar crease, slanted palpebral fissures, poor Moro reflex, and excessive skin on the neck.[38,39] Individuals with Down syndrome have a higher incidence of specific medical conditions of which physicians should be aware, including congenital cardiac disorders, thyroid disease, and hematologic disorders.[40] These are important conditions with which the neurologist should be

familiar, because side effects of several anticonvulsants may manifest in the same way.

Incidence of Down Syndrome

Down syndrome occurs in 1 of every 1,000 live births and is one of the most common known causes of mental retardation. It occurs more frequently with advancing maternal age and most commonly is a result of nondisjunction or translocation involving chromosome 21.

Incidence of Epilepsy in Down Syndrome

Seizures, particularly infantile spasms, may occur during the first year of life with an incidence of 5%.[41] More frequently, encountered seizure types include tonic-clonic, myoclonus, and febrile seizures.[42] EEG abnormalities occur in approximately 25%, and the abnormality in many of these is generalized slowing. The occurrence of epilepsy in Down syndrome individuals is more common than in the nonhandicapped population but occurs at a much lower rate than in other developmental conditions. In a comparison of institutionalized Down syndrome and matched non–Down syndrome mentally retarded individuals, the frequency of epilepsy was 6% in Down syndrome and 18% in the matched group. In addition, 1.2% in the matched cohort had daily seizures, and there were no individuals in the Down syndrome group with daily seizures.

Phenomenology of Down Syndrome

Brain size is often normal throughout gestation and the first 6 months of postnatal life before decelerating during the second half of the first year of postnatal life. Hypotonia and hyporeflexia are characteristic of all infants with Down syndrome and are probably due to dysgenesis of the cerebral cortex and cerebellum, as well as delays in myelination during the first years of life. Cortical gyri are wide, and secondary gyri are often poorly developed; the cerebellum and brain stem are frequently hypoplastic. These findings appear to be due to a generalized hypocellularity of the brain and a reduction in both neuronal number and density.[43] There is a marked reduction in the number of interneurons in cortical layer II, which use the neurotransmitter GABA and provide primary inhibitory influence to the pyramidal neuron layer IV. Ultrastructural studies of pyramidal neurons from the cerebral cortex reveal abnormalities of dendrite arborization and reduced numbers of postsynaptic spines. This lack of inhibitory input to lower cortical layers may help to explain the co-occurrence of epilepsy.

Early signs of Alzheimer's disease in individuals with Down syndrome is neuropathologically evident as early as the second decade of life[43] and by the fourth decade in almost all brains.[36] Prospective studies have shown that 11% of individuals with Down syndrome exhibit AD between the ages of 40 and 49 years and 77% between the ages of 60 and 69 years.[45] The clinical diagnosis of AD in the Down syndrome patient can be challenging to the consulting physician, because there is such a wide variation of the underlying degree of mental retardation.

Treatment of Down Syndrome

Psychomotor slowing is a prominent feature in many with Down syndrome, and vigilant monitoring for sedating side effects from AEDs is necessary. Determining the minimal effective dose is helpful. If psychomotor slowing is increased by an AED, an alternative AED should be selected. Lamotrigine infrequently causes slowing and can even be mildly activating in some individuals. Weight gain is a frequent side effect of valproate; however, in the author's experience, it is more common in individuals with Down syndrome.

Several physical conditions in persons with Down syndrome can mimic and aggravate seizures. Syncope due to cardiac defects can be difficult to differentiate from a seizure in this population, because a description of the event frequently cannot be obtained from the patient. Sleep apnea is common and can exacerbate seizures by causing sleep deprivation. The guttural sounds during this type of sleep and the lack of response to stimulation during sleep are also misinterpreted as either a seizure or a postictal phase.

Attention Deficit Hyperactivity Disorder

The core symptoms of attention deficit hyperactivity disorder (ADHD) are an inability to maintain attention and concentration for a developmentally appropriate length of time and hyperactivity and impulsivity that result in a clinically significant impairment in social or academic functioning in children and occupation functioning in adults. Symptoms begin before 7 years of age and persist for at least 6 months in at least two settings. The criteria for the age of onset of symptoms have been questioned. Although hyperactivity is usually noted before age 7 years, inattentiveness that impairs function may not appear until a later point in time.

Incidence of Attention Deficit Hyperactivity Disorder

ADHD is not considered a significant disability independently; however, it frequently is seen in individuals with DDs or epilepsy, or both. The prevalence of ADHD varies from a low of 2.0% to a high of 6.3%. The use of fourth edition *Diagnostic and Statistical Manual of Mental Disorders* criteria increases the prevalence of noted cases of ADHD.

Incidence of Epilepsy in Attention Deficit Hyperactivity Disorder

A disproportionate number of children with epilepsy have significant deficits in their ability to sustain attention for an age-appropriate length of time. It can be a challenge to determine whether the inattentiveness is an AED effect, brief subtle seizures, or an independent attentional disorder.

In a population-based study in Iceland, ADHD was found to be a risk factor for unprovoked seizures. All cases of children with an unprovoked seizure were examined over a 2-year period. Children with seizures were five to six times more likely to have been previously diagnosed with ADHD.[44] This raises the question of whether the earlier inattention was actually seizure activity or whether drugs used to treat ADHD may provoke seizures. The authors conclude that, because the children were first diagnosed with ADHD before seizures were observed, the seizure onset did not correlate with the onset of ADHD symptoms. Powell et al.[46] described a father and son who were initially diagnosed with ADHD and subsequently found to have orbitofrontal epilepsy.

Studies of brain structure have suggested a frontal subcortical etiology for ADHD. Children with dyslexia or ADHD have smaller right anterior width measurements on MRI.[47] The inferior posterior lobe of midline cerebellar structures was significantly smaller in children with ADHD than in controls.[48,49] In ADHD, a postulated cerebello-thalamo-prefrontal circuit dysfunction may impair inhibitory control of other cortical areas.

There was prefrontal hypoperfusion on high-resolution single photon emission computerized tomography imaging in 87% of children and adolescents with ADHD in a case-control study.[50] Quantitative EEG studies in adolescents showed increased anterior EEG absolute-theta activity and reduced posterior relative-beta activity when compared to controls, and there was infrequent epileptiform activity in both groups.

Phenomenology of Attention Deficit Hyperactivity Disorder

Frequent, brief episodes of either complex partial or absence seizures produce periods of apparent daydreaming, inattentiveness, or forgetfulness that may be interpreted as symptoms of ADHD. These seizures may be misinterpreted for several weeks or even months before a diagnosis of epilepsy is established and appropriate treatment is initiated. Even experienced teachers and some parents have overlooked this phenomenon. This author evaluated a 14-year-old girl with a 9-year history of "frequent forgetfulness" who was referred for a first-time convulsion. The EEG revealed persistent left temporal spike and wave complexes with focal bursts every 15–20 seconds, suggesting temporal lobe complex partial epilepsy. The forgetfulness was likely related to seizures, as it "cleared up" after initiation of carbamazepine. This example also exemplifies that a child with undetected, more subtle seizures may be interpreted as slow learning with poor concentration ability.

Treatment and Prognosis of Attention Deficit Hyperactivity Disorder

Treatment involves identification of seizure type. Absence seizures are best controlled with ethosuximide or valproate and complex partial seizures by carbamazepine in children. Phenobarbital should be avoided, because it has a higher association of behavioral and cognitive side effects. Because lamotrigine appears to have some active or stimulating properties, it would be interesting to compare the attention abilities in children with ADHD and epilepsy taking lamotrigine versus other AEDs.

Neurocutaneous Disorders

Neurofibromatosis type 1 is accompanied by epilepsy in 2–5% of individuals. The seizures are frequently associated with benign tumors and "unidentified bright objects" on MRI. Seizures can be the first neurologic symptoms that manifest in Sturge-Weber syndrome and occur in up to 90% of patients. In 75% of the individuals with Sturge-Weber, the seizures appear within the first year of life. The seizures may be partial or generalized, and the severity of the seizures often correlates with the extent of the cerebral lesions.

Seizures are also frequently the first neurologic symptoms that manifest in tuberous sclerosis and occur in up to 90% of individuals. Seizures starting in the first years of life may be partial or generalized. Infants with tuberous sclerosis complex may present with infantile spasms. The etiology of the seizures is believed to be the cortical tubers. Subcortical subependymal nodes and subependymal giant cell astrocytomas also occur. The onset of seizures is commonly associated with the decline in development.[51] Vigabatrin can be more effective in controlling seizures refractory to other AEDs, but can cause irreversible retinal damage. Vigabatrin is not currently available in the United States.

Fragile X Syndrome

Fragile X is the most common familial cause of mental retardation and is a result of amplification of a trinucleotide repeating sequence. Physical stigmata include narrow face, long prominent ears, and macro-orchidism. Seizures have been reported to occur in approximately 18% of this population. Complex partial seizures were the most common seizure type, frequently with centrotemporal spikes, and are usually well controlled.[52]

Antiepileptic Medication in the Developmentally Disabled

After the diagnosis of seizure type and epilepsy syndrome has been established, the AED that is believed to be most effective with the least chance of side effects is selected. Comorbid conditions and mode of drug delivery are prominent issues in the developmentally disabled. There is a higher incidence of behavioral and psychiatric conditions in the DD population, and AEDs are commonly used as mood stabilizers to treat these conditions. Psychiatric comorbidities occur in 25%, and severe maladaptive behavior occurs in up to 55% of those meeting criteria for mental retardation.[51] Valproate and carbamazepine are the most commonly used AEDs in the treatment of bipolar disorder, mania, and intermittent explosive disorder and in the management of aggressive behavior.[53] Therefore, when choosing a medication to treat seizures, the psychiatric history must also be obtained.

Carbamazepine is a first-line AED for partial-onset and some forms of generalized seizures. Carbamazepine is an excellent choice in the treatment of individuals with DDs, because it has minimal adverse effects on cognition and behavior. Carbamazepine is also indicated in the treatment of bipolar disorder and trigeminal neuralgia. It can be used as a single agent to treat the relatively common comorbidity of mood disorder and epilepsy. Adverse behavioral reactions occur infrequently and may be related to carbamazepine's tricyclic ring structure. This may result in mild mood elevating properties that would be problematic in a patient with hypomania that has not been detected or diagnosed. These patients may become agitated, irritable, or hyperactive. Hyponatremia is a side effect that can be exacerbated by patients who drink excessive free water (sometimes due to dry mouth as a side effect of carbamazepine, antidepressants, or antipsychotics) or receive salt-wasting diuretics.

Carbamazepine also is available in multiple formulations. The chewable tablets are helpful for patients unable to swallow tablets, and the extended-release tablets allow for less-frequent dosing. Carbatrol is a newer form of extended-release carbamazepine that is produced in a capsule that can be opened and sprinkled on food. This has allowed the use of an extended-release form in young children and impaired adults.

Valproate is a broad-spectrum agent with efficacy against primary generalized, partial, and myoclonic seizures and infantile spasms. Valproate is also indicated in the treatment of mania and migraine headaches. Additional uses in the DD population include mania, behavioral cycling,[54] aggressive behaviors, and hyperactivity or agitation in autism. This medication should be used in a limited fashion or not at all in children younger than 2 years of age with severe developmental delay who are on additional AEDs, because this group of patients has a significant risk of hepatotoxicity. Thrombocytopenia is a side effect that is rarely serious; however, if an individual's DD includes ataxia with frequent falls, caution should be used. Valproate is also available as a liquid, intravenous (IV) formulation that may be administered through a gastric tube and sprinkle capsules (divalproex sodium).

Phenytoin has a safe profile and is effective in the treatment of partial and generalized seizures. There do not appear to be any significant mood or behavioral effects. The advantage of phenytoin is that it has a long half-life and may be given once a day in those with poor compliance. It is available in liquid, chewable, and IV formulations. Phenytoin is not a first-choice AED in persons with DD, because the side effect of gingival hyperplasia is especially problematic in this population. Oral hygiene is commonly a significant problem in individuals with DD, and it is complicated. In addition, individuals with DD are often susceptible to balance disturbances, which phenytoin can exacerbate.

Phenobarbital is the oldest and one of the safest AEDs in current use. It is the drug of choice in children younger than 2 years and is effective against a wide range of seizure types. It is not commonly used in older patients, because it has been shown to slow cognition and learning and has adverse effects on mood, including irritability in children and depression in adults. However, it is a very effective AED, and there are patients who respond exceptionally well to it and are unable to be changed to other AEDs.

Felbamate was the first new-generation AED and was widely used and accepted until the post-marketing experience revealed a high incidence of hepatic failure and aplastic anemia. It had a favorable side-effect profile for many patients with DDs. It appeared to have a mild stimulant quality and therefore was beneficial for those displaying psychomotor slowing. Felbamate has a wide spectrum of antiepileptic activity and is especially effective in Lennox-Gastaut syndrome. This medication should be used only when the risk to benefit ratio has been carefully evaluated by all of those involved in the person's care.

Gabapentin can be as effective as an adjunctive therapy in partial seizures. It is widely used for neuropathic pain syndromes and occasionally refractory bipolar disorder but is only indicated for partial seizures. It is not effective in treating primary generalized seizure types. Gabapentin is only available as a capsule.

Lamotrigine also has a wide spectrum of antiepileptic activity and is effective against seizures in patients with Lennox-Gastaut syndrome. Lamotrigine may have a mild mood-elevating or stabilizing quality and is rarely sedating. This combination gives lamotrigine a favorable profile for use in individuals with DDs. However, there have been reports of adverse behavioral effects, including marked elevation of mood and agitation, in this population of patients.

Topiramate is indicated for partial seizures and Lennox-Gastaut syndrome. It has been effective in difficult-to-manage seizure disorders, is typically well tolerated, and is effective in monotherapy. Many studies have shown cognitive side effects and word-finding difficulties. This has not been a significant problem in the DD population. Topiramate is also available in sprinkle formulation.

Tiagabine is approved for adjunctive treatment of partial seizures and has not been associated with any behavioral effects. It is available in tablet forms only.

Vigabatrin is not approved in the United States, and it may not obtain approval. Changes in the white matter in animal studies and concerns about visual field deficits may prevent its approval. It is obtained from other countries and is effective and well tolerated in persons with DDs. Vigabatrin has been most useful in the treatment of infantile spasms.

Oxcarbazepine is a variant of carbamazepine and metabolically bypasses the problematic epoxide intermediate that contributes to the many side effects of carbamazepine, including sedation. Patients are therefore able to tolerate higher doses, and this results in a greater chance of successful monotherapy. This has been beneficial for use in individuals with DDs.[55]

There have been many conflicting reports regarding adverse behavioral effects of AEDs on DD persons, owing to the fact that we are unable to consistently recognize pre-existing psychiatric disorders in handicapped individuals: This results in an AED choice that might not have been used if the condition was recognized and that might aggravate a condition. In addition, DD persons often are unable to communicate side effects and may act out only when the side effects are intolerable.

Monotherapy should be attempted, because it results in fewer side effects and has been shown to be effective in up to 90% of institutionalized persons with epilepsy. Withdrawing AEDs, especially phenobarbital, can result in a marked improvement in alertness and mood. Because there is a high rate of psychiatric comorbidity in those with DDs, psychopathology can emerge during AED withdrawal. This is seen in valproate withdrawal when there is underlying mania or during carbamazepine withdrawal with an underlying bipolar disorder.

Developmental neurology is an evolving field of study. It includes understanding the unique medical needs of those patients with DDs and the constraints involved in their medical care. Further collaborative studies are required to determine the efficacy of alternative therapies, such as vagal nerve stimulation and epilepsy surgery, in individuals with DDs.

References

1. American Association on Mental Retardation. Mental retardation. Definition, classification, and systems of supports. Washington: American Association on Mental Retardation, 1992.
2. Sunder TR. Meeting the challenge of epilepsy in persons with multiple handicaps. J Child Neurol 1997;12:S38–S43.
3. Steffenberg U, Hedstrom A, Lindroth A, et al. Intractable epilepsy in a population-based series of mentally retarded children. Epilepsia 1998;39:767–775.
4. Marcus JC. Control of epilepsy in a population with mental retardation: lack of correlation with IQ, neurologic status, and the electroencephalogram. Am J Ment Retard 1993;98[Suppl]:47–51.
5. Singh BK, Towle PO. Antiepileptic drug status in adult outpatients with mental retardation. Am J Ment Retard 1993;98[Suppl]:41–46.

6. Hosford DA, Chaddick SJ, Lin FH. Generalized epilepsies: emerging insights into cellular and genetic mechanisms. Curr Opin Neurol 1997;10:115–120.

7. Berkovic SF, Scheffer IE. Genetics of human partial epilepsy. Curr Opin Neurol 1997;10:110–114.

8. Sloviter RS. Decreased hippocampal inhibition and a selective loss of interneurons in experimental epilepsy. Science 1987;235:73–76.

9. Cole AJ, Abu Shakra S, Saffen DW, et al. Rapid rise in transcription factor mRNA in rat brain after electroshock-induced seizures. J Neurochem 1990;55:1920–1927.

10. Fiore R, Murphy TH, Sanghera JS, et al. Activation of a p42 mitogen-activated protein kinase by glutamate receptor stimulation in primary cortical cultures. J Neurochem 1993;61:1626–1633.

11. Gall C, Sumikawa K, Lynch G. Levels of mRNA for a putative kainate receptor are affected by seizures. Proc Natl Acad Sci U S A 1990;87:7643–7647.

12. Saffen DW, Cole AJ, Worley PF, et al. Convulsant-induced increase in transcription factor mRNA in rat brain. Proc Natl Acad Sci U S A 1988;85:7795–7799.

13. Sutula TP, Cascino G, Cavazos J, et al. Mossy fiber synaptic reorganization in the epileptic human temporal lobe. Ann Neurol 1989;26:321–330.

14. Babb TL, Kupfer WR, Pretorius JK, et al. Synaptic reorganization by mossy fibers in human epileptic fascia dentate. Neuroscience 1991;42:351–363.

15. Cavazos JE, Golarai G, Sutula TP. Mossy fiber synaptic reorganization induced by kindling: time course of development, progression, and permanence. J Neurosci 1991;11:2795–2083.

16. Farwell JR, Lee YJ, Hirtz DG. Phenobarbital for febrile seizures: effects on intelligence and on seizure recurrence. N Engl J Med 1995;322:364–369.

17. Meador KJ, Loring DW, Allen ME. Comparative cognitive effects of carbamazepine and phenytoin in healthy adults. Neurology 1991;41:1537–1540.

18. Duncan JS, Shorvon SD, Trimble MR. Effects of removal of phenytoin, carbamazepine, and valproate on cognitive function. Epilepsia 1990;31:584–591.

19. Murphy CC, Yeargin-Ausopp M, Decoufee P, Drews CD. Prevalence of cerebral palsy among ten year old children in metropolitan Atlanta, 1985 through 1987. J Pediatr 1993;123:513–519.

20. Hadjipanayis A, Hadjichristodoulou C, Youroukos S. Epilepsy in patients with cerebral palsy. Dev Med Child Neurol 1997;39:659–663.

21. Kwong KL, Wong SN, So KT. Epilepsy in children with cerebral palsy. Pediatr Neurol. 1998;19:31–36.

22. Lipkin PH. Epidemiology of the Developmental Disabilities. In AJ Capute, PJ Accardo (eds), Developmental Disabilities in Infancy and Childhood. Baltimore: Paul H. Brookes, 1991;43–67.

23. Zahner GE, Pauls DL. Epidemiological Surveys of Infantile Autism. In D Cohen, A Donnellan (eds), Handbook of Autism and Pervasive Developmental Disorders. New York: Wiley, 1987;199–221.

24. Tuchman R, Rapin I, Shinnar S. Autistic and dysphasic children: II. Epilepsy. Pediatrics 1991;6:1219–1225.

25. Olsson I, Steffenberg S, Gillberg C. Epilepsy in autism and autistic-like conditions. A population-based study. Arch Neurol 1988;45:666–668.

26. Volkmar FR, Nelson DS. Seizure disorders in autism. J Am Acad Child Adolesc Psychiatry 1990:19:127–129.

27. Rapin I, Mattis S, Rowan J, Golden G. Verbal auditory agnosia in children. Dev Med Child Neurol 1997;19:192–207.

28. Smart SM, Smart CS. Children: Development and Relationships (3rd ed). New York: Macmillan, 1977;253–258.

29. Diagnostic and Statistical Manual of Mental Disorders: DSM-IV (4th ed). Washington: American Psychiatric Association, 1994.

30. Kugelmass IN. The Autistic Child. Springfield, IL: Thomas Publishing, 1970;154–155.

31. Soprano AM, Garcia EF, Caraballo R, Fejerman N. Acquired epileptic aphasia: neuropsychologic follow-up of 12 patients. Pediatr Neurol 1994;11:230–235.

32. Deonna T. Acquired epileptiform aphasia in children (Landau-Kleffner syndrome). J Clin Neurophysiol 1991;8:288–298.

33. Beaumanoir A, Bureau M, Deonna T, et al. Continuous Spikes and Waves during Slow Sleep—Electrical Status Epilepticus during Slow Sleep. Mariani Foundation Pediatric Neurology Series, vol. 3. London: John Libbey, 1995;260.

34. Paetu R, Granstrom M, Blomstedt G, et al. Magnetoencephalography in presurgical evaluation of children with Landau-Kleffner syndrome. Epilepsia 1999;40:326–335.

35. De Negri M. Electrical status epilepticus during sleep (ESES). Different clinical syndromes: Towards a unifying view? Brain Dev 1997;19:447–451.

36. Wisniewski KE, Wisniewski HM, Wen GY. Occurrence of neuropathological changes and dementia of Alzheimer's disease in Down syndrome. Ann Neurol 1985;17:278–282.

37. Tassinari CA, Michelucci R, Forti A. The electrical status epilepticus syndrome. Epilepsy Res 1992;[Suppl 6]:111–115.

38. Hall B. Mongolism in newborn infants. Clin Pediatr 1966;5:4–8.

39. Cooley W, Graham J. Common syndromes and management issues for primary care physicians. Clin Pediatr 1991;30:233–253.

40. Pueschel SM, Orson JM, Boylan JM, Pezzullo JC. Adolescent development in males with Down syndrome. Am J Dis Child 1985;139:236–238.

41. Adams MM, Erickson JD, Layde PM, Oakley GP. Epidemiology of Down syndrome. JAMA 1981;246:758–760.

42. Stafstrom C, Konkol R. Infantile spasms in children with Down syndrome. Dev Med Child Neurol 1994;36:576–585.

43. Malamud N. Neuropathology of Organic Brain: Syndromes Associated with Aging. In CM Gaitz (ed), Aging and the Brain (3rd ed). New York: Plenum, 1972;63–87.

44. Semrud-Clikeman M, Wical B. Components of attention in children with complex partial seizures with and without ADHD. Epilepsia 1999;40:211–215.

45. Visser FE, Aldenkamp AP, van Huffelen AC, et al. Prospective study of the prevalence of Alzheimer-type dementia in institutional individuals with Down syndrome. Am J Ment Retard 1996;101:400–412.

46. Powell AL, Yudd A, Zee P, Mandelbaum DE. Attention deficit hyperactivity disorder associated with orbitofrontal epilepsy in a father and a son. Neuropsychiatry Neuropsychol Behav Neurol 1997;10(2):151–154.

47. Hynd GW, Semrud-Clikeman M, Lorys AR, et al. Brain morphology in developmental dyslexia and attention deficit/hyperactivity. Arch Neurol 1990;47:919–926.

48. Mostofsky SH, Reiss AL, Lockhart P, Denckla MB. Evaluation of cerebellar size in attention deficit hyperactivity disorder. J Child Neurol 1998;13:434–439.

49. Berquin PC, Giedd JN, Jacobsen LK, et al. Cerebellum in attention deficit hyperactivity disorder. Neurology 1988;50:1087–1093.

50. Amen DG, Carmichael BD. High resolution SPECT imaging in ADHD. Ann Clin Psychiatry 1997;9:81–86.

51. Deb S. Mental disorder in adults with mental retardation and epilepsy. Compr Psychiatry 1997;38:179–184.

52. Musumeci SA, Hagerman RJ, Ferri R, et al. Epilepsy and EEG findings in males with Fragile X syndrome. Epilepsia 1999;40:1092–1099.

53. Mattes JA. Valproic acid for nonaffective aggression in the mentally retarded. J Nerv Ment Dis 1992,180:601–602.

54. Kastner T, FineSmith R, Walsh K. Long-term administration of valproic acid in the treatment of affective symptoms in people with mental retardation. J Psychopharm 1993;13:448–451.

55. Gaily E, Granstrom ML, Liukkonen E. Oxcarbazepine in the treatment of epilepsy in children and adolescents with intellectual disability. J Intellect Dis Res 1998;42[Suppl 1]:41–45.

Chapter 24

Epilepsy and Seizures in the Aged

A. James Rowan

Of all conditions that coexist with seizures and epilepsy, advanced age and its consequences probably present the greatest challenge. Not only does age itself profoundly influence the diagnosis and treatment of seizures, but also the many concomitant medical conditions that accompany the aging process play critical roles.

Epilepsy in the elderly is a major public health problem. Although it was well known that seizures are common in the elderly, data derived from the extensive epidemiologic studies in Rochester, Minnesota indicate that the incidence of epilepsy in the elderly increases considerably after the age of 60 years, rising more dramatically by the age of 80 years.[1] The aged have a higher annual incidence of seizures than is found in children. Given the fact that the population worldwide is rapidly aging,[2,3] physicians will encounter older patients with seizures in increasing numbers.

The treatment of seizures in the elderly differs from treatment of younger patients. Progressive changes in metabolic characteristics, alterations in pharmacokinetics and pharmacodynamics, intervening disease processes, and psychosocial factors all conspire to complicate management. Thus, the clinician cannot regard treatment of the elderly as similar to managing younger adults. This chapter aims to place in perspective the unique characteristics of epilepsy in the elderly and provide guidelines for successful management.

Etiologies and Risk Factors

The causes of seizures in the elderly population are not as diverse as those encountered in younger patients.[4] Moreover, their distribution is quite different. Cerebrovascular disease accounts for 35–40% of cases, headed by cerebral infarction but also including intracerebral hemorrhage and subarachnoid hemorrhage. Persons with evidence of arteriosclerosis without an acute cerebrovascular accident are also at higher risk, as are those with lacunar infarcts.[5] Even the presence of hypertension itself appears to confer additional risk of seizures.[6]

Alzheimer's Disease

Alzheimer's disease is associated with seizures in the elderly, although this comes as a surprise to many neurologists.[7,8] The probable reason is that neurologists tend to see these patients relatively early in the course of the disease, and seizures characteristically occur after the disease has been established for several years[9] and after the patient has entered a long-term care facility. Generalized tonic-clonic convulsions and complex partial seizures (CPSs) occur, but the latter are the most difficult to diagnose.[10] The principal characteristics of CPS include altered awareness; orofacial automatisms; automatisms of the limbs, such as rubbing or repetitive tapping;

restlessness; and to-and-fro movements. Wandering in a confused state and undressing are not uncommon. These symptoms are also seen in the dementias and probably are ascribed by staff members to the underlying disease process. The essential point is that a diagnosis of seizures in these circumstances must be suspected, and this is possible only through an intensive educational program. Such features as stereotypy of phenomenology and duration must be recognized. Changes in mental status (e.g., episodic confusion) should arouse suspicion. Confounding the problem is the observation that electroencephalogram (EEG) studies are infrequently carried out in such patients. One study found that only 5% of patients in long-stay institutions who were taking antiepileptic drugs (AEDs) for possible seizures had EEG studies during their hospital stay (AJ Rowan and RE Ramsay, *unpublished observations*, 2000). More liberal use of the EEG in these circumstances would no doubt provide evidence that some patients with fluctuating mental status or motor activity indeed experience CPSs.

Stroke

Cerebrovascular accidents (Chapter 15) are the most common cause of seizures in the elderly, accounting for up to 37% of new cases.[1,11] Arterial occlusion is most commonly seen, whether thrombotic or embolic. Cerebral hemorrhage is also a risk factor, as is subarachnoid hemorrhage.[12] Cerebral arteriosclerosis without history of stroke is also associated with a higher incidence of seizures and is often the only positive finding on imaging studies in elderly patients with new-onset seizures.[5] Many patients in epidemiologic studies who fall into the idiopathic category probably have small vessel disease or lacunes. An additional risk factor for seizures is hypertension.[6] In such cases, hypertension is likely associated with some degree of vascular disease, which in turn is the probable underlying factor in seizure precipitation.

Comorbidity is common in patients with cerebrovascular disease, leading to complications in seizure management. In particular, diabetes, heart disease, and hypertension are commonly present alone or in combination. Coexisting liver and kidney disease are also common. All of these conditions not only affect recovery from stroke but also complicate seizure diagnosis and, more particularly, pharmacologic management. These features will be discussed in subsequent sections.

Other Causes of Epilepsy in the Elderly

After cerebrovascular disease and dementing processes, brain tumors are probably third in incidence, followed by head trauma.[13] Approximately 30% of patients with brain tumors present with seizures as an initial manifestation.[14] In the elderly, brain tumors include a variety of primary tumors, such as gliomas and meningiomas, as well as metastatic lesions. Gliomas are less common than in younger subjects, whereas the incidence of meningiomas increases with age. Tumors should always be considered in patients with new-onset seizures. The diagnosis is usually made easily on historical grounds and the results of imaging studies. Remote head trauma leading to loss of consciousness, especially when associated with intracranial bleeding, may lead to seizures within the first 6 months to 1 year. Seizure onset, however, may occur years later.[15] It may be difficult to determine the role of remote head trauma in seizure causation if intercurrent disease—for example, stroke—supervenes. Furthermore, the coexistence of two potentially epileptogenic conditions increases the likelihood of seizures, although no clear data are available.

Metabolic Conditions

A wide variety of toxic and metabolic disorders lead to seizures, although in such cases the seizures are manifestations of the underlying disease process and not of epilepsy. The most common are hypoglycemia, hyponatremia, hypocalcemia, hypoglycemia, hyperosmolar state, hepatic failure, and renal failure. Seizures may occur in patients with hyperthyroidism, especially thyrotoxicosis, but also in some cases of myxedema.[16] In most of these conditions, the diagnosis is rapidly apparent, or it is revealed via routine laboratory studies. Although not unique to the elderly, two features of metabolic disorders are of particular interest. The resultant seizures are often treated with AEDs during the acute stage, although the efficacy of AEDs in these circumstances is unpredictable. Definitive treatment consists of correction of the underlying metabolic disorder. AED treatment is often continued long after the metabolic disorder has been corrected, sometimes indefinitely. This is not indicated and exposes the elderly person to the dangers of adverse AED effects and unnecessary drug interactions. Another important feature of seizures in metabolic conditions is variability.

The seizures may be stereotyped— for example, generalized tonic-clonic or focal clonic—but often are multifocal. They may be clonic or tonic, shifting from side to side. *Epilepsia partialis continua* can occur in hyperosmolar states.[17] Multifocal myoclonic jerks are common, especially in renal and hepatic failure.[18] Imaging studies reveal no focal lesions. The EEG may show multifocal epileptiform activity or simply may be disorganized and slow.

Drugs and Withdrawal States

Alcoholism is increasingly recognized as a serious problem in the elderly population, one that is often hidden, coming to light only when medical or neurologic consequences occur. Estimates of prevalence range up to 10% of the population of the United States aged 65 and older.[19] The relationship of alcohol intoxication and withdrawal to resultant seizures (alcohol-related seizures) is discussed in Chapter 8. In the elderly, covert alcoholism is epidemic. Specific inquiry is required to make the diagnosis, particularly when the cause of new-onset seizures in the aged is not apparent.

Altered mental status after withdrawal from certain prescription drugs (e.g., benzodiazepines, barbiturates, and psychotropic agents) suggests the diagnosis of nonconvulsive status epilepticus (NCSE).[20–23] NCSE can be divided conveniently into two broad subtypes: *absence status* and *complex partial status*. The former occurs mainly in children and adolescents as a complication of simple absence attacks, sometimes termed *spike-wave status*. Complex partial status, on the other hand, is a manifestation of localization-related epilepsy, often of temporal lobe origin. The condition may take the form of repeated, typical CPSs without intervening

full recovery. As such, recognition is relatively easy. On the other hand, electrographic seizure activity may be continuous or nearly so, leading to altered mental status with or without minor motor manifestations. The change in mental status varies markedly. At one end of the spectrum, the patient may be mildly confused with slow responses, still able to carry out some conversation and complex acts. At the opposite end, the patient may be unresponsive. Some patients may appear demented, with a picture similar to Alzheimer's disease. Still others may exhibit a personality change and appear subdued, with some slowing of responses, but still able to function. Indeed, the spectrum of the clinical presentation may confound diagnosis. If the patient has a clinical seizure preceding the episode or during the episode, then the diagnosis may be made quickly with the performance of an EEG. If no seizure intervenes, then diagnosis may be delayed, sometimes for weeks or months.

The EEG makes the diagnosis of NCSE, but only suspicion triggers ordering the test. Electrographic manifestations are variable, but the common denominator is the presence of bilaterally synchronous ictal activity consisting of spikes, sharp waves, rhythmic slow components, or a combination of these features. The electrographic ictal activity may be continuous, although there often is a waxing-waning pattern. EEG differentiation of NCSE from metabolic derangement, such as hepatic or renal encephalopathy, may be difficult. The wave formed in the two conditions may be quite similar. A valuable clue for the diagnosis of NCSE is brief restoration of relatively normal background activity during a temporary cessation of ictal activity. This contrasts with metabolic encephalopathies in which the EEG background rhythms are markedly disrupted.

Causes of NCSE in the elderly are varied. In many cases, there is a history of recent discontinuation of benzodiazepines or other psychotropic agents. In others, NCSE occurs in a setting of systemic illness, such as sepsis. Often, such patients have a structural lesion of the brain, such as an old infarct or tumor. Treatment with intravenous lorazepam may be highly effective, especially in the withdrawal states, and may be followed by intravenous fosphenytoin. Some patients, particularly the severely ill, show little response to this combination or only temporary cessation of ictal activity. Such patients may require general anesthesia, such as propofol or pentobarbital.[24] Morbidity and mortality may be high, especially in patients with multisystem disease. Thus, prompt diagnosis and treatment are essential.

Case Report

J.B. is a 67-year-old woman with a history of CPSs. Her geriatrician referred her for neurologic evaluation because of a progressive dementia. The patient's cognitive decline dated from a hospitalization for poorly controlled hypertension approximately 3 months earlier. During her hospital stay, she became agitated and reportedly had some form of hallucinations. No overt seizure activity was described. Her AED therapy consisted of carbamazepine and gabapentin. At the time, her carbamazepine level was within the therapeutic range.

Her agitation subsided, but, thereafter, she was noted to be confused. After discharge, her confusion worsened; she was forgetful and mentally slow and became unable to deal with activities of daily living. Haloperidol was tapered gradually over a few weeks without cognitive improvement.

Before her hospitalization, she was a retired registered nurse who had worked on a neurology floor at a large medical center in New York. For the past few years, she had been living in an adult facility but was fully independent. Her CPS disorder was diagnosed in the 1980s, but details of the early epilepsy were largely unknown. Reportedly, she had CPSs treated initially with phenytoin and later with carbamazepine, 1,200 mg per day. Recently, gabapentin, 900 mg per day, was added. There was a history of prolonged postictal psychosis in the recent and remote past. She was said to display hyperreligiosity during one such event. Her son reported a normal neuroimaging study. More detailed information on the characteristics and frequency of her seizures was not available.

One month after discharge, she was withdrawn and often noncommunicative. She was disoriented, and her level of responsiveness fluctuated. She could no longer perform simple tasks and required nearly total care. Her geriatrician noted

confusion and lethargy, psychomotor slowing, and parkinsonian features. Her carbamazepine levels remained therapeutic. An EEG was reported to show marked slowing and disorganization without epileptiform activity. She was diagnosed with progressive dementia, and plans were initiated to place her in a skilled nursing home.

A neurologic consultation was obtained 3 months after her discharge from the hospital. She was obviously confused and disoriented, did not understand why she was in a doctor's office, and wore an overcoat over her disheveled nightclothes. She could not name the U.S. president, and her recall was markedly impaired. There was paucity of speech with prolonged response latency. When she did speak, her sentences were short and fragmentary. She could follow simple commands, but there was marked psychomotor retardation. The formal neurologic examination was normal. No subtle adventitious movements were noted.

The previous EEG was available for review. It showed synchronous runs of sharply contoured rhythmic delta activity in the frontal regions, along with some sharp-slow complexes. The background was disorganized and slow. The findings were consistent with NCSE of the complex partial type. After the examination, the patient was taken to the EEG department, where the record revealed virtually continuous epileptiform activity similar to that seen on the previous EEG. Intravenous lorazepam, 0.5 mg, was administered, and within minutes the EEG began to normalize. Clinical improvement was noted as the epileptiform activity subsided—she seemed brighter and more spontaneous. Thereafter, she was started on a low dose of valproate. Within days, her family and physicians noted a remarkable improvement in her cognitive functioning. She became oriented and conversational and displayed goal-oriented behaviors. Her memory improved dramatically, and she became able to care for her needs. A follow-up EEG 2 weeks later was only mildly abnormal, owing to a mild excess of theta activity. On a subsequent visit, she reported that, during her ictal confusion, she felt as if she was in a daze or trance. She was amnestic for much of the previous 3 months. She remains well, is beautifully dressed, and hopes to return to part-time nursing.

Epilepsy in the Elderly as an Epilepsy Syndrome

The characteristics of epilepsy in the elderly lead one to the conclusion that we are dealing with an epilepsy syndrome. Syndromic diagnosis has become important. It allows characterization of clinical status combined with supportive studies, etiology, mechanism, and prognosis. Armed with a diagnosis of an epilepsy syndrome—for example, juvenile myoclonic epilepsy—the clinician is able to plan rational therapy and provide counsel to patients and care givers. Taken as a whole, the features of epilepsy in the elderly provide the framework for an epilepsy syndrome and differentiate it from epilepsy in younger population groups. The limited number of etiologies, relatively low seizure frequency, predominance of CPSs, relative ease of seizure suppression, occurrence of associated medical conditions, and multiple comedications lead to additive side effects and drug interactions. These features have clear implications for treatment and prognosis and provide the clinician with an important tool for management and counseling (Table 24-1).

Differential Diagnosis

Syncope

Seizures occur commonly in a number of medical and neurologic conditions affecting the elderly, most notably cardiac disease, metabolic disorders, cerebrovascular disease, and infectious processes. One of the most common problems is convulsive syncope. Convulsive syncope is really a complication of syncope wherein a simple syncopal attack is accompanied by convulsive activity; either clonic or tonic in character.[25,26]

The syncope itself may result from cardiac arrhythmias,[27] orthostatic hypotension,[28] or neurogenic causes.[29] When adequate history is available and a typical provocative factor or prodrome occurs, the diagnosis is not difficult. Convulsive syncope often results when, after losing consciousness, the patient does not fall. For example, if in a chair, he or she may fall to the side, the head remaining above the heart. In this circumstance, cerebral hyperperfusion may continue, leading to

Table 24-1. Comparative Features of Epilepsy in the Young and Old

	Young	Old
Seizure types	Multiple (frequently GTC)	3 (frequently CPS)
Seizure frequency	Often high	Low
Postictal state	Relatively brief	Relatively prolonged
Potential for injury	Relatively low	Relatively high
Etiology	Many	Few
Response to AEDs	Variable (poor to excellent)	Usually good (incomplete data)
Tolerance to AEDs	Variable (usually good)	Often poor (incomplete data)
Required doses of AEDs	Higher	Lower
Speed of AED titration	Higher	Lower

AED = antiepileptic drug; CPS = complex partial seizure; GTC = generalized tonic-clonic convulsion.

the convulsive movements. Differentiation from an epileptic seizure may be difficult, especially if the patient has a poor recollection of the circumstances surrounding the event. If a history of a typical prodrome and rapid recovery of consciousness is obtained, then a diagnosis of an epileptic seizure is less likely. The elderly patient may experience some confusion after a syncopal episode, with or without convulsive movements. Thus, the principle that confusion is not associated with syncope may not apply to the elderly.

Evaluation of possible syncope should include a routine EEG, followed by an activation study if there is any question concerning possible epileptiform activity. If a cardiac cause is suspected, then appropriate evaluation, including electrocardiogram and Holter monitoring in suspected arrhythmias, is indicated. Noninvasive carotid studies, as well as transcranial Dopplers, should be performed. In cases of suspected neurogenic (vasovagal) syncope, a tilt-table test may offer valuable information. Many patients with syncope are treated with AEDs, in part because historical details may be lacking and in part because a thorough evaluation was not carried out. Not only are AEDs ineffective in syncope, they also cause adverse side effects and drug interactions, both more prominent in the elderly.

Hepatic Encephalopathy

The diagnosis of hepatic encephalopathy is usually straightforward, the patient having a history of liver disease, systemic disease involving the liver, or deranged liver function tests on routine testing. Occasionally, a patient will present with altered mental status and associated seizures without available historical information. In these cases, the seizures are treated with an AED, often intravenous, in the emergency room. Only after laboratory values are obtained does the diagnosis become clear. The seizures may be generalized, focal, or multifocal, introducing diagnostic confusion. The EEG is likely to show typical triphasic waves along with random spikes. Treatment with AEDs may not be effective until the underlying metabolic defect is addressed. Long-term treatment with AEDs is not recommended.

Transient Ischemic Attacks

Differentiating transient ischemic attacks (TIAs) from seizures is usually straightforward. With respect to motor findings, TIAs are nearly always characterized by the sudden onset of negative symptoms (e.g., weakness of one side of the body). Rarely does a TIA present with tonic posturing or clonic motor activity, such as is seen in focal seizure activity. A TIA involving only sensory pathways usually presents as numbness or loss of sensation, although paresthesiae may be a principal complaint. More often, motor and sensory symptoms coexist. Occipital TIAs and occipital seizures are characterized by visual loss, although in the case of seizures vision appears to be obscured in a visual field by the positive phenomenon of scintillating scotomata or geometric shapes, not dissimilar to migraine. The typical occipital TIA involves visual loss in the appropriate visual field, either unilateral or bilateral, without accompanying scotomata. TIAs characterized by aphasia are the most difficult to discriminate from simple partial seizures characterized by isolated aphasia. In both cases, the only neurologic finding is the language disturbance, and the patient appears fully awake without clouding of consciousness. One differential point may be the more gradual development of aphasia when secondary to epileptiform activity. Investigation of one patient with isolated aphasia as a seizure manifestation was studied during such an episode with video-EEG monitoring and simultaneous neuropsychological testing.[30] This patient experienced the gradual onset of aphasia, beginning with word-finding difficulties, and progressing to neologisms, unintelligible phrases, and eventually becoming mute. The simultaneous EEG recording demonstrated a recruiting rhythm in the left frontal region, the discharge spreading to involve the whole of the left hemisphere. During the event, there was no evidence of impairment of consciousness, although it could not be stated with certainty that there was no accompanying confusion. After cessation of the discharge, language function gradually returned, reversing the course seen during its development. Without the EEG evidence, it is difficult to determine the true nature of these events. Suspecting the possibility of aphasic seizures, together with evidence of a structural lesion of the appropriate hemisphere or interictal epileptiform activity on the EEG, should lead to the correct diagnosis.

Dementias

The problem of diagnosing seizures in a setting of dementia is particularly vexing. This does not apply to generalized tonic-clonic convulsions or even focal motor seizures but rather to CPSs. A brief consideration of the symptoms of CPS will make this clear. Classically, motionless staring; orofacial automatisms, such as licking of the lips and chewing movements; other simple automatisms, such as rubbing or patting movements of the hands; tapping of the feet; or simply restless body movements are common. The patient may be completely unresponsive or partially responsive and apparently confused. A prolonged postictal confusional state is not uncommon. Indeed, CPS may be characterized by confusion with little in the way of motor activity, the postictal state blending into the ictal manifestation. Differentiation between the two is difficult without the aid of EEG recording or video-EEG monitoring. From these considerations, it is apparent that all these symptoms are seen in the dementias. Fluctuation in responsiveness and intermittent confusion are common in patients with dementia. Thus, staff members, unaware that CPSs may mimic the intermittent symptoms of dementia, are unable to suspect the presence of epilepsy in this setting. Rowan and Ramsay (*unpublished observations*, 2000), in a pilot study of nursing home residents, found that only 5% of individuals on AEDs had evidence of having had an EEG study. Given the high incidence of epilepsy in the elderly, there are probably many undiagnosed cases of CPSs. Undiagnosed seizures, even if infrequent, lead to a corresponding decrease in general functioning, given postictal consequences of seizures—that is, increased confusion and increased memory loss. Thus, quality of life cannot be maximized in such patients unless the diagnosis is made and appropriate treatment instituted.

The most important step in addressing this issue is education. This applies not only to staff members in chronic care facilities, but also to physicians who provide residential care. In-service training with lectures, seminars, and videotaped examples of seizures can be easily done with the cooperation of interested local neurologists. Materials can be provided by epilepsy organizations (Epilepsy Foundation: http://www.efa.org) that can also initiate contact with administrative personnel and facilitate planning for educational services. A second important step is increasing awareness of the value of EEG services. Any patient observed to experience episodic confusion, altered awareness, or episodic motor behaviors should have an EEG study. This can be arranged by a local hospital or clinic, or even by use of portable EEG services.

Treatment

The first decision is whether to treat a patient with newly diagnosed unprovoked seizures. As is always the case, the appropriate decision rests on balancing the risks and benefits of treatment versus the risks of seizure recurrence. In the past, this was not an easy call. Before the advent of a new series of AEDs after a 15-year hiatus, the available compounds had significant side effects that potentially disrupted overall function and compromised to some degree quality of life. Moreover, the risk of

drug-drug interactions between AEDs and commonly used compounds in the elderly was relatively high (Tables 24-2 and 24-3). A decision not to treat the first seizure in an elderly person might have been reasonable at that time, despite the potential risk of seizure recurrence.

The new generation of AEDs has changed the equation. In general, the new drugs are better tolerated than the older compounds, thanks to their low protein binding, fewer drug-drug interactions, favorable pharmacokinetic profiles, and fewer central nervous system (CNS) side effects. Tolerability of individual agents certainly varies from patient to patient, but these generalizations seem appropriate based on currently available evidence.

Thus, a decision to treat with one of the newer AEDs entails less risk to the patient. The risk of additional seizures in the elderly often outweighs the risks of treatment, leading many clinicians to recommend treatment after the first seizure in the elderly.

The next decision is choice of drug. Given the availability of seven to eight new compounds, this decision is not simple. Each patient brings a unique set of medical and other circumstances with him or her, thus requiring a tailor-made solution. In addition, the requirements of acute and chronic treatment differ. Take, for example, a patient who arrives in the emergency room having had two generalized convulsions. In most cases, that individual will be treated with intravenous phenytoin or fosphenytoin. After the acute phase has resolved, the likelihood is that chronic treatment with oral phenytoin will be recommended. Given the general reluctance to change therapy once instituted, especially if the patient has no further seizures, phenytoin may be continued for a prolonged period, despite side effects and drug interactions. In such patients, serious consideration should be given to crossing over to one of the newer drugs after the patient is stabilized. This can be done slowly and safely, thus mitigating the disadvantage of slow titration schedules for such drugs as lamotrigine, topiramate, and tiagabine. Also, if the patient presents with the new onset of a CPS, then there is little necessity for intravenous treatment. In such cases, titration with an oral agent is appropriate. The following discussion outlines the rationale for using specific drugs in specific situations.

Table 24-2. Interactions of Phenytoin with
Other Substances

Effect	Mechanism
Phenytoin concentrations decreased	
Ethanol (chronic)	Increased metabolism of phenytoin
Folic acid	Same as above
Nicotine	Same as above
Propoxyphene	Same as above
Phenobarbital	Same as above
Phenothiazines	Same as above
Rifampin	Same as above
Antacids	Decreased absorption
Diazoxide	Displacement from protein bind sites
Nonsteroidal antiinflammatory drugs	Same as above
Tolbutamide	Same as above
Salicylates	Same as above
Valproic acid	Same as above
Phenytoin concentrations increased	
Amiodarone	Decreased metabolism of phenytoin
Chloramphenicol	Same as above
Chlordiazepoxide	Same as above
Cimetidine	Same as above
Dicumarol	Same as above
Disulfiram	Same as above
Halothane	Same as above
Isoniazid	Same as above
Miconazole	Same as above
Phenylbutazone	Same as above
Propranolol	Same as above
Sulfonamides	Same as above
Trazodone	Same as above
Viloxazine	Same as above
Concentrations reduced by phenytoin	
Carbamazepine	Induction of metabolism of named compound
Dicumarol	Same as above
Doxycycline	Same as above
Folic acid	Same as above
Haloperidol	Same as above
Hormonal contraceptives	Same as above
Theophylline	Same as above
Vitamin D	Same as above

Source: Reproduced with permission from IE Leppik, D Wolf.
Drug Interactions in the Elderly with Epilepsy. In AJ Rowan,
RE Ramsay (eds), Seizures and Epilepsy in the Elderly. Boston:
Butterworth–Heinemann, 1997;291–302.

Several newer AEDs appear to be effective and safe agents for the elderly. However, relatively few data are available for use of the newer agents in the elderly population. Nonetheless, limited data on the elderly, as well as known characteristics of the compounds, allow some reasonable conclusions concerning their use in the older patient. The following is a brief summary of the characteristics of individual drugs that deserve consideration in specific cases. Felbamate, the first of the new wave of AEDs, is not discussed here because of its bone marrow and hepatic toxicity.

Gabapentin

Gabapentin is effective for the treatment of partial-onset seizures with or without secondary generalization and is now widely used not only for seizures, but also for other conditions, such as depression and pain. Gabapentin has a number of properties that augur well for its use in the elderly. It does not undergo hepatic metabolism, and more than 90% of the absorbed drug is excreted unchanged via the kidney.[31] There are few drug interactions; thus, the compound may be given safely in combination with a wide variety of AEDs and non-AEDs. Absorption occurs via a saturable L-amino acid transport system. This property results in a decreasing percentage of absorbed drugs with increasing dose. Tolerability is excellent in chronic use, and, if indicated, relatively high doses may be used without difficulty.

Side effects such as dizziness or sleepiness are not uncommon during the first weeks of titration. These are usually mild and rarely necessitate withdrawal of treatment. At this time, three-times-daily dosing is recommended because of its relatively short half-life of 6–9 hours. This may constitute a disadvantage in the elderly, in whom compliance is an important issue. Overall, however, the drug appears to be an excellent choice for the elderly patient who has infrequent seizures and takes several drugs for associated medical conditions.

Lamotrigine

Lamotrigine is widely used in the United States and abroad and has advantages over the older AEDs; some of these advantages are similar to those of gabapentin. The drug is effective in partial-onset sei-

Table 24-3. Interactions of Carbamazepine with Other Medications

Effect	Medication	Mechanism
Carbamazepine concentrations increased	Propoxyphene*	Decreased metabolism of carbamazepine
	Erythromycin*	Same as above
	Triacetylolean domycin*	Same as above
	Phenytoin	Same as above
	Verapamil*	Same as above
	Josamycin	Same as above
	Diltiazem*	Same as above
	Isoniazid	Same as above
	Cimetidine	Same as above
	Nicotinamide	Same as above
	Viloxazine	Same as above
	Imipramine	Same as above
	Fluoxetine*	Same as above
Carbamazepine concentrations decreased	Phenytoin	Increased metabolism
	Phenobarbital	Same as above
	Primidone	Same as above
	Valproate	Same as above
Concentrations of these may be decreased when used with carbamazepine	Phenytoin	Increased metabolism
	Phenobarbital	Same as above
	Valproate*	Same as above
	Coumadin	Same as above
	Doxycycline	Same as above
	Folic acid	Same as above
	Hormonal contraceptives	Same as above

*Often very clinically significant interactions.
Source: Reproduced with permission from IE Leppik, D Wolf. Drug Interactions in the Elderly with Epilepsy. In AJ Rowan, RE Ramsay (eds), Seizures and Epilepsy in the Elderly. Boston: Butterworth–Heinemann, 1997;291–302.

zures but, unlike gabapentin, has a broad spectrum of action with efficacy in primarily generalized seizures. It too has a favorable side effect profile owing to its long-term tolerability. The compound has low protein binding and few interactions with non-AEDs. It does, however, interact with other AEDs, such as phenytoin, carbamazepine, and valproate. Whereas its elimination half-life is 24 hours, when given in combination with valproate (an enzyme inhibitor) the biological half-life of lamotrigine is doubled. In contrast, as in combination with enzyme inducers such as phenytoin or carbamazepine, its half-life is decreased by approximately 50%. Lamotrigine is primarily eliminated by hepatic metabolism, with only 10% excreted in the urine.[32] A potential disadvantage is lamotrigine's rash potential. Initially reported in 10% of patients receiving the drug, recent data suggest that slow titration to target dose, say over 6 weeks, reduces rash incidence by approximately two-thirds, similar to that of carbamazepine.[33] The incidence of rash in the elderly is unknown but is likely similar to that in younger adults. Lamotrigine produces mild neurotoxicity early in treatment, but this is usually transient and does not necessitate discontinuation of therapy in most cases. Therapy must be initiated slowly, with gradual dose escalation over a 4- to 6-week period, depending on whether the patient is taking concomitant AEDs. If the patient is taking valproate and the intention is to crossover to lamotrigine monotherapy, then titration must be very slow, beginning at 25 mg every other day. This strategy will minimize the potential for lamotrigine toxicity and also reduce the incidence of rash. If the patient is taking an enzyme inducer such as phenytoin, then titration may start at 25–50 mg per day and proceed at a somewhat more rapid rate. Complete crossover will not be complete for several months, but, in most cases, this does not pose a problem. The twice-daily dosing schedule of lamotrigine is an advantage, and this plus its favorable side effect profile suggests that this drug will be useful in the elderly.

Topiramate

Topiramate is gaining a track record as an effective and safe AED. The drug has been approved as add-on therapy for CPSs but appears to have a broader spectrum of action.[34,35] Topiramate has low protein binding, demonstrates linear pharmacokinetics, and is not extensively metabolized. Its half-life permits twice-daily dosing.[36] There are few drug interactions, except for those with other AEDs. Phenytoin and carbamazepine decrease topiramate serum concentration by 40–50%, whereas topiramate decreases phenytoin concentrations by 25%. There is a small reduction in valproate concentration when given with topiramate. As with other AEDs, CNS side effects may occur during the early course of treatment; these usually subside after a few weeks. There is no major organ toxicity, although weight loss may occur. At high doses, changes in mental status have been observed. Although this property could limit the usefulness of topiramate in the elderly, it is likely that the drug will be effective at relatively low doses, thus reducing this potential problem.

Tiagabine

Tiagabine is a γ-aminobutyric acid reuptake inhibitor and therefore increases γ-aminobutyric acid accumulation in the extracellular space.[37] It is approved as add-on therapy for partial-onset seizures, but, unlike lamotrigine and topiramate, the drug has a relatively narrow spectrum of action. Although tiagabine is highly protein bound, its concentration is measured in μg/ml; thus, this feature has no practical effect. In fact, tiagabine has few important drug interactions, except for those with enzyme-inducing AEDs. When given with phenytoin or carbamazepine, the dose of tiagabine must be increased to a level approximately twice that used in monotherapy. Mild CNS toxicity may occur during the first weeks of titration, but the drug is otherwise well tolerated without major organ toxicity.[38] At very high doses, mental changes have been reported. Tiagabine is extensively metabolized in the liver. Because of its short half-life, four-times-daily dosing was initially recommended, but subsequent studies showed that twice-daily dosing is effective. There have been no systematic studies of tiagabine in the elderly, but its demonstrated tolerability suggests that it may be a good agent for the elderly.

Other New Antiepileptic Drugs

Three additional AEDs approved by the U.S. Food and Drug Administration have further increased our therapeutic options. The compounds are levetiracetam, oxcarbazepine, and zonisamide. All are effective as add-on therapy for partial-onset seizures, but only oxcarbazepine has been approved for monotherapy. In common with the above-described compounds, these drugs have favorable side effect profiles, thus suggesting they may be useful in treating the elderly. Little experience with these AEDs in older patients is available; thus, their role as effective treatment in this age group remains to be established.

Veterans Administration Cooperative Study Number 428—Treatment of Seizures in the Elderly Population

Veterans Administration (VA) Cooperative Study No. 428 is a 5-year, nationwide, multicenter study of three AEDs in the treatment of new-onset, unprovoked seizures in the elderly.[39] This research compares carbamazepine, a worldwide standard drug for the treatment of partial-onset seizures, with gabapentin and lamotrigine. The study is a three-arm, double-blind, randomized, parallel trial of the three compounds when given as monotherapy. The trial's end point is retention in the study for 12 months, a standard measure used in previous VA

Coopcrative Studies.[40] Percentage retention, in fact, is a measure of the drugs' efficacy and tolerability. Target doses for the three compounds are lower than usually used in younger subjects. Adjustments in dose are permitted depending on the patient's clinical status. Failurc to control seizures despite doses leading to side effects constitutes an end point with the patient exiting the trial. A data-monitoring board consisting of outside experts in epilepsy, geriatrics, and statistics closely scrutinizes data from the study. The trial is now in its fourth year, and all three arms continue. It is anticipated that the results of this study will contribute substantially to our concepts of seizures in the elderly and will establish specific and general guidelines for effective treatment.

Practical Guidelines for Antiepileptic Drug Treatment

Treatment of epilepsy in elderly patients with associated medical or neurologic conditions is simply the treatment of epilepsy in the elderly. This truism recognizes the fact that the majority of elderly individuals develop seizures in the context of medical or neurologic disease—in fact, associated medical conditions constitute a principal component of the syndrome itself. Thus, the choice of appropriate agents recognizes that the elderly take multiple drugs for associated conditions, many having interactions with standard AEDs. It also takes into account the increased pharmacodynamic effects of AEDs on the aging or compromised brain. Thus, the over-riding principle of AED selection for the elderly is determining which compound has the fewest drug-drug interactions and side effects. Another principle is reduction of the total daily dose as compared to that used in younger adults. Few data are available to aid in the determination of the proper AED dose for the elderly. In view of the generally lower seizure frequency in the elderly, as well as reduced tolerance for side effects, a reasonable course of action may be to target the total daily dose at approximately one-half that used in younger patients. Dose adjustment from this point can be made depending on the balance of efficacy and tolerability. Doses used in the VA Cooperative Study referred to earlier fall into this range. Yet another important principle is slow dose escalation. Many younger patients develop transitory CNS side effects, such as drowsiness or dizzi-

ness. The elderly are at greater risk for these early symptoms. A general guide would be to start any AED at approximately one-half the dose one would use in younger patients. For example, one might start carbamazepine at 100 mg per day, phenytoin at 50 mg per day, gabapentin at 300 mg per day, and lamotrigine at 25 mg per day. Incremental escalation on a weekly basis is likely to be well tolerated. This schedule should be altered as the patient's clinical status warrants.

Prognosis

Limited data at this time suggest that the outlook for elderly patients with epilepsy is quite favorable. Judging from the relatively low seizure frequency in this age group and the presumed efficacy of AEDs at relatively low dosages, the prospects for seizure freedom appear to be good. Many of the newer AEDs offer the prospect of improved tolerability as compared to the older standard agents. This combination of probable AED efficacy and improved tolerability with the newer agents suggests that elderly patients may be treated indefinitely without the attendant risk of toxic side effects. The decision to treat indefinitely is based on a balance of risks: the potential harm of recurrent seizures after discontinuation of AEDs versus the risks associated with treatment. Data on discontinuation of AEDs in seizure-free elderly patients are not available. In younger adults, the risk of seizure recurrence is on the order of 50% or more. Because seizures in an elderly person are more likely to cause injury and impaired quality of life, prolonged treatment with a relatively safe, well-tolerated AED is reasonable.

References

1. Hauser WA, Annegers JF, Kurland LT. The incidence of epilepsy in Rochester, Minnesota, 1935–1984. Epilepsia 1993;34:453.
2. Suzman R, Kinsella KG, Myers GC. Demography of Older Populations in Developed Countries. In JG Evans, TG Williams (eds), Oxford Textbook of Geriatric Medicine. Oxford, UK: Oxford University Press, 1992;3–13.
3. Manton KG, Stallard E. Cross sectional estimates of active life expectancy for the U.S. elderly and oldest old populations. J Gerontology: Social Sciences, 1991;46:S170–S182.

4. Hauser WA. Seizure disorders: the changes with age. Epilepsia 1992;[Suppl 4]:S6–S14.

5. Roberts RC, Shorvon S, Cox TCS, Gilliatt RW. Clinically unsuspected cerebral infarction revealed by computed tomography scanning in late onset epilepsy. Epilepsia 1988;29:190.

6. Ng SKC, Hauser WA, Brust JCM, Susser M. Hypertension and the risk of new-onset unprovoked seizures. Neurology 1993;43:425–428.

7. Hauser WA, Morris JC, Hewton LL, Anderson VE. Seizures and myoclonus in patients with Alzheimer's disease. Neurology 1986;36:1226–1230.

8. Hersdorffer DC, Hauser WA, Annegers JF, et al. Dementia and adult-onset unprovoked seizures. Neurology 1996;46:727–730.

9. Romanelli MF, Morris JC, Ashkin K, Coben LA. Advanced Alzheimer's disease is a risk factor for late onset seizures. Arch Neurol 1990;47:847–850.

10. Mc Areavey MJ, Ballinger BR, Fenton GW. Epileptic seizures in elderly patients with dementia. Epilepsia 1992;33:657–660.

11. Lancman ME, Golimstok A, Norscini J, Granillo R. Risk factors for developing seizures after a stroke. Epilepsia 1993;34:141–143.

12. Viitanen M, Ericksson S, Asplund K. Risk of recurrent stroke, myocardial infarction and epilepsy during long-term follow-up after stroke. Eur Neurol 1988;28:227–231.

13. Cooper KD, Tabaddor K, Hauser WA, et al. The epidemiology of head injury in the Bronx. Neuroepidemiology 1983;2:70.

14. Hauser WA. Epidemiology of Seizures and Epilepsy in the Elderly. In AJ Rowan, RE Ramsay (eds), Seizures and Epilepsy in the Elderly. Boston: Butterworth–Heinemann, 1997;7–20.

15. Annegers JF, Grabow JD, Groover RV, et al. Seizures after head trauma: a population study. Neurology 1980;30:683–689.

16. Jabbari B, Huott AD. Seizures in thyrotoxicosis. Epilepsia 1980;21:91–96.

17. Singh BM, Strobos R. Epilepsia partialis continua associated with nonketotic hyperglycemia: clinical and biochemical profile of 21 patients. Ann Neurol 1980;6:155–160.

18. Lockwood AH. Neurologic complications of renal disease. Neurol Clin 1989;7:617–627.

19. Beresford TP, Gordis E. Alcoholism and the Elderiy Patient. In JG Evans, TF Williams (eds). Oxford Textbook of Geriatric Medicine. Oxford, UK: Oxford University Press, 1992;639–645.

20. Guberman A, Cantu-Reyna G, Stuiss D, Broughton R. Nonconvulsive generalized status epilepticus: clinical features, neuropsychological testing and long-term follow-up. Neurology 1986;36:1284–1291.

21. Cascino GD. Nonconvulsive status epilepticus in adults and children. Epilepsia 1993;32[Suppl 1]:S21–S28.

22. Lee SI. Nonconvulsive status epilepticus: ictal confusion of later life. Arch Neurol 1985;42:778–781.

23. Drislane FW. Nonconvulsive status epilepticus in patients with cancer. Clin Neurol Neurosurg 1994;96:314–318.

24. Begemann M, Rowan AJ, Tuhrim S. Treatment of refractory complex-partial status epilepticus with propofol: case report. Epilepsia 2000;41:105–109.

25. Ziegler DK, Lin J, Bayer WL. Convulsive syncope: relationship to cerebral ischemia. Trans Am Neurol Assoc 1978;103:150.

26. Aminoff MJ, Scheinman MM, Griffin JC, Herre JM. Electrocerebral accompaniments of syncope associated with malignant ventricular arrhythmias. Ann Intern Med 1988;108:791–796.

27. Kapoor WN. Evaluation and management of patients with syncope. J Am Med Assoc 1992;268:2553–2560.

28. Bradshaw MJ, Edwards RTM. Postural hypotension—pathophysiology and management. QJM 1986;231:643.

29. Sra JS, Jazayeeri MR, Dhala A, et al. Neurocardiogenic syncope: diagnosis, mechanisms and treatment. Cardiol Clin 1993;11:183–191.

30. Rosenbaum DH, Siegel M, Barr WB, Rowan AJ. Epileptic aphasia. Neurology 1986;36:281–284.

31. McLean MJ. Gabapentin. Epilepsia 1995;36[Suppl 2]:S73–S86.

32. Goa KL, Ross SR, Chrisp P. Lamotrigine. A review of its pharmacological properties and clinical efficacy in epilepsy. Drugs 1993;46:152–176.

33. Richens A. Human Safety. In EH Reynolds (ed), Lamotrigine—a New Advance in the Treatment of Epilepsy. London: Royal Society of Medicine, 1993;204;35–40.

34. Biton V, Reife R, Kamin M, Bobrosky K. Topiramate as add-on therapy for patients with primary generalized epilepsy. Neurology 1996;46:A176.

35. French JA, Bourgeois BFD, Dreifuss FE, et al. An open-label multicenter study of topiramate in patients with the Lennox-Gastaut syndrome. Neurology 1995;45[Suppl 4]:A250.

36. Ben-Menachem E, Henriksen O, Dam M, et al. Double-blind, placebo-controlled trial of topiramate as add-on therapy in patients with refractory partial seizures. Epilepsia 1996;36:539–543.

37. Gustavson LE, Mengel HB. Pharmacokinetics of tiagabine, a gamma-aminobutyric acid-uptake inhibitor, in healthy subjects after single and multiple doses. Epilepsia 1995;36:605–611.

38. Uthman B, Rowan AJ, Ahmann PA, et al. Multicenter randomized dose-response trial of tiagabine adjunctive therapy in patients with complex partial seizures. Arch Neurol 1998;55:56–62.

39. Rowan AJ, Ramsay RE, Pryor F, et al. Treatment of seizures in the elderly population. Epilepsia 1997;38[Suppl 8]:89.

40. Mattson RH, Cramer JA, Collins JF, et al. Valproate for the treatment of partial and secondarily generalized tonic-clonic seizures in adults: a comparison with carbamazepine. N Engl J Med 1992;327:765–771.

Section F

Drug Issues

Chapter 25

Adverse and Beneficial Side Effects of Antiepileptic Drugs

Edward Faught and Nita A. Limdi

We think of drugs as having specific therapeutic purposes, but they are generally distributed to all body tissues, where they may have unintended results. These side effects are not all adverse effects; some of them are beneficial. In the case of antiepileptic drugs (AEDs), the most common non-therapeutic effects are on the central nervous system, whereas the most dangerous and rare adverse effects are on other organs, especially the skin, liver, and blood.

Nontherapeutic effects may occur because the drug binds indiscriminately to structures other than the targeted locus or because the binding site is common to substances or structures that perform different functions. AEDs modulate the function of ionic channels in cell membranes either directly or by influencing the actions of neurotransmitter substances. Ionic channels are universal in nervous tissue, and the major neurotransmitters are widely distributed, often serving different or even contradictory actions.

Ideally, we could direct a drug to a specific anatomic site and neurochemical mechanism tailored to the pathophysiology of a particular patient's seizures. Because we cannot at present accomplish this, we must rely on two factors to minimize unwanted effects: (1) use drugs that affect the fewest possible number of nonepileptic brain functions and systemic functions, and (2) select drug dosages that produce desirable but not undesirable effects. This is possible, because most drugs, especially central nervous system agents, have multiple concentration-dependent actions.[1] Optimally, there is an order-of-magnitude difference between a higher, "toxic" dose and a lower, "therapeutic" dose. This ratio, the therapeutic index, often is quite small for AEDs. In individual patients, it may be fractional for individual drugs: There is no therapeutic dose without toxicity.

Side effects of AEDs are common. In the Roper poll of patients with epilepsy, 61% reported medication side effects.[2] In a European study, fully 88% of patients reported at least one side effect.[3] These rates strike most physicians as high, possibly because many patients do not tell their doctors everything; 55% of patients in another study said they failed to report side effects to their physicians.[4]

Symptomatic Approach to Side Effects

The best instrument for detecting drug side effects is the ear. Neither the neurologic examination nor any battery of laboratory tests is as sensitive as a good interview with patient and family. Probing for side effects should begin with open-ended questioning—for example, "How are you feeling?" "Are you having any medication side effects?" and "Do you feel any better or worse taking this medicine?" This last question encourages patients to report beneficial as well as adverse side effects. In

Table 25-1. Common Dose Initiation Side Effects
of Antiepileptic Drugs

Drug	Side Effect
Initial sedation common	
Carbamazepine	Sedation, dysphoria, dizziness
Gabapentin	Sedation, fatigue, dizziness
Levetiracetam	Sedation, fatigue
Oxcarbazepine	Sedation, dizziness
Phenobarbital	Sedation, lethargy, depression
Phenytoin	Sedation, dizziness
Tiagabine	Sedation, dysphoria, dizziness
Topiramate	Sedation, fatigue, paresthesias
Valproic acid	Sedation, dyspepsia
Zonisamide	Sedation, dizziness
Initial stimulation common	
Felbamate	Insomnia, dyspepsia
Lamotrigine	Insomnia, irritability

clinical trials of new drugs, only open-ended questions are allowed. However, once a drug is in clinical practice, and we know the most common side effects, it makes sense to ask directed questions as well. The questions vary for each drug.

It is unusual to detect a significant unreported central nervous system side effect on neurologic examination. However, for most AEDs, it is reasonable to examine the skin and look for nystagmus, tremor, or ataxia. It is worthwhile to routinely ask about mood and emotional well-being. Much more extensive examinations on routine follow-up visits for epilepsy patients are usually not necessary, despite Medicare billing pressures to perform them.

The need for routine laboratory monitoring of AED therapy is controversial. There is no evidence that this is cost effective or that it increases patient safety.[5] Nevertheless, some testing seems prudent; we discuss this further in the section entitled Idiosyncratic Effects of Antiepileptic Drugs.

Categories of Adverse Effects

It is helpful to sort adverse effects by time of occurrence and severity. Various schemes of classification are used, but we use the following categories for AEDs: dose initiation effects, dose-limiting effects, idiosyncratic effects, long-term effects, and miscellaneous effects.

Dose Initiation Effects

Because tolerance develops to most central nervous system side effects, the highest incidence occurs soon after a drug is started. This is especially true of sedation and other global perceptions (Table 25-1). It is often true of gastrointestinal problems. Beginning with low doses and moving to gradual upward titration schedules can minimize these effects. Tell patients to expect these problems, and counsel patience if they are not intolerable.

Dose-Limiting Effects

AED doses should be increased gradually until complete seizure control or dose-limiting side effects occur.[6] These effects are more specific to each drug than are the dose initiation effects[7] (Table 25-2), although some of them may be the same as the dose initiation effects, and, similarly, patients should be told to inform the physician of them. We ask, "Do you know what too much of this drug feels like?" If the patient does not, we describe the usual limiting effects. It is important to note that some drugs tend to have easily recognized, "crisp" toxicity at a precise limiting dose for a particular patient, whereas others tend to produce graded or insidious effects without a clear dose limit (see Table 25-2). In either case, the dose should be reduced slightly and, if seizure control is not complete, a plan made for substitution or addition of a different drug.

Serum drug level measurement plays a secondary role in avoidance of adverse effects. For most drugs and for most patients, doses can be based on clinical response without the use of levels.[8] However, for individual patients, especially when their particular range of satisfactory effect is known, levels can be useful. When nonspecific toxicity occurs in a patient on more than one drug, levels may identify the culprit. In an outpatient study, measurement of serum levels led to changes in dosage in 23% of patients.[9]

Dose-limiting adverse effects are almost never dangerous, nor are "toxic" drug levels in the absence of symptoms. Patients and their primary care physicians should be educated about this as well. The incidence of dose initiation effects and, to some

Table 25-2. Common Dose-Limiting Side Effects of Antiepileptic Drugs

Drug	Effect	Timing of Appearance
Carbamazepine	Diplopia, blurred vision, dizziness	Precise
Felbamate	Ataxia, headache, nausea	Precise
Gabapentin	Dizziness (note: dose-limiting adverse effects are uncommon with gabapentin)	Gradual
Lamotrigine	Diplopia, blurred vision, dizziness	Precise
Levetiracetam	Dizziness, lethargy	Moderately precise
Oxcarbazepine	Dizziness, fatigue, nausea	Precise
Phenobarbital	Somnolence, depression, cognitive slowing	Gradual
Phenytoin	Ataxia	Moderately precise
Tiagabine	Somnolence, fatigue	Gradual
Topiramate	Dysnomia, cognitive slowing	Gradual
Valproic acid	Essential tremor, lethargy, confusion	Gradual
Zonisamide	Dizziness, cognitive slowing	Moderately precise

extent, dose-limiting effects is reflected in dropout rates in clinical trials (Table 25-3). These rates are usually lower than those seen in clinical practice after a drug is approved for general use.

Idiosyncratic Effects

Idiosyncratic effects are rare, often serious, and, for the most part, unpredictable. They are likely related to the genetic susceptibility of individual patients but are not related to dose. Because of the importance of this category of side effects, they are discussed extensively in the section Idiosyncratic Effects of Antiepileptic Drugs.

Long-Term Effects

Long-term effects vary by drug (Table 25-4). They may be cumulative and correlate with duration and dose. Agents introduced since 1993 have not been in use long enough to confirm that there are no long-term effects, but experience so far has been encouraging. *Long-term* is a purposely vague term: These effects may appear within weeks (e.g., weight gain) or years (e.g., osteoporosis).

Miscellaneous Effects

A variety of nontherapeutic effects do not fit easily into the other categories. They are neither clearly dose limiting, cumulative, or related to genetic susceptibility, nor do they always appear early in ther-

apy. Most are uncommon and peculiar to each drug (see Side Effects Classified by Organ System). Several drugs have been associated with psychosis or movement disorders: Phenytoin rarely causes pseudolymphoma or lymphoma, carbamazepine can cause cardiac dysrhythmia, and topiramate and zonisamide can cause renal stones.

Adverse Event Reporting

The adverse event percentages listed in package inserts and the Physicians' Desk Reference[10] are derived from premarketing clinical trials. There are limitations to these data. They do not differentiate between dose initiation and dose-limiting effects. Most are derived from short-term trials of 2–4 months with titration to fixed dosages. Patient reports are solicited strictly by open-ended questioning. These procedures probably result in overestimates of effects readily perceivable by patients (e.g., dizziness) and underestimates of subtle effects (e.g., depression and mild fatigue). Rare idiosyncratic effects cannot be expected to surface in these small trials. Furthermore, the typical clinical trial is not designed to detect beneficial effects, other than improved seizure control.

Overall Drug Tolerability

Tolerance to individual drugs varies tremendously between individual patients. Nevertheless, some evidence supports an inverse relationship between

Table 25-3. Adverse Events Exceeding Placebo or Control Rate by Greater Than or Equal to Ten Percent in Clinical Trials and Dropout Rates for Newer Antiepileptic Drugs When Used as Adjunctive Therapy

Drug	Event	Dropout Rate in Clinical Trials (12%)*
Felbamate	Headache, nausea, somnolence insomnia, anorexia, vomiting	12
Gabapentin	Somnolence, dizziness	7
Lamotrigine	Dizziness, diplopia, ataxia, blurred vision, headache	10
Levetiracetam	None; 10% > placebo	15
Oxcarbazepine (1,200 mg)	Diplopia, vomiting, dizziness, somnolence, nausea, nystagmus, ataxia, vertigo, abnormal vision	23
Tiagabine	Dizziness, tremor (difficulty with concentration attention at 56 mg only)	21
Topiramate (200–400 mg)	Somnolence, psychomotor slowing, dizziness, ataxia, dysarthria, paresthesia	11
Zonisamide	None; 10% > placebo	10

Note: Arranged in order of frequency. Data derived from package inserts and *Physicians' Desk Reference*[10] for each drug, except zonisamide.[135] For a slightly different view of similar data, see JA Cramer, R Fisher, E Ben-Menachem, et al. New antiepileptic drugs: comparison of key clinical trials. Epilepsia 1999;40:594.
*Averaged dropout rate for active treatment group in all clinical trials; may include some monotherapy trials. The placebo dropout rates were not always available and thus have not been subtracted.

AED efficacy and overall tolerability for populations.[11] For the new drugs, topiramate appears to be more potent but less well tolerated than lamotrigine and gabapentin, which seem to be less potent.[12] We hope that future drug development will dissociate this relationship.

Beneficial Effects of Antiepileptic Drugs

Beginning decades ago, with the use of phenytoin and carbamazepine for neuropathic pain, AEDs have been used widely for problems other than epilepsy. The newer agents are being used at accelerating rates for treatment of pain, headache, and psychiatric disorders. Although controlled trials for these indications are only now appearing, useful benefits accrue from several drugs.

For patients with epilepsy, it is sometimes hard to know whether benefits are a direct result of a new AED or result from being switched from a previous AED that caused more trouble. Felbamate and lamotrigine, in particular, are nonsedating drugs in comparison to other agents, and they may also have direct stimulatory or psychological effects.

AED selection should be based primarily on efficacy for the seizure type, but it is important to consider comorbidities as secondary selection factors. Topiramate may be a better choice than valproate for the overweight patient, and valproate better than felbamate for the patient with migraine. It is always satisfying to kill two birds with one stone.

The best-recognized beneficial effects of these drugs are on mood, neuropathic pain, headache, and weight loss.

Table 25-4. Possible Long-Term Effects of Antiepileptic Drugs

Phenobarbital	Dupuytren's contractures, osteoporosis
Phenytoin	Gingival hyperplasia, acne, hirsutism, osteoporosis, peripheral neuropathy, permanent ataxia
Valproate	Weight gain, alopecia, polycystic ovaries

Mood Effects

Patients with Epilepsy

Among patients with epilepsy taking older AEDs, such as phenytoin, phenobarbital, and carbamazepine, who are switched to gabapentin or levetiracetam, there is often a brightening of affect and increased feeling of well-being. Those who are switched to fclbamate or lamotrigine[13] often report more marked effects on mood, with increased energy and mood elevation. Sometimes this extends to undesirable stimulation with irritability or insomnia.[14]

Some physicians[15] advocate using the distinction between relatively sedating and relatively stimulating AEDs (see Table 25-1) to guide drug selection for individual patients. Either effect may be desirable for a particular patient. However, these effects are not universal, and many mood effects, especially sedative effects, are related to dose initiation and subside with time. Therefore, the classification of AEDs into sedative and nonsedative categories is somewhat misleading.

Bipolar Affective Disorder

Valproate and carbamazepine are standard treatments for bipolar affective disorder. They are most efficacious for preventing mania but may protect against depressive episodes as well.[16,17] Lamotrigine, topiramate, and gabapentin have also been used.[18]

Behavioral Disorders

AEDs do not have direct, noticeable tranquilizing effects but appear to have mood-stabilizing effects[19] and ameliorate irritability and aggressiveness in a variety of conditions. They are often prescribed for pathologic anger states, such as episodic dyscontrol,[20,21] and for aggressive behaviors in cognitively impaired individuals. Valproate may be useful in patients with Alzheimer's disease who display inappropriate hostility and outbursts of anger.[22-24]

Other Psychiatric Disorders

Clonazepam is a common treatment for panic disorder. Valproate and carbamazepine have been used for a variety of problems, including panic disorder and post-traumatic stress disorder.[25]

Neuropathic Pain

Neuropathic pain is the burning, stinging, or lancinating pain associated with pathology directly involving peripheral sensory nerves or roots. It responds poorly to standard analgesics, but several AEDs reduce the pain.[26]

Carbamazepine was first uscd for trigeminal ncuralgia, and it remains the drug of choice for this condition.[26] It is often effective for other forms of neuropathic pain, including diabetic neuropathy and postherpetic neuralgia. Oxcarbazepine may prove to be useful for the same spectrum.

Gabapentin is rapidly overtaking carbamazepine and amitriptyline as the most popular drug for all types of neuropathic pain[27-29] and seems especially helpful in diabetic neuropathic pain.[30] It has fewer side effects at the usual dosages and is at least as effective in most patients.

The mechanism of action for the pain-blocking effect of AEDs is probably sodium channel blockade or direct glutamate receptor inhibition. However, this theory does not clearly explain the action of gabapentin, and there are anecdotal reports of pain relief from AEDs with a wide variety of known mechanisms of antiepileptic action.

Headache

Valproate is the only drug approved by the U.S. Food and Drug Administration for the prophylaxis of migraine,[10] and, in 1999, it edged past propranolol and amitriptyline in popularity for this application.[31] No definite effect on muscle tension headache has been demonstrated. Gabapentin is also being prescribed for all types of headache, but controlled trials are pending.[27]

Weight Loss

Topiramate,[32] felbamate,[33] and zonisamide[34] routinely cause weight loss. The absolute magnitude of weight loss is greater in those patients who are overweight at baseline and those who switched over from valproate. In the case of topiramate, body weight tends to decline in a linear fashion for approximately a year, then levels off. For obese patients with epilepsy, this weight loss is often highly desirable. Obesity exacerbates the already poor physical self-image and social reticence of many patients with epilepsy, and eliminating it is not a trivial accomplishment for the patient and physician. Currently available AEDs are too toxic to use merely as anorectics in most patients without seizures, although topiramate is being evaluated in clinical trials for morbid obesity. In the much less common situation of patients who are underweight, valproate or gabapentin may promote caloric intake.

Idiosyncratic Effects of Antiepileptic Drugs

Idiosyncratic drug reactions (IDRs) refer to immune-mediated events that occur in susceptible individuals. Multiple predisposing factors are involved in the development of these rare and unpredictable reactions that are often associated with considerable morbidity, mortality, and cost.[35,36]

We group IDRs as dermatologic, hematologic, hepatotoxic, and teratogenic. Management of patients receiving AEDs is often a matter of balancing efficacy against toxicity.

Mechanisms of Toxicity

The mechanisms by which AEDs cause idiosyncratic toxicity may be immunologic or nonimmunologic. Nonimmunologic reactions appear owing to abnormal pharmacokinetic or pharmacodynamic factors, secondary to drug overdose, cumulative toxicity, environmental exposure, drug interactions, or metabolic changes.[37]

Immunologic reactions involve activation of the immune system via complement or antibodies. These reactions are divided into four types (types I, II, III, IV).[38] Dysregulation of the immune system results from the increased formation of reactive or toxic metabolites or deficient detoxification (e.g., epoxide hydrolase deficiency or low free-radical scavenging enzyme activity) in genetically susceptible individuals.[39,40] A schematic representation of the potential pathways involved in the pathogenesis of hypersensitivity reactions is depicted in Figure 25-1. Aromatic AEDs are metabolized by the cytochrome P-450 system to highly electrophilic arene oxides. Inefficient detoxification pathways allow these metabolites to react with cellular components. This can impair cellular function directly or indirectly by forming a hapten.[35,38]

Genetic polymorphisms that result in inadequate or inefficient detoxification pathways predispose the patient to develop idiosyncratic reactions.[39,40] Concomitant therapy with enzyme-inducing drugs leads to the formation of excessive reactive metabolites and overwhelming detoxification pathways, thereby predisposing to toxicity. Concomitant therapy with drugs that inhibit enzymes in the detoxification pathways (e.g., epoxide hydrolases) also predisposes the development of toxicity.

Dermatologic Reactions

The most common dermatologic reactions associated with AEDs are benign; however, serious rashes, such as Stevens-Johnson syndrome (SJS) and toxic epidermal necrolysis (TEN), may occur.[37]

Benign Rashes

Skin rashes are commonly encountered during initiation of phenytoin, carbamazepine, phenobarbital, and lamotrigine therapy. They usually manifest as morbilliform rashes in the first 2–8 weeks. The incidence of rash is 7–12% for carbamazepine and phenytoin and 8–10% with lamotrigine and is infrequent with valproate, topiramate, tiagabine, vigabatrin, and gabapentin.[41,42] The incidence of rash with oxcarbazepine is 6%.[43]

Dose dependency may play a role in the development of rashes. High initial doses and rapid dose escalation increase the risk of precipitating these rashes. Higher concentrations of phenytoin, carbamazepine, and lamotrigine at the onset of treatment were more prone to produce rashes compared to slow-dose escalation and low doses.[42,44]

Mild skin reactions are usually transient and resolve in 1–2 weeks after discontinuation of the drug. Unlike the morbilliform rashes associated with carbamazepine and lamotrigine, rashes due to phenytoin usually recur on rechallenge and are usually more severe. Twenty-seven percent of patients with carbamazepine-associated rashes also develop rashes to oxcarbazepine.[43]

Serious Rashes

Antiepileptic Hypersensitivity Syndrome. Antiepileptic hypersensitivity syndrome (AHS) is a

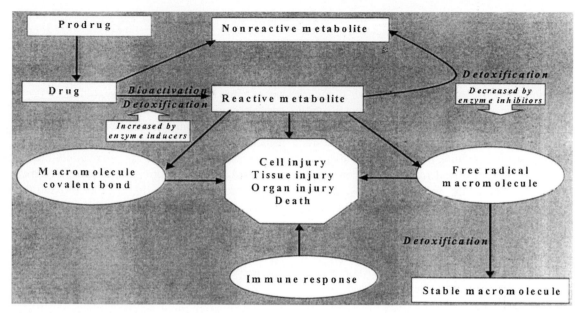

Figure 25-1. Potential mechanisms for development of idiosyncratic reactions. (Modified from TA Glauser. Idiosyncratic reactions: new methods of identifying high risk patients. Epilepsia 2000;41[Suppl 8]:S16–S29.)

rare syndrome that presents as a triad of fever, lymphadenopathy, and rash and occurs in 1 of 3,000 exposures with a 10% fatality rate. The syndrome occurs 2–6 weeks after initiation of therapy and may also present with carditis, nephritis, eosinophilia, and hepatitis with minimal mucosal involvement. Aromatic AEDs and lamotrigine cause AHS.[45,46]

Stevens-Johnson Syndrome. SJS is an immune reaction associated with drug exposure, but it often occurs without a precipitating cause. SJS produces mucosal lesions (including the respiratory and gastrointestinal tracts) and blisters but, unlike TEN, involves less than 10% of body surface. It is preceded by fever, sore throat, chills, malaise, and rash. Initially, the rash presents as small blisters or macules, which become bullous and then rupture and become infected.[47,48]

Toxic Epidermal Necrolysis. TEN is a severe rash and is fatal in 30% of cases. It is characterized by extensive skin exfoliation (more than 30% of body surface) and usually is triggered by drug exposure. The lesions appear 1–3 weeks after initiation of therapy and are similar to those seen with SJS. However, unlike SJS, TEN causes the shedding of the outer layer of the epidermis.[47,48]

Risk

The risk of serious skin reactions varies among AEDs. Phenytoin, phenobarbital, carbamazepine, and lamotrigine are associated with relative risks of 50–130 compared to controls not receiving AEDs.[49] Lamotrigine has been associated with a particularly high rate of serious skin reactions when used concomitantly with valproate,[50] but this risk can be minimized by initiating lamotrigine therapy at very low doses and escalating doses slowly.[44,51]

Cross-reactivity among aromatic AEDs with in vitro assessment of risk of AHS is reported to be around 70%,[52] but significantly lower rates are seen in clinical practice. A known allergy to a drug substantially increases the risk of skin rashes associated with lamotrigine (Mary Castigila, Glaxo, *personal communication*, May 2000).

Diagnosis and Treatment

The most critical step in optimal management is the identification of the offending agent, which is usually confounded by exposure to other potential offenders. Therefore, initial identification is based on clinical experience, laboratory findings, and experiential data from the literature, after evaluating the type of reactions, duration of AED therapy, and the dose of AED. Laboratory findings may include eosinophilia, lymphocytosis, and abnormal liver function tests (LFTs).

Although recurrence on rechallenge is considered definitive, resolution of the reactions after discontinuation of the offender is generally considered adequate to confirm the diagnosis. Usually, discontinuation of offending drug and symptomatic treatment are adequate.[37]

Antiepileptic Drug Withdrawal. Although mild reactions often resolve with dose reduction, severe reactions usually necessitate withdrawal of the offender. The risk associated with abrupt withdrawal is the precipitation of status epilepticus. Although the use of another AED is recommended, one must be aware that the second AED may again cause an IDR.[37]

Symptomatic Therapy. Patients with SJS and TEN need aggressive fluid management and nutritional support. Management of such patients in burn centers has been shown to decrease morbidity and mortality.

Arrestive Therapy. Therapy aimed at aborting IDR is largely based on anecdotal reports and small case series. Data supporting the use of corticosteroids in severe, life-threatening reactions are controversial, as corticosteroids may increase the risk of infection and sepsis. Limited data on the use of plasmapheresis, hyperbaric oxygen, and acetylcysteine make evaluation of relevance difficult.

Hematologic Reactions

Aplastic Anemia

Aplastic anemia with the use of felbamate and carbamazepine is well documented. This is a rare but serious illness with a 20–30% mortality rate. The incidence of aplastic anemia due to carbamazepine is two to five per 1 million per year, five to eight times greater than in the general popula-tion.[53] The incidence of aplastic anemia with felbamate is estimated at 1 per 4,000–5,000 patients, which is more than 100-fold greater than that seen in the general population (two of 1 million). The onset of anemia usually occurs between 5 and 30 weeks after initiation of therapy, although it can occur later in the course of therapy.[54] Toxicity may be due to a toxic atropaldehyde metabolite. Atropaldehyde undergoes glutathione conjugation and is excreted in the urine as mercapturic acids. Abnormal amounts of atropaldehyde-derived mercapturic acids indicate a higher flux through this pathway. The process of using acid carbamate or mercapturic acid ratios to predict potential toxicity is currently under investigation.[55]

Agranulocytosis

The incidence of agranulocytosis associated with carbamazepine is approximately six per 1 million per year, approximately five to eight times that seen in the general population.[53] Transient or persistent leukopenia is seen in up to 10% patients on carbamazepine. The leukopenia is usually mild and does not appear to herald the onset of severe bone marrow aplasia. Patients usually remain asymptomatic, unless the absolute neutrophil count falls below 1,500 per μl. Therefore, patients should be instructed to seek medical attention if they experience symptoms such as unexplained fever, bruising, and oral ulcers. Although routine monitoring cannot predict acute idiosyncratic aplastic anemia, it identifies patients with significant chronic leukopenia.[56]

Thrombocytopenia

The use of valproate has been associated with thrombocytopenia, inhibition of platelet aggregation, and low fibrinogen levels. Thrombocytopenia appears to be dose related. Twenty-four percent of patients receiving high doses as monotherapy had at least one low platelet count. The risk of increased as serum drug levels rose above 100 μg/ml. The incidence is approximately 1% in patients on low doses.[57] The risk of bleeding during surgical procedures has not been increased by the use of valproate. However, patients with acute head trauma treated with valproate showed an increased trend toward a higher incidence of death compared to those treated with phenytoin.[58,59]

Hepatotoxic Reactions

Effects on Liver Function Tests

The older AEDs and some newer AEDs (felbamate, oxcarbazepine, and fosphenytoin) are known to frequently induce a mild, asymptomatic elevation of liver enzymes.[60] Drugs that do not undergo hepatic metabolism have not been associated with changes in liver function. Topiramate and lamotrigine have not been associated with increases in LFTs or hepatic dysfunction, with the exception of hepatic dysfunction seen in AHS due to lamotrigine.

Monitoring the hepatotoxic effects of AEDs requires distinguishing the asymptomatic elevations in LFTs from a serious hepatotoxicity. This is confounded because several liver enzymes are elevated after a tonic-clonic seizure or may indicate hepatic dysfunction unrelated to AED therapy.[61]

LFTs reflect liver dysfunction over the prior days or weeks, not how well the liver is performing when blood is drawn. Monitoring detects hepatic damage after it has occurred. The routine monitoring of LFTs for serious adverse effects is of little predictive value in preventing potentially fatal toxicity. Serum F protein may be a better marker of liver dysfunction.[62] Careful clinical monitoring and patient education of symptoms of liver dysfunction are key to identifying serious toxicity.

Given the lack of randomized, prospective data, the clinical use of LFTs is controversial. However, experience indicates that AED-induced hepatotoxicity may, at least in part, be prevented by avoiding potential offenders in patients with pre-existing hepatic dysfunction. Therefore, LFTs (γ-glutamyltransferase, aspartate aminotransferase, alanine aminotransferase, and bilirubin) should be performed on every patient before initiating AED therapy, with the goals of screening patients before initiating AED therapy and early detection of serious toxicity. If liver dysfunction exists at baseline, potentially hepatotoxic AEDs can be avoided. Given the fact that most cases of acute AED-induced hepatic failure occur within the first 6 months, one may consider monitoring LFTs early in the course of treatment if the patient is at risk for hepatic toxicity.[61]

Hepatotoxicity

Hepatotoxicity associated with AED use can range from mild hepatitis to fulminant liver failure. An excellent review on hepatotoxicity associated with AEDs is available.[63]

Hepatotoxicity associated with aromatic AEDs is rare, occurs in fewer than 1 in 3,000 exposures, and is usually seen in patients who manifest AHS in which inflammatory processes result in liver damage. The picture resembles viral hepatitis, with elevated LFTs and decreased synthetic function, hepatomegaly, and jaundice. Laboratory values show elevated transaminases to a greater extent than alkaline phosphatase. Mortality ranges from 10% to 40% in the absence of transplantation. Because 80% of hepatotoxicity associated with carbamazepine was seen in patients over the age of 50 years,[64] LFT screening has been advocated in older patients during the early stages of therapy.

Valproate-associated hepatotoxicity is characterized by nausea, vomiting, decreased alertness, decreased synthetic function of the liver, elevated transaminases, and lipid accumulation in the liver. Valproate causes microvesicular steatosis, which is thought to be due to the production of 4-en-valproate, which, on activation, produces reactive metabolites. These metabolites bind to macromolecules, deplete glutathione, and inhibit fatty acid metabolism. The formation of 4-en-valproate is favored when the metabolism of valproate is shifted from β-oxidation to ω-oxidation, as is seen with cytochrome P-450–inducing drugs and fasting states in which fatty acids saturate the β-oxidation pathways. Valproate also produces changes in fatty acid metabolism and decreases the activity of free-radical scavenging enzymes. Hepatotoxicity most often occurs early in the treatment. Febrile illnesses and decreased food intake commonly precede the onset of hepatotoxicity.[64]

The risk is greatest in children younger than 2 years of age, patients on polytherapy with enzyme-inducing AEDs, and patients with congenital metabolic disorders, severe seizure disorders, mental retardation, or organic brain disease. Therefore, valproate is contraindicated in patients with hepatic dysfunction.[64]

Hepatotoxicity due to felbamate has been reported in 18 cases. Patients generally present with nausea, malaise, vomiting, and lethargy. Owing to the limited number of patients, the incidence of hepatotoxicity, although unknown, is estimated to approximate that associated with valproate.[54] The proposed mechanism involves the formation of reactive or toxic metabolites in genetically predisposed patients.

The newer AEDs have not been associated with hepatotoxicity. However, relatively few patients have been treated with these drugs; therefore, the occurrence and incidence of such adverse effects may not be known.[63]

Diagnosis and Treatment

Routine monitoring of LFTs is of limited value, because valproate has been associated with asymptomatic elevations in ammonia and LFTs, and the severity of initial presentation does not indicate prognosis. Treatment consists of withdrawal of valproate and supportive measures that include the management of seizure exacerbation, increased intracranial pressure, clotting abnormalities, and levocarnitine. Resolution of toxicity occurs over several weeks, but hepatic enzymes may remain elevated for several months.[63]

Hyperammonemia. Valproate causes elevation of ammonia levels in 50% of patients without associated symptoms of toxicity or abnormalities in LFTs. Valproate must be withdrawn in patients with hyperammonemia who develop lethargy, confusion, or increased seizure activity.[65,66]

Pancreatitis. Pancreatitis rarely complicates valproate therapy and occurs in 1–5% of patients.[67] Patients under the age of 20 years seem to be at a greater risk. Most cases have occurred within the first year of treatment, 76% occurred during polytherapy, and 41% occurred in association with chronic encephalopathy. Withdrawal of valproate results in rapid reversal of pancreatitis; even so, the mortality rate has been estimated to be approximately 21%.[67,68] Patients with liver failure have a

worse prognosis. Because asymptomatic elevations of amylase are often seen with valproate therapy, routine monitoring is not useful in identifying serious adverse events. Valproate should be avoided in patients with a history of pancreatic disease.

Teratogenic Effects. Children of mothers with epilepsy have a higher incidence of malformations (5.7%) compared to the general population (4.8%). The use of AEDs during pregnancy significantly increases this incidence (6–8%). The risks of teratogenicity are multifactorial and include maternal background, genetic predisposition, seizures during pregnancy, and AEDs. Malformations are mainly attributable to AED use rather than to epilepsy itself.[69]

Animal studies, although influenced by AED dose and species differences in susceptibility, indicate that most AEDs have a teratogenic potential. AED use, seizure type, maternal age at delivery, and etiology of epilepsy are identified as risk factors. AED-associated risk factors are considered to be the primary risk factors for teratogenesis. The risk of malformations due to AEDs is influenced by the individual teratogenic potential of the AED used, high drug dose, high serum concentrations, and AED polypharmacy. The mechanism by which AEDs induce teratogenesis is multifactorial, including the formation of epoxides and other reactive metabolites, inadequate detoxification, genetic predisposition, folate deficiency and impaired folate metabolism, and nutritional status.[69,70] The newer AEDs (e.g., lamotrigine, topiramate, gabapentin, tiagabine) have shown no specific trends in fetal malformations.[71] An excellent review on major malformations and drug-specific malformation syndromes is available.[72]

When treating women of childbearing potential, attempts should be directed toward the avoidance of risks before conception by switching to monotherapy, avoiding potentially teratogenic AEDs, using the lowest effective doses, and providing adequate folate supplementation.[73,74]

Side Effects Classified by Organ System

Most reviews of the side effects of AEDs provide a long list of potential effects for each drug. These are difficult to remember and even more difficult to prioritize. Patients report symptoms, so we review the most common AED side effects by symptom or organ system. Effects on skin, liver, and blood were discussed previously. This description should not be construed as comprehensive. The reader is also referred to other general reviews[12,75–77] and to reviews of specific drugs: carbamazepine,[78] felbamate,[79] gabapentin,[80,81] lamotrigine,[82,83] oxcarbazepine,[84] phenytoin,[85] tiagabine,[86] topiramate,[87] valproic acid,[88,89] and zonisamide.[34]

Central Nervous System

Cognition

In our view, this is the single most important category of AED adverse effects. It is also controversial and is the subject of extensive literature.[90–92] All AEDs can cause some degree of slowed thinking or specific cognitive impairment in some patients. However, in most patients, these effects do not occur or are not easily measurable.[93]

Of the older drugs, barbiturates are most likely to cause cognitive effects.[94,95] Of the newer drugs, topiramate was worse than gabapentin or lamotrigine in a short-term comparison among healthy adults.[96] Longer studies are needed to determine to what degree tolerance to these topiramate effects develops. Zonisamide serum levels of more than 30 μg/ml often caused cognitive effects,[97] but lower levels achieved by slower titration resulted in cognitive effects at the same frequency as or less than placebo.[79]

Cognitive adverse effects often abate with time but should be suspected even after years of therapy. It is a common event for patients to report that they feel better and think more clearly when taken off even supposedly benign drugs, such as carbamazepine and phenytoin, for inpatient seizure monitoring. In the Veterans' Administration Cooperative Studies, 11–22% of patients on carbamazepine reported problems with cognitive function.[12,98,99]

Cognitive effects of AEDs are usually global, but topiramate may produce a rather characteristic dysnomia, and phenytoin may produce specific slowing of motor coordination tasks without obvious accompanying sedation or other complaints.

Encephalopathy

Frank encephalopathy with confusion, stupor, or coma can occur with massive overdoses of most AEDs. It is important to realize that more subtle confusional states can also occur. Encephalopathy has been best described for valproate.[100,101] Valproate encephalopathy is not always associated with hyperammonemia[102] and sometimes, but not always, is associated with carnitine deficiency.[103,104]

Mood

Depression is common in epilepsy and may be caused or worsened by drugs, particularly barbiturates. A small incidence of clinically significant depression has been reported for all of the new AEDs, although lamotrigine and felbamate more commonly produce mood elevation.[13] Some AEDs are therapeutic in mood disorders (see Beneficial Effects of Antiepileptic Drugs).

Other Psychiatric and Behavioral Disorders

Psychosis, usually with paranoid features, can occur with vigabatrin, topiramate, and tiagabine.[105] It is prudent to avoid these drugs in patients with a history of psychosis. This may be an occasional consequence of γ-aminobutyric acid enhancement, but there are a few case reports with sodium channel–blocking drugs as well. The psychosis responds quickly to dose reduction and is reversible.

Mentally impaired patients may become hyperactive, irritable, aggressive, or "mean" with AEDs. This is a well-known effect of phenobarbital in children,[106] including healthy children, but can occur with other drugs and in adults. This reaction may be due to a stimulatory effect (e.g., lamotrigine) or a personality effect (e.g., topiramate). The physician needs to ask family members or caretakers to detect this effect; most patients, even those of average intelligence, do not recognize it in themselves.

Sleep

Many AEDs are sedative, at least early in therapy (see Table 25-1). There is a 33–42% incidence of sedation with AED monotherapy with older drugs.[98,99] Daytime sedation may improve if the largest dose is given at night. Some AEDs may produce insomnia. Sleeplessness may improve if the evening dose is reduced or timed to avoid a maximum concentration at bedtime; it should be given either several hours earlier or right at bedtime. Avoid chronic hypnotic use if possible. Little is known about the effects of AEDs on sleep architecture.

Headache

Headache is a common adverse effect of many medications.[107] Felbamate is the AED most likely to produce headache, especially in combination with carbamazepine.[108] Carbamazepine, lamotrigine, tiagabine, and levetiracetam also cause daily headaches in fewer than 10% of patients. In our experience, tolerance to AED-induced headache does not develop; the dose must be reduced.

Eye Movement Disorders

Nystagmus occurs with toxic levels of virtually all AEDs but is rarely apparent to patients; their visual world does not perceptibly jerk.

Diplopia, and often blurred vision—probably owing to a lesser degree of diplopia—is a routine dose-limiting effect of carbamazepine, oxcarbazepine, and lamotrigine. High levels of other drugs may also produce visual symptoms. AEDs may preferentially affect extraocular muscle function, but dysconjugate gaze cannot be observed on physical examination.

Ataxia

The usual dose-limiting effect of phenytoin is ataxia; if the patient can tandem walk, he or she is probably tolerating phenytoin satisfactorily. There is, however, a remarkable variability in the susceptibility of individual patients to this effect. Some patients with serum levels of 10 μg/ml stagger; some with 35 μg/ml do not. High doses of any AED can cause ataxia, but for other drugs, other adverse effects typically appear earlier.

Tremor

Valproate produces an essential tremor roughly proportional to dose in 20–25% of patients.[109] If disabling to handwriting or eating, the dose can be reduced, or, if absolutely necessary, propranolol can be added. Dystonia, chorea, tics, choreoathetosis, and other movement disorders are rare side effects of AEDs.[109]

Gastrointestinal Symptoms

Valproic acid often causes stomachache, nausea, or diarrhea.[110] This is usually transient but may require drug discontinuation. The divalproex sodium preparation greatly reduces these effects, and postprandial dosing also helps. Similar gastrointestinal effects occur with felbamate and ethosuximide. Postprandial dosing and antacids may be effective.

Topiramate and carbamazepine occasionally cause dyspepsia. Phenytoin, gabapentin, lamotrigine, zonisamide, and levetiracetam are usually free of gastrointestinal effects.

Nutrition

Weight Gain and Loss

Weight gain is the most common reason for patients to discontinue valproate.[111] In our experience, approximately one-half of patients gain more than 10 lb. It seems to be appetite-related, not metabolic. Prophylactic adherence to a calorie-reduced diet, especially in overweight women and men, is a good idea. Gabapentin also causes weight gain,[80,81] but it is of a lesser degree and in a lower proportion of patients.

Weight loss is a feature of topiramate, felbamate, and zonisamide therapy and is discussed in the section Beneficial Effects of Antiepileptic Drugs.

Folic Acid

Phenytoin, carbamazepine, and barbiturates induce the metabolism of folic acid.[112] This rarely results in macrocytic anemia but may increase the likelihood of birth defects from neural tube closure failures. Elevation in homocysteine levels, a risk factor for atherosclerosis, may ensue in some patients[113] and has been observed in a minority of patients taking carbamazepine, phenytoin, and lamotrigine monotherapy but not valproate monotherapy.[114]

Because folate deficiency has been associated with an increased incidence of birth defects, all women of childbearing age who take these drugs should receive daily folate supplements of at least 400 µg, the amount found in a typical multivitamin tablet, and some authorities recommend an even higher dose.[115]

Vitamin D

Metabolism of vitamin D is induced by phenytoin, carbamazepine, and barbiturates.[116] This may lead to bone demineralization and osteomalacia. Valproate may also cause osteopenia. Postmenopausal women taking these drugs should receive appropriate vitamin D and calcium nutriture.[117]

Vitamin K

Hepatic enzyme–inducing AEDs, such as phenytoin and barbiturates, have been associated with a 7% incidence of neonatal hemorrhage in infants born to mothers on these drugs, because of depletion of vitamin K–dependent clotting factors. Pregnant women should receive 10 mg of vitamin K daily during the last month of pregnancy, and newborns should receive 2 mg intramuscularly on delivery.[115,117]

Integument

Aside from rashes, phenytoin-induced gum swelling is the most common AED integumentary problem. Gum swelling and fragility can be minimized by assiduous oral hygiene,[118] but this is often not enough. Phenytoin also produces exacerbations of acne and increased facial hair growth. Avoid using it in young girls, if possible. Hair thinning is a dose-related effect of valproate, possibly because of trace metal chelation. It is rarely noticeable, except by the patient, and usually stabilizes after several months. Zinc and selenium supplementation is of unproven benefit.

Easy bruising from valproate is common because of its platelet antiaggregant properties, but this should prompt a platelet count to be sure that significant thrombocytopenia is not present. Ankle edema sometimes occurs with valproate and gabapentin, and livedo reticularis with valproate. These are not serious effects, but they may be disturbing to patients.

Peripheral Nerves

Some recipients of long-term phenytoin therapy have incurred attenuated deep tendon reflexes, but clinically significant sensory peripheral neuropathy is rare.[10,75] Peripheral nerve effects of newer agents have not been detected but might take many years to develop.

Paresthesias occur in approximately 20% of patients started on topiramate[119] and can occur with acetazolamide or zonisamide; this is, apparently, a feature of carbonic anhydrase inhibitors. *Tingling* is the word patients commonly select to describe this phenomenon; sometimes they also describe it as itching or burning. It is benign and transient, but some patients cannot tolerate it. Fosphenytoin causes a peculiar perineal itching or tingling, but because this is an intravenous, nonmaintenance drug, it is sufficient simply to inform the patient.

Cardiovascular

Hypotension can result from intravenous loading of AEDs, but the incidence did not vary between phenytoin, phenobarbital, lorazepam, or diazepam plus phenytoin in the Veterans Administration Cooperative Study of status epilepticus.[120] Except with massive overdose, oral AEDs do not affect blood pressure.

Carbamazepine, on rare occasion, produces cardiac conduction abnormalities,[121] but it is uncertain whether it is a factor in sudden death in epilepsy in some cases.[122] It is best to avoid it in patients with pre-existing myocardial conduction problems.

Endocrine

The effects of AEDs on hormones, especially sex steroids, are complex,[123] and only a few can be mentioned here. Induction of metabolism of estrogen by phenytoin, carbamazepine, barbiturates, and topiramate leads to lessened effectiveness of birth control pills.[124] Higher-dose estrogen (at least 50 µg per dose), progesterones, or other birth control methods are advisable. Amenorrhea and menstrual irregularity may be caused by drugs or by seizures.

Alterations of testosterone metabolism may contribute to common reports of impotence with AEDs.[98] Female sexual responses may also be attenuated.[115] Physicians probably grossly under-recognize these effects. It is not clear yet whether the newer agents are more benign in this regard.

Polycystic ovaries are present in up to 5–10% of healthy women of childbearing age and are probably more frequent with epilepsy, so reports of an increased incidence in women taking valproate are problematic to interpret.[125] This effect may be mediated by weight gain. Most women with polycystic ovaries are asymptomatic, although some develop amenorrhea from acyclic estrogen production, masculinization from excess testosterone production, and other effects.

Renal

AEDs are not nephrotoxic, but nephrolithiasis is a feature of carbonic anhydrase-inhibiting drugs. The incidence of kidney stones with topiramate is 1–5%[32] and was 2.8% over all clinical trials of zonisamide.[126] Stones can form during acetazolamide therapy as well.[127] Nephrolithiasis is common in middle-aged men, and the incidence may be reducible by adequate hydration and avoidance of these drugs in patients with personal or family histories of stones.

Carcinogenesis

Lymphadenopathy is a rare effect of phenytoin,[128] and there are very rare reports of frank lymphoma.[129] AEDs are generally not carcinogenic in experimental animals, and there is no other evidence for carcinogenesis in humans. Cancer rates are higher in patients with epilepsy than in control populations, but this may be because of the statistical effect of primary and metastatic brain tumors.[130]

Immune and Rheumatologic Disorders

Many AEDs have been associated with the drug-induced lupus syndrome, including phenytoin, valproate, ethosuximide, primidone, and carbamazepine.[131,132] Symptoms typically disappear gradually with drug discontinuation.[133] Vasculitis occurs rarely.

Barbiturates can cause Dupuytren's contractures and, rarely, other connective tissue disorders.[134] Aching in the joints is a complaint of some patients who take carbamazepine, but the mechanism is unknown, and serologic studies are negative.

Susceptible Populations

Certain patient populations are especially susceptible to unwanted effects of AEDs. Now that we have available a large selection of effective agents, the likelihood of side effects—adverse or beneficial—should be a major factor in the choice of therapy.

In treating children, the possibility of hypersensitivity with barbiturates, failure to gain weight with topiramate, and cosmetic problems with phenytoin are examples of things we must consider. In young women, the effects of enzyme-inducing drugs on estrogen metabolism and several drugs on fetal development must be weighed. In the elderly, cognitive dysfunction may worsen, especially with sedative drugs. Drugs likely to cause tremor or ataxia should not be prescribed to patients who already have those problems.

More important, it is critical to recognize the increased chance of dangerous idiosyncratic reactions in certain groups: valproate-induced liver failure in children younger than 2 years old, felbamate-induced aplastic anemia in patients with a previous history of blood dyscrasia or autoimmune disease, and severe cutaneous reactions to lamotrigine in patients with a history of rashes with other drugs.

Conclusion

AEDs are essential to the treatment of the 50 million patients worldwide with epilepsy. They are marvelous tools for altering brain chemistry, and physicians are finding increased clinical uses for the treatment of other disorders of the nervous system. Nevertheless, they are relatively nonselective for their intended effect and thus exhibit frequent and varied side effects. A thorough understanding of the most commonly encountered antiepileptic effects, adverse and beneficial, is essential to the proper use of AEDs.

The serious idiosyncratic effects should be respected and anticipated but not feared unduly, as they are rare. As of now, we cannot predict whether a patient may develop a serious IDR. Ongoing investigations indicate that the future may hold more promise in identifying patients at risk of developing serious IDRs. Through metabolic and genetic screening, clinicians may eventually be able to develop an "individual at-risk clinical profile" by identifying abnormal bioactivation and deficient detoxification ability.

As we increase our understanding of the mechanisms of antiepileptic action of these drugs, we should also devote resources to understanding the mechanism and prevention of their adverse effects. We can expect that such knowledge should lead to an increased ability to dissociate desirable from undesirable effects based on molecular structure and a better means of preventing serious complications.

References

1. Rogawski MA, Porter RJ. Antiepileptic drugs: pharmacological mechanisms and clinical efficacy with consideration of promising developmental stage compounds. Pharmacol Rev 1990;42:223–286.
2. The Roper Organization. Living with epilepsy: report of a Roper poll of patients on quality of life, 1992.
3. Baker GA, Jacoby A, Buck D, et al. Quality of life of people with epilepsy: a European study. Epilepsia 1997;38:353–362.
4. National Family Opinion Research, Inc. Epilepsy Awareness Study, 1996.
5. Pellock JM, Willmore LJ. A rational guide to routine blood monitoring in patients receiving antiepileptic drugs. Neurology 1991;42:223–286.
6. Mattson RH. Medical management of epilepsy in adults. Neurology 1998;51[Suppl 4]:S15–S20.
7. Troupin AS. Dose-related adverse effects of anticonvulsants. Drug Saf 1996;14:299–328.
8. Januzzi G, Cian P, Fattore C, et al. A multicenter randomized controlled trial on the clinical impact of therapeutic drug monitoring in patients with newly diagnosed epilepsy. Epilepsia 2000;41:222–230.
9. Larkin JG, Herrick AL, McGuire EM. Antiepileptic drug monitoring at the epilepsy clinic: a prospective evaluation. Epilepsia 1991;32:89–95.
10. Physicians' Desk Reference (54th ed). Montvale, NJ: Medical Economics Publishing Company, 2000.
11. Marson AG, Kadir ZA, Hutton JL, Chadwick DW. The new antiepileptic drugs: a systematic review of their efficacy and tolerability. Epilepsia 1996;38:859–880.
12. Cramer JA, Fisher R, Ben-Menachem E, et al. New antiepileptic drugs: comparison of key clinical trials. Epilepsia 1999;40:590–600.
13. Meador KJ, Baker GA. Behavioral and cognitive effects of lamotrigine. J Child Neurol 1997;12[Suppl 1]:S44–S47.
14. Jensen PK. Felbamate in the treatment of refractory partial onset seizures. Epilepsia 1993;34[Suppl 7]:S25–S29.
15. Ketter TA, Post RM, Theodore WH. Positive and negative psychiatric effects of antiepileptic drugs in patients with seizure disorders. Neurology 1999;53[Suppl 2]:S53–S67.
16. Walden J, Normann C, Langosch J, et al. Differential treatment of bipolar disorder with old and new antiepileptic drugs. Neuropsychobiology 1998;38:181–184.
17. Keck PEJ, McElroy SL, Strakowski SM. Anticonvulsants and antipsychotics in the treatment of bipolar disorder. J Clin Psychiatry 1998;59[Suppl 6]:74–81.
18. Ferrier IN. Lamotrigine and gabapentin. Alternative in the treatment of bipolar disorder. Neuropsychobiology 1998;38:192–197.
19. Bowden CL. New concepts in mood stabilization: evidence for the effectiveness of valproate and lamotrigine. Neuropsychopharmacology 1998;19:194–199.
20. Lewin J, Sumners D. Successful treatment of episodic dyscontrol with carbamazepine. Br J Psychiatry 1992;161:261–262.
21. Ryback R, Ryback L. Gabapentin for behavioral dyscontrol. Am J Psychiatry 1995;152:1399.
22. Devanand DP. Behavioral complications and their treatment in Alzheimer's disease. Geriatrics 1997;52[Suppl 2]:S37–S39.
23. Porsteinsson AP, Tariot PN, Erb R, Gaile S. An open trial of valproate for agitation in geriatric neuropsychiatric disorders. Am J Geriatr Psychiatry 1997;5:344–351.
24. Mellow AM, Solano-Lopez C, Davis S. Sodium valproate in the treatment of behavioral disturbance in dementia. J Geriatr Psychiatry Neurol 1993;6:205–209.
25. Keck PE, McElroy SL, Friedman LM. Valproate and carbamazepine in the treatment of panic and posttraumatic stress disorders, withdrawal states, and behavioral dyscontrol syndromes. J Clin Psychopharmacol 1992;12[Suppl]:S36–S41.
26. McQuay H, Carroll D, Jadad AR, et al. Anticonvulsant drugs for management of pain: a systematic review. BMJ 1995;311:1047–1052.
27. Magnus L. Nonepileptic uses of gabapentin. Epilepsia 1999;40[Suppl 6]:S66–S72.
28. Wetzel CH, Connelly JF. Use of gabapentin in pain management. Ann Pharmacother 1997;31:1082–1083.

29. Merren MD. Gabapentin for treatment of pain and tremor: a large case series. South Med J 1998;91:739–744.

30. Backonja M, Beydoun A, Edwards KR, et al. Gabapentin for the symptomatic treatment of painful neuropathy in patients with diabetes mellitus: a randomized controlled trial. JAMA 1998;280:1831–1836.

31. Abbott Laboratories. Data on file. Chicago, IL, 2000.

32. Shorvon SD. Safety of topiramate: adverse events and relationships to dosing. Epilepsia 1996;37[Suppl 2]:S18–S22.

33. Bergen DC, Ristanovic RK, Waicosky K, et al. Weight loss in patients taking felbamate. Clin Neuropharmacol 1995;18:23–27.

34. Oomen KJ, Mathews S. Zonisamide: a new antiepileptic drug. Clin Neuropharmacol 1999;22:192–200.

35. Leeder S. Mechanisms of idiosyncratic hypersensitivity reactions to antiepileptic drugs. Epilepsia 1998;39[Suppl 7]:S8–S16.

36. Schlienger RG, Oh PI, Knowles SR, et al. Quantifying the costs of serious adverse drug reactions to antiepileptic drugs. Epilepsia 1998[Suppl 7]:S27–S32.

37. Ruble J, Matsuo F. Anticonvulsant induced cutaneous reactions. CNS Drugs 1999;12:215–236.

38. Rieder MJ. Immunopharmacology of adverse drug reactions. J Clin Pharmacol 1993;33:316–323.

39. Wolkernstein P, Charue D, Laurent P, et al. Metabolic predisposition to cutaneous adverse drug reactions: role in toxic epidermal necrolysis caused by sulfonamides and anticonvulsants. Arch Dermatol 1995;131:544–551.

40. Glauser TA, Titanic-Schefft M, Pippenger CE. Racial differences in free radical scavenging enzyme activity in children. J Child Neurol 1999;14:382–387.

41. Kramlinger KG, Phillips KA, Post RM. Rash complicating carbamazepine treatment. J Clin Psychopharmacol 1994;14:408–413.

42. Chadwick D, Shaw MD, Fay P, et al. Serum anticonvulsant concentration and the risk of drug-induced skin eruptions. J Neurol Neurosurg Psychiatry 1984;47:642–644.

43. Gram L. Oxcarbazepine. In J Engel Jr, TA Pedley (eds), Epilepsy: A Comprehensive Textbook. Philadelphia: Lippincott–Raven, 1997;1544.

44. Wong IC, Mawer GE, Sander JW. Factors influencing the incidence of lamotrigine-related skin rash. Ann Pharmacother 1999;33:1037–1042.

45. Knowles SR, Shapiro LE, Shear NH. Anticonvulsant hypersensitivity syndrome. Drug Saf 1999;21:489–501.

46. Schlienger RG, Shear NH. Antiepileptic drug hypersensitivity syndrome. Epilepsia 1998;39[Suppl 7]:S3–S7.

47. Fritsch PE, Ruiz-Maldanado R. Stevens-Johnson Syndrome—Toxic Epidermal Necrolysis. In IM Freedberg, TB Fitzpatrick (eds), Dermatology in General Medicine. New York: McGraw-Hill, 1999:644.

48. Roujeau JC, Stern RS. Severe adverse cutaneous reactions to drugs. N Engl J Med 1994;331:1272–1285.

49. Rzany B, Correia O, Kelly JP, et al. Risk of Stevens-Johnson syndrome and toxic epidermal necrolysis during first weeks of antiepileptic drug therapy: a case control study. Study Group of International Case Control Study on Severe Cutaneous Adverse Reactions. Lancet 1999;353:2190–2194.

50. Schlienger RG, Knowles SR, Shear NH. Lamotrigine-associated anticonvulsant hypersensitivity syndrome. Neurology 1998;51:1172–1174.

51. Faught E, Morris G, Jacobson M, et al. Adding lamotrigine to valproate: incidence of rash and other adverse effects. Epilepsia 1999;40:1135–1140.

52. Shear NH, Spielberg SP. Anticonvulsant hypersensitivity syndrome: in vitro assessment of risk. J Clin Invest 1988;82:1826–1832.

53. Tegretol [package insert]. East Hanover, NJ: Novartis, July 2000.

54. Pellock JM. Felbamate in epilepsy therapy. Drug Saf 1999;21:225–239.

55. Thompson CD, Gulden PH, Macdonald TL. Identification of modified atropaldehyde mercapturic acids in rat and human urine after felbamate administration. Chem Res Toxicol 1997;10:457–462.

56. Wyllie E, Wyllie R. Routine laboratory monitoring for serious adverse effects of antiepileptic medications: the controversy. Epilepsia 1991;48:182–188.

57. Beydoun A, Sackellares JC, Shu V. Safety and efficacy of divalproex sodium monotherapy in partial epilepsy: a double-blind, concentration-response design clinical trial. Depakote Monotherapy for Partial Seizures Study Group. Neurology 1997;48:182–188.

58. Anderson GD, Lin YX, Berge C, et al. Absence of bleeding complications in patients undergoing cortical surgery while receiving valproate treatment. J Neurosurg 1997;87:252–256.

59. Temkin NR, Dikmen SS, Anderson GD, et al. Valproate therapy for prevention of post-traumatic seizures: a randomized trial. J Neurosurg 1999;91:593–600.

60. Camfield C, Camfield P, Smith E, et al. Asymptomatic children with epilepsy: little benefit from screening for anticonvulsant induced liver, blood, or renal damage. Neurology 1986;36:838–841.

61. Schmidt D, Siemes H. Role of liver function tests in monitoring anticonvulsant use. CNS Drugs 1998;10:321–328.

62. Foster GR, Goldin RD, Freeth CJ, et al. Liver damage in long term anticonvulsant therapy: a serological and histological study. QJM 1991;79:315–322.

63. Bryant AE, Dreifuss FE. Hepatotoxicity associated with antiepileptic drug therapy. CNS Drugs 1995;4:99–113.

64. Horowitz S, Patwardhan R, Marcus E. Hepatotoxic reactions associated with carbamazepine therapy. Epilepsia 1988;29:149–154.

65. Zaccara G, Campostrinin R, Paganini M, et al. Long-term treatment with sodium valproate: monitoring of venous ammonia concentrations and adverse effects. Ther Drug Monit 1987;9:34–40.

66. Zaccara G, Paganini M, Campostrinin R, et al. Effect of associated antiepileptic drug treatment on

valproate induced hyperammonemia. Ther Drug Monit 1985;7:185–190.

67. Asconape JJ, Penry JK, Dreifuss FE, et al. Valproate associated pancreatitis. Epilepsia 1993;34(1):177–183.

68. Binek J, Hany A, Heer M, et al. Valproic acid-induced pancreatitis. Case report and review of the literature. J Clin Gastroenterol 1991;12:690–693.

69. Sunao K, Tsuyoshi K. Antiepileptic agents and birth defects: incidence, mechanisms, and prevention. CNS Drugs 1995;3:41–55.

70. Canger R, Battino D, Canevini MP, et al. Malformations in offspring of women with epilepsy: a prospective study. Epilepsia 1999;40:1231–1236.

71. Morrell M. The new antiepileptic drug and women: efficacy, reproductive health, pregnancy, and fetal outcome. Epilepsia 1996;37[Suppl 6]:S34–S44.

72. Yerby M. Treatment of Epilepsy during Pregnancy. In E Wyllie (ed), The Treatment of Epilepsy, Principles and Practice (2nd ed). Baltimore: Williams & Wilkins, 1997;785.

73. O'Brien MD, Gilmour-White S. Epilepsy and pregnancy. BMJ 1993;307:492–495.

74. Nulman I, Laslo D, Koren G. Treatment of epilepsy in pregnancy. Drugs 1999;57:535–544.

75. Knowles SR. Adverse effects of antiepileptics. Can J Clin Pharmacol 1999;6:137–148.

76. Beghi E, Di Mascio R. Antiepileptic drug toxicity: definition and mechanism of action. Ital J Neurol Sci 1986;7:209–222.

77. Shorvon S, Stefan H. Overview of the safety of newer antiepileptic drugs. Epilepsia 1997;38[Suppl 1]:S45–S51.

78. Pellock JM. Carbamazepine side effects in children and adults. Epilepsia 1987;28[Suppl 3]:S64–S70.

79. Faught E. Felbamate. In E Wyllie (ed), The Treatment of Epilepsy, Principles and Practice (3rd ed). Baltimore: Williams & Wilkins, 2000.

80. McLean MJ. Gabapentin. Epilepsia 1995;36[Suppl 2]:S73–S86.

81. Ramsay RE. Clinical efficacy and safety of gabapentin. Neurology 1994;44[Suppl 5]:S23–S30.

82. Ramsay RE, Pellock JM, Garnett WR, et al. Pharmacokinetics and safety of lamotrigine in patients with epilepsy. Epilepsy Res 1991;10:191–200.

83. Matsuo F, Bergen D, Faught E, et al. Placebo-controlled study of the efficacy and safety of lamotrigine in patients with partial seizures. Neurology 1993;43:2284–2291.

84. Tecoma ES. Oxcarbazepine. Epilepsia 1999;40[Suppl 5]:S37–S46.

85. Wilder BJ. Phenytoin: Clinical Use. In RH Levy, RH Mattson, BS Meldrum (eds), Antiepileptic Drugs. New York: Raven Press, 1995.

86. Schachter SC. Antiepileptic drug therapy: general treatment principles and application for special patient populations. Epilepsia 1999;40[Suppl 9]:S20–S25.

87. Faught E. Clinical studies of topiramate. Drugs Today 1999;35:49–57.

88. Wallace SJ. A comparative review of the adverse effects of anticonvulsants in children with epilepsy. Drug Saf 1996;15:278–393.

89. Deckers CL, Hekster YA, Keyser A, et al. Adverse effects in epilepsy therapy. Wait and see or go for it? Acta Neurol Scand 1997;95:248–252.

90. Meador KJ, Loring DW, Allen ME, et al. Comparative cognitive effects of carbamazepine and phenytoin in healthy adults. Neurology 1991;41:1537–1540.

91. Meador K, Loring D. Cognitive Effects of Antiepileptic Drugs. In O Devinsky, W Theodore (eds), Epilepsy and Behavior. New York: Wiley, 1991;151–170.

92. Perrine K, Kiolbasa T. Cognitive deficits in epilepsy and contribution to psychopathology. Neurology 1999;53[Suppl 2]:S39–S48.

93. Prevy ML, Delaney RC, Cramer JA, et al. Effect of valproate on cognitive functioning. Comparison with carbamazepine. The Department of Veterans Affairs Epilepsy Cooperative Study 264 Group. Arch Neurol 1996;53:1008–1016.

94. Sulzbacher S, Farwell JR, Temkin N, et al. Late cognitive effects of early treatment with phenobarbital. Clin Pediatr 1999;38:387–394.

95. MacLeod C, Delzaban A, Hunt E. Memory impairment in epileptic patients: selective effects of phenobarbital concentration. Science 1978;202:1102–1104.

96. Martin R, Kuzniecky R, Ho S, et al. Cognitive effects of topiramate, gabapentin, and lamotrigine in healthy young adults. Neurology 1999;52:321–327.

97. Berent S, Sackellares C, Giordani B, et al. Zonisamide (CI-912) and cognition: results from preliminary study. Epilepsia 1987;28:61–67.

98. Mattson RH, Cramer JA, Collins JF, et al. Comparison of carbamazepine, phenobarbital, phenytoin, and primidone in partial and secondarily generalized tonic-clinic seizures. N Engl J Med 1985;313:145–152.

99. Mattson RH, Cramer JA, Collins JF, et al. A comparison of valproate and carbamazepine for the treatment of complex partial seizures and secondarily generalized tonic-clonic seizures in adults. N Engl J Med 1992;327:765–771.

100. Jones GL, Matsuo F, Baringer JR, Reichert WH. Valproic acid-associated encephalopathy. West J Med 1990;153:199–202.

101. Chadwick DW, Cumming WJ, Livingstone I, Cartlidge NE. Acute intoxication with sodium valproate. Ann Neurol 1979;6:552–553.

102. Brown JK. Valproate toxicity. Dev Med Child Neurol 1988;30:121–125.

103. Coulter DL. Carnitine, valproate, and toxicity. J Child Neurol 1991;6:7–14.

104. Triggs WJ, Bohan TP, Lin SN, Willmore LJ. Valproate-induced coma with ketosis and carnitine insufficiency. Arch Neurol 1990;47:1131–1133.

105. Khan A, Faught E, Gilliam F, Kuzniecky R. Acute psychotic symptoms induced by topiramate. Seizure 1999;3:1–3.

106. Vining EP, Mellitis ED, Dorsen MM, et al. Psychologic and behavioral effects of antiepileptic drugs in children: a double-blind comparison between phenobarbital and valproic acid. Pediatrics 1987;80:165–174.

107. Edmeads JG, Gawel MJ, Vickers J. Strategies for diagnosing and managing medication-induced headache. Can Fam Physician 1997;43:1249–1254.

108. Faught E, Sachdeo R, Remler M, et al. Felbamate monotherapy for partial onset seizures: an active-control trial. Neurology 1993;43:688–692.

109. Lang AE, Weiner WJ. Drug-Induced Movement Disorders. Mount Kisco, NY: Futura, 1992;348–349.

110. Marks WA, Morris MP, Bodensteiner JB, et al. Gastritis with valproate therapy. Arch Neurol 1988;45:903–905.

111. Sachs GS, Guille C. Weight gain associated with use of psychotropic medications. J Clin Psychiatry 1999;60[Suppl 21]:16–19.

112. Lambie DG, Johnson RH. Drugs and folate metabolism. Drugs 1985;30:145–155.

113. Mason JB, Miller JW. The effects of vitamins B_{12}, B_6, and folate on homocysteine levels. Ann N Y Acad Sci 1992;559:197–203.

114. Tamura T, Aiso K, Johnston KE, et al. Homocysteine, folate, vitamin B-12 and vitamin B-6 in patients receiving antiepileptic drug monotherapy. Epilepsy Res 2000;40:7–15.

115. Morrell MJ. Guidelines for the care of women with epilepsy. Neurology 1998;51[Suppl 4]:S21–S27.

116. Tjellesen L. Metabolism and action of vitamin D in epileptic patients on anticonvulsive treatment and healthy adults. Dan Med Bull 1994;41:139–150.

117. Zahn CA, Morrell MJ, Collins SD, et al. Management issues for women with epilepsy: a review of the literature. Neurology 1998;51:949–956.

118. Desai P, Silver JG. Drug-induced gingival enlargements. J Can Dent Assoc 1998;64:263–268.

119. Faught E, Wilder BJ, Ramsay RE, et al. Topiramate placebo-controlled dose-ranging trial in refractory partial epilepsy using 200, 400, and 600 mg daily dosages. Neurology 1996;6:1684–1690.

120. Treiman DM, Meyers PD, Walton NY, et al. A comparison of four treatments of generalized convulsive status epilepticus. N Engl J Med 1998;339:792–798.

121. Johnson CD, Rivera H, Jimenez JE. Carbamazepine-induced sinus node dysfunction. P R Health Sci J 1997;16:45–49.

122. Timmings PL. Sudden unexpected death in epilepsy: Is carbamazepine implicated? Seizure 1998;7:289–291.

123. Ramsay RE, Slater JD. Effects of antiepileptic drugs on hormones. Epilepsia 1991;32[Suppl 6]:S60–S67.

124. Herzog AG. Reproductive endocrine considerations and hormonal therapy for women with epilepsy. Epilepsia 1991;32[Suppl 6]:S27–S33.

125. Chappell KA, Markowitz JS, Jackson CW. Is valproate pharmacotherapy associated with polycystic ovaries? Ann Pharmacother 1999;33:1211–1216.

126. Faught E. Review of U.S. clinical trials of zonisamide treatment of refractory partial-onset seizures. Epilepsia 1999;40[Suppl 7]:94–95.

127. Paisley KE, Tomson CR. Calcium phosphate stones during long-term acetazolamide treatment for epilepsy. Postgrad Med J 1999;75:427–428.

128. Jeng YM, Tien HF, Su IJ. Phenytoin-induced pseudolymphoma: reevaluation using modern molecular biology techniques. Epilepsia 1996;37:104–107.

129. Olsen JH, Schulgen G, Boice JDJ, et al. Antiepileptic treatment and risk for hepatobiliary cancer and malignant lymphoma. Cancer Res 1995;55:294–297.

130. Olsen JH, Boice JD, Jensen JP, Fraumeni JF. Cancer among epileptic patients exposed to anticonvulsant drugs. J Natl Cancer Inst 1989;81:803–808.

131. Jain KK. Systemic lupus erythematosus (SLE)–like syndromes associated with carbamazepine therapy. Drug Saf 1991;6:350–360.

132. Drory VE, Korczyn AD. Hypersensitivity vasculitis and systemic lupus erythematosus induced by anticonvulsants. Clin Neuropharmacol 1993;16:19–29.

133. Adams LE, Hess EV. Drug-related lupus. Incidence, mechanisms, and clinical implications. Drug Saf 1991;6:431–449.

134. Mattson RH, Cramer JA, McCutchen CB. Barbiturate-related connective tissue disorders. Arch Intern Med 1989;149:911–914.

135. Faught E, Ayala R, Montouris G, Leppik I. Randomized controlled trial of zonisamide for refractory partial-onset seizures. The Zonisamide 922 Study Group. *(in press)*.

Chapter 26

Drug Interactions

Candace Smith

Seizure control requires continuous antiepileptic action. However, with many drugs, this is not achievable unless plasma concentrations remain within the therapeutic range. Although monotherapy with antiepileptic drugs (AEDs) is preferred, patients with multiple seizure types or refractory epilepsy generally require combinations of AEDs. Ethical concerns limit the exposure of anyone with epilepsy to monotherapy with a drug of unproven efficacy. Therefore, phase II testing of new AEDs is usually conducted as add-on therapy in refractory patients, and it leads to indications for add-on therapy and fosters polypharmacy and potential drug interactions.[1] Polypharmacy is often administered for brief periods in patients who eventually are controlled by a single drug, either during the initial selection of therapy or during periods of seizure exacerbation.[2]

Long-term treatment is common, and concurrent treatment often is prescribed by multiple health care providers during AED therapy. Thus, the risk for developing AED interactions is increased. Many patients with epilepsy take other medications for concurrent medical problems and are predisposed to drug interactions involving these drugs. Drug interactions represent a difficult dilemma for the health care provider, as they may lead to adverse outcomes in patients. However, many patients receiving potentially interacting drugs do not manifest adverse consequences.[3] Therefore, one must identify situations in which the patient is truly at risk. Knowledge of the interactive properties of drugs can enable one to predict many adverse drug interactions before they occur.

A drug interaction occurs when the effectiveness or toxicity of a drug is altered by the administration of another drug or substance.[4] Mechanisms of drug interactions can be classified as pharmacokinetic, pharmacodynamic, or both. Pharmacokinetic alterations are the most common and affect drug concentrations by altering drug absorption, distribution, metabolism, and excretion. These pharmacokinetic changes may or may not result in an altered pharmacologic response or therapeutic outcome. The most common pharmacokinetic drug interactions involve modifications in bioavailability and drug metabolism that can lead to changes in drug concentrations. In contrast, pharmacodynamic interactions occur at the site of pharmacologic effect and generally do not reflect changes in drug concentrations. The pharmacodynamic consequences may or may not closely parallel pharmacokinetic changes.

Although some pharmacokinetic interactions are clinically unremarkable and need only careful clinical monitoring, others require prompt dosage adjustment. The clinical importance of any drug interaction depends on factors that are drug, patient, and administration related, and the extent of interaction varies markedly among individuals depending on age, preexisting medical conditions, and possibly dose. Generally, a doubling or more in plasma drug concentration has the potential for an enhanced adverse effect or beneficial drug response. Less pronounced pharmacokinetic interactions may be clinically important for drugs with a narrow therapeutic range (e.g., warfarin) or nonlinear kinetics (e.g., phenytoin). Interactions may occur under single-dose conditions or only after multiple doses, when a steady state has occurred. Assessment of a drug interaction may be most apparent when a new drug is added to the regimen of a patient stabilized on the affected drug. Temporal relationships between the administration of a drug and the addition of a new drug can help determine whether a drug interaction has occurred.

Serum drug concentration monitoring, when available, is particularly useful to assess potential drug interactions and to help manage combinations of AEDs or other concurrent drugs that invariably interact. The addition or deletion of another drug, whether an AED or a drug used for another medical condition, may change the dosage requirements of either drug.

The majority of known pharmacodynamic interactions occur when drugs with additive, synergistic, or antagonistic pharmacologic effects are used therapeutically (e.g., sedatives, antihypertensives, and analgesics). In other situations, the additive or antagonistic response may produce adverse effects.[3] Although many pharmacodynamic drug interactions do not cause serious adverse effects, it is difficult to anticipate which interactions may produce clinical difficulty when a patient is receiving 5–10 drugs for various medical conditions. Therefore, clinicians should know the pharmacokinetic as well as the pharmacodynamic drug interactions to anticipate clinical effects and reduce the risk of toxicity and seizure worsening when a drug is added to or withdrawn from the patient's drug regimen.[3]

Absorption

With regard to orally administered drugs, knowledge of the extent of and factors determining the bioavailability of these substrates helps predict changes that could occur to their pharmacokinetics with the administration of interfering medications. Oral bioavailability (amount of the dose that reaches the systemic circulation) is determined by two major processes: the fraction of the dose that is absorbed from the gut and the fraction that does not undergo presystemic metabolism (i.e., occurs mainly in the small bowel and liver).

There are several mechanisms by which a drug may affect the gastrointestinal absorption of another drug: (1) binding or chelation, (2) changing gastric pH, (3) altering gastrointestinal motility, and (4) altering gastrointestinal flora (Table 26-1).

When a precipitant drug binds with or otherwise inhibits the gastrointestinal absorption of an object drug, the serum concentration of the object drug usually begins to decrease within hours of concurrent drug use.[5] However, the rate of decline in serum concentration of the object drug depends on its half-life.

Drug binding in the gastrointestinal tract occurs through mechanisms such as adsorbing drugs onto the surface and preventing passage of the drug across the wall of the intestine.[5] Examples of drugs that may interfere with drug absorption by this mechanism include activated charcoal, resins, and

Table 26-1. Common Pharmacokinetic Absorption Interactions

Mechanism	Precipitant Drug Examples	Object Drug Examples	Suggested Management
Drug binding or chelation	Antacids, iron, cholestyramine, colestipol, kaolin-pectin	Fluoroquinolones, digoxin, warfarin, tetracycline, atorvastatin	Separate drugs by 2 hrs
Gastric pH	Histamine 2 blockers, proton pump inhibitors, antacids, buffered agents (didanosine)	Iron-containing products, isoniazid, allopurinol, ketoconazole, itraconazole	Avoid concomitant use
Increased gastric motility	Metoclopramide, cisapride, laxatives	Any drug	Evaluate significance
Decreased gastric motility	Anticholinergics, antimotility agents, opioids	Any drug	Evaluate significance
Alteration in gastrointestinal flora	Antibiotics	Digoxin, oral estrogen, oral contraceptives	Monitor digoxin levels

antacids. In one study, simultaneous administration of aluminum hydroxide and magnesium hydroxide within 2 hours of a single dose of gabapentin reduced gabapentin bioavailability by approximately 10–20%.[6] Other agents are capable of forming insoluble complexes with drugs. For example, iron salts inhibit the gastrointestinal absorption of tetracycline. This mechanism may also be responsible for the ability of both antacids and sucralfate to reduce the gastrointestinal absorption of quinolones, such as ciprofloxacin, by 50–75%.[7] These types of drug interactions caused by the formation of nonabsorbable complexes can generally be prevented by separating administration times by 2 hours, with the administration of the object drug before the participant drug.

Gastric emptying can be an important determinant of drug absorption rate. Drugs that increase gastric motility (e.g., metoclopramide) can hasten the absorption of drugs, whereas drugs that slow gastric emptying, such as opioids, can delay the absorption of orally administered drugs. Although the absolute bioavailability may not be affected by altering the rate of absorption, a slowed rate of absorption could be clinically important if a rapid drug response is desired (e.g., an analgesic).[5]

Many drugs are weak acids or weak bases, and it is their nonionized form that traverses the intestinal wall. Thus, drugs that are weak acids do not dissolve well in acidic mediums, and drugs that are weak bases do not dissolve in basic mediums, leading to impaired absorption. The importance of pH on drug dissolution can be seen with drugs such as histamine 2 (H_2) receptor antagonists that alter the pH of the gastric mucosa. Ketoconazole, which requires an acidic medium to dissolve adequately for absorption, may have impaired absorption when administered with an H_2 receptor antagonist.[8]

When a patient is receiving two drugs that may potentially interact with each other in the gastrointestinal tract, it may be necessary to take action to prevent the unwanted effects of the interaction. In general, binding interactions can be minimized if the object drug is given several hours before the binding agent. However, separating the doses of the interacting drugs does not circumvent gastrointestinal motility interactions.[5] Administration of a medication after the effect of

the precipitant drug on gastrointestinal motility has dissipated may help to reduce the interaction. In many cases, interactions involving alterations in gastrointestinal pH may be avoided by adjusting the dosing times. For example, the alkalinizing effects of H_2 blockers are transient; therefore, it may be possible to administer the object drug when the effect of the H_2 blocker has minimal effect on the gastrointestinal pH.[5]

Protein Binding

Drug interactions related to protein binding result from the displacement of one drug from a protein by another drug with greater affinity.[1] Displacement interactions are usually not of clinical significance unless the displaced drug is highly protein bound (greater than or equal to 90%), is slowly eliminated, and has a narrow therapeutic range.[3] When a displaced drug possesses these properties, the enhanced pharmacologic effect may be transient, because more unbound drug is available for elimination from the body. For this reason, protein-binding displacement interactions may only be clinically significant when there is a reduction in the affected drug's elimination. In addition, displacement interactions often depend on the sequence of drug administration and dose. Phenytoin and valproate are the only AEDs involved in clinically important protein-binding interactions. The effect of valproate on phenytoin is a combination of protein-binding displacement and enzyme inhibition. The interaction can result in the total phenytoin concentrations increasing, decreasing, or not changing when valproate is added. When the serum concentration of valproic acid is less than 35 mg/liter, the displacement of phenytoin is minimal, and no dose adjustment is required.[9] However, when the valproic acid level is greater than 50 mg/liter, the extent of phenytoin displacement increases, and a dose adjustment may be required. Ideally, unbound phenytoin concentrations should be monitored in a patient receiving valproate and phenytoin.

Drug Interactions That Affect Metabolism

Pharmacokinetic interactions between AEDs and other drugs arise most frequently as a consequence of drug-induced changes in hepatic metabolism. The propensity for AEDs to interact with each other or other drugs depends on their metabolic characteristics and the action of drug metabolic enzymes.[2,10] Interactions can occur from the induction of new protein synthesis, which accelerates drug metabolism and decreases the magnitude and duration of drug response, or from inhibition, which results in elevated plasma drug concentrations with increased potential for enhanced beneficial or, in many cases, adverse effects.[4]

The *cytochrome P-450* (CYP450) *microsomal enzyme system* is the collective term for a group of related enzymes or isoenzymes that oxidize numerous drugs.[5] These metabolic enzymes are a group of heme-containing enzymes that are embedded primarily in the lipid bilayer of the endoplasmic reticulum of hepatocytes but also are present in high concentrations in enterocytes of the small intestine and in smaller quantities in extrahepatic tissues, such as the kidney, brain, and lungs.[11] Although more than 30 human metabolic CYP450 isoenzymes have been identified to date, the major ones responsible for drug metabolism are the CYP3A4, CYP2D6, CYP1A2, and CYP2C subfamilies.[11] CYP3A4 is the most abundantly expressed isoenzyme and is responsible for the majority of drug metabolism. Each isoenzyme has its own characteristic substrate affinity and is differentially affected by the inducing and inhibiting effects of other drugs (Table 26-2).[12] Drug interactions involving the CYP450 isoenzymes generally result from one of two processes—enzyme inhibition and enzyme induction. Hepatic enzyme inhibition most often occurs as a result of competitive binding at the enzyme site and results in a decrease in the rate of metabolism of the affected drug.[3] Clinically, this is associated with an increased plasma concentration of the affected drug and, potentially, an increased pharmacologic response or toxicity. The extent of inhibition is more difficult to predict than the type of interaction, because it depends on the affinity of the substrate for the enzyme and the dose of the inhibitor. The onset and offset of the drug interaction are frequently rapid but depend on the half-life of the inhibiting drug and the time needed to achieve a new steady state.[12] If the half-life of the inhibiting drug is shorter than that of the substrate, less time is required to revert to a lower steady-state concentration once the inhibitor is discontinued than when the inhibitor was initiated.[12] In drugs that are concentration dependent, such as phenytoin, stabilization of a serum concentration after the administration of an inhibitor is quite variable and may take days to occur.

Unlike competitive inhibition, enzyme induction requires time to develop after the introduction of an inducing agent. The time required depends on the time to reach the steady state of the inducing agent and the *de novo* synthesis of enzymes.[2] The mechanism of induction is generally inducer specific. Clinically, the consequences are a fall in the plasma concentration of the affected drug and a possible reduction in its therapeutic effect. If the affected drug has an active metabolite, induction can result in increased metabolite formation and, potentially, an increase in the drug's therapeutic effect or toxicity (e.g., carbamazepine). The magnitude of the effect is proportional to the dose of the inducing agent.[12] In contrast to the dose relationship, induction is not strictly additive when patients are receiving multiple inducers.[3] The offset of enzyme induction is also gradual, because it depends on elimination of the enzyme-inducing drug and an elimination of increased enzyme stores. When the inducer is removed, plasma concentrations of the affected drug increase if the dose is not reduced. In summary, enzyme inducers with long half-lives (e.g., phenobarbital; terminal half-life [$T^{1}/_{2}$], 3–5 days) usually have longer onset and offset than enzyme inducers with shorter half-lives (e.g., carbamazepine; $T^{1}/_{2}$, 8 hours). There are no known inducers of CYP2D6, but a number of agents, including phenytoin, phenobarbital, and carbamazepine, induce CYP34A.

Some drugs may be metabolized by more than one isoenzyme, as are many of the psychoactive drugs. Therefore, when one enzyme system is inhibited or induced by an interacting drug, a clinically significant interaction may or may not occur, depending on which metabolic pathway is predominant.[11] This was demonstrated in a study evaluating the interaction between phenytoin and topiramate, in which topiramate inhibited the CYP2C19 isoenzyme involved in phenytoin metabolism but did not inhibit the isoenzyme CYP2C9 (which accounts for 70–90% of the phenytoin clearance), resulting in a small, and clinically insignificant, change in phenytoin serum concentrations.[13] Few significant metabolic inter-

Table 26-2. Clinically Significant Drug Interactions

Substrate (Metabolic Isoenzyme)	Enzyme Inducer/ Increased Elimination	Enzyme Inhibitor/ Decreased Elimination	Potential Clinical Consequences/Suggested Management	Alternative
Analgesics				
Methadone (CYP3A4)		Fluvoxamine	Increased CNS depression.	—
	Carbamazepine, phenobarbital, phenytoin, primidone		Monitor for withdrawal.	Consider alternative analgesics
Meperidine	Phenobarbital, phenytoin		Monitor for withdrawal.	Consider alternative analgesic
		Ritonavir	Increased risk of seizures.	—
Morphine (oral)	Phenobarbital, phenytoin		Decreased bioavailability; monitor for increased requirements.	—
Alfentanil (CYP3A4)		Erythromycin	Monitor for oversedation; marked increase in AUC of opiate.	Azithromycin
Morphine, meperidine		Monoamine oxidase inhibitors	Marked potentiation of action; avoid combination.	—
Alfentanil, fentanyl, methadone, meperidine, oxycodone, propoxyphene		Indinavir, nelfinavir, ritonavir,* saquinavir	Avoid meperidine propoxyphene, and fentanyl; monitor for oversedation with other agents.	—
Morphine, hydrocodone, oxycodone, methadone	Rifampin, rifabutin		Monitor for withdrawal; decreased bioavailability with oral administration and increased analgesic requirements.	—
Alfentanil, meperidine, morphine, methadone		Cimetidine	Monitor for sedation; increased bioavailability with oral administration.	Famotidine, nizatidine, ranitidine
Antiarrhythmics				
Quinidine	Carbamazepine, phenytoin, phenobarbital		Increase dose; monitor serum drug concentration.	Gabapentin, lamotrigine, topiramate, valproate
Quinidine (CYP3A4)		Cimetidine	Conflicting data; up to 50% increase in serum concentration reported; monitor.	Famotidine, nizatidine, ranitidine
Quinidine		Amiodarone	Decrease dose 25–50% on initiation; monitor Q-T interval.	—
		Ketoconazole, itraconazole, miconazole IV	30-Fold increase in serum concentration after 7 days; monitor QRS wave complex.	—
		Ritonavir, amprenavir	Increase in plasma concentration.	—

Table 26-2. *Continued*

Substrate (Metabolic Isoenzyme)	Enzyme Inducer/ Increased Elimination	Enzyme Inhibitor/ Decreased Elimination	Potential Clinical Consequences/Suggested Management	Alternative
Amiodarone (CYP3A4)		Ritonavir, amprenavir	Monitor clinically.	—
Digoxin		Amiodarone, quinidine, verapamil	Increase in digoxin serum concentrations; monitor; decrease dose of digoxin 25–50%.	—
Digoxin	Topiramate		12% decrease in AUC; monitor digoxin levels.	—
		Itraconazole	Inhibition of P-glucoprotein–mediated renal tubular secretion; monitor serum concentrations.	—
Antibiotics				
Clarithromycin (CYP3A4)		Indinavir, nelfinavir, ritonavir, saquinavir, efavirenz	AUC increases with ritonavir (77%), saquinavir (45%), and indinavir (53%); decrease clarithromycin dosage.	Azithromycin
		Rifampin, rifabutin	Decreases serum concentrations of rifampin (120%) and rifabutin (50%); clinical significance unknown.	—
Erythromycin (CYP3A4)		Ritonavir	Decrease initial dose by 50% (based on in vitro data).	—
Rifabutin		Clarithromycin	Increase serum concentration; increased risk of icterus and uveitis.	—
Rifabutin		Fluconazole	Increases AUC by 80%; increased risk of icterus and uveitis; monitor for ocular side effects.	—
Rifabutin, rifampin		Indinavir, nelfinavir, saquinavir	204% increase in AUC; decrease initial rifabutin dosage by half.	—
Rifabutin		Ritonavir, nelfinavir	Fourfold increase in AUC with ritonavir; 207% increase in AUC with nelfinavir; avoid combination.	Alternative *Mycobacterium avium intracellulare* complex prophylaxis
Metronidazole		Ritonavir (liquid)	Disulfiram reaction due to alcohol; monitor.	—
Anticoagulants				
Warfarin (CYP2C9)	Carbamazepine, phenobarbital, phenytoin		Monitor INR when initiating therapy.	Gabapentin, lamotrigine, topiramate, valproate

Substrate (Metabolic Isoenzyme)	Enzyme Inducer/ Increased Elimination	Enzyme Inhibitor/ Decreased Elimination	Potential Clinical Consequences/Suggested Management	Alternative
		Erythromycin, clarithromycin	Monitor INR.	Azithromycin
		Metronidazole, cotrimoxazole	Monitor INR.	—
	Rifampin		Monitor anticoagulant response.	—
		Cimetidine, omeprazole	Monitor INR.	Ranitidine, famotidine, nizatidine, pantoprazole, rabenazole, lansoprazole
		Fluconazole, miconazole	Monitor INR.	—
	Oral contraceptives?		Monitor for hypoprothrombinemic effect.	—
		Amiodarone	Inhibition of CYP monooxygenase–dependent degradation; reduce dosage 25–50%.	—
		Ritonavir	Monitor INR.	—
Anticonvulsants				
Carbamazepine (CYP3A4)		Erythromycin, clarithromycin	Decrease dosage by 25%.	Azithromycin
Carbamazepine (CYP3A4)		Fluoxetine, fluvoxamine, nefazodone	Monitor serum concentration; monitor for adverse drug reaction.	Venlafaxine, citalopram
Carbamazepine (CYP3A4)		Risperidone,* sertindole*	—	Quetiapine
Carbamazepine		Isoniazid	More pronounced in slow acetylators; monitor serum concentrations.	—
Carbamazepine, ethosuximide (CYP3A4)		Indinavir, nelfinavir, ritonavir, saquinavir	Decrease initial dose by 50%; monitor serum concentrations.	—
Carbamazepine, ethosuximide (CYP3A4)	Rifampin		May need initial dose increase; monitor serum concentration.	—
Carbamazepine (CYP3A4)		Ketoconazole	29% increase in serum concentrations; monitor serum concentrations.	Fluconazole?
		Verapamil	40% increase in serum concentrations.	—
		Danazol	Monitor serum concentrations.	—
	Phenytoin, phenobarbital, primidone		Variable results; monitor serum concentrations.	—
	Felbamate		10–42% decrease in serum concentrations; increase in metabolite leading to adverse drug reactions; decrease dosage.	—

Table 26-2. *Continued*

Substrate (Metabolic Isoenzyme)	Enzyme Inducer/ Increased Elimination	Enzyme Inhibitor/ Decreased Elimination	Potential Clinical Consequences/Suggested Management	Alternative
	Zonisamide	Zonisamide	Variable changes in carbamazepine concentrations; monitor levels.	—
Carbamazepine	Valproic acid		Possible neurotoxicity due to epoxide metabolite.	—
Carbamazepine		Cimetidine	Monitor serum concentrations.	Ranitidine, nizatidine, famotidine
Tiagabine (CYP3A4)		Risperidone,* sertindole*	—	Quetiapine
Tiagabine (CYP3A4)		Fluvoxamine,* fluoxetine,* nefazodone*	—	Citalopram, venlafaxine
Tiagabine (CYP3A4)	Carbamazepine, phenytoin, phenobarbital		50% reduction in serum concentrations.	—
Felbamate (CYP3A4)	Phenytoin, carbamazepine		Monitor clinically; 45% decrease in serum concentration.	—
		Valproic acid	Monitor clinically.	—
Phenytoin (CYP2C9, CYP2C19)		Cimetidine, omeprazole	Monitor serum concentrations; 25% increase in serum concentrations.	Famotidine, nizatidine, ranitidine, lansoprazole, pantoprazole, rabenazole
	Rifampin		Monitor serum concentrations when initiating and discontinuing therapy.	—
		Isoniazid	More pronounced with slow acetylator.	—
		Fluconazole, chloramphenicol, ciprofloxacin	Increase in serum concentrations; monitor conflicting data.	Ketoconazole, other antimicrobial agents
		Amiodarone	25–50% increase in serum concentration after 3–4 wks.	—
Phenytoin (CYP2C9, CYP2C19)		Fluoxetine, fluvoxamine, sertraline	Avoid if possible.	Nefazodone, venlafaxine
		Topiramate	25% increase in serum concentration when phenytoin concentrations are near saturation.	—
		Clozapine*	Monitor serum concentrations.	—
Phenytoin (CYP2C9, CYP2C19)	Phenobarbital		Unpredictable response; monitor serum concentrations.	—

Substrate (Metabolic Isoenzyme)	Enzyme Inducer/ Increased Elimination	Enzyme Inhibitor/ Decreased Elimination	Potential Clinical Consequences/Suggested Management	Alternative
	Vigabatrin		Monitor serum concentrations.	—
	Clonazepam	Clonazepam	Variable; monitor serum concentrations.	—
		Felbamate, oxcarbazepine	Decrease dosage by 20%.	—
	Carbamazepine		Unpredictable response; monitor serum concentrations.	—
	Valproic acid		Concentration dependent changes in phenytoin protein binding; follow free phenytoin serum concentrations.	—
Phenobarbital (CYP2C9, CYP2C19)	Phenytoin		Monitor serum concentrations.	—
		Valproic acid, felbamate	Decrease phenobarbital dosage 20%.	—
Topiramate	Carbamazepine, phenytoin, valproate		40% decrease, 50% decrease, 10% decrease in serum concentrations.	—
Valproic acid		Erythromycin	Increase in serum concentration; monitor.	—
Valproic acid		Cimetidine	Increase in serum concentration.	—
	Rifampin		40% decrease in serum concentrations; increase dosage.	—
	Phenytoin, phenobarbital, carbamazepine		50% decrease in serum concentration; monitor serum concentrations.	—
		Felbamate	Decrease dosage 20%.	—
Ethosuximide (CYP3A4)		Fluoxetine,* fluvoxamine,* nefazodone*	Monitor.	Citalopram
		Risperidone,* sertindole*	Monitor.	Quetiapine
	Phenytoin, phenobarbital, carbamazepine		Increase dosage 25%.	—
Lamotrigine	Phenytoin, phenobarbital, carbamazepine, primidone		Increase dosage by 50%.	—
		Valproic acid	Decrease dosage by 50%.	—
	Verapamil		20% decrease in serum concentration.	—

Table 26-2. *Continued*

Substrate (Metabolic Isoenzyme)	Enzyme Inducer/ Increased Elimination	Enzyme Inhibitor/ Decreased Elimination	Potential Clinical Consequences/Suggested Management	Alternative
Oxcarbazepine	Carbamazepine, phenytoin, phenobarbital, valproic acid		Decreased AUC 40%, 30%, 25%, 18%; adjust dosage accordingly.	—
Zonisamide (CYP3A4)		Fluoxetine,* fluvoxamine,* nefazodone*	Monitor clinically.	Citalopram
		Risperidone,* sertindole*	Monitor clinically.	Quetiapine
	Phenytoin, carbamazepine, phenobarbital		Monitor clinically; decrease in terminal half-life.	—
Antianxiety drugs				
Buspirone		Monoamine oxidase inhibitors	Avoid combination.	—
		Nefazodone, fluvoxamine	Use a low dosage of buspirone.	—
		Itraconazole, erythromycin	Use a low dosage of buspirone.	—
Antidepressants				
Amitriptyline, desipramine, doxepin, imipramine, nortriptyline, trazodone	Carbamazepine		Monitor clinical response.	—
Citalopram (CYP2C19, CYP3A4)	Carbamazepine, phenytoin,* phenobarbital,* felbamate*	Felbamate,* oxcarbazepine*	Monitor clinically.	—
Venlafaxine (CYP2D6)		Risperidone, clozapine,* sertindole*	Monitor clinical response.	—
		Fluoxetine, paroxetine,* sertraline*	Monitor clinical response.	—
Amitriptyline (CYP1A2)		Fluvoxamine, fluoxetine, paroxetine	—	—
Fluvoxamine, fluoxetine (CYP2D6)		Paroxetine*	Monitor for adverse effects.	—
		Risperidone	Monitor for adverse effects.	—
Paroxetine (CYP2D6)		Fluoxetine,* sertraline*	Monitor for adverse effects.	Citalopram, venlafaxine
Nefazodone (CYP3A4)	Carbamazepine,* phenytoin,* phenobarbital,* felbamate,* oxcarbazepine,* topiramate*		Monitor decreased clinical response.	—

Substrate (Metabolic Isoenzyme)	Enzyme Inducer/ Increased Elimination	Enzyme Inhibitor/ Decreased Elimination	Potential Clinical Consequences/Suggested Management	Alternative
		Fluvoxamine, fluoxetine*	Monitor for adverse effects.	—
Citalopram, sertraline, nefazodone (CYP3A4)		Erythromycin, clarithromycin	Monitor for adverse effects.	Azithromycin
Desipramine, amitriptyline, doxepin, imipramine, nortriptyline		Paroxetine, fluoxetine, fluvoxamine, citalopram, sertraline	Severe adverse effects; avoid concomitant use.	—
Nefazodone, sertraline, trazodone, desipramine		Indinavir, nelfinavir, ritonavir, saquinavir	Decrease initial dose 50%.	—
Antiemetics				
Dronabinol, ondansetron		Indinavir, nelfinavir, ritonavir, saquinavir	Decrease initial dose 50%.	—
Antifungal agents				
Ketoconazole		Ritonavir, indinavir, saquinavir	Ketoconazole levels increased threefold; indinavir increased 67%; saquinavir increased threefold; do not exceed 200 mg per day of ketoconazole.	—
Itraconazole, ketoconazole	Carbamazepine, phenobarbital, phenytoin		Therapeutic failures reported.	Fluconazole
	Rifampin		Consider dosage increase; poor clinical response reported.	Fluconazole
Antihistamines				
Loratadine		Indinavir, ritonavir, saquinavir, amprenavir	Decrease initial loratadine dose 50%; therapeutic monitoring; no cardiac side effects reported.	Cetirizine
Antipsychotics				
Haloperidol		Lithium	Monitor adverse effects.	—
	Carbamazepine, phenytoin, phenobarbital		Monitor for increased or decreased effect.	—
		Fluoxetine, fluvoxamine, buspirone, nefazodone, paroxetine	Monitor clinically for adverse effects.	—
Sertindole (CYP3A4, CYP2D6)	Carbamazepine, phenytoin, phenobarbital,* felbamate,* topiramate,* oxcarbazepine*		Increased clearance; monitor for decreased effect.	—

Table 26-2. *Continued*

Substrate (Metabolic Isoenzyme)	Enzyme Inducer/ Increased Elimination	Enzyme Inhibitor/ Decreased Elimination	Potential Clinical Consequences/Suggested Management	Alternative
Olanzapine (CYP1A2)		Fluvoxamine	Decreased clearance; monitor for adverse effects.	—
	Carbamazepine, phenytoin, phenobarbital*		Increased clearance; monitor for decreased effect.	—
Clozapine (CYP1A2, CYP2D6, CYP3A4 [minor])	Carbamazepine, phenytoin, valproic acid, primidone, felbamate,* topiramate,* phenobarbital*		Increased clearance; monitor for decreased effect.	—
		Fluvoxamine, paroxetine, sertraline	—	—
		Ritonavir	Increased risk of agranulocytosis, electrocardiogram changes, and seizures.	—
Risperidone (CYP2D6, CYP3A4)	Carbamazepine, felbamate,* phenytoin,* phenobarbital,* oxcarbazepine*		Increased clearance; monitor clinically.	—
		Clozapine	Monitor clinically for adverse effects.	—
Quetiapine (CYP3A4, CYP2C19)	Carbamazepine, phenytoin, thioridazine, felbamate,* topiramat,* oxcarbazepine*	Felbamate,* oxcarbazepine*	Monitor for decreased or increased response.	—
Benzodiazepines				
Midazolam, triazolam, alprazolam		Itraconazole, ketoconazole	27-Fold increase in concentration with sedation; decreased psychomotor abilities.	Fluconazole
		Erythromycin	Decrease initial triazolam dose 50%; monitor for oversedation.	Azithromycin
Diazepam (CYP3A4)		Cimetidine	Some CNS effects documented.	Famotidine, nizatidine, ranitidine
Diazepam		Omeprazole	Monitor clinically.	Pantoprazole, lansoprazole, rabenazole
Diazepam, alprazolam, midazolam, triazolam (CYP3A4)		Fluoxetine, fluvoxamine, nefazodone	Decrease initial alprazolam dose by 50% and triazolam dose by 75%; monitor for oversedation.	Temazepam, lorazepam

Substrate (Metabolic Isoenzyme)	Enzyme Inducer/ Increased Elimination	Enzyme Inhibitor/ Decreased Elimination	Potential Clinical Consequences/Suggested Management	Alternative
Alprazolam, midazolam, triazolam		Indinavir, nelfinavir, ritonavir, saquinavir, efavirenz, delavirdine, amprenavir	Avoid concomitant use.	Temazepam, lorazepam
	Rifampin		Hypnotic effects substantially diminished; monitor and give higher initial doses of benzodiazepine.	—
Calcium channel blockers				
Felodipine	Carbamazepine		Decreased serum concentrations.	—
		Erythromycin	Monitor for adverse effects.	Azithromycin
Amlodipine, felodipine, nicardipine, nifedipine, nimodipine, nisoldipine, verapamil, diltiazem		Itraconazole, ketoconazole	Decrease initial calcium channel blocker dose 50%; monitor for adverse effects.	Azithromycin, fluconazole?
		Indinavir, nelfinavir, ritonavir, saquinavir	Monitor clinically for adverse effects.	—
Amlodipine, felodipine, nicardipine, nifedipine, nimodipine, verapamil, diltiazem	Rifampin, rifabutin		May need initial dose increase; monitor clinical effects; best documented with diltiazem, verapamil, and nifedipine.	—
Nifedipine, felodipine, verapamil	Phenobarbital		Bioavailability may be decreased.	—
Nifedipine, verapamil, diltiazem, nicardipine, felodipine		Cimetidine	Conflicting results; some reports of decreased blood pressure, heart rate.	Famotidine, nizatidine, ranitidine
Bepridil		Amprenavir, ritonavir	Avoid combination.	Other antiretrovirals
Gastrointestinal agents				
Cisapride (CYP3A4)		Grapefruit juice	Avoid >200 ml per day.	Orange juice, other juices
		Fluoxetine, fluvoxamine, nefazodone, sertraline	Avoid combination.	Paroxetine, venlafaxine
		Fluconazole, itraconazole, ketoconazole, miconazole IV	Avoid use.	Metoclopramide
		Metronidazole	Avoid combination.	Metoclopramide
		Clarithromycin, erythromycin	Avoid these combinations.	Metoclopramide,* azithromycin

Table 26-2. *Continued*

Substrate (Metabolic Isoenzyme)	Enzyme Inducer/ Increased Elimination	Enzyme Inhibitor/ Decreased Elimination	Potential Clinical Consequences/Suggested Management	Alternative
Cisapride		Indinavir, ritonavir saquinavir, nelfinavir, amprenavir, delavirdine, efavirenz	Avoid these combinations.	Metoclopra-mide
Hepatic hydroxyme-thylglutaryl coen-zyme A reductase inhibitors				
Lovastatin, atorvasta-tin, pravastatin, sim-vastatin, cerivastatin (CYP3A4)		Nefazodone	Monitor for adverse effects.	—
		Erythromycin, clarithromycin	Monitor for myopathy; most common with lova-statin.	Azithromycin
Simvastatin, lovastatin, atorvastatin (CYP3A4)		Itraconazole, ketoconazole	Monitor for myopathy.	Fluvastatin, pra-vastatin, cerivastatin
Lovastatin, simvastatin		Indinavir, nelfi-navir, ritonavir, saquinavir, amprenavir, delavirdine	Avoid use.	Pravastatin, flu-vastatin, cerivastatin, atorvastatin
Fluvastatin (CYP2C9)	Phenytoin		—	—
Fluvastatin (CYP2C9)	Rifampin		Monitor.	Simvastatin, lova-statin, ator-vastatin
Pravastatin (CYP3A4)		Cyclosporin	Increased bioavailability due to decrease in first-pass metabolism; reduce pravastatin dosage.	—
Immunosuppressants				
		Synercid	Increased AUC; monitor for adverse effects.	—
Cyclosporine tacroli-mus (CYP3A4)	Rifampin		May need initial dose increase; monitor serum concentrations.	—
		Amiodarone	Decrease clearance by 50%; monitor serum concentrations.	—
		Erythromycin, clarithromycin	Avoid combination or reduce dosage by 50%; can see within 2 days; monitor trough concen-tration 2–3 times per week.	Azithromycin

Substrate (Metabolic Isoenzyme)	Enzyme Inducer/ Increased Elimination	Enzyme Inhibitor/ Decreased Elimination	Potential Clinical Consequences/Suggested Management	Alternative
Cyclosporine tacrolimus (CYP3A4)		Fluconazole, itraconazole, ketoconazole	Consider 50% dosage reduction when starting azole; monitor trough concentration more carefully.	—
		Nicardipine, nifedipine, diltiazem, verapamil	Monitor trough concentration.	Amlodipines
		Methylprednisolone	Competitive metabolism; monitor trough concentration.	—
	Carbamazepine, phenobarbital, phenytoin		—	Gabapentin, lamotrigine, topiramate, valproate
		Oral contraceptives	Not well documented; may need dosage decrease; monitor trough concentration.	—
Miscellaneous Theophylline (CYP1A2)		Fluvoxamine	Monitor serum concentrations.	Paroxetine, citalopram, sertraline
	Carbamazepine, phenobarbital, phenytoin		Monitor serum concentrations; can see within a couple of days	Gabapentin, lamotrigine, topiramate, valproate
		Clarithromycin, erythromycin, ciprofloxacin	Increased serum concentrations; monitor.	Azithromycin, gatifloxacin, levofloxacin
	Ritonavir		Increased glucuronyl transferase; 40% decrease in AUC of theophylline; monitor serum concentrations.	—
Oral contraceptives	Benzodiazepines		Use alternative contraception for short courses; for long courses use higher dosages.	Medroxyprogesterone acetate
Oral contraceptives (CYP3A4)	Rifampin, rifabutin		Use alternative contraception or increase estradiol dosage.	—
	Carbamazepine, ethosuximide, phenobarbital, phenytoin, primidone, topiramate?, felbamate		40% reduction in serum levels; monitor for breakthrough bleeding; alternative contraception (e.g., medroxyprogesterone) desirable.	Gabapentin, lamotrigine, topiramate, valproate

Table 26-2. *Continued*

Substrate (Metabolic Isoenzyme)	Enzyme Inducer/ Increased Elimination	Enzyme Inhibitor/ Decreased Elimination	Potential Clinical Consequences/Suggested Management	Alternative
	Ritonavir, efavirenz		Decrease AUC (40%) of ethinyl estradiol.	Increase estradiol or alternative contraceptive agent
		Indinavir	Increase in ethinylestradiol 24%, 37%.	—
Protease inhibitors Indinavir, nelfinavir, ritonavir, saquinavir, amprenavir	Rifabutin, rifampin		40% decrease in saquinavir AUC with rifabutin and 80% decrease with rifampin; rifampin decreases ritonavir AUC 35%; 82% decrease with nelfinavir; may need dosage increase.	—
	Carbamazepine, phenobarbital, phenytoin		Use cautiously; monitor serum concentrations.	Gabapentin, lamotrigine, topiramate, valproate
		Nefazodone, fluvoxamine, fluoxetine	Potential for increased concentrations based on inhibition of P-450 enzymes.	Use antipsychotic without CYP3A4 inhibition
Indinavir		Clarithromycin, erythromycin	Increases AUC 30%.	Azithromycin
Indinavir, saquinavir		Ketoconazole	Ketoconazole increases AUC by 150%; with ketoconazole, decrease initial indinavir dose to 600 mg q8h; decrease saquinavir dosage if ketoconazole dosage is >200 mg per day.	—
Nelfinavir		Indinavir	AUC increased 83%.	—
Indinavir		Nelfinavir	AUC increased 53%.	—
Saquinavir		Nelfinavir	AUC increased 393%.	—
Nelfinavir		Ritonavir	AUC increased 152%.	—
Saquinavir		Ritonavir	Increases concentration by 18-fold to improve saquinavir absorption.	—

AUC = area under the concentration curve; CNS = central nervous system; INR = international normalized ratio.
*Potential interaction based on metabolism.
Source: Modified from references 1, 2, 10–12, 17, 18, 37–39, 52, 58, 69, 71, 78, 79, 101–106, 119, 123, 124.

actions occur with phenobarbital, because each elimination pathway is responsible for no more than 20% of its clearance, and only drugs affecting more than one pathway are likely to produce clinically relevant effects.[2] The metabolism of felbamate appears to be contradictory in terms of the role of CYP34A. The clearance of felbamate can be increased with inducers of the CYP34A isoenzyme, but CYP34A inhibitors have little effect on its pharmacokinetics. This is because, under normal conditions, the metabolic pathway is relatively minor. However, it is capable of being induced, leading to clinically significant effects on felbamate's clearance.[14] Additionally, a drug may inhibit or induce the activity of a specific isoenzyme, even though it is not a substrate or metabolized by that particular isoenzyme. As an example, phenytoin, despite being a potent inducer of CYP34A, is not metabolized by this isoenzyme but rather by CYP2C9.[15]

Some of the most important factors involved in drug biotransformation include age, nutrition, stress, hepatic disease, and genetic polymorphisms.[11] Genetic polymorphism is a functional expression of some CYP450 isoenzymes (i.e., CYP2D and CYP2C) that can contribute to marked interpatient variability in drug metabolism and lead to significant drug interactions.[11] Individuals can be characterized as extensive (rapid) or poor (slow) metabolizers. Poor metabolizers are at risk for drug accumulation and toxicity. The CYP2D6, for example, occurs in a relatively inactive form in 5–10% of white persons and in 1–3% of Asians and black persons.[16] The wild type CYP2C19 gene is absent in 2–6% of white populations and up to 20% of Asian populations.[16] Therefore, poor metabolizers might experience adverse events that result from high concentrations of drugs that are metabolized by these pathways, including many of the psychoactive drugs that are metabolized via both CYP2D6 and CYP2C19.

Because of the anatomic relationship of the liver to the gastrointestinal tract and the systemic circulation, metabolism of an orally administered drug can occur before it reaches the systemic circulation. This is referred to as *first-pass metabolism*. The efficiency with which the liver removes a drug is referred to as the *extraction ratio*. Drugs with a low hepatic extraction (low extraction ratio) tend to be more available to the systemic circulation, whereas drugs that are efficiently removed by the liver (high extraction ratio) have a low bioavailability after oral administration.

For enzyme induction and enzyme inhibition, systemic clearance of low extraction ratio drugs (e.g., phenytoin and phenobarbital) is generally affected to a greater extent than that of high extraction ratio drugs (e.g., morphine), because the clearance of high extraction ratio drugs depends on hepatic blood flow, not the intrinsic clearance of the liver. However, the bioavailability of a high extraction ratio drug is affected by enzyme induction or enzyme inhibition due to alterations in first-pass metabolism.[11] As a result, drugs that induce the CYP450 enzyme, such as phenytoin, should be avoided in patients who take a drug that undergoes extensive first-pass metabolism, such as saquinavir, which can lead to a decreased bioavailability and subsequent therapeutic failure.[17]

Therapeutic Implications of Drug Metabolism

Many known inhibitors or inducers of metabolism are of uncertain clinical relevance. However, particular attention must be paid to specific drugs or drug classes that are strong inducers or inhibitors of other drugs. Specific drug classes that deserve mention because they are potent inhibitors and have been associated with clinically relevant interactions include specific anticonvulsants, antifungal agents, antibiotics, protease inhibitors, cardiovascular drugs, psychopharmacologic agents, and gastrointestinal agents. Specific drugs, such as rifampin, isoniazid, carbamazepine, phenytoin, and phenobarbital, are examples of strong inducers of hepatic metabolism. Some drug classes are relatively homogeneous, and all members of the class interact with other drugs in essentially the same way. However, for most drug classes, pharmacokinetic differences can result in differing interaction patterns for individual members of the same class. Therefore, as some of the most notable drug classes for altering drug metabolism are discussed, note the differences in the propensity for one drug to cause an interaction relative to another.

Antiepileptic Drugs and Their Effects on Other Antiepileptic Drugs and Classes of Drugs

Clinically significant drug interactions that involve hepatic metabolism are observed with all the AEDs except gabapentin, levetiracetam, and tiagabine (Table 26-3). Of the AEDs, phenobarbital, phenytoin, and carbamazepine are strong inducers of the

Table 26-3. Effects of Antiepileptic Drugs on Metabolic Drug Processes and Their Corresponding Antiepileptic Drugs

Drug	Protein Binding (%)	Metabolic System Affected	Enzyme Mechanism	Drugs Affected
Felbamate (FLB)	22–36	CYP2C19	Inhibitor	Phenytoin (PHT), phenobarbital (PB)
		CYP3A4	Inducer	Carbamazepine (CBZ)
		β-Oxidation	Inhibitor[a]	Valproic acid (VPA)
Lamotrigine (Lm)	55	Glucuronidation	Weak inducer	VPA
		Epoxide-hydrolase	Inhibitor	CBZ[b]
Gabapentin (Gaba)	0	None	None	None
Oxcarbazepine (OX)	40	CYP2C19	Inhibitor[a]	PHT
		Glucuronidation	Inducer	Lm
Tiagabine (Tgb)	96	None	None	None
Vigabatrin (VIG)	0	Unknown	Unknown	PHT
Topiramate (TOP)	15	CYP2C19	Inhibitor[a]	PHT
		β-Oxidation	Inducer	VPA[b]
Phenytoin	90	CYP2C9	Inducer	PB, TOP
		CYP3A4	Inducer	CBZ, FLB, Tgb, Zonisamide (Zon), Ethosuximide (Eth), Oxcarbazine (OX)-MHD
		Glucuronidation	Inducer	VPA, Lm
Carbamazepine	75	CYP3A4	Inducer	PB, FLB, Tgb, OX-MHD, Zon, Eth
		CYP2C	Inducer	PHT,TOP
		Glucuronidation	Inducer	VPA, Lm
Phenobarbital	40–60	CYP2C9	Inducer	PHT
		CYP34A	Inducer	OX-MHD, Zon, CBZ
		Glucuronidation	Inducer	Tgb, FLB, Eth VPA, Lm
Valproic acid	80–90	CYP2C9	Protein binding	PHT
		CYP2C19	Displace/inhibitor	Eth
		Glucuronidation	Competition	Lm
Levetiracetam (Le)	<10	None	None	None
Zonisamide	40	None	None	None
Ethosuximide	0	None	None	None

[a]Dose related.
[b]Pharmacodynamic interaction.
Source: Modified from references 1, 10–12, 14, 18, 26, 37, 108–118, 120.

P-450 enzyme system and therefore are involved in many drug interactions. Phenytoin, as well as carbamazepine and phenobarbital, increases the metabolism of drugs that are metabolized by the CYP2C9 and CYP3A subfamilies and UGT enzymes.[2]

In addition to inducing the same isoenzymes as phenobarbital and phenytoin, carbamazepine induces its own metabolism via CYP3A4 catalyzed metabolism to carbamazepine-10,11-epoxide (CBZ-E).

CBZ-E is pharmacologically active and contributes to the therapeutic effects of carbamazepine as well as to its systemic toxicity and neurotoxicity. Patients who receive co-medications with enzyme-inducing agents, such as phenobarbital and phenytoin, have an increased ratio of CBZ-E to carbamazepine in the plasma because of the CYP3A4-mediated conversion of carbamazepine to the epoxide metabolite.[18–20] This interaction has also been demonstrated with concurrent use of carbamazepine with felbamate or valproic acid, with a 50% increase in the epoxide metabolite of carbamazepine.[21,22] Therefore, one should also consider the effects on the active metabolite of carbamazepine when other enzyme-inducing agents are administered concurrently. Maximal induction or deinduction occurs approximately 1–2 weeks after initiation or removal of drug therapy but depends on the drugs' half-lives.

Although phenytoin and phenobarbital induce hepatic metabolism, competition at the site of metabolism can occur with other drugs metabolized by the same isoenzyme. Because phenytoin and phenobarbital are metabolized by the same isoenzyme, the combined use of phenytoin and phenobarbital may have a variable response. Individually, phenytoin and phenobarbital accelerate the elimination of carbamazepine, probably by stimulating the CYP3A4 isoenzyme, resulting in a significant reduction in carbamazepine concentrations.[18] However, adding phenobarbital to the dosage of patients stabilized on a combination of carbamazepine and phenytoin is of little consequence, because the metabolism of carbamazepine is maximally induced.[23]

Certain drugs can affect the metabolism of some drugs in one way and affect other drugs in the opposite direction. For example, when carbamazepine and phenytoin are given concurrently, the serum concentrations of both drugs can often be affected in opposite directions. The simultaneous effect of inhibition of phenytoin metabolism by carbamazepine and induction of carbamazepine metabolism by phenytoin can result in toxicity of phenytoin and subtherapeutic levels of carbamazepine.[19,24,25]

Plasma concentrations of felbamate are increased during co-administration with valproic acid and decreased with phenytoin and carbamazepine.[26] Furthermore, plasma concentrations of phenytoin, phenobarbital, and valproic acid are increased during co-administration with felbamate, whereas those of carbamazepine are decreased and those of CBZ-E are increased.[26–28]

Some AEDs may be the affected drug or the cause of a drug interaction, depending on which metabolic pathway controls the elimination of the drug. For example, after the addition of erythromycin, carbamazepine serum concentrations are elevated owing to inhibition of its hepatic metabolism by the isoenzyme CYP3A4. However, the erythromycin serum concentrations are decreased owing to the enhancement of erythromycin's metabolism via CYP3A4 induction by carbamazepine. In contrast, patients on 3,000 mg of felbamate per day reported no changes in plasma concentrations when 333 mg of erythromycin 3 times a day for 10 days was added.[29] This lack of drug interaction may be explained by felbamate's metabolic pathway, which is controlled by CYP3A4 and represents less than 20% of the clearance.[14] Because tiagabine is extensively metabolized by the CYP3A pathway, its metabolism is inhibited (demonstrated in vitro) by CYP3A inhibitors, such as erythromycin.[30]

Some AEDs, such as valproic acid, affect the hepatic metabolism of the P-450 enzyme system but also affect protein binding, glucuronyl transferases, and epoxide hydrolase. Valproate does not inhibit cyclosporin or oral contraceptives, suggesting a lack of inhibition of CYP34A-metabolized drugs. However, the glucuronide conjugation of lamotrigine and zidovudine is inhibited by valproate, as are the protein binding alterations of phenytoin.[2,31]

Some AEDs have the advantage of minor or no interference with the metabolism of other drugs, as is the case for gabapentin, lamotrigine, tiagabine, levetiracetam, and vigabatrin.[32] Although lamotrigine and tiagabine are drugs that do not interfere with the metabolism of many drugs, they are strongly induced or inhibited by other AEDs.

Oral Contraceptives

Breakthrough bleeding and unintended pregnancies due to drug interactions between AEDs and oral contraceptives can occur.[11] Clinically significant drug interactions with oral contraceptives occur secondary to CYP34A isoenzyme induction with phenytoin, carbamazepine, phenobarbital, and other enzyme inducers of this P-450 system. With these interactions, a higher dose of oral contraceptive, alternative AEDs (e.g., gabapentin and lamotrigine), or a nonhormonal alternative method of contraception is recommended.

Warfarin

Clinically used warfarin is a racemic mixture with the S-isomer primarily responsible for pharmacologic activity. The anticoagulant activity of the S-warfarin is mediated by CYP2C9 hepatic metabolism, whereas the formation of R-10-hydroxy warfarin is mediated by CYP34A. AEDs, including phenobarbital, carbamazepine, and phenytoin, can induce the metabolism of warfarin, leading to a reduction in prothrombin time.[33] Because warfarin and phenytoin are CYP2C9 substrates, competitive inhibition of warfarin metabolism can occur, whereas decreased warfarin concentrations are the result of hepatic enzyme induction and an alteration in protein binding.[34] Thus, one may observe an initial increase in the effect of S-warfarin, the pharmacologically active component, followed by a decline in plasma concentration over 1–2 weeks after phenytoin is added, which indicates a biphasic interaction with sustained induction of CYP2C9 metabolism. The management of patients should be an initial decrease in the warfarin dose followed by an increase in the warfarin dose as indicated by the international normalized ratio (INR) to maintain the anticoagulant effect desired.[2] The INR should be closely monitored when warfarin is used concomitantly with AEDs that induce CYP2C9.

Cyclosporin

The major pathway for elimination of cyclosporin involves hydroxylation and demethylation by the CYP3A family of enzymes, and interference with the oxidative metabolism of this drug is clinically significant because of its narrow therapeutic range and concentration-dependent efficacy. Any interaction that changes the cyclosporin concentration is of potential clinical importance, as it may lead to transplant organ rejection or nephrotoxicity. Phenytoin, carbamazepine, and phenobarbital can affect the pharmacokinetics of cyclosporin.[35] Alternative AEDs that do not affect cyclosporin levels include gabapentin, lamotrigine, topiramate, and valproate.

Psychopharmacologic Agents

With the increasing use of psychotropic drugs in the treatment of psychiatric disorders associated with epilepsy, potential drug interactions exist, because both of these classes of drugs, psychotropic agents and antiepileptics, are primarily metabolized by the P-450 microsomal enzyme system, with some antiepileptic agents (e.g., carbamazepine, phenytoin, phenobarbital, felbamate) acting as inducers of metabolism and some psychotropics (particularly selective serotonin reuptake inhibitors [SSRIs]) inhibiting metabolism of AEDs.[36]

Interactions between Selective Serotonin Reuptake Inhibitors and Antiepileptic Drugs

From the data presented in Table 26-4, it appears that the potential for an individual SSRI to inhibit the metabolism of an AED is greatest for fluvoxamine, fluoxetine, and nefazodone (a weak SSRI) and least for sertraline, paroxetine, and citalopram. In vivo, the SSRIs fluoxetine and fluvoxamine are common in their ability to inhibit CYPIA2, CYP2C19, and CYP3A4 isoenzymes. The better-recognized CYPIA2 inhibitor fluvoxamine, however, exhibits moderate CYP2C enzyme-inhibitory effects, similar to fluoxetine, that can result in phenytoin toxicity.[1,37] On the basis of in vitro studies, the rank order, from greatest to least, of potency for inhibition of CYP3A4 is nefazodone, fluvoxamine, fluoxetine, paroxetine, and sertraline, which can result in clinically meaningful increases in blood levels of AEDs that are metabolized via this enzyme system. Nefazodone's effects on CYP1A, CYP2C19, and CYP2D6 are not clinically significant.[38] However, paroxetine and fluoxetine are equipotent inhibitors of CYP2D6, whereas sertraline has less pronounced inhibition, and fluvoxamine is almost devoid of inhibitor effects on this isoenzyme.[38–40] On this basis, the concomitant administration of the SSRIs fluvoxamine and fluoxetine with carbamazepine have the potential to increase plasma concentrations of carbamazepine, leading to adverse effects. Case reports have shown variable effects on carbamazepine serum concentrations or its metabolite, ranging from no effect to a 70% increase when fluvoxamine was co-administered.[39,41] Similar to fluvoxamine, fluoxetine either increased carbamazepine's serum concentrations or had no effect.[41–43] In contrast, neither sertraline nor paroxetine altered carbamazepine concentration, indicating their lack of effect on CYP34A.[44,45] The better-recognized IA2 inhibitor flu-

Table 26-4. Potential Interactions of Antidepressant Medications with Antiepileptic Medications

Relative Rank	CYP1A*	CYP2C*	CYP2D6*	CYP3A*
High	Fluvoxamine	Fluvoxamine Fluoxetine	Paroxetine Fluoxetine	Nefazodone
Moderate		Sertraline	Secondary tricyclic antidepressant	Fluvoxamine Fluoxetine (metabolite)
Low to minimal	Fluoxetine Bupropion Sertraline Paroxetine Citalopram Nefazodone Venlafaxine	Venlafaxine Paroxetine Nefazodone	Sertraline Fluvoxamine Citalopram (metabolite) Bupropion Nefazodone Venlafaxine	Fluoxetine Paroxetine Sertraline
Substrates	Carbamazepine (minor)	Phenytoin Phenobarbital		Carbamazepine Tiagabine Felbamate Zonisamide Ethosuximide

*Selective serotonin reuptake inhibitors listed in descending order of magnitude.
Source: Modified from references 2, 11, 37–39, 44, 107, 121, 122.

voxamine, however, exhibits moderate CYP2C enzyme-inhibitory effects similar to fluoxetine that can result in phenytoin toxicity. Symptoms of toxicity, including nausea and ataxia, have been reported with patients receiving fluvoxamine and concomitant phenytoin.[39] Case reports involving patients on phenytoin reported a 67–309% increase in serum concentration with the addition of inhibitor fluoxetine.[46,47] In several case reports, fluoxetine also increased valproic acid levels to the toxic range.[48,49] Paroxetine does not appear to significantly affect the metabolism of carbamazepine, valproic acid, or phenytoin.[45] In conclusion, it is likely that fluoxetine and fluvoxamine will affect AED serum concentrations to a greater extent than paroxetine, sertraline, or citalopram because of the pathways used.

There is little data describing the effects of AEDs on SSRIs. There is evidence that phenobarbital and phenytoin may cause a 25% decrease in plasma concentrations of paroxetine,[45] whereas valproic acid may increase plasma paroxetine concentrations. However, these pharmacokinetic alterations were not associated with any observable clinical effects. Because fluoxetine and sertraline are substrates of the isoenzyme CYP3A4, there is a theoretical poten-

tial for phenytoin and carbamazepine to affect these drugs' serum concentrations.

Interactions between Antiepileptic Drugs and Antipsychotics

Because of the metabolic induction caused by many AEDs, notably carbamazepine, phenytoin, and phenobarbital, there is generally an increase in the clearance rate of many of these antipsychotic medications, which leads to clinical failure.[50] The principal isoenzymes of significance with antipsychotics are CYP2D6, CYP3A4, and CYP1A2. Potential drug interactions of clinical significance that affect the clearance of antipsychotic agents might result at the CYP2D6 and CYP3A4 systems for sertindole, at CYP1A2 and CYP3A4 for clozapine, at CYP1A2 for olanzapine, at CYP3A4 for risperidone, at CYP3A4 and CYP2D6 for quetiapine, and at CYP2D6 for haloperidol.[51,52] In the presence of multiple metabolic pathways, the chance that an inducer or inhibitor may cause significant effects is reduced, because the alternate pathway can often compensate for the alterations in the primary pathway. For instance, because sertindole is metabolized by CYP2D6 and CYP34A, inhibition of the primary pathway should not cause the same degree of toxicity that would occur if a drug had only one pathway of metabolism. However, those patients who are genotypic poor metabolizers at CYP2D6 might demonstrate an increased risk of a drug interaction when taking sertindole and quetiapine.[51]

In the presence of carbamazepine, phenytoin, or phenobarbital, doses of sertindole, clozapine, olanzapine, quetiapine, risperidone, and haloperidol may require up to a 50% increase in dose. Valproic acid has been shown to either increase or decrease clozapine levels.[53,54]

Data on the effects of the new antipsychotics on AEDs are lacking. Because most of the AEDs are not substrates of CYP2D6, there is a low potential for any drug interactions.[50,51] In contrast, the potential exists for a drug interaction between clozapine, a CYP2C19 inhibitor; risperidone, a CYP3A4 inhibitor; phenytoin; and carbamazepine, respectively.[51]

Interactions between Antiepileptic Drugs and Benzodiazepines

Benzodiazepines are a large class of drugs that are used in the treatment of epilepsy as adjunctive therapy. In particular, diazepam, lorazepam, and midazolam are used for acute seizures, whereas clonazepam and clobazam are used for adjunctive chronic antiepileptic therapy.[2]

In general, benzodiazepines exhibit a low capacity to alter the disposition of the majority of AEDs.[2] However, because both diazepam and phenytoin are metabolized by the CYP2C19 isoenzyme system, competition for this pathway may cause a change in the pharmacokinetics of both drugs. Diazepam has been shown to inhibit the metabolism of phenytoin, leading to increased serum concentrations.[55] Additionally, reports of serum concentrations of phenytoin after the initiation of clonazepam have been variable; some show a doubling in serum concentration as well as a 50% decrease in serum concentration of phenytoin.[56] Therefore, monitoring plasma phenytoin concentrations may facilitate dose adjustments if an interaction with a benzodiazepine has occurred.

In contrast, because benzodiazepines are primarily metabolized by the CYP isoenzyme system and are highly protein bound, interactions are expected with enzyme inducers and inhibitors. Carbamazepine induces the metabolism of alprazolam, resulting in a marked lowering in its plasma concentrations.[57] Because felbamate and topiramate are inhibitors of CYP2C19, a reduction of diazepam clearance by these two drugs is expected.[2] Monitoring of plasma concentrations of AEDs and clinical signs and symptoms of toxicity aids in the evaluation of a potential drug interaction between these two pharmacologic classes.

Interactions between Antiepileptic Drugs and Antidepressants

Anticonvulsant drugs, including carbamazepine, phenytoin, and phenobarbital, may increase the rate of tricyclic antidepressant metabolism, thereby decreasing the antidepressant effect.[58] A 60% reduction in nortriptyline levels that required a doubling of the nortriptyline dose to achieve therapeutic levels was reported after the addition of carbamazepine.[59,60] In addition, lower desipramine, amitriptyline, nortriptyline, protriptyline, imipramine, and clomipramine levels have been reported with co-administration of these anticonvulsants.[44,60-62]

In contrast, the tricyclic antidepressants have been shown to have an inhibitory effect on the elimination of some AEDs. Phenytoin levels were reported to be increased with the use of nortriptyline, imipramine, and trazodone.[44,63]

Some anecdotal reports have indicated that chlorpromazine, prochlorperazine, and thioridazine may cause increased phenytoin concentrations.[1] However, most patients tolerate the combination of the two drug classes.

Selective Serotonin Reuptake Inhibitors and Their Effects on Benzodiazepines

Benzodiazepines are frequently administered to patients with psychiatric disorders, including those receiving long-term antidepressant therapy; therefore, the potential for drug interactions between SSRIs and benzodiazepines is an important clinical concern (Table 26-5).

Table 26-5. Likelihood That Select Antidepressants May Interact with P-450 Substrates

Relative Likelihood	Antidepressant (Substrate)	Clinically Significant Substrate Interactions
Most	Fluvoxamine (CYP1A2, CYP2D6)	CYP1A2 > CYP2C19/C9 > CYP3A4 >> 2D6
	Fluoxetine (CYP2C9, CYP2D6)	CYP2D6 >> CYP2C9/2C19 >> CYP3A4
	Paroxetine (CYP2D6)	CYP2D6 >> CYP1A2 = CYP34A = CYP2C9/2C19
	Nefazodone (CYP34A)	CYP3A4
Less	Sertraline (CYP2D6, CYP34A)	CYP2C19/2C9 > CYP2D = CYP1A2 = CYP34A
Least	Venlafaxine (CYP2D6)	2D6 (weak)

Source: Adapted from references 37–40, 122.

Fluoxetine is a potent inhibitor of the many isoenzymes and, through inhibition, increases serum concentrations of many benzodiazepines, except lorazepam and oxazepam, which are not metabolized by the P-450 enzyme system. The half-life of fluoxetine and its active metabolite, norfluoxetine, further increases its impact on drug metabolism.

Alprazolam, midazolam, temazepam, and triazolam are among the currently known substrates of CYP3A4, whereas diazepam is a substrate of CYP3A4, CYP1A2, and CYP2C19.[11] Pharmacokinetic studies with diazepam and alprazolam demonstrated increased serum concentrations when given with fluoxetine as well as with fluvoxamine. In a study of eight healthy volunteers, the clearance of diazepam was reduced by 65%, with a prolongation in diazepam half-life (51–118 hours), leading to an increase in the area under the curve (AUC) from 70% to 390% after the initiation of fluvoxamine.[64] Additionally, 100 mg per day of fluvoxamine produced a twofold increase in alprazolam plasma concentrations.[11] Co-administration of 60 mg of fluoxetine for 8 days produced a 40% increase in the diazepam AUC, also indicating that fluoxetine inhibits the metabolism of diazepam.[65] However, the drug interaction was minor, because psychomotor responses were unaffected, demonstrating the low inhibitory effect of fluoxetine on CYP34A and the possibility of an alternate pathway's being used.[65] In another study, fluoxetine only resulted in a 25% decrease in the clearance of alprazolam, but because of fluoxetine's active metabolite, norfluoxetine, the effects of alprazolam persisted for weeks after the discontinuation of the offending drug.[66] In the same study, fluoxetine did not alter the clearance of clonazepam.

In contrast to fluoxetine's inhibition of the metabolism of diazepam, the results of a study conducted in healthy male volunteers demonstrated that sertraline at maximum recommended doses is unlikely to exert significant inhibitory effects on the CYP2C19 and CYP34A isoenzymes responsible for diazepam's metabolism.[67] Although not an SSRI but an atypical antidepressant, nefazodone was shown to increase alprazolam and triazolam serum concentrations twofold and induce clinical adverse effects, but it had no effect on lorazepam.[68] Because of the frequent coprescription of benzodiazepines and SSRIs, it is recommended that a nonoxidized benzodiazepine, such as lorazepam or oxazepam, be used when there is uncertainty of a drug interaction.

Selective Serotonin Reuptake Inhibitors and Warfarin

Although the R-isomer of warfarin is less pharmacologically active, significant drug interactions involving the CYP3A4 and CYP1A2 isoenzyme systems have resulted from inhibition of its metabolism. Fluvoxamine, sertraline, and paroxetine can increase prothrombin time with reports of bleeding.[38,39] The effect of sertraline on warfarin, however, is modest even with high doses.[41] Nonetheless, the manufacturer of sertraline suggests careful monitoring of the prothrombin time in patients who take warfarin concomitantly with this SSRI.

Health care professionals must assess drug combinations on a case-by-case basis when using psychiatric medications. Vigilant pharmacodynamic monitoring should accompany therapy with these agents, especially SSRIs, to avoid adverse events and minimize the clinical impact of potential drug interactions (see Table 26-5).

Antifungal Agents and Their Effects on Other Classes of Drugs

All of the azole antifungal agents are inhibitors of the CYP enzymes, particularly CYP3A4 and CYP2C9, albeit with different potencies.[69] Ketoconazole and itraconazole are selective and highly potent inhibitors of CYP3A activity, whereas the potency of fluconazole as a CYP3A inhibitor is much lower and generally observed only with dosages of greater than or equal to 200 mg per day. Therefore, these agents may produce clinically significant interactions with specific anticonvulsants, benzodiazepines, hepatic hydroxymethylglutaryl coenzyme A (HMGCoA) reductase inhibitors, cyclosporin, and warfarin.

The interactions between azole antifungal agents and AEDs, such as carbamazepine and phenytoin, may be complicated by their bidirectional nature, because phenytoin and carbamazepine induce hepatic oxidative drug metabolism. In agreement with in vivo findings that CYP2C9 metabolism is affected by fluconazole, doses of fluconazole greater than or equal to 200 mg per day increase phenytoin serum concentrations by an average of 130%, indicating a significant impairment of phenytoin's clearance.[70,71] In contrast, ketoconazole, a relatively specific inhibitor of CYP34A, does not appear to affect phenytoin pharmacokinetics but does increase carbamazepine plasma concentration by 29% with no effect on the epoxide metabolite.[70-72] This is consistent with CYP34A's being the primary enzyme responsible for carbamazepine metabolism. Although itraconazole does not significantly decrease in phenytoin clearance, this combination should be avoided, because phenytoin-induced drug metabolism decreases the AUC of itraconazole by 10-fold.[73]

Ketoconazole and itraconazole are potentially hazardous when combined with benzodiazepines, such as triazolam, midazolam, and, to a lesser extent, alprazolam. Pharmacokinetic interactions of triazolam and midazolam with fluconazole are of smaller magnitude as is expected by its less potent effect on the CYP3A isoform.[69]

HMGCoA reductase inhibitors have been associated with myalgia and myopathy to severe rhab-domyolysis that may be associated with high serum concentrations of the parent drug or its metabolite.[4] These effects most frequently occur when HMG-CoA reductase inhibitors are combined with CYP34A isoenzyme inhibitors or drugs that compete for their metabolism. CYP3A4 plays a major role in the metabolism of lovastatin, simvastatin, atorvastatin, and cerivastatin, and CYP2C9 is responsible for metabolizing fluvastatin. CYP3A4 is involved in a minor metabolic pathway for pravastatin.[4] The in vivo data indicate that itraconazole and possibly ketoconazole can significantly impair the clearance of simvastatin, lovastatin, and atorvastatin, whereas the pharmacokinetics of fluvastatin, pravastatin, and cerivastatin are largely unaffected.[69]

To avoid the risk of nephrotoxicity, the co-administration of ketoconazole with cyclosporin requires a dose reduction of cyclosporin by 70–80%.[69] The impact of fluconazole and itraconazole on cyclosporin pharmacokinetics remains controversial, and the clinical significance of such an interaction may vary between individuals.[69,74] The potent selective inhibition of CYP2C9 over CYP34A by fluconazole explains the pharmacokinetic interactions involving warfarin that can result in a clinically significant increase in INR.[69] The effects in humans of ketoconazole and itraconazole on the clearance of warfarin are unclear.[69]

Antibiotics and Their Effects on Other Classes of Drugs

Cotrimoxazole

Cotrimoxazole and warfarin can interact.[75] The interaction is reversed either by discontinuation of warfarin or reduction of dosage. The findings are consistent with CYP2C9's being primarily responsible for S-warfarin clearance and with inhibition by cotrimoxazole on the clearance of this CYP substrate. This interaction may be more pronounced with escalating doses, as is used in the treatment of *Pneumocystis carinii* pneumonia.

Macrolides

The macrolide antibacterials produce slow, reversible, noncompetitive inhibition of the CYP3A4 isoenzyme as well as the CYP1A2 isoenzyme. Interactions with macrolides are fairly well documented, with erythromycin and clarithromycin having the most effect. One report recommended that the dose of carbamazepine be reduced by 25% when beginning clarithromycin therapy, followed by further dose modification as suggested by clinical observation and drug monitoring.[75] The dose of drugs such as theophylline should be reduced, and serum concentrations should be monitored when initiating a macrolide antibiotic. Azithromycin is considered an alternative agent for patients with a suspected or documented mycobacterial infection. Daily erythromycin doses as low as 500 mg orally can increase trough cyclosporin concentrations within 24–72 hours.[35] The mechanism of this interaction probably involves enhanced oral absorption and impaired metabolism of cyclosporin.

Fluoroquinolones

The fluoroquinolones differ in their ability to inhibit CYP1A2 isoenzyme metabolism. Interactions with theophylline occur with several fluoroquinolones. The greatest effect has been seen with enoxacin, which reduced theophylline clearance by approximately 50–65% at high doses.[77] Ciprofloxacin reduces theophylline clearance by approximately 25%, although there is marked interindividual variation. Clinically significant interactions with ofloxacin, levofloxacin, and gatifloxacin are unusual, making them alternative agents.

Quinupristin or Dalfopristin (Synercid)

In vitro interaction studies have shown that Synercid significantly inhibits CYP3A4 metabolism of midazolam, nifedipine, and cyclosporin. After 2 days of therapy, Synercid increased cyclosporin AUC by 63% and T$^{1}/_{2}$ by 77%.[78] It is reasonable to expect that concomitant administration of Synercid and other drugs primarily metabolized by the CYP3A4 enzyme system (e.g., carbamazepine, diazepam) may result in increased plasma concentrations of these drugs and may lead to prolonged therapeutic or adverse effects.

Protease Inhibitors and Their Effects on Other Drugs

The pharmacokinetic or pharmacodynamic drug interactions involving protease inhibitors remain an important factor in their clinical use. The protease inhibitors are metabolized in the liver primarily by the isoenzyme CYP3A4. Thus, they are prone to significant drug interactions. Saquinavir, ritonavir, indinavir, and nelfinavir may act as substrates of cytochrome-mediated drug metabolism or as inhibitors of the CYP3A4 microsomal system.[11] Ritonavir is also a potent inhibitor and inducer of the CYP2D6 isoenzyme system and may also induce the CYP1A2, CYP2C9, and CYP2C19 isoenzymes.[11,17] When comparing these agents, ritonavir is a more potent inhibitor and indinavir a less potent and reversible inhibitor of the CYP3A4 isoenzyme.[79]

Ritonavir, a powerful inhibitor of the CYP450 metabolic pathway, can produce large increases in the plasma concentrations of various antiarrhythmic drugs (e.g., amiodarone, flecainide, and quinidine) and potentially lead to fatal cardiac arrhythmias.[17] Thus, use of these agents with ritonavir is contraindicated. Owing to the potential for oversedation with agents such as alprazolam, triazolam, and midazolam, concurrent administration with the protease inhibitors, especially ritonavir, should be avoided. Although not contraindicated, other agents metabolized by CYP3A4 isoenzyme (e.g., methadone, erythromycin, carbamazepine, fluoxetine, ketoconazole, lovastatin, simvastatin, and haloperidol) may require dosage modification and drug level monitoring when administered with ritonavir.

Despite indinavir's being a less-potent inhibitor of the CYP3A4 isoenzyme system, concomitant administration of indinavir affects the metabolism of some drugs, such as rifabutin, by increasing its AUC by 204%, requiring the rifabutin dose to be reduced by 50% when the two drugs are used concurrently.[79]

One of the most serious drug interactions caused by the inhibition of hepatic metabolism involves the concomitant use of cisapride and inhibitors of the CYP3A4 isoenzyme system. Combinations of cisapride and protease inhibitors of this isoenzyme system (e.g., ritonavir, indinavir, nelfinavir, and saquinavir) should be avoided to prevent serious cardiac arrhythmias.

The protease inhibitors can also inhibit the metabolism of other protease inhibitors. Administration of the combination of ritonavir and saquinavir can increase the peak plasma concentration of saquinavir by 18-fold.[80] The clinical usefulness of this combination is under further investigation.

The protease inhibitors may act as inhibitors of drug metabolism as well as substrates for drug metabolism that lead to clinically significant outcomes. The addition of the antifungal agent ketoconazole increases the AUCs of saquinavir (150%) and indinavir by inhibiting their hepatic metabolism.[17,79] Therefore, if a patient requires ketoconazole, the dose of the protease inhibitor should be reduced to avoid any adverse effects. Another major interaction of the protease inhibitors is with enzyme inducers, such as rifampin. Rifampin decreases the concentrations of saquinavir by 80% and ritonavir by 35%.[79] The clinical significance of this decrease in the protease inhibitor concentrations is unknown, but because resistance is associated with suboptimal plasma levels of these drugs, the consequences may be serious.[11]

Cardiovascular Drugs

The CYP34A isoenzyme plays a significant role in the metabolism of cardiac drugs, including quinidine, amiodarone, and the calcium antagonists. Hence, drug interactions may occur when cardiovascular agents are used with CYP3A4 inhibitors or inducers. The half-life of quinidine, for example, can be reduced by up to 50% by combining it with phenobarbital.[81,82] Rifampin increases the elimination rate of quinidine by nearly threefold while reducing its bioavailability by almost sixfold.[83] A frequent but often unnoticed drug interaction is the combination of an inducer with a high extraction ratio drug, such as verapamil, that is a substrate for the CYP3A4 isoenzyme. Rifampin decreases the bioavailability of verapamil significantly by increasing the first-pass metabolism, which leads to treatment failures that may not be seen with the administration of intravenous verapamil.[84] Therefore, during concurrent therapy with rifampin, patients with atrial arrhythmias may respond to intravenous verapamil, but oral administration may fail to prevent recurrences.[84]

Quinidine

Digoxin

Quinidine and amiodarone significantly increase serum digoxin concentrations and place the patient at a higher risk of digoxin toxicity. Quinidine approximately doubles serum digoxin concentrations in patients who receive both agents. The magnitude of this interaction depends on the concentration of quinidine—that is, the higher the dose of quinidine, the greater the increase in digoxin concentration.[81] Because quinidine decreases digoxin's volume of distribution, digoxin serum concentrations begin to rise within hours of quinidine administration, making an alteration in the loading dose of digoxin imperative when using concomitant quinidine. Quinidine also reduces the renal and nonrenal clearance of digoxin, resulting in an approximately 50% increase in digoxin serum concentrations when a new steady state is achieved in up to 5–7 days.

Amiodarone

Amiodarone increases the serum concentrations of several drugs, including quinidine, phenytoin, warfarin, procainamide, digoxin, and flecainide.[85-89] The major mechanism of amiodarone's drug interactions is inhibition of hepatic metabolism, but it can also affect the bioavailability, protein binding, and renal excretion of co-administered drugs.[85] In most cases, a 20–50% reduction in doses of the affected drugs is necessary to minimize the pharmacokinetic alterations caused by amiodarone.

Phenytoin. Phenytoin serum concentrations increase during co-administration of amiodarone secondary to hepatic microsomal inhibition,[87,89] not changes in serum protein binding.[87] A 25–50% reduction in the dose of phenytoin is recommended when amiodarone therapy is initiated. All changes in phenytoin regimens should be guided by monitoring serum phenytoin concentrations and clinical status. In addition, phenytoin induces the metabolism of amiodarone, a substrate of the CYP34A isoenzyme.[89] The clinical significance of this interaction remains uncertain.

Warfarin. Amiodarone enhances the anticoagulant effect of warfarin by direct and indirect mechanisms, including changes in protein binding, inhibition of hepatic metabolism (65%), and inhibition of vitamin K–dependent clotting factor synthesis.[33,85,86] Inhibition of warfarin hepatic metabolism which reduces the metabolic clearance of the S- and R-warfarin enantiomers in a dose-dependent manner.[86] Potentiation of warfarin effects occurs in the first 2 weeks of amiodarone therapy, with variable increases of prothrombin by 22–108%, and the warfarin requirement is lowered by 25–50%.[86] After discontinuation of amiodarone, its effect on prothrombin activity can persist for weeks or months as a result of its extensive tissue accumulation and slow elimination.[86] To minimize potential elevations in prothrombin time and bleeding complications associated with this drug interaction, the dose of warfarin should be reduced by 25–50% on initiation of amiodarone therapy. Weekly monitoring of INR should be performed initially for the first month and monthly thereafter.

Digoxin.   The amiodarone-digoxin interaction is similar to the digoxin-quinidine interaction.[85] Amiodarone reduces the renal and nonrenal clearance of digoxin, but it may also displace digoxin from tissue binding sites.[85] The drug interaction can be of clinical significance, because a doubling in digoxin steady-state serum concentrations is commonly seen.[90] Baseline digoxin serum concentration should be monitored on initiation of amiodarone and weekly until the digoxin serum concentration ceases to rise. Thereafter, digoxin concentrations should be repeated periodically because of the extended time necessary for amiodarone to reach a steady state, which could take up to 1 year.

Cyclosporin.   Introduction of amiodarone can cause a 30–50% increase in blood cyclosporin concentrations after the introduction of amiodarone.[91,92] Cyclosporin trough concentrations should be monitored closely on the initiation of amiodarone.

Gastrointestinal Drugs and Their Effects on Other Drugs

Cisapride

Cisapride can cause tachycardia, palpitations, and extrasystoles when combined with inhibitors of the isoenzyme CYP34A. Postulations about the cause of these cardiac aberrations include activation of serontonin-4 receptors on the myocardium and prolonged atrioventricular conduction due to cisapride's structural similarity to procainamide.[93] The first report of an arrhythmic drug interaction with cisapride was in a patient who received concomitant erythromycin.[94] The patient developed a prolonged Q-T interval with progression to polymorphic nonsustained ventricular tachycardia. Once the dosage of cisapride was reduced from 40 mg to 5 mg every 6 hours, the Q-T interval returned to baseline. Cisapride is not recommended for patients with a history of coronary disease and arrhythmia, renal insufficiency, and electrolyte imbalance or for patients on other medications that prolong Q-T interval (e.g., amiodarone) or isoenzyme inhibitors of CYP34A, such as macrolides, azole antifungals, antiretrovirals, or metronidazole. An alternative agent for these patients is metoclopramide. Because cisapride's profound drug interactions lead to serious adverse effects, it was removed from the market in July, 2000, and is available only through an investigational limited-access program.

Histamine 2 Antagonists

Of the current four H_2 blockers (ranitidine, famotidine, nizatidine, and cimetidine), cimetidine is the only one that significantly affects the metabolism of concurrent drugs. Cimetidine contains an imidazole ring that contributes to its inhibitory effects on CYP34A and CYP1A2 isoenzymes and its mild inhibitory effects on the CYPC29 isoenzyme.

Antiepileptic Drugs

Owing to the inhibition of the various isoenzymes, cimetidine potentially may inhibit the drug metabolism of carbamazepine or phenytoin, resulting in an increase in their plasma concentrations.[2,18] Although it may be difficult to detect, in patients with nonlinear pharmacokinetic metabolism of phenytoin, generally seen at higher serum levels, the risk of a drug interaction with cimetidine is increased. Therefore, patients who require an H_2 antagonist should be treated with a drug such as ranitidine, famotidine, or nizatidine, which is less likely to cause metabolic inhibition.

Theophylline

Probably the most notable drug interaction that occurs with cimetidine is with theophylline. Similar to phenytoin, theophylline demonstrates nonlinear pharmacokinetics at high serum concentrations, placing patients at risk for theophylline toxicity. It is therefore recommended that an initial dosage adjustment be considered in patients whose baseline theophylline level is greater than 12 mg/liter or who change to another H_2 antagonist.

Proton Pump Inhibitors

Omeprazole, lansoprazole, rabeprazole, and pantoprazole are all metabolized by the P-450 enzyme system, leading to potential drug interactions.

Omeprazole has a benzimidazole moiety similar to the imidazole ring of cimetidine and is also a competitive inhibitor of CYP2C19 and CYP1A2 isoenzymes, and possibly the CYP34A isoenzyme. It inhibits the metabolism of diazepam (27%), warfarin, and phenytoin (19%) in a dose-related manner.[95] In vivo, the elimination half-life of benzodiazepine is increased by an average of 130%.[96] The effects appear a few days after initiation of omeprazole and do not abate immediately on discontinuation of the drug.[96] Low doses of omeprazole of 20 mg per day do not alter steady-state plasma concentrations of phenytoin.[97] A clinically significant interaction between warfarin and omeprazole (20 mg daily) occurred in one patient who developed widespread bruises and hematuria, with a prothrombin time of 48 seconds.[98] Lansoprazole may slightly increase the clearance (6%) of theophylline, but it is probably not significant. Rabeprazole does not interact with theophylline, warfarin, or phenytoin, possibly owing to low affinity to the CYP2C19 isoenzyme.[99] However, rabeprazole may increase digoxin serum concentrations.[100] Pantoprazole, in contrast to the other proton pump inhibitors, is also metabolized by a cytosolic sulfotransferase that appears to interact less with drugs that are in competition for the same P-450 system. This may explain the lower potential for drug interactions.

Clinical Management

Drug interactions are notoriously difficult to detect in the clinical setting, making personal clinical impressions one of the least reliable methods of assessing potential drug interactions. Nevertheless, personal clinical impressions can provide valuable information if applied in the context of clinical studies and appropriate assessment.

Underestimation of the clinical importance of specific drug interactions is more common than overestimation, because most patients who receive potentially interacting drugs do not develop observable adverse effects.[7] Therefore, the clinical outcome of most drug interactions is highly situational, and the potential to cause serious consequences is patient specific. Identifying patients who are actually at significant risk and who would benefit from appropriate preventive measures is imperative. Failure to assess the risk of a particular patient before taking action often results in the institution of unnecessary precautions that may not be in the best interest of the patient. If a patient is at risk for a potential drug interaction, precautions to minimize the likelihood of an adverse consequence should be taken.

The potential for drug interactions rises as the number of medications taken concomitantly increases. Some interactions may produce adverse effects but are avoidable, whereas some drug combinations do not produce any observable adverse effect. Knowledge of potential interactions and their mechanisms is the best preparation for the health care provider. Management strategies may differ depending on the type of drug interaction. In general, if a drug interaction is contraindicated, avoid the combination. Some interactions can be avoided simply by administering them at separate times (e.g., ciprofloxacin and antacids). Some potential drug interactions can be avoided by close monitoring of serum concentrations, clinical outcome, and adjusting doses. Table 26-2, although not inclusive, is a tool that can be used to aid in assessing the potential for many clinically significant drug interactions involving alterations in hepatic metabolism or clearance. Alternative therapies are recommended if the risk is greater than the benefit for the concomitant use of two drugs.

References

1. Elwes RD, Binnie CD. Clinical pharmacokinetics of newer antiepileptic drugs. Clin Pharmacokinet 1996;30:403–415.
2. Riva R, Albani F, Contin M, et al. Pharmacokinetic

interactions between antiepileptic drugs. Clin Pharmacokinet 1996;31:470–493.

3. Hansten PD. Drug Interactions. In LL Young, M Koda-Kimble (eds), The Clinical Use of Drugs (6th ed). Vancouver, WA: Applied Therapeutic Inc, 1995;1–8.

4. Dresser GK, Spence DJ, Bailey DG. Pharmacokinetic-pharmacodynamic consequences and clinical relevance of cytochrome P450 3A4 inhibition. Clin Pharmacokinet 2000;38:41–57.

5. Drug Interaction Mechanisms and Clinical Characteristics. In PD Hansten (ed), Drug Interactions. Vancouver, WA: Applied Therapeutic Inc, 1990:1–27.

6. Busch JA, Radulovic LL, Bockbrader HN, et al. Effect of Maalox TC on single-dose pharmacokinetics of gabapentin capsules in healthy subjects. Pharm Res 1992;9:S315.

7. Schentag JJ, Watson WA, Nix DE, et al. Time dependent interactions between antacids and quinolone antibiotics. Clin Pharmacol Ther 1988;43:135.

8. Van der Meer JW, Keuning JJ, Scheijgrond HW, et al. The influence of gastric acidity on the bio-availability of ketoconazole. J Antimicrob Chemother 1980;6:552–554.

9. Winters ME. Phenytoin. In M Koda-Kimble (ed), Basic Clinical Pharmacokinetics (3rd ed). Vancouver, WA: Applied Therapeutics Inc., 1994;312–347.

10. Rambeck B, Specht U, Wolf P. Pharmacokinetic interactions of the new antiepileptic drugs. Clin Pharmacokinet 1996;31:309–324.

11. Michalets EL. Update: clinically significant cytochrome P450 drug interactions. Pharmacotherapy 1998;18:84–112.

12. Anderson GD. A mechanistic approach to antiepileptic drug interactions. Ann Pharmacother 1998;32:554–563.

13. Levy RH, Bishop F, Streeter AJ, et al. Explanation and prediction of drug interactions with topiramate using a CYP450 inhibition spectrum. Epilepsia 1995;36[Suppl 4]:47.

14. Glue P, Banfield CR, Perhch JL, et al. Pharmacokinetic interactions with felbamate. Clin Pharmacokinet 1997;33:214–224.

15. Bajpai M. Roles of cytochrome P4502C9 and cytochrome P4502C19 in the stereoselective metabolism of phenytoin to its major metabolite. Drug Metab Dispos 1996;24:1401–1403.

16. Brosen K. Recent developments in hepatic drug oxidation. Clin Pharmacokinet 1990;18:230–239.

17. Deeks SG, Smith M, Holodniy M, et al. HIV-1 protease inhibitors. JAMA 1997;277:145–153.

18. Spina E, Pisani F, Perucca E. Clinically significant pharmacokinetic drug interactions with carbamazepine. Clin Pharmacokinet 1996;31:198–214.

19. Zielinski JJ, Haidukewych D, Leheta BJ, Carbamazepine-phenytoin interaction: elevation of plasma phenytoin concentrations due to carbamazepine comedication. Ther Drug Monit 1985;7:51–53.

20. Spina E, Martines C, Fazio A. Effect of phenobarbital on the pharmacokinetics of carbamazepine-10,11-epoxide, an active metabolite of carbamazepine. Ther Drug Monit 1991;13:109–112.

21. Albani F, Theodore WH, Washinton P, et al. Effect of felbamate on plasma levels of carbamazepine and its metabolites. Epilepsia 1991;32:130–132.

22. Pisani F, Caputo M, Fazio A, et al. Interaction of carbamazepine-10, 11-epoxide, an active metabolite of carbamazepine, with valproate: a pharmacokinetic study. Epilepsia 1990;312:339–342.

23. Tomson T, Spina E, Wedlund J. Minor additive inducing effects of phenobarbital on carbamazepine clearance in patients on combined carbamazepine-phenytoin therapy. Ther Drug Monit 1987;9:117–119.

24. Zielinski JJ, Haidukewych D. Dual effects of carbamazepine-phenytoin interaction. Ther Drug Monit 1987;9:21–23.

25. Browne TR, Szabo GK, Evans JE, et al. Carbamazepine increases phenytoin serum concentration and reduces phenytoin clearance. Neurology 1988;38:1146–1150.

26. Palmer KJ, McTavish D. Felbamate. A review of its pharmacodynamic and pharmacokinetic properties and therapeutic efficacy in epilepsy. Drugs 1993;45:1041–1065.

27. Hooper WD, Franklin ME, Glue P, et al. Effect of felbamate on valproic acid disposition in healthy volunteers: inhibition of beta-oxidation. Epilepsia 1996;37:91–97.

28. Reidenberg P, Glue P, Banfield CR. Effects of felbamate on the pharmacokinetics of phenobarbital. Clin Pharmacol Ther 1995;58:279–287.

29. Montgomery PA, Sachdeo RJ, Narang-Sachdeo SK, et al. Felbamate pharmacokinetics after coadministration of erythromycin. Epilepsia 1994;35[Suppl 8]:113(abst).

30. Boop BA, Nequist GE, Rodrigues AD, et al. Role of the cytochrome P450 #A subfamily in the metabolism of C-tiagabine by human hepatic cicroosomes. Epilepsia 1995;36[Suppl 3]:S159(abst).

31. Anderson GD, Yau MK, Gidal BE. Bidirectional interaction of valproate and lamotrigine in healthy subjects. Clin Pharmacol Ther 1996;60:145–156.

32. Gram L. Pharmacokinetics of new antiepileptic drugs. Epilepsia 1996;37[Suppl 6]:S12–S16.

33. Harder S, Thurmann P. Clinically important drug interactions with anticoagulants. Clin Pharmacokinet 1996;30:416–440.

34. Panegyres PK. Fatal phenytoin warfarin interaction. Postgrad Med J 1991;67:98.

35. Campana C, Regazzi MB, Buggia I, et al. Clinically significant drug interactions with cyclosporin. Clin Pharmacokinet 1996;30:141–179.

36. Alldredge BK. Seizure risk associated with psychotropic drugs: clinical and pharmacokinetic considerations. Neurology 1999;53[Suppl 2]:S68–S75.

37. Flockhart DA. Drug interactions and the cytochrome P450 system. Clin Pharmacokinet 1995;29[Suppl 1]:45–52.

38. Richelson E. Pharmacokinetic drug interactions of new antidepressants: a review of the effects on the metabolism of other drugs. Mayo Clin Proc 1997;72:835–847.

39. Wagner W, Vause EW. Fluovaxamine: a review of global drug-drug interactions data. Clin Pharmacokinet 1995;29[Suppl 1]:26–32.

40. Ereshefsky L, Riesenman C, Francis YW. Antidepressant drug interactions and the cytochrome P450 system: the role of cytochrome P450 2D6. Clin Pharmacokinet 1995;29[Suppl 1]:10–19.

41. Spina E, Avenoso A, Pollicino, et al. Carbamazepine coadministration with fluoxetine or fluovoxamine. Ther Drug Monit 1993;15:247–250.

42. Gidal BE, Anderson GD, Seaton TL, et al. Evaluation of the effect of fluoxetine on the formation of carbamazepine epoxide. Ther Drug Monit 1993;15:405–409.

43. Grimsley SR, Jann MW, Carter JG, et al. Increased carbamazepine plasma concentrations after fluoxetine coadministration. Clin Pharmacol Ther 1991;50:10–15.

44. Monaco F. Cicolin A. Interactions between anticonvulsant and psychoactive drugs. Epilepsia 1999;40[Suppl 10]:571–576.

45. Dechant KL, Clissold SP. Paroxetine. Drugs 1991;41: 225–253.

46. Nemeroff BC, DeVane L, Pllock BG. Newer antidepressants and the cytochrome P450 system. Am J Psychiatry 1996;153:311–317.

47. Darley J. Interaction between phenytoin and fluoxetine. Seizure 1994;3:151–152.

48. Lucena MI, Blanco E, Corrales M, et al. Interaction of fluoxetine and valproic acid. Am J Psychiatry 1998;155:575–576.

49. Sovener R, Davis JM. A potential drug interaction between fluoxetine and valproic acid. J Clin Psychopharmacol 1991;11:389.

50. Ereshefsky L. Pharmacokinetics and drug interactions. Update for new antipsychotics. J Clin Psychiatry 1996;579[Suppl 11]:12–25.

51. Ereshefsky L, Riesenman C, Lam F. Serotonin selective reuptake inhibitor drug interaction and the cytochrome P450 system. J Clin Psychiatry 1996;57[Suppl 8]:16–23.

52. Ring B, Binkley S, Vandenbranden M, et al. In vitro interaction of the antipsychotic agent olanzapine with human cytochromes P450 CYP2C9, CYP2C19, CYP2D6 and CYP3A. Br J Clin Pharmacol 1996;41:181–186.

53. Costello L, Suppres TA. Clinically significant interaction between clozapine and valproate. J Clin Psychopharmacol 1995;15:139–141.

54. Longo LP, Salzman C. Valproic acid effects on serum concentrations of clozapine and norclozapine. Am J Psychiatry 1995;152:650.

55. Bajda FJ, Prineas RJ, Lowell RRH. Interaction between phenytoin and the benzodiazepines. BMJ 1971;1:346.

56. Saavedra IN, Aguilera LI, Faure E, et al. Phenytoin/clonazepam interaction. Ther Drug Monit 1985;7:481–484.

57. Arana GW, Epstein S, Molloy M, et al. Carbamazepine-induced reduction of plasma alprazolam concentrations: a clinical case report. J Clin Psychiatry 1989;49:448–449.

58. Bernstein JG. Drug Interactions. In L DeYoung (ed), Handbook of Drug Therapy in Psychiatry (3rd ed). St. Louis: Mosby, 1995:328–364.

59. Jerling M, Bertilsson L, Sjoqvist F. The use of therapeutic drug monitoring data to document kinetic drug interactions: an example with amitriptyline and nortriptyline. Ther Drug Monit 1994;16:1–12.

60. Braithwaite RA, Flanagan RA, Richens A. Steady-state plasma nortriptyline concentrations in epileptic patients. Br J Clin Pharmacol 1975;2:469–471.

61. Moody JP, Whyte SF, McDonald AJ, et al. Pharmacokinetic aspects of protriptyline plasma level. Eur J Clin Pharmacol 1977;11:51–56.

62. Hewich DS, Sparks RG, Stevenson IH, et al. Induction of imipramine metabolism following barbiturate administration. Br J Clin Pharmacol 1977;3:399.

63. Perucca E, Richens A. Interaction between phenytoin and imipramine. Br J Clin Pharmacol 1977;4:485–486.

64. Perucca E, Giuliana G, Gipolla G, et al. Inhibition of diazepam metabolism by fluvoxamine: a pharmacokinetic study in normal volunteers. Clin Pharmacol Ther 1994;56:471–476.

65. Lemberger L, Rowe H, Bosomworth J. The effect of fluoxetine on the pharmacokinetics and psychomotor responses of diazepam. Clin Pharmacol Ther 1988;43:412–419.

66. Greenblatt DJ, Preskorn SH, Cotreau MM. Fluoxetine impairs clearance of alprazolam but not clonazepam. Clin Pharmacol Ther 1992;52:479–486.

67. Gardner MJ, Baris BA, Wilner KD. Effect of sertraline on the pharmacokinetics and protein binding of diazepam in healthy volunteers. Clin Pharmacokinet 1997;32[Suppl 1]:43–49.

68. Greene DS, Dockens RC, Salazar DE, et al. Coadministration of nefazodone and benzodiazepines; pharmacokinetic assessment. Am Soc Clin Pharm Ther 1995;74:141.

69. Venkatakrishman K, von Moltke L, Greenblatt DJ. Effects of the antifungal agents on oxidative drug metabolism. Clin Pharmacokinet 2000;38:111–180.

70. Blum, RA, Wilton JH, Hilligoss DM, et al. Effect of fluconazole on the disposition of phenytoin. Clin Pharmacol Ther 1991;49:420–425.

71. Touchette MA, Chandrasekar PH, Milad MA, et al. Contrasting effects of fluconazole and ketoconazole on phenytoin and testerone disposition in man. Br J Clin Pharmacol 1992;34:75–78.

72. Spina E, Arena D, Scordo MG, et al. Elevation of plasma carbamazepine concentrations by ketoconazole in patients with epilepsy. Ther Drug Monit 1997;19:535–538.

73. Ducharme MP, Slaughter RL, Warbasse LH, et al. Itraconazole and hydroitraconazole concentrations are

reduced more than ten-fold by phenytoin. Clin Pharmacol Ther 1995;58:617–624.

74. Canafax DM, Graves NM, Hilligoss DM, et al. Interaction between cyclosporine and fluconazole in renal allograft recipients. Transplantation 1991;51:1014–1018.

75. Errick JK, et al. Co-trimoxazole and warfarin: case report of an interaction. Am J Hosp Pharm 1978;35:1399–1401.

76. Fiorenzo A, Riva R, Baurzzi A. Clarithromycin-carbamazepine interaction: a case report. Epilepsia 1993;34:161–162.

77. Marchbanks CR. Drug-drug interactions with fluoroquinolones. Pharmacotherapy 1993;13:23S–28S.

78. Synercid [package insert]. Bridgewater, NJ: Aventis Pharmaceuticals, Inc.

79. Piscitelli ST, Flexner C, Minor JR. Drug interactions in patients infected with human immunodeficiency virus. Clin Infect Dis 1996;23:685–693.

80. Cohen C, Sun E, Cameron W, et al. Ritonavir-saquinavir combination treatment in HIV-infected patients. In Program and Abstracts of the 36th Interscience Conference on Antimicrobial Agents and Chemotherapy, American Society for Microbiology; September 15–18, 1996; New Orleans, LA. Abstract LB7b.

81. Bauman JL, Sanoski CA, Chan LN. Pharmacokinetic and pharmacodynamic drug interactions with antiarrhythmic agents. Cardiol Rev 1997;5:292–304.

82. Data JL, Wilkinson GR, Niew AS. Interaction of quinidine with anticonvulsant drugs. N Engl J Med 1976;294:699–702.

83. Twum-Barima Y, Carruthers SG. Quinidine-rifampin interaction. N Engl J Med 1981;304:1466–1469.

84. Fromm MF, Busse D, Kroemer HK, et al. Differential induction of prehepatic and hepatic metabolism of verapamil by rifampin. Hepatology 1996;24:796–801.

85. Lesko LJ. Pharmacokinetic drug interactions with amiodarone. Clin Pharmacokinet 1989;17:130–140.

86. Nolan PE, Erstad BL, Hoyer GL, et al. Steady-state interaction between amiodarone and phenytoin in normal subjects. Am J Cardiol 1990;65:1252–1257.

87. Kerin NZ, Blevins RD, Goldman L, et al. The incidence, magnitude and time course of the amiodarone-warfarin interaction. Arch Intern Med 1988;148:1779–1781.

88. Nolar PE, Marcus FI, Karol MD, et al. Effect of phenytoin on the clinical pharmacokinetics of amiodarone. J Clin Pharmacol 1990;30:1112–1119.

89. Nademanee K, Kannan R, Hendrickson J, et al. Amiodarone-digoxin interaction: clinical significance, time course of development, potential pharmacokinetic mechanisms and therapeutic implications. J Am Coll Cardiol 1984;4:111–116.

90. O'Reilly RA, Trager WF, Rettie AE, et al. Interaction of amiodarone with racemic warfarin and its separated enontiomorphs in humans. Clin Pharmacol Ther 1987;42:290–294.

91. Chitwood KK, Abdul-Haqq AJ, Heim-Duthoy KL. Cyclosporine-amiodarone interaction. Ann Pharmacother 1993;27:569–571.

92. Mamprin F, Mullins P, Graham T, et al. Amiodarone-cyclosporine interaction in cardiac transplantation. Am Heart J 1992;123:1725–1726 [Letter].

93. Olsson S, Edwards IR. Tachycardia during cisapride treatment. BMJ 1992;305:748–749.

94. Bran S, Murray W, Hirsch IB, et al. Long QT syndrome during high-dose cisapride. Arch Intern Med 1995;155:765–768.

95. Andersson T, Lagerstrom PO, Unge P. A study of the interaction between omeprazole and phenytoin in epileptic patients. Ther Drug Monit 1990;12:329–333.

96. Cederberg C, Anderson T, Skanberg I. Omeprazole: pharmacokinetics and metabolism in man. Scan J Gastroenterology 1989;28[Suppl 166]:33–40.

97. Saltiel E. Proton pump inhibitors: a comparative review. US Pharmacist 1997;22(12):HS21–HS29.

98. Ahmad S. Omeprazole-warfarin interactions. South Med J 1991;84:674–675 [Letter].

99. Humphries TJ, Nardi RV, Spera AC, et al. Coadministration of rabeprazole sodium does not affect the pharmacokinetics of anhydrous therophylline or warfarin. Gastroenterology 1996;11:A138(abst).

100. Humphries TJ, Nardi RV, Lazar JD, et al. Drug-drug interaction evaluation of rabeprazole sodium: a clean/expected slate? Gut 1996;39[Suppl 297]:A47(abst).

101. Wetzel H, Harter S, Szegedi A, et al. Fluvoxamine comedication to tricyclic antidepressants: metabolic interactions, clinical efficiency and side effects. Pharmacopsychiatry 1993;26:211–214.

102. Hartter S, Szegedi A, Wetzel H, et al. Differential interactions of fluvoxamine and paroxetine with the metabolism of tricyclic antidepressants. Pharmacopsychiatry 1993;26:156–159.

103. Tomson T, Svensson JO, Hilton-Brown P. Relationship of intraindividual dose to plasma concentration of carbamazepine: indication of dose-dependent induction of metabolism. Ther Drug Monit 1989;11:533–539.

104. Zielinski JJ, Lichten EM, Haidukewych D. Clinically significant danazol-carbamazepine interaction. Ther Drug Monit 1987;9:24–27.

105. Fauci AS, Bartlett JG, Goosby EP, et al. Guidelines for the use of antiretroviral agents in HIV-infected adults and adolescents; January 28, 2000. Washington, DC: Department of Health and Human Services, 2000.

106. Bertz RJ, Granneman RG. Use of in vitro and in vivo data to estimate the likelihood of metabolic pharmacokinetic interactions. Clin Pharmacokinet 1997;32:220–240.

107. Caccia S. Metabolism of the newer antidepressants. Clin Pharmacokinet 1998;34:281–302.

108. May TW, Rambeck B, Jurgens U. Influence of oxcarbazepine and methsuximide on lamotrigine concentrations in epileptic patients with and without valproic acid comedication: results of a retrospective study. Ther Drug Monit 1999;175–181.

109. Bottiger Y, Svensson J, Stahle L. Lamotrigine drug interactions in a TDM material. Ther Drug Monit 1999;21:171–174.

110. Kellermann RA, May T, Boenigk H. Influence of ethosuximide on valproic acid serum concentrations. Epilepsy Res 1997;26:345–349.

111. Sachdeo RC. Topiramate. Clin Pharmacokinet 1998;34: 335–346.

112. Rey E, Pons G, Olive G. Vigabatrin. Clin Pharmacokinet 1992;23:267–278.

113. Gustavson LE, Cato A, Guenther HJ, et al. Lack of clinically important drug interactions between tiagabine and carbamazepine, phenytoin, or valproate. Epilepsia 1995;36[Suppl 3]:S159.

114. Brodie MJ. Tiagabine pharmacology in profile. Epilepsia 1995;36[Suppl 6]:S7–S9.

115. Rambeck B, Wolf P. Lamotrigine clinical pharmacokinetics. Clin Pharmacokinet 1993;25:433–443.

116. Perucca E, Bialer M. The clinical pharmacokinetics of the newer antiepileptic drugs. Clin Pharmacokinet 1996;31:29–46.

117. Johannessen SI, Pharmacokinetics and interaction profile of topiramate: review and comparison with other newer antiepileptic drugs. Epilepsia 1997;38[Suppl 1]:S18–S23.

118. Hamer HM, Knake S, Schomburg MA. Valproate-induced hyperammonemic encephalopathy in the presence of topiramate. Neurology 2000;54:230–232.

119. Albani F, Riva R, Baruzzi A. Clarithromycin-carbamazepine interaction: a case report. Epilepsia 1993;34:161–162.

120. Levy RH. Cytochrome P450 isoenzyme and antiepileptic drug interactions. Epilepsia 1995;36[Suppl 5]:S8–S13.

121. Brosen K. Are pharmacokinetic drug interactions with the SSRIs an issue? Int Clin Psychopharmacol 1996;11[Suppl 1]:23–27.

122. Greenblatt D, von Moltke L, Harmatz J, et al. Human cytochromes and some newer antidepressants: kinetics, metabolism, and drug interactions. J Clin Psychopharmacol 1999;19[Suppl 5]:S23–S35.

123. Lee DO, Lee CD, et al. Serotonin syndrome in a child associated with erythromycin and sertraline. Pharmacotherapy 1999;19:894–896.

124. Gisclon LG, Curtin CR, Kramer LD. The steady-state (SS) pharmacokinetics (PK) of phenytoin (Dilantin) and topiramate (Topamax) in epileptic patients on monotherapy and during combination therapy. Epilepsia 1994;35[Suppl 8]:54.

Section G

Procedures and Emergency Situations in Epilepsy

Chapter 27

Procedures in Epilepsy Patients

Souhel Najjar, Orrin Devinsky,
Andrew D. Rosenberg, and Douglas R. Nordli, Jr.

Patients with epilepsy are often considered at high risk for routine medical and dental procedures. This designation is based primarily on the risk of seizures occurring during or shortly after the procedure and, to a lesser degree, the potential interaction between drugs for the procedure and for seizure control. Although few procedures have been documented to have increased risks among patients with epilepsy, an increased level of concern is often present. Procedures in children and adults with epilepsy raise the following issues: (1) steps that can be taken before the procedure to reduce the risk of seizures associated with the procedure, (2) education of health care workers involved in the procedure about a patient's seizures and medications and first aid for seizures, (3) defining the risks of the procedure for patients with epilepsy, (4) defining the effects of anesthetics or analgesics used for the procedure on seizure threshold and the potential for interaction with antiepileptic drugs (AEDs), which is the focus of this chapter, and (5) differential diagnosis of paroxysmal behavioral events that occur around the time of procedures.

Epileptic seizures during medical and dental procedures can be more dangerous (e.g., onset of uncontrolled clonic movements in an extremity in which a microsurgical procedure is being performed under local anesthesia) or less dangerous (e.g., onset of status epilepticus in a physician's office) than seizures occurring at other times (e.g., while sleeping alone in bed). Some simple precau-

tions should be used before a person with epilepsy undergoes a procedure. First, factors that can precipitate seizures should be avoided. Because missed medications are a common cause of breakthrough seizures,[1] emphasize compliance and ensure that patients continue taking medication up until shortly before the procedure (see following discussion). Although patients are instructed not to eat or drink for at least 8 hours before surgery, medications are often administered with sips of water within a few hours of surgery. Antiepilepsy medications should be given at this time as well. Sleep deprivation, common before many procedures, should be avoided. When needed, low doses of chloral hydrate or benzodiazepines can be safely used for insomnia the night before a procedure. Patients with epilepsy, who should always avoid excessive alcohol intake (i.e., greater than two beverages per day), should avoid alcohol for a week before surgery.[2]

Much of the concern regarding patients with epilepsy results from perceived as well as real risks associated with seizures. Health care workers often receive little education concerning seizure classification, phenomenology, duration, and first aid. This lack of understanding fosters fear and conservatism that can lead to excessive precautions and restrictions and management errors. Induced labor and cesarean section are examples in which interventions and procedures may be undertaken more often in women with epilepsy—two to four times more often than in other pregnancies—than medical reasons alone would justify.[3] Epilepsy alone is not an indication for either of these interventions. However, in selected cases, labor should be induced and a cesarean section should be performed on an elective (e.g., weekly tonic-clonic seizures during the last trimester) or emergency (e.g., tonic-clonic seizure during labor or lack of active maternal contribution) basis.[4]

Physicians, nurses, dentists, technicians, and other health care workers involved with procedures in patients with epilepsy should have a basic understanding of the patient's seizure types, medications, and first aid for the seizures. A complex partial seizure during a routine dental procedure can frighten the dentist and the technologist. If previously informed of the possibility and educated about the need for calm observation as opposed to intervention, fears and chances of inappropriate responses can be reduced. For example, restraint during a complex partial seizure or after a tonic-clonic seizure can provoke an aggressive reaction, which leads to a dangerous cycle that requires greater restraint. In such cases, restraint should be removed, and the patient should be reassured in a comforting manner.

Paroxysmal behavioral events that occur during or after procedures have a differential diagnosis that extends well beyond epileptic seizures.[5] Occasionally, a patient with psychogenic seizures has events mainly around the time of medical procedures. More commonly, patients with convulsive syncope develop symptoms during painful or emotional procedures. In such cases, which can occur in procedures such as venipuncture, excision of moles under local anesthesia, and electromyography, the patient experiences a tonic-clonic seizure secondary to a fall in heart rate or blood pressure.[6] These seizures are typically brief, lasting less than 2 minutes, but they may be followed by prominent postictal confusion. No specific therapy is required, and AEDs should not be prescribed. In selected cases of recurrent convulsive syncope associated with medical procedures, an anticholinergic agent may be beneficial.

Perioperative seizures have numerous potential etiologies. Postoperative seizures are more commonly due to nonanesthetic causes. Seizures are a frequent occurrence after operation and irradiation for supratentorial gliomas, and anticonvulsants may be effective in reducing the incidence of those

seizures.[7] Cardiac surgery is also associated with a higher incidence of perioperative epileptic paroxysms owing to the complex and sometimes severe metabolic, hemodynamic, or blood modifications that are induced by cardiopulmonary bypass and may alter cerebral electrogenesis.[8] It seems that normothermic light hemodilution and elimination of neuroleptic drugs for analgesia prevent pre- and postoperative epileptic paroxysms. One study showed that administration of calcium chloride minimizes the hemodynamic effects of propofol in patients who undergo coronary artery bypass grafting, and thereafter it may potentially reduce postoperative epileptic paroxysms in these patients.[9]

Premedication and Anesthesia

During the preoperative interview, the anesthesiologist determines and prescribes premedication for the patient. The choice of premedication can have major implications for the patient with epilepsy. Considerations include

1. Continuing the patient's prescribed daily medications. Administering medications either orally with a sip of water, or via an acceptable alternate route (intravenously, intramuscularly, or rectally) can avoid decreasing serum levels into the subtherapeutic range. AEDs are included in this category as, well as antihypertensives and cardiac, diabetic, and asthma medications. When oral or parenteral administration of AEDs cannot be administered (e.g., hyperemesis, gastrointestinal procedures, AEDs without parenteral forms), some may be given rectally (Table 27-1). Although clonazepam has an intermediate absorption rate,[10] the injectable forms of diazepam and lorazepam are rapidly absorbed rectally.[11,12] A gel formulation of diazepam (Diastat) is rapidly absorbed rectally, with an absolute bioavailability of 90% relative to injectable diazepam. Diazepam rectal gel is an effective and safe treatment that is used to abort an episode of acute repetitive seizures in children.[13] Carbamazepine can be given rectally with 80% absorption.[14] Ninety percent of rectal phenobarbital (liquid parenteral form) is absorbed in 4.4 hours.[11] Phenytoin (liquid parenteral form) given rectally is slowly absorbed in dogs.[15] Rectal absorption of oral

Table 27-1. Antiepileptic Drugs Available for Rectal Administration

Drug	Treatment Usefulness	Dose (mg/kg/dose)	Preparation	Pharmacokinetics	Comments
Carbamazepine	Maintenance	Same as oral	Oral suspension (dilute with equal volume of water) Suppository gel (carbamazepine powder dissolved in 20% alcohol and methyl hydroxy cellulose)*	Peak concentration 4–8 hrs; 80% absorbed	Cathartic effect.
Clonazepam	?Acute	0.02–0.10 mg	Suspension	Peak concentration 0.1–2.0 hrs	Onset may be too slow for acute use.
Diazepam	Acute	0.2–0.5 mg	Parenteral solution	Effect in 2–10 mins; peak concentration 2–30 mins	Well tolerated. Nordiazepam accumulates with repeated doses.
Lorazepam	Acute	0.05–0.10 mg	Parenteral solution	Peak concentration 0.5–2.0 hrs	Well tolerated.
Paraldehyde	Acute	0.3 ml	Oral solution (dilute with equal volume of mineral oil)	Effect in 20 mins; peak concentration 2.5 hrs	Moderate cathartic effect; use glass syringe.
Phenobarbital	?Acute	10–20 mg	Parenteral solution	Peak concentration 4–5 hrs; 90% absorbed	Onset may be too slow for acute use.
Secobarbital	Acute	5 mg	Parenteral solution	Peak concentration 0.5–1.5 hrs	—
	Maintenance	Same as oral	Same as acute	Same as acute	
Valproic acid	Acute	5–25 mg	Oral solution (dilute with equal volume of water)	Peak concentration 1–3 hrs	Cathartic effect.
	Maintenance	Same as oral	Valproic acid liquid from capsules mixed into Supocire C lipid base	Peak concentration 2–4 hrs; 80% absorbed	Well tolerated.

*Extemporaneously prepared using commercial products; all other preparations are commercial products given rectally.
Source: Adapted from NM Graves, AL Kriel. Rectal administration of antiepileptic drugs in children. Pediatric Neurol 1987;3:321–326. These data are based largely on pediatric studies.

forms of sodium valproate is complete, with peak concentrations occurring approximately 2 hours after administration.[16] In *non per os* patients, alternative routes of anticonvulsant administration (parenteral or rectal) can be considered. There is a need for close clinical monitoring during parenteral administration of antiepileptic medications in patients with renal, hepatic, or cardiac diseases. To minimize the incidence of adverse effects in this population, antiepileptic medications need to be administered at lower doses or infused more slowly. Monitoring therapeutic levels is essential to prevent postoperative seizures. The incidence of subtherapeutic anticonvulsants in patients dying as a direct result of their epilepsy is significantly greater than it is in those dying of unrelated causes.[17]

2. Administering premedication for sedative or analgesic purposes, or both. To calm the patient for transport to the operating room and to smooth induction, benzodiazepines (e.g., diazepam, midazolam, lorazepam), antihistamines (e.g., hydroxyzine), barbiturates, and narcotics (e.g., meperidine, morphine) may be administered. Pro- and anticonvulsant considerations of these medications are addressed in the following discussion.

3. Diminishing risks of perioperative problems or complications, such as aspiration, hemorrhages, or postoperative nausea and vomiting. Complications associated with aspiration are related to the volume (greater than 25–30 ml) and acidity (pH of less than 2.5) of the aspirated gastric fluid. Medications are administered based on their ability to increase gastric pH or decrease gastric volume. Histamine 2 antagonists (e.g., cimetidine, ranitidine, and nizatidine) increase gastric pH and are often administered to patients who are at high risk for aspiration (e.g., obesity, hiatal hernia). Although histamine 2 antagonists do not have proconvulsant activity, cimetidine can increase phenytoin plasma levels, and serum phenytoin blood levels should be monitored. Metoclopramide is also prescribed for patients at risk for aspiration, because it increases low esophageal sphincter tone, facilitates gastric emptying, and has an antiemetic effect. This medication works both centrally and peripherally as a dopaminergic antagonist. Metoclopramide should be used cautiously in epilepsy patients, because it may increase the frequency and severity of seizures.[18]

Sodium valproate can cause thrombocytopenia and platelet dysfunction. The mechanism that underlies these effects is unknown. Bleeding time and platelet count are essential in the presurgical evaluation of patients on sodium valproate. Specific platelet function tests, such as platelet adhesiveness or aggregation, may also be helpful. The role of valproate-induced hemorrhage or exacerbation of surgically induced blood loss is not clearly defined. However, valproate has been suspected in the pathogenesis of hemorrhagic complications of surgery. There was a significant increase in the number of patients with abnormal bleeding times and a significant difference ($p < .001$) in blood loss during spine surgery in patients who took valproic acid as monotherapy.[19] Other studies showed that valproic acid apparently did not increase complications of hemostasis during therapeutic surgical resections for epilepsy, and these studies did not recommend routinely discontinuing valproic acid before craniotomy.[20] For major surgical procedures, another AED should be substituted, if possible. When valproate is used, dosages over 40 mg/kg per day should be avoided, because the hematologic effects of sodium valproate may be dose related.[21]

Topiramate is a novel antiepileptic medication with several mechanisms of action, including inhibition of carbonic anhydrase, which may result in a normal anion-gap metabolic acidosis. The latter side effect can become clinically significant during surgery, especially with concomitant use of another carbonic inhibitor.[22]

Anesthesia

In general, when seizures occur during surgery, their onset often coincides with the introduction of a specific anesthetic or analgesic drug. However, there have been reports of postoperative convulsions that appeared to be caused by anesthetic or analgesic drugs administered intraoperatively via injection or inhalation. Some anesthetics may possess proconvulsant or anticonvulsant properties, or both. One possible factor is an inherent pharmacodynamic variability in the responsiveness of inhibitory and excitatory target tissues in the central nervous system (CNS).[23] The effects of local and general anesthetics on seizure threshold have been examined to determine intrinsic pharmacologic properties and mechanisms of action; interictal and ictal effects on surface, depth, or cortical electroencephalogram (EEG) recordings; and behavioral effects in animals and humans.

General Anesthetics

Inhalation and intravenous anesthetics possess proconvulsant and anticonvulsant properties. The mechanisms of these contrasting neural effects are not fully understood. Biological differences in responses, bioavailability, effect on excitatory and inhibitory neurons, and these neurons' responses to the agents may result from delivery of varying concentrations or doses. With deepening levels of anesthesia, there are characteristic EEG changes, beginning with increased beta activity and followed by progressive slowing of the background until a flat-line or burst-suppression record is obtained (Table 27-2). Postoperatively, slowing often persists for several days or, occasionally, for several weeks. As general anesthetics, all halogenated inhalational agents have anticonvulsant properties and can terminate status epilepticus.[24]

Among the volatile anesthetics, methoxyflurane and halothane produce the least CNS irritability; enflurane produces the most irritability, and isoflurane and desflurane produce intermediate levels of irritability.[25,26] Changes in the basicity of these compounds, which depends on the degree of fluorination of the carbon atoms adjacent to the ether oxygen, may parallel effects on cortical excitability. Isoflurane, the least fluorinated and most basic of these ethers, produces the least amount of cortical reactivity.[25] The mechanism of enflurane-induced hyperexcitability in humans is unclear. In animals, enflurane inhibits synapses and stimulates excitatory neuronal transmission in cortical and subcortical areas.[27]

Enflurane

Enflurane is the major inhalation agent that anesthesiologists usually avoid when caring for epilepsy patients, because it lowers seizure threshold. In children and adults with no history of epilepsy, enflurane can cause epileptiform activity with concomitant facial or appendicular myoclonus or generalized tonic-clonic movements.[28-30] In epilepsy patients, the extent but not the frequency of spike activity on the electrocorticogram is increased.[29] Epileptogenic foci may be activated during epilepsy surgery.[23,31] As the depth of anesthesia is increased with enflurane, the EEG demonstrates high-voltage spikes and spike and slow-wave complexes, the spikes with burst suppression. Although low enflurane concentrations (1.0–1.5%) administered to a normocarbic patient (arterial partial pressure of carbon dioxide [$PaCO_2$] equals 40 mm Hg) are not frequently associated with seizure activity,[32] increasing enflurane concentrations (2–3%) or hyperventilating an anesthetized patient enhances seizure activity. Hyperventilation to a $PaCO_2$ of 20 mm Hg from 40 mm Hg is associated with seizure activity at a 1% lower enflurane concentration. Because hyperventilation is frequently used by neuroanesthesiologists to decrease cerebral blood flow and intracranial pressure, enflurane is avoided when hyperventilation is indicated. An increase in $PaCO_2$ from 40 mm Hg to 60 mm Hg increases the minimum enflurane concentration at which seizures occur by 1%.[27]

Generalized tonic-clonic and myoclonic seizures can occur within the immediate postoperative period and, potentially, a few days after enflurane anesthesia. The role of other CNS active drugs remains uncertain in these cases.[33] The convulsant effects may result from enflurane's organic and inorganic nonvolatile fluorinated metabolites.[34]

Although anesthesiologists consider diazepam and thiopental anticonvulsant agents and use them extensively to treat seizure activity, there is some evidence that these drugs may potentiate enflurane-related epileptiform activity in humans.[35] Nitrous oxide (N_2O) does not alter epileptiform activity induced by enflurane.[32]

Halothane

Halothane has anticonvulsant properties and can terminate status epilepticus. When used alone, halothane does not cause CNS irritability.[36] In the few reports of halothane-related seizures, N_2O was also administered.[37] Rarely, sharp waves that are maximal over the vertex can appear during the first postoperative week, usually on the first 2 postoperative

Table 27-2. Anesthetic Drugs and the Electroencephalogram (EEG)

Drug	Effect on EEG Frequency	Effect on EEG Amplitude	Burst Suppression?
Isoflurane			Yes, >1.5 MAC
Subanesthetic	Loss of α, ↑ frontal β	↓	
Anesthetic	Frontal 4- to 8-Hz activity	↑	
Increasing dose >1.5 MAC	Diffuse θ and δ → burst suppression → silence	↑ → 0	
Enflurane			Yes, >1.5 MAC
Subanesthetic	Loss of α, ↑ frontal β	↓	
Anesthetic	Frontal 7- to 12-Hz activity	↑	
Increasing dose >1.5 MAC	Spikes/spike and slow waves → Burst suppression; hypocapnia → Seizures	↑↑	
Halothane			Not seen in clinically useful dose range
Low dose	↑ Frontal 10- to 20-Hz activity	↓	
Moderate dose	Frontal 10- to 15-Hz activity	↑	
Increasing dose >1.5 MAC	Diffuse θ, slowing with increasing dose	↑	
Desflurane	Similar to equi-MAC dose of isoflurane	Similar to equi-MAC dose of isoflurane	Yes, >1.2 MAC
Nitrous oxide (alone)	Frontal fast oscillatory activity (>30 Hz)	↑, especially with inspired concentration >50%	No
Barbiturates			Yes, with high doses
Low dose	Fast frontal β activity	Slight ↑	
Moderate dose	Frontal α frequency spindles	↑	
Increasing high dose	Diffuse δ → burst suppression → silence	↑↑↑ → 0	
Etomidate			Yes, with high doses
Low dose	Fast frontal β activity	↓	
Moderate dose	Frontal α frequency	↑	
Increasing high dose	Diffuse δ → burst suppression → silence	↑↑ → 0	
Propofol			Yes, with high doses
Low dose	Loss of α, ↑ frontal β	↓	
Moderate dose	Frontal δ, waxing-waning α	↑	
Increasing high dose	Diffuse δ → burst suppression → silence	↑↑ → 0	
Ketamine			No
Low dose	Loss of α, ↑ variability	↑↓	
Moderate dose	Frontal rhythmic θ	↑	
High dose	Polymorphic δ, some β	↑↑ (β is low amplitude)	
Benzodiazepines			No
Low dose	Loss of α, increased frontal β activity	↓	
High dose	Frontally dominant δ and θ	↑	
Opiates			No
Low dose	Loss of β, α slows	↔ ↑	
Moderate dose	Diffuse θ, some δ	↑	
High dose	δ, often synchronized	↑↑	

α = alpha (8–13 Hz) frequency; β = beta (>13 Hz) frequency; δ = delta (<4 Hz) frequency; MAC = minimum alveolar concentration; θ = theta (4–7 Hz) frequency.

Note: Arrows indicate direction of change; number of arrows indicates the magnitude of change.

Source: Adapted from Black S, Mahla ME, Cucchiara RF. Neurologic Monitoring. In RD Miller. (ed). Anesthesia. New York: Churchill Livingstone,1994:1323.

days. Persistence of an epileptogenic halothane metabolite (e.g., trifluoroacetic acid) may contribute to this sharp activity.[36]

Isoflurane

Isoflurane, a commonly used inhalation agent, is an isomer of enflurane and contains little or no epileptogenicity.[26] In the few cases of isoflurane-related seizures, N_2O was also administered.[38] Isoflurane has anticonvulsant properties; it suppresses drug-induced convulsions in animals[39] and terminates status epilepticus in patients at inspired concentrations from 0.5% to 3.0%.[40,41] Isoflurane reduces the frequency and field of spikes on the electrocorticogram of epilepsy patients.[29,40]

Desflurane

Desflurane is a recently introduced inhalation agent that is structurally similar to isoflurane. Compared to isoflurane, it has a more rapid onset of action and recovery. The EEG patterns for desflurane are similar to those seen with equipotent doses of isoflurane. Burst suppression is easily achieved. There was some concern that EEG tolerance may develop to desflurane. However, this has not been demonstrated in humans.[42,43]

Sevoflurane

Sevoflurane is an inhalation agent currently in use in Japan. Two pediatric patients with epilepsy had EEG but no clinical evidence of seizure activity with sevoflurane induction.[44]

Nitrous Oxide

N_2O has very low epileptogenic potential and has been used extensively in epileptic and nonepileptic patients.[23,45] N_2O does not significantly affect neuronal firing in the human limbic areas.[46] Among 11 epilepsy patients who underwent dental procedures, there were no EEG changes during anesthesia in nine patients, and there was a decreased frequency of paroxysmal discharges in two patients.[45]

Barbiturates

Barbiturates are anticonvulsants that can also have proconvulsant actions. Slight structural changes of a barbiturate (e.g., sulfuration or methylation of the 1 position) can convert it from an anticonvulsant to a convulsant.[47] Depending on the dose used, some barbiturates can have pro- and anticonvulsant properties, with low doses associated with seizure activity in epilepsy patients[48] and higher doses leading to burst suppression.

Thiopental (Pentothal) and Ultra Short–Acting Barbiturates

Thiopental is used to stop seizures, including those due to local anesthesia overdose. The proconvulsant action of thiopental is low compared to methohexital.[49] This drug is less effective than methohexital in activating existing epileptogenic activity on the electrocorticogram in epilepsy patients. Thiopental may be a safer induction agent than methohexital for patients with epilepsy.[50] Other ultra short–acting thiobarbiturates, such as thiamylal sodium, buthalitone, and thialbarbitone, share common pharmacologic properties as thiopental.

Methohexital

Methohexital is an ultra short–acting methyl barbiturate that does not cause seizure activity in patients without epilepsy. However, it can be associated with some excitatory phenomena, such as hiccoughing, tremors, and abnormal muscle movements.[23] In patients with epilepsy, electrographic and clinical seizures can occur after intravenous (0.5–1.0 mg/kg), intramuscular (10 mg/kg), and rectal (25 mg/kg) administrations.[50,51] Low-dose methohexital (less than 0.5 mg/kg) can activate interictal and ictal discharges among epilepsy patients during electrocorticography.[49] The activating effect of methohexital may be largely restricted to patients with partial epilepsy, occurring in up to 72% of such patients.[52] Methohexital does not appear to cause seizures during anesthetic induction of patients with generalized epilepsy.[50,52] In higher doses, methohexital can suppress epileptogenic foci and cause electrical silence. This suppressive effect is used in the methohexital suppression test, which has been recommended as an adjunctive tool to distinguish the primary focus in patients with secondary bilateral synchrony or multifocal discharges.[53] This is most valuable in the investigation of temporal lobe epilepsy. Methohexital is administered in incremental doses of 0.5–1.0 mg/kg until EEG silence is obtained or only a single focus remains. If total EEG silence is obtained, as the EEG returns, it is hoped that a single focus becomes evident.

Etomidate

Etomidate is a hypnotic nonbarbiturate, ultra short–acting anesthetic agent associated with involuntary muscle movements in 10–70% of patients. These movements can be violent and mimic seizure activity. Etomidate is often administered because of its cardiovascular stabilizing effect. In patients without epilepsy, surface electrode recordings during the myoclonic movements are not associated with epileptiform activity.[54]

Etomidate (0.2 mg/kg) can activate seizure foci in epilepsy patients within 30 seconds[55] and has been used intraoperatively for this purpose. Despite the lack of evidence that etomidate causes seizures in nonepileptic patients, epileptiform activity occurred in 6 of 30 nonepileptic patients who were induced with etomidate for heart valve replacement.[54]

Benzodiazepines

Benzodiazepines are potent anticonvulsants that are commonly used intravenously and, occasionally, rectally to treat status epilepticus.[23] Diazepam, midazolam, clonazepam, and lorazepam are all used as AEDs.[48] Diazepam rectal gel is effective in controlling acute repetitive seizures (clusters). Intravenous midazolam drip may be more effective for refractory status than other benzodiazepines[56] and may represent a substantial improvement over other therapeutic approaches, such as pentobarbital anesthesia.[57] Paradoxically, diazepam may induce seizures in patients with Lennox-Gastaut syndrome and lower the seizure threshold in epilepsy patients receiving enflurane.[58]

Opioids

Patients without epilepsy are not at risk for seizures when administered typical anesthetic doses of narcotics. However, high-dose opioids can elicit seizures. What practitioners observe as seizure activity may actually be myoclonic jerks, rigidity, and other nonepileptic drug–induced movements.[23] Simultaneous scalp EEG and electromyography recordings do not reveal epileptiform activity during abnormal movements. In epilepsy patients, high-dose narcotics may elicit seizure activity in isolated cases (see discussion of fentanyl in the section Fentanyl, Sufentanil, and Alfentanil). However, scalp EEG recordings may not be adequate to determine this, and electrocorticographic recordings may be required to detect narcotic-induced seizure activity in epilepsy patients.[59]

Morphine

In humans, routine oral or intravenous morphine doses have little or no effect on seizure threshold.[23] Seizures have occurred after epidural administration of morphine in an epilepsy patient[60] and after inadvertent intrathecal administration of a high dose to a cancer patient without prior seizures.[61] In animals, high doses of intravenous morphine can cause epileptic seizures.[59]

Meperidine

Myoclonus, seizures, jitteriness, and tremors are neurotoxic effects of meperidine. Myoclonus generally precedes seizures, but both resolve over several days with discontinuation of meperidine adminstration.[62] These neurotoxic effects are directly related to blood levels of normeperidine, the N-demethylated active metabolite of meperidine.[62,63] Because the half-life of normeperidine (14–21 hours) is longer than that of meperidine (3–4 hours), continued use can result in high systemic normeperidine levels.[62,63] In patients receiving oral meperidine, normeperidine levels may increase at a faster rate owing to hepatic metabolism.[64] AEDs that induce microsomal hydroxylation (e.g., phenytoin, phenobarbital) increase the conversion of meperidine to normeperidine.

If meperidine causes significant neurotoxicity, it should be discontinued. A short course of a benzodiazepine may help to control jitteriness and tremors, although myoclonus can be refractory.[65] Patients with renal disease have decreased normeperidine clearance and an increased risk of toxicity.[63] Patients with sickle cell anemia and malignancy are also at increased risk.[62,63] Seizures have been reported in patients who receive long-term or high-dose meperidine via patient-controlled analgesia pumps.[66]

Seizurelike movements have not been reported in epileptic patients during acute or chronic meperidine administration. It is unknown whether acute or chronic meperidine use activates epileptogenic EEG foci in epilepsy patients. Neither meperidine nor its metabolites have anticonvulsant properties.[23] EEG changes in otherwise healthy individuals in whom seizures have occurred after repeated meperidine administration include diffuse slow activity and epileptiform discharges.[2,67]

Fentanyl, Sufentanil, and Alfentanil

Myoclonic movements and rigidity occurring with fentanyl, sufentanil, and alfentanil prompted reports that high doses of narcotics can cause seizures. However, these reports have not been substantiated with EEG documentation of seizure activity.[68,69] Simultaneous EEG and electromyography recordings during fentanyl, sufentanil, and alfentanil induction did not reveal epileptiform activity during intense rigidity and associated movements that might be interpreted as seizures.

Eight of nine patients with complex partial epilepsy had fentanyl-induced epileptiform activity on the electrocorticogram.[59] In four of these patients, epileptiform activity was recorded beyond the seizure focus. Alfentanil increases the mean temporal lobe spike frequency during temporal lobe electrocorticography.[70]

Neuroleptic-Opioid Combination (Innovar [Droperidol plus Fentanyl])

Among 104 patients receiving neuroleptic anesthesia for various neurodiagnostic procedures using metrizamide, there was no clinical or EEG evidence of seizures.[71]

Dissociative Anesthesia (Ketamine Hydrochloride)

Ketamine hydrochloride (HCl) has proconvulsant and anticonvulsant properties. Of eight epilepsy patients who underwent dental work, two had focal motor seizures and another had a generalized tonic-clonic seizure with ketamine. In some patients with epileptiform activity on their baseline EEGs, particularly those receiving 2–4 mg/kg intravenous doses, the activity progressed to electrical seizure.[72] EEG recordings in all of these patients returned to their preanesthetic baseline within a week.[73] Ketamine should be used with caution in epilepsy patients. If a clinical seizure occurs during ketamine use, further administration of ketamine to deepen anesthesia should be avoided. Instead, a CNS depressant, such as a barbiturate or benzodiazepine, should be used.[3]

In other studies, ketamine did not increase epileptiform or seizure activity in epilepsy subjects.[74,75] Owing to the mixed depressant-stimulant effects of ketamine, epilepsy patients should be adequately premedicated with anticonvulsants and sedatives.

Propofol

Spontaneous movements can occur during induction with propofol without associated epileptiform abnormalities. These movements include dystonia, chorea, athetosis, twitches, and opisthotonus. Abnormal movements may mimic tonic and clonic movements during seizures, especially during the postoperative period.[76] In several cases, cortical epilepsy was activated during electrocorticography, with epileptiform activity beginning 20–30 seconds after a bolus of intravenous propofol.[77] Seizures may recur for 7–23 days after propofol anesthesia, suggesting a proconvulsant metabolite.[78,79] Propofol also has anticonvulsant properties in animals[80] and humans.[81] Continuous propofol infusion can terminate status epilepticus refractory to other therapies.[82]

In epilepsy patients who underwent dental procedures, administration of propofol in subanesthetic doses to achieve conscious sedation did not provoke seizures or enhance any interictal epileptiform activity.[45] Recent studies indicate that the synergetic sedation with propofol and midazolam in intensive care patients after coronary artery bypass grafting reduces hemodynamic impairment, which is implicated in the pathogenesis of postoperative seizures.[83]

Local Anesthesia

Differences in CNS effects of local anesthetics are attributable to differences in potency, systemic rate of absorption from the site of injection, speed of passage through the blood-brain barrier, rate of biotransformation, and speed of intravascular injection of the anesthetic.[84] CNS stimulation with some local anesthetics may result from selective depression of inhibitory neurons. Rapid administration or large doses can depress all neuronal activity with only transient or no CNS signs of stimulation.[85]

Lidocaine

Lidocaine has proconvulsant and anticonvulsant effects, with CNS effects related to blood concentrations. Low doses of lidocaine (2–3 mg/kg) can terminate status epilepticus. With increasing blood levels, CNS symptoms and signs of toxicity occur from perioral numbness, lightheadedness, dizziness, tinnitus, and fine tremors to generalized seizures and coma. In animals, lidocaine produces epileptiform activity that is limited to the amygdala and hippocampus.[86]

Lidocaine doses that are commonly used for local anesthesia can cause CNS toxicity if they are inadvertently administered intravenously. For example, when administering epidural anesthesia, total doses of 5–8 mg/kg are commonly injected into the epidural space.[84] Accidental intravascular injection of this dose can cause epileptic seizures. In addition to direct intravascular injection and immediate toxicity, systemic lidocaine levels can rise to toxic levels by rapid systemic absorption from the area of injection. This can occur 10–20 minutes after injection. Anesthesiologists often add 5 mg/ml of epinephrine to the local anesthetic to decrease systemic absorption and peak serum lidocaine levels. Efforts should be made to deliver minimum amounts of lidocaine to the lower respiratory tract in airway anesthesia (e.g., for bronchoscopy), because its pharmacokinetics at that site are similar to those with intravenous administration.[87] When a regional anesthesia block is successful, early reinjection of local anesthesia can cause toxicity (including seizures), because peak absorption of the first injection occurs while additional medication is injected.

High doses of lidocaine cause sedation. Increasing the partial pressure of carbon dioxide decreases the dose of lidocaine needed to produce a generalized electrical seizure.[88] Higher partial pressure of carbon dioxide levels increases cerebral blood flow, thus increasing the amount of anesthetic reaching the brain, and may directly excite the amygdala. In contrast to hyperventilation to activate seizure activity, by decreasing cerebral blood flow, hyperventilation may prevent seizures from occurring in patients with lidocaine overdose.

Lidocaine is injected intravenously to provide local anesthesia (intravenous regional anesthesia or Bier blocks). In this technique, after an extremity is exsanguinated, and the blood supply is arrested by a tourniquet, lidocaine is injected into a vein to provide anesthesia. Doses of lidocaine up to 3 mg/kg of 0.5% solution without preservatives or epinephrine are used. Premature tourniquet release (less than 20 minutes) can result in high systemic lidocaine levels and possible seizure activity. Release after 20 minutes can also be associated with toxicity. Some physicians cycle the deflation of the tourniquet with an intermittent inflation-deflation-inflation cycle in an attempt to decrease rapid absorption of lidocaine from the extremity.

Etidocaine HCl, a long-acting derivative of lidocaine, as well as mepivacaine and prilocaine HCl share common pharmacologic properties with lidocaine HCl. Seizures induced by lidocaine can be terminated with barbiturates.

Bupivacaine

Bupivacaine causes CNS toxicity at plasma levels greater than 4 µg/ml. Seizures can occur with plasma levels of 2.3 µg/ml and 3.0 µg/ml after accidental intravenous injection during obstetric epidural anesthesia.[89] A more dangerous concern with bupivacaine toxicity is intractable ventricular fibrillation.

Cocaine

Cocaine produces electrical and clinical seizure activity in animals. Electrographic discharges arise in the amygdala. Protection against such cocaine-induced seizures is afforded by dibenamine, chlorpromazine, reserpine, pyridoxine, and hydroxylamine, but not with traditional anticonvulsants. Thus, cocaine may cause seizures by potentiating noradrenergic or dopaminergic activity in the amygdala.[90]

Seizures occurred in an 11-week-old infant who received intranasal installation of a 4% cocaine solution[91] and in a child who received topical cocaine solution through a bronchoscope.[92] Edematous and inflamed mucosa may absorb excessive amounts of anesthetic. In these settings, administering benzodiazepines or short-acting barbiturates, using local vasoconstrictors, and rinsing the mucosal surface with water or normal saline to prevent further drug absorption have been recommended for the management of cocaine-induced seizures in children.[91]

Procaine

At low doses, procaine has anticonvulsant properties.[93] Procaine given at 18–29 mg/kg causes generalized tonic-clonic seizures. In one study, thiopental pretreatment failed to prevent procaine-induced seizures, but it increased the dose of procaine necessary to produce seizures. Thiopental given during a procaine-induced seizure stopped the seizure.[84] Para-aminobenzoic acid is a procaine metabolite that can prevent seizures induced by local anesthetics.[94] This metabolite might explain the low incidence of generalized convulsions reported during the continuous infusion of intravenous procaine.

Chloroprocaine, a halogenated derivative of procaine, shares the same pharmacologic properties as procaine. Tetracaine HCl, a derivative of para-aminobenzoic acid, is 10 times more active and potent than procaine after intravenous injection.

Anesthetic Adjuvants

Muscle Relaxants

None of the muscle relaxants used in clinical anesthesia has been reported to cause epileptiform activity or seizures, nor have there been reports regarding the anticonvulsant properties of these drugs in humans. Accumulation of laudanosine, a metabolite of atracurium, may

slightly decrease the seizure threshold.[95] Resistance to metocurine[96] and atracurium or vecuronium-induced[97] neuromuscular blockade has been demonstrated in patients who chronically receive phenytoin. Patients treated with chronic anticonvulsant therapy recovered from pipecuronium more rapidly than nonmedicated patients. Furthermore, there seems to be a dose-effect relationship between the number of anticonvulsants received and a decreased time to recovery from pipecuronium neuromuscular blockade.[98]

Anticholinesterases

Anticholinesterases used in clinical anesthetic practice have not been reported to cause or stop seizures.

Anticholinergics

Atropine can reduce abnormal discharges of the EEGs of epileptic patients.[99] It can also block spontaneous and hyperventilation-induced petit mal seizures.[100] These effects are probably related to its central anticholinergic action.

Analgesia

Non-Opiate Analgesics

Acetaminophen. Phenytoin facilitates the elimination of acetaminophen by accelerating its biotransformation,[57] whereas phenobarbital induces acetaminophen metabolism, which can result in an increase in toxic metabolites.[101] This may increase the risk of acetaminophen overdose.

Salicylates. Salicylates compete with phenytoin for plasma protein–binding sites. One study showed an increase from 10% to 16% in the unbound fraction of phenytoin. Changes were proportional to the acetylsalicylic dose, which ranged from 900 mg to 3,600 mg per day.[102] Although high and repeated doses may cause a slight increase in free phenytoin and a decrease in the total phenytoin level, there is usually no need to adjust the phenytoin dose.[103] An increase of the free fraction but not the total valproate concentration can occur in patients who receive 15–30 mg/kg of acetylsalicylic acid. This increase is not clinically significant in most cases.

Ibuprofen. Ibuprofen has not been reported to cause any significant interaction with anticonvulsants or to affect the seizure threshold.

Surgery and Recovery

Neurologists may be asked to provide clearance for an epilepsy patient to have surgery. A good history with particular emphasis on seizures types and frequency is important. History of status epilepticus should be sought, as it may place the patient in a higher risk group. Seizure etiology should be identified, and progressive neurologic disorder should be excluded. Medication history, including reactions, tolerance, side effects, and efficacy, should be obtained. Current medical problems that require medications should be defined, anticipating possible interactions with the antiepileptics and anesthetics.

Serum drug levels should be obtained before surgery, and additional doses should be given to attain desired and steady-state drug levels before the procedure. Oral doses can be administered the morning of surgery with a small sip of water. Some AEDs can be administered intravenously when surgical time exceeds the half-life of the maintenance AED. The decision to use an intravenous AED in patients maintained on AEDs that only can be given orally depends on several factors, including degree of preoperative seizure control and the anticipated surgical time. The risk of seizures is minimal if adequate blood levels are attained before surgery. Intraoperative or postoperative seizures can occur in undiagnosed or undertreated epilepsy patients.[104]

Serum drug levels may be significantly altered by anesthetics and the physiologic changes resulting from surgery. These changes include AED distribution, enzyme saturation and competition, binding competition at the neuroreceptor level and carrier substances, pharmacokinetics and pharmacodynamics, and blood loss and volume changes. Carbamazepine levels can increase up to twofold after surgery and return to normal in 7–10 days. Phenytoin levels can also increase. Serum drug levels should be obtained after surgery to see this pattern. Clinical toxicity from an AED can cause a

significant delay in postoperative recovery, although seizures may occur as a result of a decrease in drug levels.[48]

Dental Procedures

Before a dental procedure, drug levels should be obtained and adjusted based on the individual patient's history. Precipitating factors, such as sleep deprivation or alcohol intake, should be avoided before the procedure. The dental team should be informed about the patient's seizure type and first aid.

Methohexitone was compared to local anesthetic in conservative dental procedures. Although a seizure occurred in only 1 out of 200 patients, the main disadvantage of its use over local anesthetic is side effects, including tongue movements, coughing, hiccoughs, and prolonged lethargy after the procedure.[105] Seizures that occur during or after a dental procedure can occur with N_2O[104] and methohexital.[51] In these studies, seizures most often occur in undiagnosed epilepsy patients or those who missed a dose of their antiepileptic medications on the day of the dental procedure. Other studies demonstrate that N_2O and propofol in subanesthetic doses for conscious sedation are safe for mentally handicapped epilepsy patients who undergo dental procedures.[45] N_2O and propofol are almost always safe in epilepsy patients who are adequately treated with AEDs.

Summary

Proper history taking with attention to the seizure type and frequency as well as medication compliance and response is of basic importance. Factors that may precipitate seizures must be identified. The health care provider should be able to identify different seizure types and understand principles of first aid for seizures. AEDs should be obtained before and after a procedure and adjusted individually (if needed) to minimize the risk of seizures or side effects. Drug interactions should be considered in adjusting maintenance doses.

Most general and local anesthetics have pro- and anticonvulsant properties. Except for enflurane, which has been associated with a higher risk for seizures, all of the anesthetics in use may be safely administered to epilepsy patients if the proper approach in epilepsy patient care is observed. The risk of seizures during or after a surgical or dental procedure is minimal when routine precautions and guidelines are followed.

References

1. Mattson RH. Emotional Effects on Seizure Occurrence. In D Smith, D Treiman, M Trimble (eds), Advances in Neurology vol. 55. New York: Raven Press, 1991;453–460.
2. Andrews HL. Cortical effects of demerol. J Pharmacol Exp Ther 1956;117:414–419.
3. Winter WD. Epilepsy or anesthesia with ketamine. Anesthesiology 1972;36:309–312.
4. Hiilesma VK. Pregnancy and birth in women with epilepsy. Neurology 1992;42[Suppl 5]:8–11.
5. Morrell MJ. Differential diagnosis of seizures. Neurol Clin 1993;11:737–754.
6. Lin JT-Y, Ziegler DK, Lai CW, Bayer W. Convulsive syncope in blood donors. Ann Neurol 1982;11:525–528.
7. Boarini DJ, Beck DW, VanGilder JC. Postoperative prophylactic anticonvulsant therapy in cerebral gliomas. Neurosurgery 1985;16:290–292.
8. Serbanesco F, Mermet B, Vicat J, Serbanesco-Ventila F. Epilepsy and cardiac surgery. J Cardiovasc Surg (Torino) 1991;32:814–819.
9. Tritapepe L, Voci P, Marino P, et al. Calcium chloride minimizes the hemodynamic effects of propofol in patients undergoing coronary artery bypass grafting. J Cardiothorac Vasc Anesth 1999;13:150–153.
10. Jensen PK, Abild K, Poulsen MN. Serum concentration of clonazepam after rectal administration. Acta Neurol Scand 1983;68:417–420.
11. Graves NM, Kriel RL. Bioavailability of rectally administered lorazepam. Clin Neuropharmacol 1987;10:555–559.
12. Moolenaar F, Bakker S, Visser J, et al. Biopharmaceutics of rectal administration of drugs in man. IX: comparative biopharmaceutics of diazepam after single rectal, oral, intramuscular and intravenous administration in man. Int J Pharm 1980;5:127–137.
13. Kriel RL, Cloyd JC, Pellock JM, et al. Rectal diazepam gel for treatment of acute repetitive seizures. The North American Diastat Study Group. Pediatr Neurol 1999;20:282–288.
14. Graves NG, Kriel RL, Jones-Saete C, et al. Relative bioavailability of rectally administered carbamazepine suspension in humans. Epilepsia 1985;26:429–433.
15. Fuerst RH, Graves NM, Kriel RL, et al. Absorption and safety of rectally administered phenytoin. Eur J Drug Metab Pharmacokinet 1988;13:257–260.
16. Holmes GB, Rosenfeld WE, Graves NM, et al. Absorption of valproic acid suppositories in human volunteers. Arch Neurol 1989;48:906–909.
17. George JR, Davis GG. Comparison of anti-epileptic drug levels in different cases of sudden death. J Forensic Sci 1998;46:598–603.
18. Bredahl C. Seizures and opisthotonos after propofol anaesthesia. A possible connection. Ugesks Laeger 1990;152:748–749.
19. Chambers HG, Weinstein CH, Mubarak SJ, et al. The effect of valproic acid on blood loss in patients with cerebral palsy. J Pediatr Orthop 1999;19:792–795.
20. Ward MM, Barbaro NM, Laxer KD, Rampil IJ. Preoperative valproate administration does not increase blood loss during temporal lobectomy. Epilepsia 1996;37:98–101.
21. Loiseau P. Sodium valproate, platelet dysfunction, and bleeding. Epilepsia 1981;22:141–146.
22. Wilner A, Raymond K, Pollard R. Topiramate and metabolic acidosis. Epilepsia 1999;40:792–795.
23. Modica PA, Tempelhoff R, White PF. Pro- and anticonvulsant effects of anesthetics (part I and II). Anesth Analg 1990;70:433–444.
24. Opitz A, Marschall M, Degan R, Koch D. General Anesthesia in Patients with Epilepsy and Status Epilepticus. In AV Delgado-Escueta, CG Wasterlain, DM Treiman, RJ Porter (eds), Status Epilepticus: Mechanisms of Brain Damage and Treatment. New York: Raven Press, 1983;531–535.
25. Clark DL, Rosner BS. Neurophysiologic effects of general anesthesics. I. The electroencephalogram and sensory evoked responses in man. Anesthesiology 1973;38:564–582.
26. Clark DL, Hosick EC, Adam N, et al. Neural effects of isoflurane (forane) in man. Anesthesiology 1973;39:261–270.
27. Burchiel KJ, Stockard JJ, Myers RR, et al. Metabolic and electrophysiologic mechanisms in the initiation and termination of enflurane-induced seizures in man and cats. Electroencephalogr Clin Neurophysiol 1975;38:555.
28. Burchiel KJ, Stockard JJ, Calverly RK, Smith NT. Relationship of pre- and postanesthetic EEG abnormalities to enflurane-induced seizure activity. Anesth Analg 1977;56:509–514.
29. Ito BM, Sato S, Kufta CV, Tran D. Effect of isoflurane and enflurane on the electrocorticogram of epileptic patients. Neurology 1988;38:924–928.
30. Lebowitz MH, Blitt CS, Dillon JB. Clinical investigation of compound 374 (ethrane). Anesth Analg 1970;49:1–10.
31. Flemming DC, Fitzpatrick J, Fariello RG, et al. Diagnostic activation of epileptogenic foci by enflurane. Anesthesiology 1980;52:431–433.
32. Neigh JL, Garman JK, Harp JR. The electroencephalographic pattern during anaesthesia with ethrane: effects of depth of anaesthesia, $PaCO_2$, and nitrous oxide. Anesthesiology 1971;35:482–487.
33. Ohm WW, Cullen BF, Amory DW, Kennedy RD. Delayed seizure activity following enflurane anesthesia. Anesthesiology 1975;42:367–368.

34. Chase RE, Holaday DA, Fiseroua-Bergerouva V, et al. The biotransformation of ethrane in man. Anesthesiology 1971;35:262–267.

35. Darimont PC, Jenkins LC. The influence of intravenous anesthetics on Enflurane-induced central nervous system seizure activity. Canad Anaesth Soc J 1977;24:1:42–56.

36. Burchiel KJ, Stockard JJ, Calvery RK, et al. Electroencephalographic abnormalities following halothane anesthesia. Anesth Analg 1978;57:244–251.

37. Smith PA, McDonald TR, Jones CS. Convulsions associated with halothane anaesthesia. Anaesthesia 1966;21:229–233.

38. Harrison JL. Postoperative seizures after isoflurane anesthesia. Anesth Analg 1986;65:1235–1236.

39. Kofke WA, Snider MT, O'Connell BK, et al. Isoflurane stops refractory seizures. Anesthesiol Rev 1987;15:58–59.

40. Kofke WA, Snider MT, Young RSK, Ramer JC. Prolonged low flow isoflurane anesthesia for status epilepticus. Anesthesiology 1985;62:653–656.

41. Ropper AH, Kofke WA, Bromfield EB, Kennedy SK. Comparison of isoflurane, halothane, and nitrous oxide in status epilepticus [Letter]. Ann Neurol 1986;19:98–99.

42. Rampil IJ, Lockhart SH, Eger EI 2nd, Yasuda N, Weiskopt RB, Calahan MK. The electroencephalographic effects of desflurane in humans. Anesthesiology 1991;74:434–439.

43. Young WL. Effects of desflurane on the central nervous system. Anesth Analg 1992;75:S32–S37.

44. Konatsu H, Taie S, Syoiti E, et al. Electrical seizure during sevoflurane anesthesia in two pediatric patients with epilepsy. Anesth Analg 1994;81:1535–1537.

45. Oei-Lim VL, et al. A comparison of the effects of propofol and nitrous oxide on the electroencephalogram in epileptic patients during conscious sedation for dental procedures. Anesth Analg 1992;75:708–714.

46. Babb TL, Ferrer-Brechner T, Brechner VL, Crandall PH. Limbic neuronal firing rates in man during administration of nitrous oxide-oxygen or sodium thiopental. Anesthesiology 1975;43:402–409.

47. Knoefel PK. Stimulation and depression of the central nervous system by derivatives of barbituric acid. J Pharmacol Exp Ther 1945;84:26.

48. Kofke WA, Templehoff R, Dasheiff RM. Anesthesia for Epileptic Patients and for Epilepsy Surgery. In JE Cotrell, DS Smith (eds), Anesthesia and Neurosurgery. St. Louis, MO: Mosby, 1994;495–524.

49. Paul R, Harris R. A comparison of methohexitone and thiopentone in electrocorticography. J Neurol Neurosurg Psychiatry 1970;33:100–104.

50. Rockoff MA, Goudsouzian NG. Seizures induced by methohexital. Anesthesiology 1981;54:333–335.

51. Ryder W. Methohexitone and epilepsy. Br Dent J 1969;126:343.

52. Musella L, Wilder BJ, Schmidt RP. Electroencephalographic activation with intravenous methohexital in psychomotor epilepsy. Neurology 1971;21:594–602.

53. Smith MC, Whisler WW, Morrell F. Neurosurgery of epilepsy. Semin Neurol 1989;9:231–248.

54. Kreiger W, Copperman J, Laxer DL. Seizures with etomidate anesthesia. Anesth Analg 1985;64:1226–1227.

55. Ebrahim ZY, DeBoer GE, Luders H, et al. Effect of Etomidate on the electroencephalogram of patients with epilepsy. Anesth Analg 1986;65:1004–1006.

56. Parent JM, Lowenstein DH. Treatment of refractory generalized status epilepticus with continuous infusion of midazolam. Neurology 1994;44:1837–1840.

57. Perucca E. Pharmacokinetic interactions with antiepileptic drugs. Clin Pharmacokinet 1982;7:57–84.

58. Tassinari CA, Dravet C, Roger J, Cano JP, Gastaut H. Tonic status epilepticus precipitated by intravenous benzodiazepine in five patients with Lennox-Gastaut syndrome. Epilepsia 1972;13:421–435.

59. Templehoff R, Modica PA, Bernardo KL, Edwards I. Fentanyl-induced electrographic seizures in patients with complex partial epilepsy. J Neurosurg 1992;77:201–208.

60. Borgeat A, Biollaz J, Depierraz B, Neff R. Grand mal seizures after extradural morphine analgesia. Br J Anaesth 1988;60:733–735.

61. Landow L. An apparent seizure following inadvertent intrathecal morphine. Anaesthesiology 1985;62:545–562.

62. Kaiko RF, Foley KM, Grabinsky PY. Central nervous system excitatory effects of meperidine in cancer patients. Ann Neurol 1983;13:180–185.

63. Szeto HH, Inturrisi CE, Houde R, et al. Accumulation of normeperidine, an active metabolite of meperidine in patients with renal failure and cancer. Ann Intern Med 1977;86:738–741.

64. Mather LE, Tucker GT. Systemic availability of orally administered meperidine. Clin Pharmacol Ther 1976;20:535–540.

65. Hochman MS. Meperidine associated myoclonus and seizures in long term hemodialysis patients. Ann Neurol 1983;14:593.

66. Hagmeyer KO, Mauro LS, Mauro VF. Meperidine-related seizures associated with patient controlled analgesia pumps. Ann Pharmacother 1993;27:29–32.

67. Goetting MG, Thirmam MJ. Neurotoxicity of meperidine. Ann Emerg Med 1985;14:1007–1009.

68. Rao TLK, Mummaneni N, El-Etr AA. Convulsions: An unusual response to intravenous fentanyl administration [Letter]. Anesth Analg 1982;61:1020–1021.

69. Safwat AM, Daniel D. Grand mal seizure after fentanyl administration [Letter]. Anesthesiology 1983;59:78.

70. Cascino GD, So EL, Sharbrough FW, et al. Alfentanil-induced epileptiform activity in patients with partial epilepsy. J Clin Neurophysiol 1993;10:520–525.

71. Rudehill A, Gordon E, Grepe A, Widen L. The epileptogenicity of neurolept anesthesia in patients during and after neuroradiological examinations with metrizamide. Acta Anaesthesiol Scand 1983;27:285–288.

72. Ferrer-Allado T, Brechner VL, Dymond A, et al. Ketamine induced electroconvulsive phenomena in the

human limbic and thalamic regions. Anesthesiology 1973;38:333–344.

73. Bennett DR, Madsen JA, Jordan WS, Wiser WC. Ketamine anesthesia in brain damaged epileptics. Neurology 1973;23:449–460.

74. Celesia GG, Chen RC, Bamforth BJ. Effects of ketamine in epilepsy. Neurology 1975;25:169–172.

75. Corseen G, Little S, Tavakoli M. Ketamine and epilepsy. Anesth Analg 1974;53:319–335.

76. Cameron AE. Opisthotonos again. Anaesthesia 1987;42:1124.

77. Hodkinson BP, Frith RW, Mee EW. Propofol and the electroencephalogram. Lancet 1987;8574:1518.

78. Brunton LL. Agents Affecting Gastrointestinal Water Flux and Motility, Digestants and Bile Acids. In A Gillman, TW Rall, AS Neis, P Talor (eds), Goodman and Gillman's The Pharmacological Basis of Therapeutics (8th ed). New York: McGraw-Hill, 1990;914–932.

79. Hopkins CS. Recurrent opisthotonos associated with anaesthesia. Anaesthesia 1988;43:905.

80. Lowson S, Gent JP, Goodchild CS. Anticonvulsant properties of propofol and thiopentone: comparison using two tests in laboratory mice. Br J Anaesth 1990;64:59–63.

81. Bone ME, Wilkins CJ, Lew JK. A comparison of propofol and methohexitone as anaesthetic agents for electroconvulsive therapy. Eur J Anaesthesiol 1988;5:279–286.

82. Miller-Pitt PL, Elcock BJ, Maharaj M. The management of status epilepticus with continuous propofol infusion. Anesth Analg 1994;78:1193–1194.

83. Carrasco G, Cabre L, Sobrepere G, et al. Synergistic sedation with propofol and midazolam in intensive care patients after coronary artery bypass grafting. Crit Care Med 1998;26:844–851.

84. Usubiaga JE, Moya F, Wikinski JA, et al. Relationship between the passage of local anesthetics across the blood-brain barrier and their effects on the central nervous system. Br J Anaesth 1967;39:943–947.

85. Ritchie JM, Greene NM. Local Anesthetics. In A Gillman, TW Rall, AS Neis, P Talor (eds), Goodman and Gillman's The Pharmacological basis of Therapeutics (8th ed). New York: McGraw-Hill, 1990;311–331.

86. de Jong RH, Wagman IH. Cortical and subcortical electrical effects of IV lidocaine and inhalation anesthetics. Fed Proc 1963;22:187.

87. Wu FL, Razzaghi A, Souney PF. Seizure after lidocaine for bronchoscopy: case report and review of the use of lidocaine in airway anesthesia. Pharmacotherapy 1993;13:72–78.

88. Wagman IH, de Jong RH, Prince DA. Effects of lidocaine on the central nervous system. Anesthesiology 1967;28:155–169.

89. Ryan DW. Accidental intravenous injection of bupivacaine: a complication of obstetrical epidural anaesthesia. Br J Anaesth 1973;45:907–908.

90. Erdelberg E, Lesse H, Gault FL. Convulsant effects of cocaine. Fed Proc 1960;20:322.

91. Schubert CJ, Wason S, Cocaine toxicity in an infant following intranasal instillation of a four percent cocaine solution. Pediatr Emerg Care 1992;8:82–83.

92. Schou H, Krogh B, Knudsen F. Unexpected cocaine intoxication in a 14 month old child following topical administration. Clin Toxicol 1987;25:419–422.

93. Berry CA, Sanner JH, Keasling HH. A comparison of the anticonvulsant activity of mepivacaine and lidocaine. J Pharmacol Exp Ther 1961;133:357–363.

94. Richards RK. New concepts on the mechanisms of convulsive and anticonvulsive action. Arch Neurol Psychiat 1963;13:346.

95. Beemer GH, Dawson PJ, Bjorksten AR, et al. Early postoperative seizures in neurosurgical patients administered atracurium and isoflurane. Anaesth Intens Care 1989;17:504–509.

96. Ornstein E, Matteo RS, Young WL, Diaz J. Resistance to metocurine-induced neuromuscular blockade in patients receiving phenytoin. Anesthesiology 1985;63:294–298.

97. Ornstein E, Matteo RS, Schwartz AE, et al. The effects of phenytoin on the magnitude and duration of neuromuscular block following atracurium or vecuronium. Anesthesiology 1987;67:191–196.

98. Jellish WS, Modica PA, Tempelhoff R. Accelerated recovery from pipecuronium in patients with chronic anticonvulsant therapy. J Clin Anesth 1993;5:105–108.

99. Grob D, Harvey AM, Langworthy OR, Lilienthal JL Jr. The administration of di-isopropyl fluorophosphate (DFP) to man. 111. Effect on central nervous system with special reference to the electrical activity of the brain. Johns Hopkins Hosp Bull 1947;81:257–266.

100. Toman JEP, Davis JP. The effects of drugs upon the electrical activity of the brain. Pharmacol Rev 1949;1:425–492.

101. Prescott LF, Critchley JA, Balali-Mood M, Pentland B. Effects of microsomal enzyme inductions on paracetamol metabolism in man. Br J Clin Pharmacol 1981;12:149–154.

102. Fraser DG, Ludden TM, Evens RP, Sutherland EW. Displacement of phenytoin from plasma binding sites by salicylate. Clin Pharmacol Ther 1980;27:165–169.

103. Paxton JW. Effects of aspirin on serum phenytoin kinetics in healthy subjects. Clin Pharmacol Ther 1980;27:170–178.

104. Galley AH. Unforeseen complications during dental anesthesia: fits and faints. Proc R Soc Med 1966;59:734–738.

105. Mann PE, Hatt SD, Dixon RA, et al. A minimal increment methohexitone technique in conservative dentistry. A comparison with treatment under local analgesia. Anaesthesia 1971;26:3–21.

Chapter 28

Management of Epilepsy and Comorbid Disorders in the Emergency Room and Intensive Care Unit

Stephen J. Kolb and Brian Litt

In this chapter, we present practical approaches and a basic clinical guide for the management of individuals with epilepsy in the emergency department (ED) and intensive care unit (ICU) settings. The chapter highlights the methods to approach individuals with seizures in these settings and complements the other chapters in this book, which delve into individual diseases and conditions in more detail. The chapter is divided into sections on the ED and ICU.

Epilepsy, Comorbid Disorders, and the Emergency Department

The ED, although providing the first line of care to individuals with epilepsy, is also a place in which experience with and knowledge of chronic epilepsy care and antiepileptic drugs (AEDs) can be greatly beneficial. The evaluation and treatment of a patient with seizures in the ED can vary dramatically, depending on whether the patient has a history of epilepsy or presents with his or her first seizure. Care may be too aggressive in many cases, such as when an individual with poorly controlled epilepsy arrives by ambulance after a habitual seizure, and, even though the patient has recovered to his or her normal interictal state of health, is aggressively evaluated (e.g., lumbar puncture) or treated (e.g., pheny-

toin load). Alternatively, abnormal findings, such as fever, focal weakness, or altered awareness, may be casually attributed to the postictal state. These findings may signal new or deteriorating disorders. Individuals with epilepsy are still subject to the medical problems that unaffected individuals may have. To highlight these points, we consider the following ED presentations:

- The patient with epilepsy who is admitted emergently for reasons other than seizures
- The patient with a history of seizures who presents to the ED after a seizure
- The patient who presents to the ED after a first seizure or with an unknown seizure history
- The patient who is actively seizing in the ED

Seizure Threshold

Many factors can affect an individual's propensity to have seizures. The contribution of multiple factors to the generation of seizures is expressed as *seizure threshold*. The seizure threshold is a limit beyond which anyone can be made to seize when subjected to a sufficient number or degree of epileptogenic factors. These factors include sleep deprivation; hypoglycemia; hyponatremia; exposure to epileptogenic compounds, such as alcohol; phenothiazines; withdrawal from AEDs; benzodiazepines; alcohol; fever; infection; and other factors.

A guiding principle of seizure prophylaxis and treatment is to minimize the number of factors that lower the seizure threshold. All precipitants, such as normal psychological stress, cannot be completely eliminated; therefore, the goal of AED therapy is to raise the seizure threshold sufficiently to allow individuals to lead normal lives, subject to normal stresses and epileptogenic factors, without having seizures. Also, there are factors that can lower the seizure threshold against which no AED regimen can fully protect, such as repeated alcohol binges and withdrawal.

Patients with Epilepsy Who Are Admitted Emergently for Reasons Other Than Seizures

The care of individuals with epilepsy who are admitted emergently for reasons other than seizures shares a number of aspects with the care provided to those admitted electively to the ICU postoperatively or after some type of invasive procedure. The first concerns of the ED staff are to ensure the patient's overall stability and to verify a stable airway, adequate breathing, and circulation. Normoglycemia should be documented by glucometer and verified by serum assay. When there is any doubt about possible hypoglycemia, dextrose and thiamine should be administered per ED protocol. After these acute issues are addressed, the focus should shift to protecting brain function. Any disease process that can lower the seizure threshold may provoke seizures in individuals with a history of epilepsy. Thus, suspected infection should be treated aggressively, fever controlled, and metabolic issues addressed promptly.

After addressing acute, potentially life-threatening issues, the caregiver next focuses on maintaining a stable AED regimen and minimizing other less-acute factors that may reduce the patient's seizure threshold. A common error in this situation is not giving the patient his or her usual AED on time. Waiting periods of hours are common in many EDs, and there may be considerable delays to assessment, prescription orders, and medication delivery. We recommend that this issue be addressed at triage or ED registration, if at all possible. Patients should be asked if they have their AEDs and encouraged to take them on time. Serum AED levels, electrolytes, and liver function studies should be drawn as soon as possible to provide a baseline. If the patient is physically unable to take his or her usual AEDs on time, immediate attention must be given to alternative strategies to prevent medication withdrawal seizures. These strategies include administration of medications through tubes inserted into the stomach or intestinal tract (e.g., nasogastric tubes [NGTs]) and intravenous (IV) administration. If the patient is unable to continue his or her standard AED regimen for a prolonged period of time, then a suitable substitute medication, which can be administered in a loading dose and then continued after hospital admission, should be chosen. If the period is short or an appropriate alternative medication specific to the patient's seizure type and history cannot be chosen immediately, another alternative is to administer periodic low-dose benzodiazepines, such as lorazepam, chlorazepate, or clonazepam, as bridge therapy to suppress seizures for relatively short periods of time. If necessary, this approach can be used for several weeks, although initial sedation from benzodiazepines can be problematic or even contraindicated—for example, when the neurologic exam must be followed closely in the case of head injury or stroke. Although diazepam is a reasonable choice of medication for the acute suppression of seizures, it is not desirable as bridge therapy. It has an antiepileptic half-life of usually approximately 30 minutes after IV administration, owing to redistribution out of the brain, whereas its sedative half-life may be much longer. The antiepileptic half-life of lorazepam, in comparison, may be more than 4–6 hours.[1]

Factors that could potentially lower seizure threshold should be minimized when individuals with epilepsy present for emergent care. Medications such as butyrophenones (e.g., haloperidol), phenothiazines (e.g., chlorpromazine), antihistamines, xanthines (e.g., aminophylline), meperidine (particularly in the setting of renal dysfunction), and tricyclic antidepressants should be administered with care, and attempts should be made to keep doses closely in line with the manufacturer's recommendations. Electrolytes, such as sodium, calcium, and magnesium, should be monitored closely and abnormalities treated aggressively. Clinically significant hyperammonemia and hypo- or hyperglycemia should be treated.

The ED staff should remain cognizant of factors that may alter AED absorption, metabolism, distribution, or excretion. Administration of antacids, histamine 2 blockers, or sucralfate (Carafate), for example, may affect levels of AEDs that require an acidic pH for absorption (e.g., phenytoin). Antibiotics, such as erythromycins, antifungal agents, and quinolone antibiotics, can raise the level of AEDs, resulting in dramatic toxicity, often delayed several days after the patient is given a prescription in the emergency room. When treating epilepsy patients in the ED, potential drug interactions with newly prescribed medications should be quickly researched. A few minutes proactively spent in this manner may prevent a second ED visit several days later.

Two underlying themes for the care of individuals with epilepsy treated in the ED are communication and follow-up. Equally important as changes in regimen made by the emergency physician is the need to ensure that these changes are communicated effectively to the patient or the patient's family or caregivers and the physician who treats the patient after the ED discharge. If appropriate follow-up is arranged and changes are communicated rapidly and effectively, many difficulties can be avoided and, often, exacerbations prevented. For example, we have seen patients placed on medications in the ED that rapidly elevated AED levels. On occasions in which these changes were communicated, we were able to avoid toxicity in the patient by monitoring levels and adjusting AED doses appropriately. On occasions in which these changes were not communicated, we discovered the changes only when patients presented to the ED for acute toxicity or when, as in status epilepticus, the patients were taken off their medications owing to acute toxicity.

Patients with a History of Epilepsy Who Present after Seizures

Almost one-third of individuals with epilepsy do not gain complete control by standard therapy[2]; often, such individuals frequently present to the ED after typical seizures. The ED physician must determine whether the patient has merely had a typical seizure, which may require no acute therapy, or whether the seizure was atypical or due to some other condition that might require immediate evaluation and treatment. As with many aspects of neurology, the key to appropriate diagnosis and treatment is the history. However, history is often lacking in this setting, as individuals with epilepsy are often confused after seizures, reliable historians are often hard to contact in the ED, and patients are usually brought in by ambulance, leaving witnesses behind.

The simplest scenario is the one in which the patient is brought to the ED after a seizure and returns to his or her normal interictal baseline by the time of assessment by the ED physician. If the patient is completely normal, recounts a typical aura before seizure onset, has a normal examination and no fever, and has appropriate medical care in place, then the visit may only require sending serum for electrolytes, complete blood count (CBC), and AED levels and calling the patient's physician to arrange appropriate follow-up. It is also preferable in such circumstances to discharge the patient into the care of family, friends, or caretakers who can observe the patient and initiate a return to the ED at the first sign of any recurrence, illness, or unusual change in behavior. Such clear-cut cases are relatively rare. A large percentage of individuals with seizures are unaware of the seizure's occurrence or of any of the events that transpired during the event. They usually become cognizant of their seizures and the events that surround them after hearing about the seizures from witnesses or surmising that they have occurred after awakening in the ED with sore muscles, a lacerated tongue, or urine incontinence. This complicates the ED care of individuals with epilepsy and decisions about whether to release or admit these patients to the hospital.

Issues that complicate the care of epilepsy patients in the ED after seizures usually pertain to one of the following deviations from their typical seizures:

- Seizure duration, frequency, or type (e.g., prolonged seizures, clustering or change from complex partial to generalized convulsive seizures)
- Abnormal postictal examination (e.g., focal weakness, altered awareness, fever, and visual or sensory, language, or behavioral abnormalities)

- Abnormal laboratory findings (e.g., leukocytosis, low sodium, magnesium, and calcium, "abnormal" AED levels; and cerebrospinal fluid [CSF] pleocytosis)
- Abnormal neuroimaging

When deviations from the previously mentioned perfect scenario occur, always err on the side of caution; admit the patient if there is any significant concern or unexplained findings. Although this approach likely results in admitting individuals to the hospital who could probably go home, it is unlikely that serious conditions remain untreated.

Seizure Duration

Seizures are usually brief, lasting one to several minutes at most. Seizures that are prolonged, occur with increased frequency (new clustering of events), or change in type from the patient's usual seizures may indicate a significant change in the patient's condition. In this setting, the ED physician should search carefully for factors that can lower the seizure threshold or changes in the patient's neurologic status. These factors might be as simple as decreased bioavailability of medication (e.g., recent changes to another medication preparation, generic substitution), a lapse in compliance, or an addition of a new medication that alters absorption or metabolism. Alternatively, this change in pattern might portend a more serious problem, such as systemic illness, electrolyte abnormality, infection, or a new brain lesion. Thus, a thorough history, physical examination, and serologic evaluation should be undertaken. The patient should also be observed until at least AED levels can be evaluated and treatment given, if necessary. If any concerns are raised by the history (e.g., complaints of new neurologic symptoms) or significant abnormalities on laboratory or physical examination are found, then a more complete evaluation should ensue, and hospital admission should be contemplated (see following discussion). If no abnormalities are found, then a plan for altering the patient's AED regimen should be made in conjunction with the patient's neurologist, if the contact can be made. Alternatively, immediate outpatient follow-up should be arranged with the patient's treating physician, or a

new physician should be found if the patient is not under continued care. If there are no contraindications, consideration should be given to prescribing, as needed, treatment with an oral benz- odiazepine, such as lorazepam (usually 1 mg up to 3 times a day), clonazepam (0.5–1.0 mg by mouth up to 2 times a day), or chlorazepate (up to one-half of a 3.75-mg tablet by mouth up to 2 times a day) for clusters. Alternatively, diazepam gel for rectal administration (Diastat) can help individuals who are unable to recover sufficiently or otherwise cooperate to take an oral medication between seizures during a cluster. The patient or caretakers should be instructed not to use these medications regularly but only as needed, as their efficacy wears off over a period of weeks to a few months, and it is sometimes difficult to taper off these medications without withdrawal seizures. Only a small number of doses should be provided, and the patient should be encouraged to obtain refills from his or her treating physician, if needed.

Should the patient have low serum levels of his or her AEDs, efforts should be made to determine the reason for the low levels. Noncompliance often results from medication side effects. Low levels may also be due to rapid metabolism of some drugs. However, almost-nonexistent levels, despite prescribed high doses, strongly suggest noncompliance not rapid metabolism. Usually, some significant, although perhaps inadequate, blood level is apparent in these individuals. If no other potential cause for the seizure is found, doses should be increased in individuals with low serum AED levels who are compliant, with close follow-up arranged. However, doses should be increased only if the patient has not previously failed higher-dose therapy with this agent in the past. If the prescribed medication is intolerable to the patient, consider starting a new AED, as outlined in the following discussion.

Abnormal Postictal Neurologic Examination

Seizure activity may be followed by a period of decreased function in regions controlled by seizure focus and the surrounding brain. This period of decreased activity is the postictal period and usually lasts less than 48 hours, although after status epilepticus, deficits may take several days to resolve. A transient deficit that results from seizure activity is usually called a *postictal state*. Postictal phenomena might include transient blindness after an occipital seizure and loss of memory after a complex partial seizure that originates in one or both temporal lobes. Generalized convulsive seizures may be followed by minutes to hours of sleep, confusion, or unresponsiveness. A postictal state that is characterized by a motor weakness in the distribution of muscles controlled by seizing neurons is called *Todd's paralysis*.[3]

In the ED, it is critical to determine whether a postictal neurologic deficit is owing to a postictal state, which resolves spontaneously, or another process that may require immediate treatment. This task is complicated by the fact that fever, headache, disorientation, and focal weakness may be normal sequelae of seizures. Attribute abnormal postictal neurologic findings to a postictal state as a diagnosis of exclusion. This rule should be violated only in cases in which there is a clear history of identical postictal deficits after typical seizures, no other significant abnormalities are found on physical and laboratory examination, and the patient can be discharged into the care of reliable individuals who rapidly return to the ED if symptoms do not resolve typically or new symptoms emerge. Other causes of postictal neurologic deficits must be investigated, especially when any postictal state lasts for more than 24 hours. If there is any question about the nature of the patient's deficits, the patient should be admitted to the hospital, and an appropriate neuroimaging study, preferably a magnetic resonance imaging (MRI) scan with and without contrast, should be performed. Todd's paralysis extends to other brain regions, where persistent focal deficits can result from focal brain lesions or physiologic dysfunction.

In the ED, we investigate any fever in the postictal period as a new fever and assume that it is unrelated to the seizure until no other source is found. Blood should be sent for CBC, electrolytes, and blood cultures from two independent sites. Lumbar puncture should be performed whenever a central nervous system infection is suspected. This should occur on most occasions when patients present with a new-onset seizure. One may forgo the lumbar puncture if the patient returns rapidly to

normal baseline and the fever rapidly abates, as long as the patient can be observed by someone reliable. A strong recommendation is made for performing a lumbar puncture, because it is, in competent hands, a relatively painless and low-morbidity procedure, and because the consequences of missing a meningitis or encephalitis can be devastating. In cases when there is a postictal fever and the patient refuses lumbar puncture, the patient should be admitted for observation for at least 24 hours. Further studies should include urinalysis; urine culture, when appropriate; a thorough lung examination; and a chest x-ray, if indicated. Patients who are febrile postictally and immunocompromised (e.g., patients with human immunodeficiency virus or on chemotherapy, chronic alcoholics, individuals with chronic renal failure) or are cognitively impaired, particularly those who cannot communicate well, should undergo aggressive, thorough evaluations, including lumbar puncture, in this setting unless there is a contraindication.

Abnormal Postictal Laboratory Studies

Abnormal laboratory studies of general concern to the patient with epilepsy who presents with seizures are AED levels, CBC, electrolytes, glucose, CSF studies, and urinalysis. Assuming that the patient has an adequate airway, breathing, and circulation, several laboratory tests must be assessed in the postictal period.

AED levels are frequently misinterpreted in the ED. A guiding therapeutic principle here is to "treat the patient and not the level." If a patient presents with seizures and the levels are not unusually high, it is reasonable to increase the patient's dose to improve control, although not in large amounts abruptly. Most epileptologists increase AED doses until the patient stops having seizures or develops significant side effects (e.g., clinical symptoms or laboratory abnormalities). Most would not reduce a patient's medication dose if the serum level was slightly higher than the top of the average therapeutic range (e.g., phenytoin level of 20, carbamazepine level of 12, valproic acid level of 100), provided that the patient was not having significant side effects. Before increasing a medication dose in this setting, however, inquire if the patient was previously tried on this dose of the drug and whether it was tolerated. Again, changes in medication regimen must always be complemented by communication with the patient's primary physician or neurologist, and a close follow-up must be arranged.

Electrolytes, particularly calcium, magnesium, and sodium, must be assessed and corrected when a significant abnormality is found. Glucose should be rapidly assessed and abnormalities corrected promptly. CBCs help to assess possible infection. Differential counts help in this circumstance, as postictal leukocytosis is common owing to demargination of white blood cells, although in this setting no "left shift" is found. If there are elevated bands or immature white blood cell forms in the setting of an elevated white blood cell count, consider systemic infection as a cause of the patient's seizure. CSF abnormalities should be noted. CSF pleocytosis can occur after an acute seizure. Although white blood cells in the CSF after seizures may be reported of significant numbers of cells (e.g., over 20 white blood cells),[4] our experience relates that cell counts of more than 10 are quite unusual after acute seizures. We initiate broad-spectrum antibiotic therapy and hospital admission for presumed CNS infection for white blood cell counts of more than six to eight in the setting of an acute seizure, for any number of polymorphonuclear white blood cells in the CSF, or for fewer cells with abnormal CSF protein or glucose. The threshold for therapy is lower for immunocompromised individuals. Treatment is continued only until CSF cultures are negative at 24 hours.

Abnormal Neuroimaging

Abnormal neuroimaging results in the setting of a known seizure disorder rarely require acute intervention. Exceptions to this include when an acute hemorrhage is found, suggestive of a possible aneurysm or arteriovenous malformation rupture, and when acute hydrocephalus or imminent brain stem herniation due to mass effect is seen. In most cases, ED physicians do not have access to old brain images, and it is rare that intervention needs to be undertaken in the ED, unless the patient becomes unstable. In most cases, if the patient's treating physician cannot be reached, patients with worrisome lesions should be admitted overnight for observation and for formulation of a treatment plan by the next day. See Use of Neuroimaging.

Patients Who Present after a First Seizure or with Unknown Seizure History

The presentation of an adult with a first generalized seizure is a common cause of admission to the ED, accounting for nearly 1% of all ED visits.[5] In one retrospective study of a 3-year period during which 247 patients were admitted for a first generalized seizure, the principal etiologies were unknown (23.9%), secondary to alcohol abuse (19.8%), stroke (13.4%), tumor (10.4%), and intoxication (9.3%).[6] When a patient presents with a first seizure, he or she actually may have had seizures in the past that had not generalized or were not noticed. The vast majority of new-onset seizures seen in the ED are due to factors that lower the seizure threshold, not epilepsy. This necessitates a thorough and immediate workup for the cause of the seizure.

The evaluation of a patient after a first known seizure should proceed as described previously, except that few tests are routinely omitted. Another test that is important to consider in these patients is the evaluation of the patient for pregnancy[7] to determine limits on testing, such as computed tomography scanning, as well as the evaluation for hemorrhage or ischemia related to arteriovenous malformations, cavernous angiomata, or venous thrombosis, all of which are more likely to present in pregnancy. A toxicology screen is indicated if there is a suspicion of drug abuse. Testing for human immunodeficiency virus and syphilis should be considered, if suggested by the patient's history.

If the patient is not actively seizing at the time of evaluation, obtain a clear history of the event, preferably in person and from a witness, so as to be able to distinguish the event from syncope, fainting, hyperventilation, psychogenic nonepileptic seizures, and other types of events that can mimic epileptic seizures. If the event cannot be clearly determined by the history, as is often the case, initial screening can help to determine whether the event was an acute symptomatic seizure or an idiopathic event. The focus of the initial evaluation is to look for a focal brain lesion, infection, inflammatory process, toxic exposure, trauma, systemic disorder, or other acute medical conditions that could have precipitated the event. If such a condition is found, rapid admission to the hospital, evaluation, and treatment are indicated.

If the patient provides a good history, it is common in those who present with idiopathic seizures to find a history of multiple prior events that have gone unreported.[8] These events might be as subtle as brief episodes of morning myoclonus after sleep deprivation, occasional auras of déjà vu, a rising abdominal sensation, or unusual smells or tastes. The patient should be screened for epilepsy risk factors, such as head trauma resulting in loss of consciousness or amnesia, premature birth, history of febrile seizures (especially prolonged or focal ones), family history of seizures, cognitive dysfunction, or other causes of an abnormal neurologic examination. Laboratory study, (see Abnormal Postictal Laboratory Studies), including lumbar puncture if indicated, and a seizure protocol MRI scan should be performed. If the patient rapidly returns to normal and the neurologic examination, screening blood work, and screening neuroimaging (e.g., computed tomography scan) are normal, it is reasonable to discharge the patient from the emergency room without prescribing medication, provided that the patient can be seen promptly by a neurologist to complete the evaluation. In this setting, we inform the patient that, statistically, AEDs reduce the risk of seizure recurrence by approximately 50% over 2 years, with an almost 100% chance of at least some minor side effects once therapy is initiated.[9–11]

If therapy is initiated, the new AED should treat the patient's seizure type, or, if there is uncertainty, a broad-spectrum agent should be chosen. Such agents include levetiracetam, lamotrigine, zonisamide, topiramate, and valproic acid. If there is no clear family history and the patient presented with a generalized convulsive seizure, most ED physicians are still inclined to start therapy with phenytoin. We do not disagree with this choice and advocate physicians' using medications with which they feel comfortable. In many of these patients, this medication is eventually discontinued, either without replacement medication or with another agent that may have fewer long-term side effects.

Acutely Seizing Patients

Every ED should have a published protocol or critical pathway for treating status epilepticus (Table 28-1)[12] in adults and children. ED physicians must be familiar with patient assessment and treatment as outlined in these protocols and apply that knowledge whenever confronted with an acutely seizing patient. Status epilepticus is defined by many as continuous seizure activity or periodic seizures that last 30 minutes or more without recovery to baseline consciousness between seizures. It is a retrospective diagnosis, which means that by the time one identifies that the patient has been seizing for 30 minutes, valuable time for treatment has been lost. The ED's status epilepticus protocol should be initiated for every patient who is acutely seizing. The protocol is then aborted at the point when seizing stops and the patient's condition comes under control. Nonconvulsive status epilepticus (NCSE), in which there may be few or no outward signs that the patient is seizing, differs from the acute, life-threatening emergency of the convulsive status[13] with regard to the urgency and aggressiveness of treatment. This entity is discussed in the Intensive Care Unit section.

The most common cause of status epilepticus in individuals with epilepsy is acute medication withdrawal related to noncompliance,[14] and the clinical outcome in status epilepticus is determined by its cause.[12] In this way, patients with easily treatable toxic, metabolic, or other nonstructural causes of status epilepticus usually experience a good clinical outcome, whereas those with devastating structural, infectious, or other catastrophic causes usually have a poor prognosis for meaningful recovery.

Special Cases

Myoclonic Seizures

Myoclonic seizures are a type of generalized seizure and can be seen in patients with a history of myoclonic epilepsy and patients with toxic or metabolic disorders or after global hypoxic or ischemic injury, such as cardiac arrest. In patients with a history of myoclonic epilepsy, seizures consist of focal or generalized, rapid, uncontrolled

Table 28-1. Protocol for Treatment of Status Epilepticus

Time (mins)	Intervention
0	Recognition
	Airway, breathing, circulation
	History, trauma survey
	Establish intravenous access
	Oxygen
5	Send blood sample for lab tests
	Dextrose 50%, 50 ml IV
	Naloxone 2 mg IV
	Thiamine 100 mg IV
10	Benzodiazepines*
	Phenytoin load
30	Phenobarbital or benzodiazepine infusion (midazolam or diazepam)
	Electroencephalogram monitoring (if not yet begun)
60	Pentobarbital coma
80	General anesthesia, neuromuscular blockade

*Treatment with benzodiazepines should be initiated as rapidly as possible after addressing earlier items in the protocol, and always by 10 minutes, if possible.
Source: Reproduced with permission from B Litt, GL Krauss. Pharmacologic Approach to the Acute Seizure Patient. In B Chernow (ed), Pharmacologic Approach to the Critically Ill Patient (2nd ed). Baltimore: Williams & Wilkins, 1988;484–506.

muscle movements that are usually synchronous. Consciousness may or may not be impaired. The prognosis for full recovery is generally good with proper treatment when these patients present with uncontrolled seizures.[15] Usually, these patients are exquisitely sensitive to treatment with IV benzodiazepines, although the addition of IV valproate preparations is sometimes required.

Approximately 17% of patients who experience hypoxic or ischemic injury that results in coma develop focal, multifocal, or generalized periodic myoclonic movements, often, manifested by eye blinking, chewing movements, or multifocal twitching.[16] When this type of seizure activity is seen after a global ischemic event, the prognosis for a meaningful recovery is poor. Most experts in the field believe that, with rare exception, this clinical presentation more likely represents an agonal neurologic event in an irreparably injured brain rather than an electrical dysfunction in salvageable tissue. Postanoxic myoclonus is also notoriously difficult

to control and may be continuous, giving rise to myoclonic status epilepticus. Management may include the use of paralytic agents to eliminate myoclonic movements, but this is not recommended. This may be done purely for cosmetic reasons, in cases in which prognosis for survival is poor, to make the patient's death easier for the family. In this case, nothing is done to treat the agonal discharges of the dying brain, and electrical status epilepticus persists. Benzodiazepines and other AEDs have been used to treat postanoxic myoclonus but generally with poor results.

Absence Seizures

Childhood absence usually begins in the first or second decade of life and is marked by multiple, brief episodes of staring, up to 100 times per day, without loss of body tone. Automatisms are sometimes seen. Childhood absence seizures often resolve by late adolescence, but they may persist into adulthood. Occasionally, absence seizures develop in elderly patients with no prior history of seizures.[17,18] Patients with this condition appear confused, are variably responsive, and may express automatisms. This state may persist for long periods of time (weeks or months) before it is detected,[19] is easy to miss in the ED unless one is aware of its presentation, and usually responds to low-dose IV benzodiazepines.[20,21] It is usually diagnosed in elderly individuals who are confused, sometimes with a low-grade fever and no other obvious cause of altered sensorium. Diagnosis of this type of absence seizure requires urgent, bedside electroencephalogram (EEG).

Nonepileptic Psychogenic Seizures

Nonepileptic psychogenic seizures are episodes of clinical seizurelike activity that do not result from abnormal electrochemical activity in the brain. NESs can be potentially life threatening, owing to iatrogenic morbidity from futile attempts to control the seizurelike activity. Patients with this type of seizure may have a history of psychiatric disease, an unusual medical history, or an atypical response to AEDs. Clinically, they may present with unresponsiveness and minor movements, although sometimes they may present with generalized convulsive movements. Features that sometimes identify NESs include side-to-side head movements, asynchronous motor movements, pelvic thrusting, and forced eye closure and guarding the face when presumed to be unresponsive and alerting to stimuli during convulsive movements. Approximately 20% or more of patients with NESs also have epileptic seizures.[22,23] Diagnosis and treatment of this condition are usually beyond the ED setting, although its presentation often results in hospital admission, owing to the difficulty with diagnosing and treating this condition. A review of this disorder by Glosser and Litt gives more information on diagnosis, treatment, and prognosis for nonepileptic seizures.[24]

Communication and Driving

Review issues of compliance with the patient, and inform him or her about the state laws that pertain to driving. Also, ask the patient to contact the physician who manages his or her seizures. In states where the physician is required by law to inform the Department of Motor Vehicles of acute seizures (e.g., Pennsylvania, New Jersey, Delaware, California), this should be done by form from the ED. Contacting the patient's treating physician is vital to good quality and continuity of care. In one study, AED therapy was altered by the ED in nearly 20% of epilepsy patients who were evaluated and discharged from an ED, but documentation that these changes were discussed or communicated to the primary treating physician was lacking in 85% of these patients.[5]

Neck Immobilization

Spinal immobilization in individuals after seizures is rarely necessary. In one retrospective study, 1,656 cases over a 10-year period were reviewed, and no spinal injuries were found.[25]

Use of Neuroimaging

Neuroimaging is a useful tool in the ED in evaluating patients with seizures. An emergent neuroimage should be taken in patients who have epilepsy with recurrent seizures whenever the physician suspects a serious structural lesion.[26,27] There is evidence supporting a higher frequency of life-threatening lesions in patients with new focal deficits, persistent altered mental status (with or without intoxication), fever, recent trauma, persistent headache, history of cancer, history of anticoagulation, or suspicion of acquired immunodeficiency syndrome.[26] Any change in the patient's seizure pattern or type warrants an emergent scan, as do patients with prolonged postictal confusion or worsening mental status.

A patient who has completely recovered from his or her seizure and for whom no clear-cut exacerbating factor has been identified should be scheduled for a scan as part of the disposition from the ED. The patient may be asked to follow up within the week of the ED visit to the primary physician after obtaining a scan to ensure the absence of a new or developing structural lesion. If the patient has an MRI scan, it should be done using a seizure protocol, which includes thin coronal cuts through the amygdala, hippocampus, and mesial temporal regions, using T1, T2, and flair pulse sequences.

Many patients with epilepsy do not require neuroimaging in the ED. These are seizure patients with typical febrile or recurrent seizures related to previously treated epilepsy who recover completely from their seizure. Often, these patients are brought to the ED when they seize in a public place and are alone. They can report that their seizure was typical.

Intensive Care Unit

The ICU presents a potentially treacherous environment for individuals with a history of epilepsy. It is a milieu that commonly precipitates seizures even when there is no prior history. Stresses to every organ system in the body are common in the ICU. Fluid and electrolyte abnormalities, cerebral edema, hypoxia, cerebral hypoperfusion, metabolic failure, and many other conditions that can exacerbate epilepsy or cause seizures are relatively common. Patients are subject to a variety of medications that can lower seizure threshold or cause dramatic changes in the levels of AEDs. Sleep deprivation and poor nutrition occur in almost all ICU patients. Hypoglycemia is common. Although estimates of the overall incidence of seizures in the ICU vary, the risk of seizures is higher in this area than in any other place in the hospital, perhaps with the exception of the ED.[28–30] The risk of seizures for individuals with epilepsy is extremely high. The ICU environment often disrupts stable AED regimens through altered absorption and metabolism, and loss of ability to administer drugs orally. Endotracheal intubation, paralytic agents, and altered awareness due to critical illness and sedation can make it extremely difficult to assess clinically whether patients are seizing, necessitating close observation and liberal use of the EEG. ICU physicians should understand the nuances of caring for individuals with seizures and concomitant illness in the ICU. We summarize the major considerations in this area and relate a few "clinical pearls of wisdom."

Managing Patients with Epilepsy Who Are Admitted to the Intensive Care Unit for Other Reasons

Patients with epilepsy are admitted to the ICU electively and emergently. When admissions are elective, such as for a brief stay postoperatively after surgery for an invasive procedure, there is time to plan the approach in advance (see Chapter 27). Several issues should be considered:

- How long is the operation or procedure, and are doses of medication missed during that time?
- Is the patient *non per os* before and after the procedure, and if so, for how long?
- Can the patient swallow; is there some form of access to the gastrointestinal (GI) tract (e.g., nasogastric, jejunostomy, or some other type of nonoral enteric access)?
- Is enteral nutrition given postoperatively in the form of NGT feedings?
- Does the patient require medications that can alter the seizure threshold or the absorption, metabolism, or excretion of AEDs?
- Has the patient previously received phenytoin, valproic acid, benzodiazepines, phenobarbital, or other AEDs that can be administered IV? What has been the patient's reaction to these medications (e.g., unusual responses, allergies)?

Patients should be instructed to take their AEDs with sips of water before surgery, even during the period when they are instructed to refrain from eating or drinking (e.g., *non per os* past midnight the day before surgery). If the surgery and postoperative period involve a prolonged period when the patient cannot use his or her GI tract, consider changing his or her regimen to an IV AED. The lack of IV forms for many outpatient oral AEDs complicates ICU care. IV choices in the United States include phenytoin, valproic acid, phenobarbital, or benzodiazepines. If possible, a gradual transition to oral administration of one of these medications before elective surgery is often preferable to an abrupt transition to the IV form postoperatively. If the time period off of medications is brief, then another option is to place the patient on round-the-clock doses of benzodiazepines as bridge therapy, after which the patient's AED can be resumed. This may only involve a few doses of lorazepam, chlorazepate, or clonazepam. If it is not practical to make the transition to a new AED before an elective procedure, it is common to load patients with the IV AED before or during surgery. During lengthy procedures that cause the patient to miss one or several doses of an AED, consider administering an IV AED during the procedure. Again, if transition to an IV agent is not required for more than a few hours, intermittent doses of a benzodiazepine with a relatively long antiepileptic half-life, such as lorazepam, may be best. The type of IV access available is critical for certain kinds of therapy. IV phenytoin should best be given via high-flow and, preferably, central venous access, owing to the risk of thrombophlebitis with peripheral IV administration.[31,32] Central access is not required for administration of fosphenytoin, which can be injected more rapidly IV or intramuscularly, has a lower reported incidence of thrombophlebitis and other adverse reactions, and is preferable to IV phenytoin in all circumstances.

Postprocedure Period

Once the patient has been moved out of the operating or procedure room and into the recovery or more central ICU area, the choice of AED remains a function of how long the patient's typical AED regimen is interrupted and which routes of therapy are available for administration. Using the patient's normally functioning GI tract is almost always preferable to IV administration, but there are several potential pitfalls. NGT feedings, for example, raise stomach pH and can interfere with absorption of AEDs that require an acidic environment. For example, phenytoin levels can plummet after NGT feedings are initiated.[33] One solution for this problem is to bolus feed the patient when possible, limiting the patient to a number of boluses of nutrition per day, more closely mimicking normal eating. Holding continuous NGT feedings for several hours before and after administration of phenytoin elixir can help, but serum levels must be monitored carefully to assess the effect on absorption. Administration of AED preparations through feeding tubes can pose difficulties. Elixirs (e.g., phenytoin, valproic acid, and carbamazepine) must be vigorously shaken before they are administered. We have encountered several cases in which AED levels have plummeted, because suspensions were not carefully shaken before dosing. Crushing and administering the patient's normal oral medication can be accomplished but may result in widely fluctuating levels if the appropriate preparation is not used. Preparations of AEDs that are designed to be chewed or mixed in with food, such as valproate (Depakote) sprinkles and the coated carbamazepine beads emptied out of Carbatrol capsules, can be given via tubes inserted into the stomach and intestines, usually with good results.[34] These preparations of valproic acid and carbamazepine are preferable to attempts to pulverize enteric-coated oral preparations of these drugs. Whether they are preferable to the elixir form of these medications is not clear. Table 28-2 lists preparations of standard AEDs that can be crushed and administered through gastric or intestinal tubes with reasonable expectations of absorption. In general, sustained-release and enteric-coated preparations should not be used for this purpose. Chewable preparations are acceptable for crushing and administering through enteric tubes, although they may result in more rapid serum peak levels than slower-to-dissolve preparations. Specific medication preparations need to be judged individually. Those marked "Do not crush, chew, or break" on the package insert can be assumed to result in erratic absorption when these directions are ignored. Flushing feeding tubes is also vital to be sure that the full dose of medication is delivered to the patient. Proximity of dosing medications to NGT-feeding administration is important for AEDs that require an acidic pH for absorption.

Table 28-2. Medication Preparations That Can Be Delivered via Nasogastric or Other Enteric Tubes with Reliable Kinetics

Drug	Form
Phenytoin	Elixir
Carbamazepine	Elixir; can empty capsule contents from Carbatrol brand and inject with water
Valproic acid	Elixir; administer valproate (Depakote) sprinkles and inject with water
Lamotrigine[a]	Pulverize chewable 25 mg tabs and inject with water
Topiramate	Administer sprinkles (25 mg) and inject with water
Phenobarbital	Elixir
Gabapentin[b]	Empty capsules into solution and inject, or liquid (now available)
Levetiracetam	Efficacy via nasogastric tube is currently being determined
Oxcarbazepine	Unknown (may substitute 200 mg of carbamazepine for each 300 mg of oxcarbazepine, if no contraindication)
Zonisamide	Unknown (beware of sulfa allergies)

[a]From BE Gidal, GD Anderson, A Lanning, et al. Lack of effect of VPA concentration on lamotrigine pharmacokinetics in developmentally disabled patients with epilepsy. Epilepsy Res 2000;42:23–31.
[b]BE Gidal, *personal communication*, July 2001.

Pharmacologic Considerations: Absorption in Electively Admitted Patients

Several medications can affect absorption of AEDs into the blood stream through the alimentary tract, most commonly antacids and histamine 2 blockers. Through lowering gastric pH, these medications can interfere with absorption of many AEDs, most notably phenytoin. In this case, AED dosing should be timed away from the administration of these agents, when possible. If this does not help to maintain levels, it may be necessary to change to an IV agent. Increasing the dose of medication may be useful in some cases, but the response should be assessed through peak serum levels after a dose of medication. A common problem with assessing the efficacy of AED delivery strategies in the ICU is waiting for changes in the daily level, as it often results in pro-

Table 28-3. Common Drugs That Can Lower
Seizure Threshold

Aminophylline or other xanthines
Butyrophenones (e.g., haloperidol)
Phenothiazines (e.g., Thorazine, Compazine)
Tricyclics (less potent)
Penicillin antibiotics
Quinolone antibiotics
Narcotic analgesic (Demerol; epileptogenic metabolite
  accumulates in higher levels in renal failure)
Cyclosporine (when causes seizures, often associated
  with parietooccipital white matter abnormalities)

---

longed periods of underdosing medications while
assessing a variety of ineffective strategies for their
administration.

Seizures in Epilepsy Patients Who Are Admitted Electively to the Intensive Care Unit

If an ICU patient with a history of epilepsy has a seizure postprocedure, response should be rapid. First,
assess whether the seizure is due to the patient's epilepsy, a new problem (e.g., difficulties with airway,
breathing, or circulation; acute brain injury; metabolic disturbance; or other direct result of a procedure), the patient's underlying illness, or ICU
treatment. The patient should be treated with the
hospital's status epilepticus protocol if a tonic-
clonic seizure persists for more than 3–5 minutes.
Rapid treatment with low-dose benzodiazepines,
such as 1 mg of lorazepam, may protect the patient
for a brief period while the initial assessment takes
place. IV diazepam, although effective for treating
acute seizures, undergoes rapid redistribution in
body fat after initial rapid penetration into the brain.
It has an effective antiepileptic half-life of approximately 30 minutes, whereas lorazepam's half-life
lasts hours.[35] If brief altered consciousness due to
benzodiazepines may interfere with assessment,
such as in neurosurgical patients, then the patient
must be carefully evaluated before this medication is
administered. Alternatively, a long-term AED can be
administered first. AED levels should be sent immediately, and a bolus of the patient's standing medication should be given if there is strong suspicion of
medication withdrawal as a cause of seizures. The
downside, a transiently elevated AED level, usually

has a low morbidity in the ICU setting. Immediate
bedside serum glucose testing is required in such
circumstances. It is vital to send serum for electrolytes, particularly sodium, magnesium, and calcium,
CBC, glucose, coagulation studies, and any laboratories that may be pertinent to the patient's particular condition. Low serum AED levels are often the
cause of such seizures. Assess other possible causes
of seizures, such as withdrawal from alcohol and
nonprescription medications (perhaps not reported,
e.g., chronic benzodiazepines, infection, and illicit
drug use). Concomitant medications should be
assessed for the potential to lower the seizure threshold (Table 28-3) or interactions with AEDs. If the
patient does not rapidly recover to baseline, consider
NCSE (see Nonconvulsive Status Epilepticus). If
seizures recur, treat for status epilepticus if the
appropriate criteria are met.

Prophylaxis with Antiepileptic Drugs

The topic of AED prophylaxis in the ICU is controversial, often driven by tradition, not data. There are
several primary scenarios in which AED prophylaxis
is used often in this setting: (1) after procedures or
injuries with penetrating head injury or invasive procedures affecting the brain, (2) in closed head trauma
during the first week after injury, and (3) when the
potential morbidity associated with a single seizure
is high. Most neurosurgeons routinely administer
prophylactic AEDs during and after resective surgery
for focal lesions (e.g., tumors, vascular anomalies,
evacuation of hematomas) or other procedures associated with potential injury (e.g., prolonged retraction) of cortical structures. In these cases, AED
therapy is usually tapered off after weeks to a few
months after the procedure. Temkin et al. reported
that AED prophylaxis after closed head trauma significantly reduces the incidence of seizures during
the first week after head injury but not after that
point.[36] Occasions in which the potential morbidity
associated with a single seizure is high enough to
require prophylactic AED therapy include subarachnoid hemorrhage due to aneurysm rupture before
surgical repair and conditions in which intracranial
pressure is elevated with coincident risk of seizure.
In the first case, an increase in arterial blood pressure
during a seizure may induce rebleeding from the
aneurysm. In the second case, increased intracranial

pressure due to a single seizure could cause brain stem herniation. In these settings, prophylactic AED therapy is usually tapered within weeks to months after the acute period, unless side effects or adverse reactions dictate termination. Even in cases in which a single acute seizure occurs during high-risk states, tapering of AED therapy usually proceeds in a similar fashion. Should seizures be repetitive, particularly even after the acute phase of the illness, medication taper is often delayed. The timing of when to stop prophylactic AED treatment is arbitrary. Many epileptologists advocate using the EEG to help to predict the probability of relapse, which is increased when focal epileptiform activity is found.

Emergently Admitted Patients with Epilepsy Who Are Admitted for Reasons Other Than Seizures

The principles of care previously described also apply to emergent ICU admissions. Efforts should be made to continue the patient's outpatient AED regimen. Some of the newer agents may be administered via NGTs or other alimentary tubes (see Table 28-2). The choices of IV substitutes for newer AEDs are limited, and it may be necessary to deliver periodic doses of benzodiazepines in the short-term interval while loading the patient with an acceptable IV medication preparation. Targets for serum levels should be in the therapeutic range (e.g., 10–20 mg/dl for phenytoin, 10–20 mg/dl for phenobarbital, and 50–100 mg/dl for valproic acid). Rarely, AEDs are chosen that do not interact with other medications, particularly those that are hepatically metabolized or that induce metabolism of other agents that are specifically required for urgent therapy (e.g., immunosuppressant agents given after organ transplant), although these considerations are usually more important during chronic treatment than in the ICU. Acutely, it is usually more important to establish rapidly adequate levels of a therapeutic AED than to make an optimal choice for long-term therapy.

Important Pharmacologic Principles

Several pharmacologic principles must be taken into account when treating individuals with epilepsy in the ICU.

Medications That Can Lower Seizure Threshold

The point here is not to avoid absolutely medications that can lower seizure threshold, but rather to be aware of this association during their use. See Table 28-3, which lists several drugs and drug classes that can lower seizure threshold and are encountered commonly in the ICU.

Protein Binding

Many AEDs are highly protein bound (e.g., phenytoin, phenobarbital, valproic acid), and most agents have some protein binding. Free levels of these agents are increased in the setting of low albumin, which frequently occurs in the setting of malnutrition in the ICU. In addition, medications or conditions that compete with these medications for binding to albumin increase free levels. The most common of these conditions is uremia, in which blood urea nitrogen displaces other agents bound to albumin. In these settings, monitor free serum levels of AEDs to adjust medication doses. Notable exceptions to this rule are gabapentin and levetiracetam, which are not metabolized hepatically or significantly protein bound.

Increased Metabolism, Autoinduction, and Tolerance

Increased metabolism, autoinduction, and tolerance are usually phenomena that occur after a number of days and, more commonly, after weeks of AED therapy. This is not usually a major concern in the ICU, except for individuals with tremendous hepatic induction or tolerance induced before ICU admission. Drugs such as phenytoin, carbamazepine, and phenobarbital cause autoinduction of hepatic enzymes, and individuals with a recent history of taking these medications may require higher-than-typical doses of these medications. Subjects with a history of significant chronic alcohol or benzodiazepine use often require much higher doses of benzodiazepines than usual to achieve an antiepileptic effect. Finally, many patients are rapid acetylators, in whom it can be difficult to achieve therapeutic AED levels, despite large doses.[37] This condition is usually apparent early after initiation of therapy and usually is best addressed by changing to another AED that is not dependent on the affected enzyme system for metabolism. Large increases in medication dose help in this situation, but doses may be difficult to titrate, with shifts from subtherapeutic to toxic levels. In our experience, this often results in wasted time and prolonged periods in which the patient experiences low serum levels of AED.

Difficulties Associated with Specific Antiepileptic Drugs

Vigilant monitoring for particular side effects or difficulties that are associated with the use of specific AEDs is important in the ICU. All AEDs can cause allergic reactions, hepatic dysfunction, and encephalopathy. More specific side effects or medication-associated challenges of which the ICU physician must be aware include

- Valproic acid can cause thrombocytopenia and increased risk of bleeding. This agent is often avoided when active bleeding, or increased risk of bleeding is a problem, although the magnitude of these risks is difficult to assess.[37] Valproate also carries with it an increased risk of hyperammonemia and encephalopathy in the elderly, which can be difficult to recognize in ICU patients unless one is specifically aware of this difficulty.[38,39]
- Carbamazepine and oxcarbazepine can cause leukopenia and hyponatremia. These side effects may be dose related or idiosyncratic. Both types of side effects may be severe, but usually are not. Hyponatremia, when due to carbamazepine, is usually due to inappropriate antidiuretic hormone section and may respond, to some degree, to fluid restriction.
- Phenytoin can cause zero-order kinetics after a level of more than 10–12 μg/ml. The metabolizing enzyme becomes saturated, and levels may rise dramatically in response to a small increase in dose. Phenytoin is highly protein bound. Monitor free levels in uremia, hypoalbuminemia, and pregnancy.
- Topiramate can cause acute psychosis, depression, decreased ability to speak clearly, and nephrolithiasis.
- Lamotrigine: rapid titration may result in a rash that leads to erythema multiforme. This problem is exacerbated by simultaneous admin-

istration of valproic acid. Risks of severe allergic reaction leading to erythema multiforme are increased in those 16 years of age and younger.
- Phenobarbital can cause prolonged sedation at high levels owing to its long half-life. Large amounts of protein binding may result in elevated free levels in uremia and hypoalbuminemia. The half-life may be prolonged in hepatic failure.
- Benzodiazepines: extended infusion may result in prolonged sedation due to storage and slow release from adipose tissue.

Treating Seizures in the Intensive Care Unit

Treating seizures in the ICU and in the ED share a great deal (see previous discussion). In contrast to the ED, however, seizure care in the ICU branches out from acute assessment, emergent therapy, and triage to more prolonged care, in-depth diagnosis, prognostication, and definitive care planning. The goal of therapy in the ICU is to suppress seizures and obtain a good patient outcome. The over-riding principle of ICU seizure care is that, barring therapeutic misadventure, the outcome ultimately is determined by how sick the patient is rather than by nuances of care. The ICU patient is subjected to factors that lower the seizure threshold. Although aggressive AED treatment reverses this, some conditions (e.g., end-stage organ failure) can only be treated by improving or compensating for decreased organ function. This is the case in acute renal failure, in which rapid recovery of function or emergent hemodialysis must be performed if seizures are to be stopped. In cases in which recovery or replacement of function is not an option, such as status epilepticus and fulminant hepatic failure in patients who are not candidates for liver transplantation, physicians may still choose to follow treatment protocols for status epilepticus, although with little hope of ultimately affecting outcome.

The addendum on treating status epilepticus and Tables 28-1 and 28-4 cover the treatment of the patient with acute seizures in the ICU. The following sections cover challenges to seizure care that are uncommon outside of the ICU.

Specific Conditions

Sepsis

When seizures occur in the septic patient, they most commonly originate from hypotension, metabolic dysfunction, electrolyte disturbances, infection, or other factors that are directly related to the cause or consequences of the underlying disorder. In many cases, a patient may have an underlying predisposition to seizures, such as an old cerebral infarct, small-vessel vascular disease, or, less commonly, a neurodegenerative disorder. As with all ICU patients, the focus should be on addressing the underlying cause or sequela of sepsis rather than on the seizures themselves. The specific choice of AED in these patients is not usually as crucial as the care with which the AED is given. These patients may be exquisitely sensitive to the hypotensive side effects of IV phenytoin or benzodiazepines, and these agents must, in general, be given much more slowly than in individuals who do not have sepsis. Interactions with steroid medications must be considered, if they have been prescribed. Finally, it is important to be aware of hepatic dysfunction in these individuals early in the course of treatment, as it may alter the choice of AED.

Acute Brain Injury

Seizures are frequently seen in the ICU in the setting of acute brain injury. Prophylactic therapy with an AED reduces the incidence of seizures, although only in the first week after acute head trauma.[36] Other types of brain injury that are associated with a higher incidence of seizures include intracranial hemorrhage, embolic stroke, abscess, meningitis, and encephalitis. It is not common to administer prophylactic therapy to patients with these conditions, unless the risk of harm from a single seizure is quite high (e.g., cerebral edema). The risks of administering AEDs to these individuals outweigh the benefits. However, each patient's case must be considered individually. There has been some interest in investigating the use of AEDs in acute brain injury to interfere with epileptogenesis and inhibit the development of spontaneous seizures, although these studies have not yielded encouraging results in most cases. Studies

Table 28-4. Pentobarbital-Induced Anesthesia in Refractory Generalized Tonic-Clonic Status Epilepticus[a]

General guidelines for pentobarbital infusion:
    Loading dose[b]: 5–20 mg/kg IV at infusion rate of 25 mg per min
    Initial maintenance: 2.5 mg/kg per hr
    For breakthrough seizures: 59-mg bolus and increase maintenance by 0.5–1.0 mg/kg per hr
    Begin tapering 24 hrs after last seizure
    Tapering rate (every 4–6 hrs): 1.0 mg/kg per hr if pentobarbital level is >50 mg/liter or 0.5 mg/kg per hr if pentobarbital level is <50 mg/liter
    For seizures during tapering: 50-mg pentobarbital bolus, then increase maintenance to closest preseizure dose
General guidelines for patient management:
    Endotracheal intubation; assisted ventilation
    Continuous blood pressure monitoring (arterial line)
    Hemodynamic monitoring (Swan-Ganz) optional
    Hypotension[c]: fluids and dopamine up to 12 μg/kg per min
    Prophylaxis of decubiti and venous thrombosis
    Daily complete blood count
    Maintenance of high therapeutic antiepileptic drug serum concentrations
    Obtain serum at least once daily
    Electroencephalogram monitoring
        Baseline
        Continuous electroencephalography monitoring for the first 2–6 hrs of anesthesia
Ten-minute strips every 30–60 mins for duration of treatment

[a]Separation of the cardiorespiratory complications of refractory generalized tonic-clonic status epilepticus from the effects of pentobarbital may be difficult.
[b]In most patients, 5 mg/kg was effective for induction anesthesia.
[c]Defined as a decrease in systolic blood pressure by 10 mm Hg as compared with preanesthetic blood pressure. Decrease or discontinue pentobarbital temporarily if dopamine requirements exceed 12 μg/kg per minute.
Source: Adapted from I Osorio, RC Reed. Treatment of refractory generalized tonic-clonic status epilepticus with pentobarbital anesthesia after high-dose phenytoin. Epilepsia 1989;30:464–471.

of newer AEDs for cerebral protection, such as topiramate, are under consideration.

Patients with Single or Multisystem Organ Failure

Individuals with single and multiple organ system failure are common in the ICU. This group is at a significantly increased risk of acute seizures. Considerations regarding therapy must be carefully considered with respect to the particular systems affected, particularly with regard to choice, dose, and metabolism of AEDs. Individuals with intermittent, involuntary jerking movements; impaired consciousness and EEG patterns exhibiting rhythmic, sharp, and other patterns suggestive of seizures; and NCSE have been previously discussed.[40–42] Like convulsive status epilepticus, survival in these patients is primarily dictated by the underlying causes of the conditions and how ill the patients are (e.g., the number of organ systems failing) and not by the aggressiveness of treatment.[41] In the most ill patients, benzodiazepine use was statistically associated with an increased mortality. We recommend treating convulsive or definitive partial seizures with adequate levels of a single AED, with add-on therapy if necessary. Aggressive pharmacologic treatment of more nonspecific, generalized EEG patterns in these patients is not recommended, as it has not been demonstrated to improve clinical outcome.

Comatose Patients

The comatose patient provides a great challenge to clinicians, particularly in diagnosing and treating seizures. Mechanical ventilators, continuous sedation, and paralytic agents make it difficult to diagnose seizures, although one study has indicated that the prevalence of undetected seizures and status epilepticus is high.[43] The threshold for ordering routine EEGs and bedside, continuous EEG monitoring should be low in these patients, particularly in the case of those predisposed to or with a history of epilepsy. Therapy is aimed first toward suppressing clinical seizures. Then, suppression of electrographic seizures is accomplished, when possible. In our experience, escalating therapy to suppress interictal epileptiform activity on the EEG is generally considered counterproductive in these patients. Periodic lateralizing epileptiform discharges usually fall into this category, unless they evolve into frank clinical seizures. When isolated electrographic seizures are focal, are limited to brief periods of time, are not associated with clinical signs, and occur in the setting of severe critical illness, the clinician is encouraged to weigh the risk of aggressive treatment (e.g., AED-induced hypotension and cardiac dysrhythmias, rash) against potential benefits.

Addendum: Treating Status Epilepticus

Convulsive Status Epilepticus

Seizure activity that lasts for more than 30 minutes or that continues intermittently during this period of time without recovery of alertness is defined as *status epilepticus*. Practically, a treatment regimen begins when a seizure lasts for more than a few minutes. Bilateral motor activity with preserved consciousness is rare in epilepsy, with the exception of epileptic myoclonus and supplementary motor seizures. Motor signs may become subtle during prolonged seizures, as the neurons subserving motor function become fatigued and refractory to activation. Animal data suggest that 30 minutes of sustained seizure activity results in irreversible neuronal injury.[44] Our approach closely follows the recommendations of the Epilepsy Foundation of America's Working Group on Status Epilepticus, with a few exceptions.[12,45,46]

The initial priority is given to the airway, breathing, and circulation. Oxygen is given by nasal cannula, and the patient is often placed on his or her side to minimize the chance of aspiration. Objects should not be placed in the patient's mouth. Within the first 5 minutes of a seizure, two reliable IV lines should be established. Venous blood is sent for electrolytes, glucose, and hematology studies and determination of AED levels. If there is any question of hypoglycemia, give 100 mg thiamine followed by 50 ml of 50% glucose by direct push into the IV line.

The pharmacologic approach to status epilepticus begins with treatment with a benzodiazepine, followed by phenytoin and then, if needed, barbiturates for refractory seizures. Diazepam and lorazepam are acceptable initial treatments of status epilepticus; however, lorazepam is preferred because of its longer duration of action. We begin by giving 2 mg IV of lorazepam and then repeating every 5 minutes up to a total dose of 0.1 mg/kg. If the status is stopped, we then load phenytoin to prevent recurrent status.

Phenytoin often controls those seizures not effectively terminated by benzodiazepines. For most adults, the loading dose of 20 mg/kg is sufficient to produce blood levels of 10–15 mg/liter. If the initial dose of phenytoin is not effective, a second dose of 10 mg/kg can be given, which increases the blood level to approximately 25 mg/liter. Phenytoin must be given at a rate no faster than 50 mg per minute in adults, and cardiac monitoring should be used to watch for cardiac arrhythmias and hypotension. Fosphenytoin, a phenytoin prodrug, is preferred when available, as it does not require a glycol diluent that renders phenytoin incompatible with glucose-containing solutions. This compound carries a much lower incidence of thrombophlebitis, can be given at a faster IV rate than phenytoin, and can be loaded intramuscularly when IV access is not available.

Seizures that are refractory to benzodiazepines and adequate doses of phenytoin can be treated with barbiturates. Barbiturates, when given in adequate doses, lead to hypotension and respiratory depression. For these reasons, dopamine should be present at the bedside when therapy with barbiturates is begun, and assisted ventilation should be readily accessible. Phenobarbital is given with an initial loading dose of 20 mg/kg at a rate of no more than 50 mg per minute.

EEG testing is required when the patient does not stop seizing. Continuous EEG is necessary to guide the degree of cerebral electrical suppression. Anesthetic doses of pentobarbital are initiated if the patient remains in status epilepticus. All patients are intubated before this step, if this has not been done before this time. A loading dose of pentobarbital is 10 mg/kg, which is followed by a continuous infusion at a rate of 0.5 to 4.0 mg/kg per hour. This infusion is titrated to maintain the EEG in a three to one burst-suppression pattern. More recent evidence may suggest that titrating therapy to complete suppression of the EEG background may be more effective than titrating to burst suppression.[47] Once suppression of epileptiform discharges is achieved, we allow 12–24 hours to pass and then lighten the amount of sedation with EEG guidance. If seizures recur, a small bolus of pentobarbital is given to return the EEG to burst suppression or complete suppression, and the infusion is continued for another 48–60 hours. If seizures recur after this period of time, the prognosis for meaningful recovery is often poor, although many centers have pursued prolonged drug-induced coma, some for durations lasting up to 50 days, which results in the survival of patients with significant neurologic impairment.[48]

There are numerous relatively small studies of other medications for the treatment of status epi-

lepticus, including IV midazolam and propofol infusions.[49] In general, these therapies may be useful in certain circumstances, but their absolute indications have yet to be determined in the setting of convulsive status epilepticus.

Tables 28-1 and 28-4 summarize protocols for treating convulsive status epilepticus; Table 28-1 details the general approach to the patient, and Table 28-4 details how to initiate and manage pentobarbital coma.

Nonconvulsive Status Epilepticus

The treatment of NCSE is similar in the initial approach to the patient to that outlined previously for convulsive status epilepticus. Philosophically, the difference here is in deciding when and how to proceed to aggressive treatment after initial trials of benzodiazepines and phenytoin (or, preferably, fosphenytoin). Prolonged complex partial status epilepticus may cause brain injury, although this is controversial.[50–52] There is not, however, convincing evidence that the benefits always outweigh the risks of further treating these individuals aggressively with barbiturate-induced coma. The decision must be made on a case-by-case basis. When approaching these patients, consider the patient's overall medication condition and the circumstances responsible for its occurrence. For example, in the patient with severe anoxic-ischemic encephalopathy and continuous seizure activity, the use of aggressive therapy is unclear and, perhaps, less likely to definitively affect outcome in most cases. Alternatively, the patient with well-controlled complex partial epilepsy who presents with complex partial status epilepticus after an acute precipitant may well benefit from more aggressive therapy. In this case, therapy is similar for convulsive status epilepticus. Between these two cases might be a more frail elderly person with NCSE who is at high risk for potentially fatal complications if intubated and placed into barbiturate coma. In this case, one might try a more gradual approach, with gradually escalating oral or lower-dose IV therapy, even over days, if required, in the hope of stopping seizures and, at the same time, preventing iatrogenic complications.

Electroencephalogram in the Intensive Care Unit and Emergency Department

Although 24-hour-per-day EEG technologist availability is expensive, the service can be very important in evaluating patients in the ICU and ED. Important indications for such studies are to distinguish successful resolution of convulsive status epilepticus from a conversion to "subtle" status epilepticus, to identify potential causes of cryptic coma in the ICU, to rule out seizures as a cause of unusual behavior or movements in the ED or ICU, and to identify individuals with NCSE. When muscle and movement artifacts present difficulty in interpreting these events, video-EEG can be extremely useful. An urgent EEG service should only be used selectively. In many cases, one should provide treatment based on the clinical impression at odd hours and wait until morning to obtain a standard EEG. Resist the temptation to use the EEG (or other tests) as a substitute for clinical acumen. With prolonged studies that last more than 1–2 days, be aware that electrode paste can abrade the scalp. In these cases, a more chronic solution, such as affixing electrodes to the scalp with collodial adhesive, is often preferable.

References

1. Greenblatt DJ, von Moltke LL, Ehrenberg BL, et al. Kinetics and dynamics of lorazepam during and after continuous intravenous infusion. Crit Care Med 2000;28:2750–2757.
2. Kwan P, Brodie MJ. Early identification of refractory epilepsy. N Engl J Med 2000;342:314–319.
3. Todd RB. Clinical Lectures on Paralysis, Disease of the Brain and Other Affections of the Nervous System. Philadelphia: Lindsay & Blakiston, 1855.
4. Edwards R, Schmidley JW, Simon RP. How often does a CSF pleocytosis follow generalized convulsions? Ann Neurol 1983;13:460–462.
5. Krumholz A, Grufferman S, Orr ST, et al. Seizures and seizure care in an emergency department. Epilepsia 1989;30:175–181.
6. Tardy B, Lafond P, Convers P, et al. Adult first generalized seizure: etiology, biological tests, EEG, CT scan, in an ED. Am J Emerg Med 1995;13:1–5.
7. Dalessio D. Seizure disorders and pregnancy. N Engl J Med 1984;312:559–563.
8. Hauser WA, Annegers JF, Kurland LT. Incidence of epilepsy and unprovoked seizures in Rochester, Minnesota: 1935–1984. Epilepsia 1993;34:453–468.
9. Beghi E. Randomized clinical trial of the efficacy and safety of the treatment of the first unprovoked epileptic seizure. First Seizure Trial Group. Neuroepidemiology 1992;11:50.
10. Beghi E, Ciccone A. Recurrence after a first unprovoked seizure. Is it still a controversial issue? First Seizure Trial Group (first). Seizure 1993;2:5–10.
11. Randomized clinical trial on the efficacy of antiepileptic drugs in reducing the risk of relapse after a first unprovoked tonic-clonic seizure. First Seizure Trial Group (FIR.S.T. Group). Neurology 1993;43:478–483.
12. Lowenstein DH, Alldredge BK. Status epilepticus. N Engl J Med 1998;338:970–976.
13. Degiorgio CM, Tomiyasu U, Gott PS, et al. Hippocampal pyramidal cell loss in human status epilepticus. Epilepsia 1992;33:23–27.
14. Aminoff MJ, Simon RP. Status epilepticus. Causes, clinical features and consequences in 98 patients. Am J Med 1980;69:657–666.
15. Jumao-as A, Brenner RP. Myoclonic status epilepticus: a clinical and electrographic study. Neurology 1990;40:1199–1202.
16. Krumholz A, Sung GY, Fisher RS, et al. Complex partial status epilepticus accompanied by serious morbidity and mortality. Neurology 1995;45(8):1499–1504.
17. Schwartz MS, Scott DF. Isolated petit mal status presenting de novo in middle age. Lancet 1971;2:1399–1402.
18. Van Zandycke M, Orban LC, Vander Eecken H. Acute prolonged ictal confusion (resembling petit mal status) presenting "de novo" in later life. Acta Neurol Belg 1980;80:174–179.
19. Yeo PT, Wodak J, Roe CJ, et al. Absence status: a report of two cases. Aust N Z J Med 1984;14:53–55.
20. Kaplan P. Nonconvulsive status epilepticus in the emergency room. Epilepsia 1996;37:643–650.
21. Kaplan P. Nonconvulsive Status Epilepticus. In S. Reich (ed), Zebras and Rare Birds. New York: Thieme Medical Publishers Inc, 1996;33–40.
22. Meierkord H, Will B, Fish D, et al. The clinical features and prognosis of pseudoseizures diagnosed using video-EEG telemetry. Neurology 1991;41:1643–1646.
23. Leis AA, Ross MA, Summers AK. Psychogenic seizures: ictal characteristics and diagnostic pitfalls. Neurology 1992;42:95–99.
24. Glosser G, Litt B. Nonepileptic Seizures. In J Griffin, J McArthur (eds), Current Therapy in Neurologic Disease. 2001 (in press).
25. McArthur CL 3rd, Rooke CT. Are spinal precautions necessary in all seizure patients? Am J Emerg Med 1995;13:512–513.
26. Greenberg MK, Barsan WG, Starkman S. Neuroimaging in the emergency patient presenting with seizure. Neurology 1996;47:26–32.
27. Committee QS. Practice parameter: neuroimaging in the emergency patient presenting with seizure—summary statement. Quality Standards Subcommittee of the

American Academy of Neurology in cooperation with American College of Emergency Physicians, American Association of Neurological Surgeons, and American Society of Neuroradiology. Neurology 1996;47:288–291.

28. Sheth RD. Frequency of neurologic disorders in the neonatal intensive care unit. J Child Neurol 1998;13:424–428.

29. Young GB, Jordan KG, Doig GS. An assessment of nonconvulsive seizures in the intensive care unit using continuous EEG monitoring: an investigation of variables associated with mortality. Neurology 1996;47:83–89.

30. Bleck TP, Smith MC, Pierre-Louis SJ, et al. Neurologic complications of critical medical illnesses. Crit Care Med 1993;21:98–103.

31. Jamerson BD, Dukes GE, Brouwer KL, et al. Venous irritation related to intravenous administration of phenytoin versus fosphenytoin. Pharmacotherapy 1994;14:47–52.

32. White M, Yalkowsky SH, Studies in phlebitis. III. Evaluation of diazepam and phenytoin. Pharm Res 1991;8:1341–1342.

33. Bauer LA. Interference of oral phenytoin absorption by continuous nasogastric feedings. Neurology 1982;32:570–572.

34. Garnett W, Huffman J, Welsh S. Administration of Carbatrol (Carbamazepine Extended-Release Capsules) Via Feeding Tubes. Paper presented at American Epilepsy Society Meeting, Miami, Florida; 1999.

35. Appleton R, Sweeney A, Choonara I, et al. Lorazepam versus diazepam in the acute treatment of epileptic seizures and status epilepticus. Dev Med Child Neurol 1995;37:682–688.

36. Temkin NR, Dikmen SS, Wilensky AJ, et al. A randomized, double-blind study of phenytoin for the prevention of post-traumatic seizures. N Engl J Med 1990;323:497–502.

37. Clark DW. Genetically determined variability in acetylation and oxidation. Therapeutic implications. Drugs 1985;29:342–375.

38. Duarte J, Macias S, Coria F, et al. Valproate-induced coma: case report and literature review. Ann Pharmacother 1993;27:582–583.

39. Panikkar GP, Gilman SM. Valproate-induced hyperammonemia in the psychiatric setting: 2 cases. J Clin Psychiatry 1999;60:557–559.

40. Young G, Jordan K, Doig G. An assessment of nonconvulsive seizures in the intensive care unit using continuous EEG monitoring: an investigation of variables associated with mortality. Neurology 1996;47:83–89.

41. Litt B, Wityk RJ, Hertz SH, et al. Nonconvulsive status epilepticus in the critically ill elderly. Epilepsia 1998;39:1194–1202.

42. Treiman DM, Meyers PD, Walton NY, et al. A comparison of four treatments for generalized convulsive status epilepticus. Veterans Affairs Status Epilepticus Cooperative Study Group. N Engl J Med 1998;339 (12):792–798.

43. Towne AR, Waterhouse EJ, Boggs JG, et al. Prevalence of nonconvulsive status epilepticus in comatose patients. Neurology 2000;54:340–345.

44. Lothman E. The biochemical basis and pathophysiology of status epilepticus. Neurology 1990;40[Suppl 2]:13–22.

45. Treatment of convulsive status epilepticus. Recommendations of the Epilepsy Foundation of America's Working Group on Status Epilepticus. JAMA 1993;270:854–859.

46. Yaffe K, Lowenstein DH. Prognostic factors of pentobarbital therapy for refractory generalized status epilepticus. Neurology 1993;43:895–900.

47. Krishnamurthy KB, Drislane FW. Depth of EEG suppression and outcome in barbiturate anesthetic treatment for refractory status epilepticus. Epilepsia 1999;40:759–762.

48. Mirski MA, Williams MA, Hanley DF. Prolonged pentobarbital and phenobarbital coma for refractory generalized status epilepticus. Crit Care Med 1995;23:400–404.

49. Bleck TP. Management approaches to prolonged seizures and status epilepticus. Epilepsia 1999;40[Suppl 1]:S59–S63;discussion S64–S66.

50. Rabinowicz AL, Correale JD, Bracht KA, et al. Neuron-specific enolase is increased after nonconvulsive status epilepticus. Epilepsia 1995;36:475–479.

51. Wasterlain CG, Fujikawa DG, Penix L, et al. Pathophysiological mechanisms of brain damage from status epilepticus. Epilepsia 1993;34[Suppl 1]:S37–S53.

52. Drislane FW. Evidence against permanent neurologic damage from nonconvulsive status epilepticus. J Clin Neurophysiol 1999;16:323–331; discussion 353.

Index

Note: Page numbers followed by *f* indicate figures; numbers followed by *t* indicate tables.